Phlebotomy Handbook

Blood Specimen Collection from Basic to Advanced

NINTH EDITION

Diana Garza, EdD, MLS (ASCP)^{CM}
Medical Writer/Editor
Health Care Consultant
Houston, Texas

Kathleen Becan-McBride, EdD, MASCP, MLS (ASCP)^{CM}
Director, Community and Educational Outreach
Medical School Professor in the Department of Family & Community Medicine
The University of Texas Health Science Center at Houston
Texas Medical Center, Houston, Texas

Contributing Authors

Donna Hermis, MHA, FACHE, MT(ASCP)SC
Director, Laboratory Services and Hospital Safety Officer
Houston Methodist Sugar Land Hospital
Sugar Land, Texas

Passion Sparrow Lockett, Dr.PH, MBA, MT (ASCP) DLM^{CM}, CCRC
Laboratory Manager
Clinical & Translational Research Center (CTRC) Laboratory
University of Texas M. D. Anderson Cancer Center
Houston, Texas

PEARSON

Boston   Columbus   Indianapolis   New York   San Francisco   Upper Saddle River
Amsterdam   Cape Town   Dubai   London   Madrid   Milan   Munich   Paris   Montreal   Toronto
Delhi   Mexico City   Sao Paulo   Sydney   Hong Kong   Seoul   Singapore   Taipei   Tokyo

To my husband, Peter McLaughlin; my daughters, Lauren and Kaitlin, and my son, Kevin; and my parents for their affection, patience, and constant support.

—Diana Garza

To my husband, Mark; my sons, Patrick and Jonathan, and my daughter-in-law, Danielle; my grandsons, Finnaveir and Mitchell; my granddaughter, Madeleine, my parents; my sister; and my parents-in-law for their support and devotion.

—Kathleen Becan-McBride

Publisher: Julie Levin Alexander
Publisher's Assistant: Regina Bruno
Editor in Chief: Marlene McHugh Pratt
Executive Editor: John Goucher
Editorial Program Manager: Jonathan Cheung
Editorial Assistant: Ericia Vivani
Development Editor: Cathy Wein
Director of Marketing: David Gesell
Marketing Manager: Katrin Beacom

Marketing Specialist: Michael Sirinides
Project Management Lead: Cynthia Zonneveld
Project Manager: Patricia Gutierrez
Operations Specialist: Nancy Maneri-Miller
Art Director: Mary Siener
Text and Cover Designer: Eva Ruutopold
Cover Art: angellodeco
Media Director:

Lead Media Project Manager: Lorena Cerisano
Full-Service Project Management: Bruce Hobart, Laserwords
Composition: Laserwords
Printer/Binder: Courier Kendallville
Cover Printer: Courier Kendallville
Text Font: 10/12 Palatino LT Std

Credits and acknowledgments for content borrowed from other sources and reproduced, with permission, in this textbook appear on appropriate page within text.

Notice: The author and the publisher of this book have taken care to make certain that the information given is correct and compatible with the standards generally accepted at the time of publication. Nevertheless, as new information becomes available, changes in treatment and in the use of equipment and procedures become necessary. The reader is advised to carefully consult the instruction and information material included in each piece of equipment or device before administration. Students are warned that the use of any techniques must be authorized by their medical advisor, where appropriate, in accordance with local laws and regulations. The publisher disclaims any liability, loss, injury, or damage incurred as a consequence, directly or indirectly, of the use and application of any of the contents of this book.

Many of the designations by manufacturers and seller to distinguish their products are claimed as trademarks. Where those designations appear in this book, and the publisher was aware of a trademark claim, the designations have been printed in initial caps or all caps.

Library of Congress Cataloging-in-Publication Data
Garza, Diana, author.
  Phlebotomy handbook: blood specimen collection from basic to advanced/Diana Garza, Kathleen Becan-McBride; contributing authors, Donna Hermis, Passion Sparrow Lockett. — Ninth edition.
    p. ; cm.
Includes bibliographical references and index.
ISBN 978-0-13-314456-7 — ISBN 0-13-314456-9
I. Becan-McBride, Kathleen, 1949- author. II. Hermis, Donna, author. III. Sparrow Lockett, Passion, author. IV. Title.
[DNLM: 1. Phlebotomy—Handbooks. QY 39]
RB45.15
616.07'561—dc23

2014011620

Pearson® is a registered trademark of Pearson plc

Pearson Education Ltd., London.
Pearson Education Singapore, Pte. Ltd.
Pearson Education Canada, Inc.
Pearson Education—Japan
Pearson Education Australia PTY, Limited
Pearson Education North Asia Ltd., Hong Kong
Pearson Educación de Mexico, S.A. de C.V.
Pearson Education Malaysia, Pte. Ltd.
Pearson Education Upper Saddle River, New Jersey

10 9 8 7 6 5 4 3 2 1

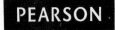

ISBN-13: 978-0-13-314456-7
ISBN-10: 0-13-314456-9

Contents

Contents

CHAPTER 10   Venipuncture Procedures   299

CHAPTER 11   Capillary Blood Specimens   359

CHAPTER 12   Specimen Handling, Transportation, and Processing 381

PART IV   Point-of-Care Testing and Special Procedures

CHAPTER 13   Pediatric and Geriatric Procedures 405

CHAPTER 14   Point-of-Care Collections 440

About the Authors

Diana Garza received her Bachelor of Science degree in Biology from Vanderbilt University in Nashville, Tennessee, followed by an additional year to complete her Medical Laboratory Science certification requirements at Vanderbilt University Medical Center. Her interest in laboratory sciences and in teaching led her to earn a Masters in Science Education at the Peabody School of Vanderbilt University. She worked at Vanderbilt Medical Center in the Microbiology Department while a graduate student. A move back to her home state of Texas led her to a collaborative graduate program with Baylor College of Medicine at the University of Houston, and resulted in her Doctorate of Education in Allied Health Education and Administration, all while she worked in the Microbiology Laboratory at the University of Texas M. D. Anderson Cancer Center (MDACC). Her laboratory and teaching experience continued at the University of Texas Health Science Center at Houston and for many years at MDACC, where she later became the Administrative Director of the Division of Laboratory Medicine. While in Houston, Drs. Garza and Becan-McBride were involved in numerous courses for technologists, nurses, and physicians to teach phlebotomy techniques. As young faculty members, they began to develop curriculum materials for their own use, and in 1984 collaborated in publishing one of the first comprehensive textbooks focused solely on phlebotomy pracitices. Their successful coauthoring partnership has endured for over two decades. In 1990, Dr. Garza joined the faculty of Texas Woman's University–Houston Center, where she taught Internet-based quality improvement courses and became editor of several journals and continuing education publications. She has taught extensively; been a reviewer/inspector in many regulatory processes; participated in accreditation procedures; and authored, edited, and published numerous manuscripts in the field of phlebotomy, health care, and quality management. She has been on numerous health care advisory boards and nationwide committees, including those for certification examinations, and served as a consultant for companies and health care organizations. She continues her writing and editorial pursuits primarily in the field of phlebotomy.

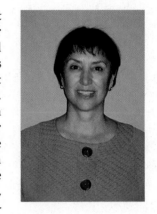

Kathleen Becan-McBride is Director of Community and Educational Outreach at The University of Texas Health Science Center at Houston (UTHealth) and tenured Medical School Professor in the Department of Family and Community Medicine at UTHealth. She received her Bachelor of Science degree in Biology from University of Houston with completion of her medical laboratory science education at St. Luke's Episcopal Hospital in Houston, Texas, and national board certification as a Medical Laboratory Scientist. While working at St. Luke's Episcopal Hospital Clinical Laboratory, she received a full scholarship to the University of Houston/Baylor College of Medicine collaborative Masters in Allied Health Education and Administration Program. This inspired her to continue her studies and she completed her Doctorate in Higher Education and Administration while teaching in the Medical Laboratory Science program and Physician Assistant program at University of Texas Medical Branch Galveston and Medical Laboratory Technician program at Houston Community College. She then became a faculty member and Chair of the Clinical Laboratory Science Department at the University of Texas Health Science Center at Houston (UTHealth). And in more recent years, she has become the Director of Community and Educational Outreach, Director of Workforce and Resource Development, and Professor in the Medical School Department of Family and Community Medicine.

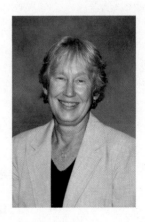

She has published 24 books and more than 55 articles and has been on numerous national and international health care advisory boards and several editorial boards for health care journals. Dr. Becan-McBride has had research projects related to the medical laboratory sciences and also community (i.e., UV/TB Prevention Research Project in Homeless Shelters in Houston). Most recently, she has received a National Institute of Health (NIH) grant in research on new point-of-care (POC) technology as defined through blood collection techniques. She is on educational advisory boards for medical laboratory science educational programs and community outreach programs. She has had invitational medical laboratory science presentations nationally and internationally to countries including Singapore, China, Russia, France, South America, New Zealand and more recently, Croatia. She was the elected Chair of the ASCP Board of Certification Board of Governors from 2008 to 2010 and received the ASCP Mastership Award in 2012 and ASCP Board of Certification Distinguished Service Award in 2012.

During her years at UTHealth, she has been fortunate to have the opportunity to receive several grants for phlebotomy training programs. Drs. Becan-McBride and Garza became involved in developing curricular materials to teach phlebotomy students as well as nursing and other health professional students. These two faculty developed one of the first comprehensive textbooks devoted strictly to phlebotomy and its importance in the health care settings. Drs. Becan-McBride and Garza have been collaborators for over 31 years on numerous phlebotomy textbooks and curricular materials and as presenters at national and international meetings.

Preface

Phlebotomy Handbook: Blood Specimen Collection from Basic to Advanced, **9th edition,** is designed for health care students and practitioners who are responsible for blood and specimen collections (i.e., nurses, phlebotomists, medical laboratory technicians, medical laboratory scientists, respiratory therapists, and others). The primary goal of this book is to link the phlebotomist (blood collector) to the latest safety information, techniques, skills, and equipment for the provision of safe and effective collection procedures, for the improvement of diagnostic and therapeutic laboratory testing, for enhancement of customer satisfaction, and ultimately, for the promotion of better health outcomes. This award-winning textbook provides the most up-to-date comprehensive compilation of information about phlebotomy available. It covers a wide range of competencies, including communication, clinical, technical, and safety skills that any health care worker will use in the practice of phlebotomy and other specimen collection procedures. The equipment chapter (ch. 8) emphasizes the most recent and comprehensive safety features of phlebotomy supplies and equipment. This edition also includes the latest information about standards from the Clinical and Laboratory Standards Institute (CLSI), error reduction, patient and worker safety, updates linked to needlestick prevention, and The Joint Commission National Patient Safety Goals. The content also addresses generational traits, age-specific considerations, transcultural communication, and patients with special needs. In addition, the chapters provide extensive information and insights about quality issues to support and improve technical skills.

This book highlights the professional role that phlebotomists play as essential members of the health care team. Part of being an effective member of the health care community is learning to communicate effectively, so this edition has a greater focus on medical terminology, roles of other health care providers, and health literacy. The scope of work for the blood collector has expanded to encompass additional patient care duties and clinical responsibilities, a more patient-sensitive role, and improved interpersonal communication skills to deal effectively with patients, treat their families with respect, handle any special needs, and establish effective collaborations with other members of the health care teams. These roles and responsibilities are important and applicable around the world.

The order in which the material is presented generally follows the way in which a phlebotomist approaches the patient (i.e., beginning with important communication skills, knowledge of ethical behavior and legal implications, and a basic understanding of physiologic aspects, then moving to safety and infection control considerations in preparation for the phlebotomy procedure, preparation of supplies and equipment, actual venipuncture or skin puncture, and potential complications). Specialized specimen collection procedures, point-of-care testing, pediatric care, and considerations for the elderly are included. Problem-solving cases, Action in Practice cases, and Check Yourself sections integrate the information into real-life situations. The Competency Assessments provide a Check Yourself feature or can be used by instructors for evaluation. And the Glossary has been updated and expanded to include key words and other words important to phlebotomists. The appendices provide useful procedures (such as taking vital signs) and important terms, phrases, and symbols.

The content is divided into four major parts:

- **PART I: Overview, Safety Procedures, and Medical Communication**—provides a knowledge base of the roles and functions of a phlebotomist in the health care industry and presents information about safety and infection control in the workplace.
- **PART II: Anatomy and Physiology of the Human Body**—provides the basics of anatomy and physiology with an emphasis on the circulatory system.
- **PART III: Phlebotomy Equipment and Procedures**—provides comprehensive coverage on the latest equipment and supplies, the most updated information and comprehensive description of the actual techniques used in phlebotomy, and documentation and transportation procedures needed for safe handling of biohazardous specimens. Clinical and technical complications that may occur during the procedure are also reviewed.
- **PART IV: Point-of-Care Testing and Special Procedures**—provides information about pediatric phlebotomy procedures, blood culture collections, arterial and IV collections, and special considerations for the elderly, homebound, and long-term care patients. In addition, topics such as donor phlebotomy and drug and forensic laboratory testing are reviewed.

Key Features of the Ninth Edition

- **Objectives** at the beginning of each chapter list the important concepts discussed in the chapter.
- **Key Terms** list the vocabulary introduced and defined in the chapter. These terms also appear in boldface type within the body of the chapter so that they are easier to find.
- **Clinical Alerts** indicate procedures or concepts that have vitally important clinical consequences for the patient. Each Clinical Alert! indicates that extra caution should be taken by the health care worker to comply with the procedure, thereby avoiding adverse outcomes for the patient.
- **Procedures** throughout the text provide step-by-step instructions with an "on-the-job" perspective.
- **Colorful photographs** illustrate important concepts and show procedural steps and equipment.
- **Study questions** at the end each chapter help test your knowledge of the chapter content.
- **Case Studies** help you develop problem-solving and troubleshooting skills.
- **Action in Practice** presents an additional case study with questions to test your critical thinking skills.
- **Check Yourself** presents a brief description of a procedure to be performed along with questions to test your knowledge of the requirements and steps to perform to complete the procedure.
- **Competency checklists** provide a list of competencies you should master relevant to the chapter content and the National Accrediting Agency for Clinical Laboratory Sciences (NAACLS) competencies.
- **References** correlate to the endnotes in the chapter.
- **Resources** provide additional readings and websites related to the chapter content.
- The **Glossary** has been updated to include more terms as a valuable reference.
- A full-color **Tube Guide chart** provides a list of the types of blood collection tubes and shows the appropriate color codings with additives.
- The **Appendices** include a guide to NAACLS phlebotomy competencies coverage in the text, essential elements for finding a job, basic procedures for taking vital signs, hand hygiene recommendations, laboratory tests and blood requirements, blood

donation procedures, units of measurement and symbols, formulas and calculations used in laboratories, military time, Spanish phrases, and several other topics.

Video Program

A four-hour DVD video library is available for separate purchase, serving as the most complete skills collection of its kind. The series contains 38 segments demonstrating a wide array of blood specimen collection procedures and patient interactions (including pediatrics and adults in both clinic and hospital settings). The video is based on current Clinical and Laboratory Standards Institute (CLSI) guidelines and standards, and emphasizes safety, infection control, effective communication, quality assessment, and avoiding errors. The footage correlates directly with the procedures shown in *Phlebotomy Handbook,* **9th edition,** and was filmed in collaboration with the authors. The video series is ideal for independent self-study or review for those aiming to enhance their understanding and performance. It is also an excellent classroom teaching tool for instructors who wish to supplement their teaching with dynamic footage of experts in action. The series helps fulfill National Association for Accreditation of Clinical Laboratory Sciences competencies for accredited programs in Phlebotomy. Educators should contact their Pearson sales representative to learn about special offers and institutional pricing.

Additional Resources for Educators

This ninth edition has digital companion resources that are cross-referenced to the text. The *Instructor's Resource Manual* contains a wealth of material to help faculty plan and manage their course. It includes a detailed lecture outline, a complete test bank, teaching tips, and more for each chapter. For instructors, log on to www.pearsonhighered.com to access the complete test bank and PowerPoint lectures that contain discussion points with embedded color images from the book.

An Accompanying Guide
for Examination Review

Available for separate purchase is Pearson's *SUCCESS! in Phlebotomy: Q&A Review,* 7th edition. This is an aid to students and health care workers preparing for a certification examination. It has over 850 exam-type questions and an accompanying access to www.myhealthprofessionskit.com multiple-choice questions, flashcards, and an audio glossary.

In summary, the authors have created a book with several audio and visual learning tools that health care professionals and students will use as a central authority on blood collection practices. Instructors can also use this as the central text for teaching specimen collection skills.

Acknowledgments

We are grateful to many generous individuals, product suppliers, manufacturing companies, professional organizations, and health care organizations for their assistance in preparing the previous editions of this text. The first edition was conceptualized in the 1980s, when phlebotomy was learned in an apprentice-type situation and teaching materials were scarce. As licensing, credentialing, manufacturing of new products, procedures, competencies, hazards, and safety regulations expanded, so did our text. Each edition used previous editions as a framework for updating, redesigning, and improving the next. In 2006, *Phlebotomy Handbook*, 7th edition, won a first-place Book Award from the American Medical Writers Association in the Allied Health Category, and we are proud to continue the tradition of excellence in this ninth edition with the participation of so many talented people. Thus, we thank many phlebotomists, medical technicians and technologists, artists, photographers, and educators who have given us countless editorial tips and practical advice over the years. We also thank health care workers around our country and the world who have taken the time to read about new and better ways of improving the practice of phlebotomy.

We are particularly grateful to BD Vacutainer Systems, Greiner Bio-One, Marketlab, the American Society for Clinical Pathology, The University of Texas M. D. Anderson Cancer Center (MDACC), Memorial Hermann Health Care System, and The University of Texas Houston Health Science Center for their support throughout many stages of our previous and current editions. We thank Donna Hermis and Dr. Passion Lockett for their assistance and expertise as contributing authors. We also thank the many students, faculty, and staff of the Diagnostic Center at the University of Texas M. D. Anderson Cancer Center who were models for the photographs and technical experts, especially Dr. Brandy Greenhill, Program Director, Clinical Laboratory Science Program; Kimberly Murray; and Peter McLaughlin, MD. Thanks also go to photographer Patrick Watson for his patience, effieicncy, and organizational skills.

We greatly appreciate our positive working relationships with editors and copyeditors, past and present, who have encouraged us and improved our writing through eight editions. Special thanks go to Jane Licht, Cheryl Mehalik, Lin Marshall, Mark Cohen, Melissa Kerian Bashe, Cathy Wein, and Amy Peltier.

Last, and most important, we gratefully acknowledge our families, who have proudly grown up with this text as part of their lives. They have continued to encourage us and have supportively tolerated the thousands of hours over many years that we have spent writing the previous and current edition of this textbook. They will always hold a special place in our hearts.

Diana Garza
Kathleen Becan-McBride

Reviewers

Thank you to the following reviewers for their valuable contributions:

Pamela Audette, MBA, MT, RMA
Program Chair, Medial Assistant
 Program
Finlandia University
Hancock, Michigan

Jerry Barton, MLS (ASCP)
Phlebotomy Program Director
Cape Fear Community College
Wilmington, North Carolina

Doris Beran, MPH, MT (ASCP)
Allied Health Instructor
Coconino Community College
Flagstaff, Arizona

Jimmy Boyd, MLS (ASCP)
Program Director
Arkansas State University Beebe
Beebe, Arkansas

Jennifer Elenbaas
Instructor
Davenport University
Grand Rapids, Michigan

Penny Ewing, BS, CMA (AAMA)
Instructor
Gaston College
Dallas, North Carolina

**Michelle Mantooth, MSc., MLS
 (ASCP)^{CM}, CG(ASCP) ^{CM}**
Instructor
Trident Technical College
North Charleston, South Carolina

Kimberly Meshell
Instructor
Angelina College
Lufkin, Texas

Margaret Oliver, MT (ASCP)
Instructor
Neosho County Community College
Ottawa, Kansas

Evelyn Paxton, MS, MT (ASCP)
Program Director
Rose State College
Midwest City, Oklahoma

**Pam Tully, MHS, MT (ASCP), PBT
 (ASCP)**
Phlebotomy Program Director
Bossier Parish Community College
Bossier City, Louisiana

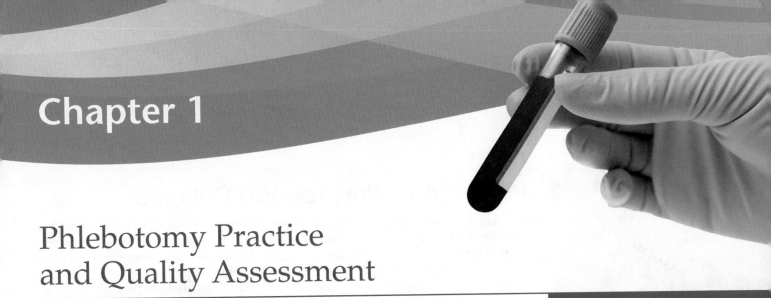

Chapter 1

Phlebotomy Practice
and Quality Assessment

Chapter Objectives

Upon completion of Chapter 1, the learner is responsible
for doing the following:

1. Define phlebotomy and identify health professionals who perform phlebotomy procedures.

2. Identify the importance of phlebotomy procedures to the overall care of the patient.

3. List professional competencies for phlebotomists and key elements of a performance assessment.

4. List members of a health care team who interact with phlebotomists.

5. Describe the roles of clinical laboratory personnel and common laboratory departments/sections.

6. Describe health care settings in which phlebotomy services are routinely performed.

7. Explain components of professionalism and desired character traits for phlebotomists.

8. Describe healthy behaviors, fitness, and coping skills to reduce stress in the workplace.

9. List the basic tools used in quality improvement activities and give examples of how a phlebotomist can participate in quality improvement activities.

10. Define the difference between quality improvement and quality control.

KEY TERMS

accuracy
acute care
aliquot
ambulatory care
American Society for Clinical
    Laboratory Science (ASCLS)
American Society for Clinical Pathology
    (ASCP)
anatomic pathology
Centers for Medicare & Medicaid
    Services (CMS)
clinical decisions
clinical pathology
competency statement
continuing education (CE)
continuous quality
    improvement (CQI)
examination (analytical phase)
Food and Drug Administration (FDA)
home health personnel
hospital- or health care-acquired
    infections (HAIs)
inpatients
International Organization for
    Standardization (ISO)
long-term care
nanotechnology
National Phlebotomy
    Association (NPA)
personal protective equipment (PPE)
phlebotomist
phlebotomy
CONTINUED

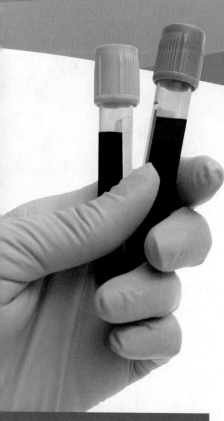

Phlebotomy Practice and Definition

Clinical decisions are based on medical standards of practice, diagnostic testing (e.g., laboratory tests and x-rays), a patient's history, and observation of signs and symptoms. Therefore, before physicians can make clinical decisions, they need laboratory test results for the patient. The development of modern diagnostic techniques, clinical laboratory automation, computer technology, standardization, globalization, and changes in the delivery of health care services have increased the variety and number of laboratory test options available for clinical decisions. Since laboratory test results influence the majority of medical decisions and play such an important role in the clinical management of patients, many health care workers are taking greater roles in the specimen collection process. Among those who perform phlebotomy tasks are clinical or medical laboratory personnel (including certified phlebotomists), nurses and nurse aides, respiratory therapists, medical assistants, home health personnel, and others. Regardless of specific job backgrounds, common elements about the practice of phlebotomy should be known by all who are responsible for blood specimen collections.

The term **phlebotomy** is derived from the Greek words, *phlebo*, which relates to veins, and *tomy*, which relates to cutting. In ancient times, phlebotomy was practiced to withdraw blood using various means, including knives, crude lancets, leeches, blood cups or bowls, pumps, and glass syringes. In some cultures, phlebotomy was thought to cleanse or purify the body and/or get rid of unwanted spirits. However, today, modern phlebotomy equipment and practices are very advanced. The current definition of *phlebotomy* can be summarized as the incision of a vein for collecting a blood sample (a portion of blood removed that is small enough so as not to cause harm) for laboratory testing or other therapeutic purposes (e.g., blood donations). Synonymous words are *venesection* or *venisection,* and the **phlebotomist,** or blood collector, is the individual who performs phlebotomy. The term *phlebotomist* will be used throughout this text even though it is interchangeable with *blood collector*. Phlebotomists often assist in the collection and transportation of specimens other than venous blood (e.g., arterial blood, urine, tissues, sputum) and may perform clinical, technical, or clerical functions. However, the primary function of the phlebotomist is to assist the health care team in the accurate, safe, and reliable collection and transportation of specimens for laboratory analyses.

In this text, numerous phlebotomy procedures and practices are covered, ranging from the most basic to more advanced procedures. However, the two most common phlebotomy techniques are extensively covered and are the essence of all phlebotomy practices:

- **Venipuncture**—Withdrawing a venous blood sample (from a vein, not an artery) using a needle attached to an evacuated tube system or other collection devices (covered in Chapters 8 and 10).

- **Skin Puncture**—Puncturing a finger with a specially designed safety lancet to withdraw a smaller amount of capillary blood (covered in Chapters 8 and 11).

- Advanced and/or specialized procedures are covered in Chapters 13, 15, 16, and 17.

Patients' blood specimens are discrete portions of blood taken for laboratory analysis of one or more characteristics to determine the character of the whole body.[1] Laboratory analyses of a variety of specimens are used for *three* important clinical purposes:

- **Diagnostic and Screening Tests**—To figure out what is wrong with the patient (e.g., tests that detect abnormalities) or to detect irregularities that require more extensive follow-up testing.

- **Therapeutic Assessments**—To develop the appropriate therapy or treatment of the medical condition (e.g., tests that predict the most effective treatment or the drug of choice)

- **Monitoring**—To make sure the therapy or treatment is working to alleviate the disease or illness (e.g., tests to confirm that the abnormality has returned to normal or that the drug is reaching its effective dosage)

Thus, the requirement for a high-quality specimen that is correctly identified, collected, and transported is vital to the overall care of a patient. Phlebotomists' duties vary in scope and range, depending on the setting. They may have duties related to all phases of laboratory analysis or may be assigned to only specimen collection duties in one area of a hospital. Technology has enabled laboratory testing to be performed closer to the **point-of-care (POC)**; for example, at the patient's bedside, at ancillary or mobile clinic sites, in the home, or even in an ambulance (**BOX 1–1**). Phlebotomists' duties have become more coordinated with other health care processes. In some cases, health professionals—such as nurses, respiratory therapists, patient care technicians, medical assistants, and others—have been cross-trained to assume phlebotomy duties; in other cases, traditional laboratory-based phlebotomists have been cross-trained to assume expanded clerical or patient care duties—for example, performing electrocardiograms and low-risk laboratory procedures. Whatever the case, the workplace settings and roles and responsibilities of the health care professional who performs phlebotomy procedures will continue to evolve and change.

HEALTH CARE SETTINGS AND HEALTH CARE TEAMS

Health care organizations in the United States vary widely but most fit into two categories: **inpatient,** where patients are in a hospital for more serious conditions and care and outpatient or **ambulatory care,** where patients's conditions are less critical and can be treated without hospitalization. Traditional hospitals are organized into departments according

---

BOX 1–1

Potential Job Sites for Phlebotomists

Hospital (Inpatient) Settings

Acute-care hospitals (urban or rural)	Hospital-based clinics
Specialty hospitals (cancer, psychiatric, long-term care, pediatric)	Hospital-based emergency centers

Ambulatory Care (Outpatient) Settings

Health department clinics	Health maintenance organizations (HMOs)
Community health centers (CHCs)	Insurance companies
Rural health clinics	Physician group practices
Community-based mental health centers	Individual or solo medical practices
School-based clinics	Specialty practices
Prison health clinics	Rehabilitation centers
Dialysis centers	Mobile vans for blood donations
Screening centers	Mobile vans for primary care delivery
Home hospice	Free-standing surgical centers
Durable medical equipment suppliers	Reference laboratory collection sites
Physician's office laboratories (POLs) (in medical clinics)	Drug screening sites
	Mobile mammography units
Home health care (provided in the patient's home)	

to medical/surgical specialties and/or around organs systems as shown in **TABLE 1–1**. Sometimes, departments are organized by therapy services or procedures offered to the patient. Phlebotomists should become knowledgeable about these areas of the hospital and the personnel who work there because patients spend time in them prior to, during, and/or after their phlebotomy procedures. Some factors that relate to these departments may affect the outcome of the laboratory test, and they all involve members of the health care team.

HOSPITALS IN THE UNITED STATES

There are over 5,700 hospitals in the United States. They vary according to the following factors:

- Mission (patient care, education, research)
- Number of staffed beds (over 920,000 beds in the United States)[2]
- Admissions (a total of over 37 million per year)[2]
- Ownership (public or nonprofit, governmental, for profit [investor owned or proprietary])
- Length of stay (short term [e.g., less than 30 days] or long-term [e.g., greater than 30 days])
- Type of care (e.g., **acute care** [short term treatment for an urgent injury or medical condition], cancer center, psychiatric, **long-term care** [treatment for chronic conditions], pediatric, rehabilitation, etc.)
- Location (urban or rural)
- Relationship to other health facilities (e.g., hospital system-managed by a central organization or a network of providers that work together to coordinate care and may or may not be affiliated with each other)

TABLE 1–1

Medical, Surgical, and Ancillary Service Departments in Large Health Care Facilities

Health care professionals make up one of the largest workforce segments in the United States. For every one physician, there are approximately 16 health care workers who provide direct and support services to the patient and physician. The following list is only a partial listing of common clinical departments and personnel. There are many levels of education, experience, credentialing processes, and licensing requirements for the health care industry, and it is beyond the scope of this text to cover all the important individuals. There are also a variety of specialties and subspecialties for physicians (medical doctors, MDs), scientists, biomedical engineers, nurses, physician assistants (PAs), social workers, pharmacists, therapists, technical individuals, and spiritual support personnel who are valuable members of the health care team but too numerous to mention here.

Department	Functions	Personnel
Allergy	Diagnosis and treatment of persons who have allergies or "reactions" to irritating agents.	Physicians, nurses, medical assistants
Anesthesiology	Pain management before, during, and after surgery.	Anesthesiologist, nurse anesthetist
Cardiology	Medical diagnosis and treatment of conditions relating to the heart and circulatory conditions.	Cardiologist (MD)
Cardiovascular	Surgical diagnosis and treatment of heart and blood circulation disorders.	Cardiovascular surgeon (MD), surgical nurse
Dermatology	Diagnosis and treatment of skin conditions.	Dermatologist (MD), nurse, medical assistant
Diagnostic Imaging or Radiology	Uses ionizing radiation for treating disease, fluoroscopic and radiographic x-ray instrumentation and imaging methods for diagnosis, and radioisotopes for both diagnosing and treating disease. Sometimes patients are injected with dye that might interfere with some laboratory tests. The phlebotomist should document the circumstances as appropriate. In addition, the phlebotomist should be aware of applicable safety requirements.	Radiologist, radiologic technician/technologist
Electrocardiography	Uses the electrocardiograph (ECG or EKG) to record the electric currents produced by contractions of the heart. This assists in the diagnosis of heart disease.	Cardiologist, nurse, medical assistant, EKG technician
Electroencephalography	Uses the electroencephalograph (EEG) to record brain wave patterns.	Neurologist (MD), nurse
Endocrinology	Diagnosis and treatment of disorders in the organs and tissues that produce hormones (e.g., estrogen, testosterone, cortisol).	Endocrinologist (MD), nurse
Family medicine/General practice	Care of general medical problems of all family members.	Family practice or primary care physician (MD)

TABLE 1–1

Medical, Surgical, and Ancillary Service Departments in Large Health Care Facilities (continued)

Department	Functions	Personnel
Gastroenterology	Diagnosis and treatment of conditions relating to esophagus, stomach, and intestines.	Gastroenterologist
Geriatrics/Gerontology	Diagnosis and treatment of the elderly population.	Gerontologist
Hematology	Diagnosis and treatment of conditions relating to the blood.	Hematologist
Immunology	Diagnosis and treatment of conditions relating to the immune system	Immunologist
Internal Medicine	General diagnosis and treatment of patients for problems of one or more internal organs	Internist (MD) or doctor of osteopathic medicine (DO), nurse, physician assistant (PA)
Laboratory Medicine/Pathology	Uses sophisticated instrumentation to analyze blood, body fluids, and tissues for pathological conditions. Laboratory results are used in diagnosis, treatment, and monitoring of patients' health status.	Pathologist, pathology assistant, laboratory personnel (Box 1–2)
Neonatal/Perinatal	Study, support, and treatment of newborn and prematurely born babies and their mothers.	Neonatologist
Nephrology	Kidneys.	Urologist
Neurology	Nervous system.	Neurologist, neurosurgeon
Nuclear Medicine	Uses radioactive isotopes or tracers in the diagnosis and treatment of patients and in the study of the disease process. The radioactive substance is injected into the patient and emits rays that can be detected by sophisticated instrumentation. Phlebotomists should be knowledgeable of special safety requirements for entering this area. Also, the radioisotopes may interfere with laboratory testing, so documentation of this therapy may be required.	Radiotherapist (MD)
Nutrition and Dietetics	Perform nutritional assessments and patient education, and design special diets for patients who have eating-related disorders (e.g., diabetes, obesity, anorexia).	Nutritionist, dietician
Obstetrics/Gynecology	Diagnosis and treatment relating to the sexual reproductive system of females, using both surgical and nonsurgical procedures.	Obstetrician, gynecologist (MD)
Occupational Therapy	Assists the patient in becoming functionally independent within the limitations of the patient's disability or condition. Occupational therapists (OTs) collaborate with the health care team to design therapeutic programs of rehabilitative activities for the patient. The therapy is designed to improve functional abilities or activities of daily living (ADLs).	Occupational therapist (OT)
Oncology	Diagnosis and treatment of malignant (life-threatening) tumors (i.e., cancer).	Oncologist (MD)
Ophthalmology	Diagnosis and treatment of the eyes and vision-related medical problems.	Ophthalmologist (MD), optometrist (DO)
Orthopedics	Care of medical concerns related to bones and joints.	Orthopedic Surgeon (MD), physical therapist
Otolaryngology	Diagnosis and treatment of medical problems related to ears, nose, and throat (ENT).	Otolaryngologist, speech pathologist, audiologist
Pathology	*See* Laboratory Medicine/Pathology	
Pediatrics	General diagnosis and therapy for children.	Pediatrician (MD)
Pharmacy	Dispenses medications ordered by physicians. Pharmacists also collaborate with the health care team on drug therapies. Phlebotomists may collect blood specimens at timed intervals to monitor the level of the drug in the patient's bloodstream.	Doctor of Pharmacy (Pharm. D), pharmacist
Physical Medicine	Diagnosis and treatment of disorders of the neuromuscular system.	Physical therapist (PT), occupational therapist (OT)
Physical Therapy	Assists in restoring physical abilities that have been impaired by illness or injury. Rehabilitation programs often use heat/cold, water therapy, ultrasound or electricity, and physical exercises designed to restore useful activity.	PT and OT
Plastic Surgery	Cosmetic surgery or surgical correction of the deformity of tissues, including skin.	Plastic surgeon (MD)
Proctology	Diagnosis and treatment of diseases of the anus and rectum.	Proctologist (MD)
Psychiatry/Neurology	Diagnosis and treatment for people of all ages with mental, emotional, and nervous system problems, using primarily nonsurgical procedures.	Psychiatrist/Neurologist (MD)
Pulmonary	Diagnosis and treatment of conditions relating to the respiratory system.	Pulmonologist (MD)
Radiotherapy	Uses high-energy x-rays, such as from cobalt treatment, in the treatment of disease, particularly cancer. Safety precautions are important to avoid unnecessary irradiation.	Radiotherapist (MD), nuclear medicine technician
Rheumatology	Diagnosis and treatment of joint and tissue diseases, including arthritis.	Rheumatologist (MD)
Surgery	Diagnosis and treatment in which the physician physically alters a part of the patient's body.	General surgeon, specialty surgeon (orthopedic, cardiovascular, etc.) (MD)
Urology	Diagnosis and treatment of medical conditions related to sexual/reproductive system in men, and renal system for men and women.	Urologist, nephrologist (MD)

BECOMING A PART OF THE HEALTH CARE TEAM

All health care workers are expected to be valuable members of a health care team (**FIGURE 1–1**). Even though there are many levels and types of health care teams (self-directed work groups, manager-led group, etc.) and roles/responsibilities that are assigned to each, there are important questions to ask in each situation:

What do I need to do to maximize team/group effectiveness?
How can I be a better team member?

In high-performance teams, every team member should:

- Understand the mission of the organization, the goals of the group, and/or the project
- Know basic skills for group processes (listening skills, setting norms for the team, etc.)
- Show reliability and dependability in work assignments
- Communicate one's own ideas and feelings
- Actively and respectfully participate in decision making
- Learn how to be flexible in decision making (give and take)
- Constructively manage conflicts
- Contribute to the cohesion of the team
- Contribute to problem-solving strategies
- Support and encourage other team members

Individuals should reflect on this list periodically as they go through this text and through their careers. To make it a self-assessment, simply add the words "Do I . . ." to each phrase in the list. Professional growth and maturity occur if one can honestly answer these questions and strive for improvement if there are deficits. Additional resources for team development and communication are listed at the end of this chapter and in Chapter 2.

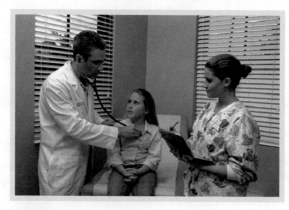

FIGURE 1–1
Health Care Team

Daily communication with a health care team is part of the job. Discussions that occur within a patient's hearing range must be highly professional.

The Clinical Laboratory and Specimen Collection Services

A typical hospital-based clinical laboratory has two components: clinical pathology and anatomic pathology. In the **clinical pathology** area (also called the *clinical laboratory* or *medical laboratory*), blood and other types of body fluids and tissues are analyzed (e.g., urine, cerebrospinal fluid [CSF], sputum, gastric secretions, and synovial fluid). In the **anatomic pathology** area, autopsies are performed, histologic and cytologic procedures are utilized for tissue and fluid specimens, and fine-needle aspirates and surgical biopsy tissues are analyzed.

Laboratories can also be independently owned and operated outside the hospital setting i.e., physicians office laboratories. Large hospital laboratories typically have organizational structures that have an administrative/management hierarchy, a central specimen processing area, and divisions or sections for the testing processes (**FIGURE 1–2**). Each section may have a pathologist as the director and supervisors who oversee the technical procedures and troubleshoot issues that arise in that section.

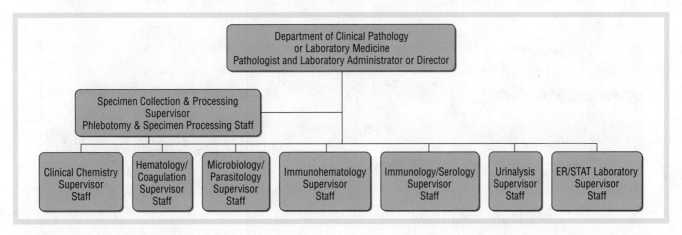

FIGURE 1–2

Example of an Organizational Chart for a Clinical Laboratory

This figure shows an overview of the major sections of a hypothetical hospital-based clinical laboratory.

Regardless of the type or size of the clinical laboratory, it is important to understand that the phlebotomist plays a vital role early in the process of producing laboratory results/reports. **Reliability** (reproducibility and consistency) and **accuracy** (the degree of correctness) of *all* patient test results depend on the **preexamination process (preanalytical phase)** of specimen collection—that is, the part of the process that occurs from the time laboratory tests are ordered through the time that specimens are actually delivered to the laboratory and then processed and/or transported to a referral laboratory (i.e., before the actual testing and analysis is performed). The preexamination process is the fundamental and crucial domain of every phlebotomist. **FIGURE 1–3** depicts the functional phases of laboratory testing, the preexamination (preanalytical phase), the **examination (analytical phase),** and the **postexamination (postanalytical phase).**[1]

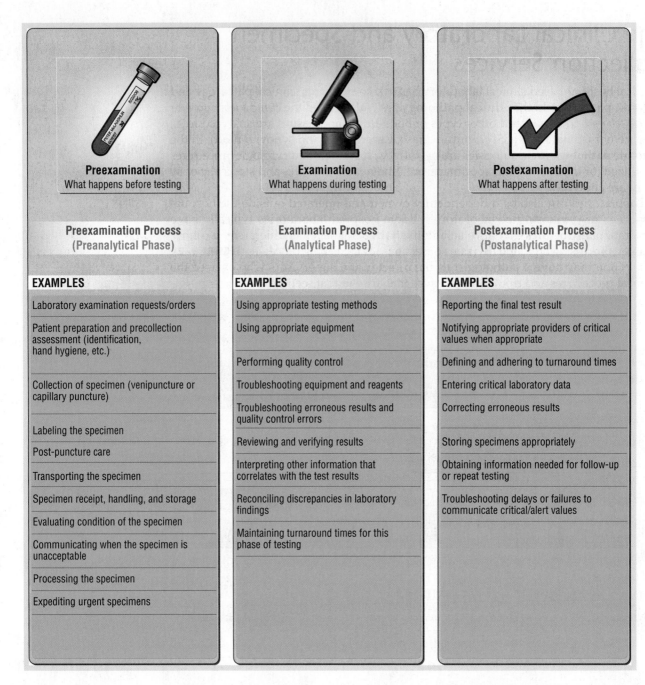

FIGURE 1–3

The Clinical Laboratory's Workflow Pathway

The Clinical and Laboratory Standards Institute (CLSI) describes the basic workflow of a clinical laboratory as beginning with a request for a laboratory test and ending with laboratory examination results and their interpretation by a health care provider. The workflow concept is depicted here in general terms and in reality involves many steps and actions; only a few examples are listed under each heading. The importance of these processes cannot be overstated because any failure to perform them correctly or completely can result in harm to patients, medical errors, waste of resources, and repeated work. All steps in each of these domains must be done according to standards of practice and must be traceable to the individual who performs the tasks. **Standards of practice** are procedural guidelines set by governmental, accreditation, certification agencies; professional organizations; and/or manufacturing and equipment requirements.

Smaller clinical laboratories can be located in remote locations or in clinics, physicians' offices, and mobile vans. Health care workers who perform the testing must maintain the same high standards of quality as are found in larger, high-volume laboratories.

The federal government has several agencies that regulate and oversee all clinical laboratories; they include the U.S. **Food and Drug Administration (FDA),** the **Centers for Medicare & Medicaid Services (CMS)** in the federal Department of Health and Human Services, the Occupational Safety and Health Administration (OSHA) in the Department of Labor, and the Department of Transportation (DOT). Some of these will be discussed more extensively in later chapters. Other regulatory agencies also have oversight of clinical laboratories, depending on the health care setting, the type and complexity of the testing they do, and employee certification. Among these are the International Association of Blood Banks, the American Society for Clinical Pathologists (ASCP), the College of American Pathologists (CAP), and The Joint Commission.

Also, some states (including California, New York, and Florida) have licensure/certification regulations and/or testing requirements for laboratory personnel. Phlebotomists should be knowledgeable about the licensure requirements when applicable because they may be allowed to perform certain procedures in one state but not in another. For example, many phlebotomists are allowed to perform basic point-of-care tests in most states, but they are not allowed to do so in California. Also, in California, the Department of Public Health requires specific proficiency areas for three different levels of licensed phlebotomists: Limited Phlebotomy Technician, Phlebotomy Technician I, and Phlebotomy Technician II. Refer to the Resources at the end of the chapter for more information.

CLINICAL/MEDICAL LABORATORY DEPARTMENTS

Clinical laboratories, especially those that are hospital based, typically have an administrative office headed by a pathologist and/or a director who oversees the many financial and operational aspects of the laboratory. Administrative responsibilities include all financial matters, such as cost accounting and budgeting, as well as human resources, strategic planning, operational issues, and regulatory issues. Depending on the size of the organization, the laboratory may have multiple supervisory/management personnel and/or physicians or scientists overseeing specific areas of the clinical laboratory. Large clinical laboratories usually cluster similar testing processes according to the sections listed in the organizational chart in Figure 1–2.

CLINICAL/MEDICAL LABORATORY PERSONNEL

Laboratory personnel work as a team to provide essential clinical data to physicians for diagnosing, treating, and monitoring patients. They provide the many pieces of a complex puzzle that make up a patient's condition. Laboratory professionals have some common characteristics: They like to solve problems, they strive for accuracy and reliability in their job tasks, they communicate well, they work under pressure and follow through on complex tasks, and they set high-quality standards for themselves and their work. Regardless of the level of education, health care workers involved with phlebotomy should familiarize themselves with various members of the clinical laboratory team (**BOX 1–2**).

Competencies, Certification, and Professionalism for Phlebotomists

The requirements for a phlebotomist vary across health care settings and regions of the country. A high school diploma or its equivalent is most often required to enter a phlebotomy training program in hospitals, community colleges, or technical schools. Typically, the length of training ranges from a few weeks to months, depending on the location, size of the facility, and the complexity of patients being served. Prior to

BOX 1–2

Clinical/Medical Laboratory Personnel

- **Pathologists**—Physicians (medical doctors, MDs) who have extensive training in pathology (the study and diagnosis of disease).
- **Administrative/Management Staff**—Individuals who may have a graduate degree in health care administration or business.
- **Technical supervisors**—Medical laboratory scientists with additional experience and education in a laboratory specialty area, such as hematology, microbiology, or clinical chemistry.
- **Medical Laboratory Scientists (MLS)**—Certified professionals with a bachelor's degree in a biological science. Educational requirements include one or more years of study in an MLS program. Licensing is required in some states. Roles and responsibilities include performing chemical, microscopic, microbiologic, or immunologic tests pertaining to patient care; recording and reporting test results; participating in research and development of new test methods; performing preventive maintenance, troubleshooting, and quality control of instruments and reagents; maintaining safety in the clinical laboratory; and teaching residents and fellows in pathology and laboratory sciences.
- **Medical Laboratory Technicians (MLT)**—Individuals who have a two-year certificate or associate's degree. The MLT may perform designated tests and procedures, prepare specimens for testing and transport, prepare reagents, perform quality control measures, and assist the MLS in numerous preanalytic and postanalytic processes and in performing limited analytical processes.
- **Phlebotomists or Phlebotomy Technicians**—Individuals with a high school diploma and specialized phlebotomy educational and clinical training; most phlebotomists take a certification examination. More information is presented in the next section.
- **Medical Assistants (MA)**—Individuals who have completed a medical assisting certificate, often in conjunction with an associate's degree. The MA in a laboratory setting may perform phlebotomy procedures, specified low-risk laboratory tests, basic patient assessments (blood pressure, etc.), specimen processing and handling, and clerical duties.
- **Certified Specialists**—Individuals who complete required experiences and a certification examination in a specified area of the laboratory such as blood banking, hemapheresis, microbiology, clinical chemistry, hematology, laboratory safety, or laboratory management.
- **Other Laboratory Personnel**—Doctoral-level scientists who specialize in specific areas such as immunology or microbiology, laboratory information systems (LIS) operators and programmers, clerical staff, quality management staff, infection control officers, and biomedical equipment specialists.

acceptance and/or employment, screening requirements may be requested, including a criminal background check, a drug screen, and/or evidence of specific immunizations, including the Hepatitis B vaccination series. Employers often require phlebotomy certification, which is accomplished by passing a national certification examination and/or attending **continuing education (CE)** programs in the field. Certification provides career advantages through job opportunities, career advancement, and portability (i.e., recognized from state to state). Since some state requirements vary, double-checking the educational requirements in a specific area prior to beginning the curriculum will prevent any misunderstandings.

Professional organizations that recognize phlebotomists include those listed in **BOX 1–3**. Many of these organizations have developed **competency statements** to describe the entry-level skills, ability level, aptitude, tasks, and/or roles performed

BOX 1–3

Professional Organizations for Phlebotomists

The organizations listed here have an interest in promoting and improving the practice of phlebotomy. They differ slightly in their membership requirements, fees, member benefits, continuing education courses, availability of certification examinations specifically for phlebotomists, and their profit motives (some are nonprofit and others are for-profit or proprietary; i.e., commercial, private ownership). The eligibility requirements and documentation for each certification also differ among these groups. Before applying for one or more of the certification examinations, double-check to see which ones are more reputable, secure, and accepted in the local community or state. Sometimes health care organizations have preferences for specific certifications and will adjust salaries accordingly. Likewise, local community colleges and universities can also provide recommendations about which certification examination to take. Since some states have credentialing or continuing education requirements for phlebotomists, it is important to know which organizations are approved by the state health departments to provide the examination or CE programs. Keep in mind that this is not an exhaustive list; in addition to the organizations listed here, there are other groups that market phlebotomy-related products and may offer continuing education programs as well.

Nonprofit Organizations

The American Society for Clinical Laboratory Science (ASCLS)

1861 International Drive, Suite 200
McLean, VA 22102
(571) 748-3370
www.ascls.org

ASCLS has recognized clinical laboratory personnel for more than 50 years. Several types of memberships are available, depending on the education and experience of the individual. Phlebotomists may join ASCLS as associate members in the Phlebotomy Section.

American Society for Clinical Pathology (ASCP)

33 W. Monroe Street, Suite 1600
Chicago, IL 60603
(312) 541-4999; (800) 267-2727
(312) 541-4998 (fax)
www.ascp.org

ASCP offers many levels of certification for laboratory personnel through the Board of Certification (BOC), including a Phlebotomy Technician Examination (PBT), a Donor Phlebotomy Technician (DPT), and an international certification examination for PBT (ASCP[i]). It also provides educational programs, teleconferences, webinars, workshops, phlebotomy scholarships, and online CE for phlebotomists. The certification exam covers the entry-level skills of a phlebotomist and uses taxonomy levels that assess recall (recognize facts), interpretive skills (use knowledge to interpret numeric data), and problem-solving skills (use applications of specific information to solve problems). Over 13,000 phlebotomists have been certified by ASCP since 1989.

American Society of Phlebotomy Technicians (ASPT)

P.O. Box 1831
Hickory, NC 28603
(828) 294-0078
(828) 327-2969 (fax)
www.aspt.org

ASPT offers a CPT (ASPT) certification examination. It also offers certification examinations for point-of-care technician, EKG technician, drug collection specialist, paramedical insurance examiner, and patient care technician.

(continued)

BOX 1–3 (*continued*)

National Accrediting Agency for Clinical Laboratory Sciences (NAACLS)
5600 N. River Road, Suite 720
Rosemont, IL 60018-5119
(773) 714-8880
(773) 714-8886 (fax)
www.naacls.org

NAACLS accredits educational programs in clinical laboratory sciences, including phlebotomy. No certification examinations are provided.

National Phlebotomy Association (NPA)
1901 Brightseat Road
Landover, MD 20785
(301) 386-4200
(301) 386-4203 (fax)
www.nationalphlebotomy.org

NPA was established in 1978 to recognize the phlebotomist as a distinctive and identifiable part of the health care team. The association has established professional standards, a code of ethics, educational opportunities, and an annual certification examination resulting in a CPT (NPA). NPA has trained and certified approximately 15,000 phlebotomists in all 50 states and abroad and has accredited 75 teaching programs. Accredited programs must include the following topic areas: Historical Perspective, Medical Terminology, Anatomy and Physiology, Communication, Phlebotomy Practical, Cardio-Pulmonary Resuscitation (CPR), Stress Management, Phlebotomy Techniques, Human Relations, Legal Aspects, Infection Control, and Drug Awareness.

Commercial Organizations
American Certification Agency (ACA)
P.O. Box 58
Osceola, IN 46561
(574) 277-4538
(574) 277-4624 (fax)
Contact: Shirley Evans, Testing Specialist or Carole Mullins, Director
E-mail: info@acacert.com.
www.acacert.com

The ACA provides certification examinations for phlebotomy technicians and instructors.

American Medical Technologists (AMT)
10700 W. Higgins Road, Suite 150
Rosemont, IL 60018
(847) 823-5169 or (800) 275-1268
(847) 823-0458 (fax)
www.amt1.com

AMT offers several certification examinations, including Phlebotomy Technician, Medical Laboratory Technician, Medical Laboratory Assistant, Medical Assistant, Medical Administrative Specialist, Allied Health Instructor, and Clinical Laboratory Consultant.

National Center for Competency Testing (NCCT/MMCI)
7007 College Boulevard, Suite 385
Overland Park, KS 66211
(800) 875-4404
(913) 498-1243 (fax)
www.ncctinc.com

The NCCT provides certification and CE for phlebotomy technicians and instructors.

BOX 1–3 (*continued*)

National Healthcareer Association (NHA)
National Headquarters
7 Ridgedale Avenue, Suite 203
Cedar Knolls, NJ 07927
(973) 605-1881 or (800) 499-9092
(973) 644-4797 (fax)

Established in 1989, NHA was formed to create a network for health care professionals. NHA provides a certification examination for phlebotomists, CPT.

by designated health care workers. Some offer convenient continuing education opportunities via conferences, online coursework, webinars, or podcasts. In addition, some professional organizations require CE to maintain certification and/or states may have specific CE licensure requirements through their respective public health departments.

The following list identifies competencies for entry-level phlebotomy technicians adapted from the American Society for Clinical Pathology and the National Accrediting Agency for Clinical Laboratory Sciences. In general, phlebotomists should have basic knowledge of anatomy of the arms and hands, physiology related to the circulatory system and basic body systems, specimen collection, specimen processing and handling (for blood and non-blood specimens), quality assessment tools, and laboratory operations related to phlebotomy. At career entry, a phlebotomist should be able to accomplish the tasks listed here. Also refer to Appendix 1 for a more detailed list of competencies from the National Accrediting Agency for Clinical Laboratory Sciences (NAACLS).

Fundamental knowledge of:

- principles of basic and special blood collection procedures
- basic anatomy and physiology and biological aspects of the human body
- preanalytic (preexamination) variables
- standard operating procedures (SOPs) for laboratories
- medical terminology
- regulatory requirements
- patient and personal safety
- infection control

Decision-making skills related to:

- the correct course of action
- selecting equipment/methods/reagents/samples
- applying quality control procedures
- selecting the most appropriate site for blood collection

Ability to prepare the following for a phlebotomy procedure:

- patients
- phlebotomy supplies and equipment

Evaluation skills related to:

- specimen and patient situations
- care of the patient after the procedure
- quality control procedures
- actions during adverse patient reactions
- sources of preanalytic (preexamination) variables
- common procedural/technical problems
- corrective action

At *minimum,* **BOX 1–4** shows the types of competencies that an employer might assess for the phlebotomist's performance evaluation. Competency statements describe the entry-level skills and tasks performed by phlebotomy technicians and measured on certification examinations. However, professional practice, experience, and continuing education contribute to a well-rounded, successful career in phlebotomy. Employee performance evaluations are important to both the employee and the employer because they provide feedback, identify problems early on, encourage employees to improve their skills and knowledge of policies, target specific improvements, and document that employees are competent in their job duties. Evaluations play a key role in determining who gets a raise or promotion when those opportunities are present. Box 1–4 describes examples of typical job duties for phlebotomists.

BOX 1–4

Typical Clinical, Technical, and Clerical Duties and Attributes of Phlebotomists

What are the clinical duties of phlebotomists?

- Communicate professionally with patients and coworkers.
- Identify the patient correctly.
- Assess the patient before blood collection.
- Prepare the patient accordingly.
- Perform the puncture.
- Withdraw blood into the correct containers/tubes.
- Assess the degree of bleeding and pain.
- Assess the patient after the phlebotomy procedure.

What kind of technical duties do phlebotomists have to perform?

- Manipulate small objects, tubes, and needles.
- Select and use appropriate equipment.
- Perform quality control functions.
- Transport the specimens correctly.
- Prepare/process the sample(s) for testing/analysis.
- Assist in laboratory testing procedures, washing glassware and cleaning equipment.

What clerical duties are expected of phlebotomists?

- Print/collate/distribute laboratory requisitions and reports.
- Work on secure computers, faxes, printers, and telephones.
- Answer all queries as appropriate.
- Demonstrate courtesy in all patient encounters.
- Always respect privacy and confidentiality (on and off the job).

BOX 1–4 (*continued*)

What kinds of policies must a phlebotomist adhere to?

- Safety in the laboratory and in patients' rooms.
- Infection control, gowning/gloving, and hand hygiene.
- Fire prevention and control.
- Dress codes.
- Attendance, sick leave, and vacation.

What kind of communication skills do phlebotomists need?

- Verbal skills.
- Nonverbal skills.
- Listening skills.
- Telephone etiquette.
- Written communication.
- Use of medical terminology appropriate for patients and coworkers.
- Management of angry or difficult patients.

How is the quality and productivity of a phlebotomist's work measured?

- Quality can be measured by waiting times, lack of complications or mistakes, contamination rates, etc.
- Workload metrics are often used to evaluate efficiency such as the amount of work processed in a given period of time.
- Productivity is also measured by the time and attention given to patients and to detailed procedures, and by the throughput of work based on how much work is completed during specified amounts of time.

Professionalism is the skill, competence, or character expected of an individual in a trained profession. It is hard to describe without sounding like one must achieve perfection. However, health care workers can use four categories to "frame" their concept of professionalism.[3] Refer to **FIGURE 1–4**.

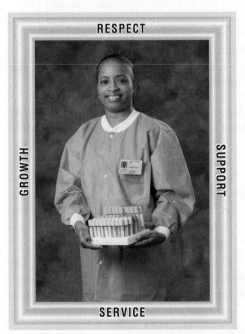

FIGURE 1–4

Four Categories of Professionalism

This health care worker is the "picture of professionalism." Each side of the frame is an important aspect of her career:

- **Respect**—For others, in personal appearance and in organizational policies/procedures such as patient confidentiality; for coworkers; and of cultural and/or racial differences
- **Service**—Shift focus from oneself to others; commit to one's job duties and to effective communication
- **Support**—Maintain a clean workspace; report errors and damaged equipment or supplies; exhibit courteous behavior; engage one's employer by respectfully disagreeing and offering solutions to problems
- **Growth**—Learning more about one's job and other aspects of the organization and employees who help run it

Throughout the remaining chapters of this text, the reader will be exposed to many aspects of professionalism and professional standards of practice. A job in the health care profession is not an "entitlement to a paycheck" and is not compatible with a "me-me-me" attitude. It is a commitment to respectfully serve others in an honest, meaningful, and highly professional manner.[3]

As mentioned earlier in this chapter, some states require that laboratory personnel be licensed before working in the field. State licensing may require an additional test or the state may utilize one of the certification examinations provided by a professional organization such as those listed in Box 1–3. To maintain licensing and/or certification credentials, phlebotomists must also participate in continuing education activities. In addition, some health care organizations prefer specific certifications over others, so it may be beneficial to check with local employers and state health departments before applying for a certification examination.

Specific competencies required of a phlebotomist can vary by employer but most are likely to include those listed above. There are many ways for supervisors to assess competency—for example, direct observation, video recording, reviewing worksheets or log books, reviewing quality control records, providing simulations of real-life situations, and providing written examinations.

ETHICAL STANDARDS AND CHARACTER TRAITS FOR PHLEBOTOMISTS

Within the health professions, organizations such as the American Society for Clinical Pathology (ASCP) and the National Phlebotomy Association (NPA) have developed standards of ethical conduct and behavior for members, and members are expected to adhere to those standards of performance. The major points common to most ethical standards for phlebotomists are:

- Do no harm to anyone intentionally.

- Perform according to sound technical ability and good judgment.

- Respect patients' rights (confidentiality, privacy, the right to know about their treatment, and the right to refuse treatment).

For phlebotomists, professional and ethical conduct involves responsibilities for accuracy and reliability of laboratory specimen integrity, respect for patient confidentiality and privacy, honesty, integrity, and regard for the dignity of all human beings. Many hospitals and health service organizations across the country have also established specific codes of ethics for their employees and/or statements of organizational values. For further discussion of ethical issues in phlebotomy, refer to Chapter 3.

Before entering the field of phlebotomy, one should reflect on the important character attributes for this career. Generally speaking, they include the following:

- **Sincerity and Compassion**—Phlebotomists should possess an intense desire to serve people and a sincere interest in learning about blood and specimen collection practices.

- **Emotional Stability and Maturity**—Phlebotomists must cope daily with seeing others in pain, handling blood and body fluids, facing injury and trauma, seeing disease sites, and the possibility of observing death. Patients are often fearful and anxious at the thought of having their blood collected. Responses of health care workers to harsh situations must be prompt, professional, compassionate, and reassuring to the patients, their families, and the health care team.

- **Accountability for Doing Things Right**—Personal integrity, veracity (telling the truth), and "doing what's right when no one is looking" (e.g., hand hygiene between patient collections, observing infection control precautions, reporting one's own mistakes, and collecting timed tests at the proper time) reflect a health care worker's personal responsibility for actions.

- **Dedication to High Standards of Performance and Precision**—Phlebotomists must continually upgrade and maintain the quality of their skills and seek out knowledge about new techniques and safety procedures, new supplies and equipment, and computer technology through CE. They should be willing to ask for assistance when dealing with a difficult patient or procedure and have the desire to follow rigid standards of performance. Also, they must collect only the specimens ordered and only those that they have been trained and authorized to collect.

- **Respect for Patients' Dignity, Privacy, Confidentiality, and the Right to Know**—Phlebotomists have an obligation to respect all patients' rights regardless of their personal opinions and biases. All patients must be treated with dignity and respect regardless of race, culture, religion, gender, age, or disabling conditions. Phlebotomists should have a full understanding of patients' rights to privacy and confidentiality and to knowing which procedures are being performed and by whom.

- **Acute Attention to Cleanliness**—Phlebotomists must protect themselves and patients by accepting that sterile techniques, good personal hygiene, and cleanliness affect safety and the quality of health care. Slacking off in this area can result in serious health hazards for both patients and health care workers. Maintaining cleanliness is more important than cutting corners to save time or money.

- **Pride, Satisfaction, and Self-Fulfillment in the Job**—Phlebotomists can attain professional satisfaction from continually improving their professional skills and knowledge, from knowing that others are dependent on the quality of their work, and from knowing that their skills contribute to the betterment of patients. The most successful, highly regarded phlebotomists are those who are most gratified with their work.

- **Working with Team Members**—Phlebotomists are obliged to be flexible enough to work with a variety of professionals in a wide range of settings. Teams can improve skills (more talent, expertise, and technical competence), communication (more ideas, mutual respect, crossing departmental lines), collaboration (valued above individual efforts), and effectiveness (solutions are more likely to be implemented; the team has ownership of the shared decisions).

- **Take Pleasure in Communicating with Patients**—The quality and ease of collecting blood specimens depends both on the technical skills of the health care worker and successful interactions with the patient. Phlebotomists should learn about transcultural communication strategies, communication barriers, special needs, and gender- or age-related issues that affect communication.

The decision to become a phlebotomist requires a special person with multiple talents and internal drive. The choice of this career path should not be taken lightly. Refer to **BOX 1–5** for help with this decision.

APPEARANCE, GROOMING, AND PHYSICAL FITNESS

Most health care organizations have rigid policies about what to wear in the workplace. Keep in mind that style and creativity are not key goals of most dress codes in the health care field. Rather, the focus is usually on safety, cleanliness, professionalism, and consistency. There are many examples of dress codes available online, a few of which are listed in the resources at the end of the chapter. **BOX 1–6** is an example of a typical dress code policy.

Posture

Phlebotomists usually perform their work while standing. There are occasions, however, particularly with ambulatory patients, when it is more effective to sit adjacent to the patient for the blood collection procedure. Erect posture conveys a sense of confidence and pride in job performance. Slouching conveys a sense of laziness and apathy.

Phlebotomy Career Self-Assessment

To consider a career in phlebotomy, ask yourself the following questions. If there are doubts in your mind about your answers, think about whether you are willing to change or learn new ways of behaving and working. These are important to your success and happiness with this career.

1. Do I pay attention to details?
2. Do I like to work with small objects such as needles and test tubes?
3. Do I follow procedures exactly or do I like to do things my own way?
4. Does it bother me if I am closely watched or supervised?
5. Do I mind seeing blood, sick patients, body tissues, or fluids or smelling unpleasant odors?
6. Can I help people calm down when they are fearful or show signs of anxiety?
7. What is my reaction to inflicting the pain of a needle-stick on someone?
8. Will I focus on keeping myself healthy and fit so that I can give my best effort at work every day?
9. Am I willing to admit my own mistakes?
10. Do I like working with a team? Do I get along well with other people?
11. Am I willing to stand for long periods of time, walk extensively, reach, stoop, lift, or carry equipment?
12. Am I willing to work on holidays and weekends occasionally?

Example of Dress Code Policy

Purpose—Presenting a consistent, professional, and positive image to all patients, customers, and members of the community is a goal of this health care organization. Professional dress, good grooming, and personal cleanliness are important aspects in helping customers and employees feel safe, confident, and comfortable.

To establish a standard appearance, the following guidelines will be enforced. Please note that these are minimum guidelines and that individual departments may have more rigid requirements as a result of safety, infection control, or patient preferences. Consult your supervisor regarding any questions you may have regarding these guidelines.

Policy—This policy applies to any employee who is at work as part of his or her regular duties and is representing the organization to the public. Employees who appear inappropriately dressed or groomed will be sent home. Failure to comply with this policy will result in disciplinary action up to and including termination.

Identification	■ Name badges will be visibly worn at all times.
	■ Stickers, pins, or other types of tokens should not cover the employee or department name.
Daily hygiene	■ Having clean teeth, hair, clothes, and body is a basic daily requirement.
	■ Breath should not be offensive.
	■ Clean, wrinkle-free clothes, scrubs, or uniforms that are in good condition should be worn.
	■ Lab coats should be clean and not frayed or worn-out.
Hair	■ Hair should be clean, neat, and trimmed. Conservative styles are recommended. Hair colors should be natural tones. (Extreme trends such as spiked hair or non-natural colors such as pink or blue are not acceptable.)
	■ Well-groomed, closely trimmed beards, sideburns, and mustaches are allowed.
	■ Shoulder-length or longer hair should be pulled back and secured to avoid patient contact or interference with equipment.

BOX 1-6 (*continued*)

Nails	■ Nails should be clean and neatly manicured, conservative in color of nail polish, and not more than one-fourth inch past the fingertip. ■ Artificial nails are not acceptable.
Fragrances/ Scents	■ Perfumes, aftershaves, and fragrances cannot be excessive. (Some patients are allergic to fragrances and/or they can be nauseating to patients who are ill.) ■ Minimize or eliminate the use of fragrances.
Make-up	■ Make-up should be conservative and lightly applied. ■ Extreme or excessive make-up is not allowed. (Frosted, bright colored eye shadow or bright or thick eyeliner is not acceptable.)
Clothing	■ Wear hospital-approved uniform/scrubs or other suitable attire. ■ Denim clothing of any type or style will not be allowed except on special occasions announced by the hospital administration. ■ Tight-fitting clothing, tank tops, lacy or sequined camisole-type tops or clothes that are sheer or revealing are not permitted. ■ Shirts should be buttoned up to the second button. ■ Shirttails (not scrubs) should be tucked in. (T-shirts with logos or athletic prints will not be allowed. Wrinkled or faded tops are not acceptable.) ■ Proper undergarments should be worn at all times. ■ Skirts and dresses should not be shorter than 3 inches above the knee. (Shorts, sundresses, back-less or strapless dresses are not permitted.) ■ Pants/slacks should be worn with a belt if they have belt loops. Pants should be tailored slacks or trousers and made of a firm fabric such as wool, cotton, and twill to maintain a professional appearance. (Baggy pants worn below the hips or that expose underwear is not permitted. Faded, torn, or stained pants or yoga, sweat pants, or leather pants are not permitted.) ■ Tight-fitting leggings are not permitted. ■ It is recommended that male employees who are not involved in patient care wear neckties.
Shoes	■ Shoes should be comfortable, safe in the work environment (close toed), clean, and polished. ■ Consideration should be made to minimizing noise when walking. ■ Socks and/or proper hosiery in neutral colors should be worn. ■ Sandals and flip-flops are not permitted.
Jewelry	■ Excessive jewelry is not allowed. Limits include 2 small rings per hand, 2 earrings per lobe. (Large rings or earrings are not acceptable.) ■ Because safety is a major concern, chains must be worn inside the collar, and long dangling earrings are not acceptable. ■ Other types of exposed jewelry (facial or body piercings such as eyebrow, tongue, cheek, lip, nose, chest, etc.) may also pose hazards and/or may become irritated with the use of personal protective equipment; therefore, they are not acceptable.
Tattoos	■ Clothing styles should cover visible tattoos.
Head Gear	■ No hats or head coverings may be worn inside (except for approved departments and for those worn for religious or medical purposes). ■ Reading glasses in neutral colors may be worn. (Sunglasses worn inside are not acceptable.)

Good posture is helpful for both the phlebotomist and the patient. It minimizes the health care worker's back and neck strain, promotes better breathing, and eases the patient's mind about the confidence of the phlebotomist. Relaxed hands, arms, and shoulders enable the health care worker to work more freely; this also provides an example to patients about how to relax their arms and shoulders.

If a health care worker is experiencing soreness in the neck and shoulder area as a result of poor posture, the worker should try to stretch his or her arms toward the ceiling periodically throughout the day. Massage therapy or medical assistance may be required in severe conditions.

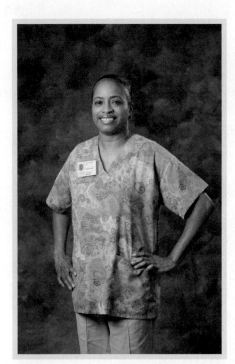

FIGURE 1–5

Stay Healthy, Look Professional

This health care worker has a colorful smock that is appropriate for her work area. Notice her erect posture, relaxed shoulders and arms, and the smile on her face. She appears to be professional, confident, clean, and approachable.

Grooming and Personal Hygiene

Physical appearance communicates a strong impression about an individual. Neatly combed hair; clean fingernails; a clean, pressed uniform; protective garb; and an overall tidy appearance communicate a commitment to cleanliness and infection control, and instill confidence in a person. This is particularly important in today's health care environment, in which patients and employees are deeply concerned about the spread of infectious diseases.

Employers of health care workers are legally required to provide **personal protective equipment (PPE)** or barrier protection for workers handling biohazardous, infectious substances. This type of garb includes gowns, gloves, masks, laboratory coats or aprons, and face shields. Because of latex sensitivities and allergies, employers must provide an array of sizes and styles of gloves and gowns in order to protect their employees. Careful compliance with safety standards minimizes the risk of occupational exposures to blood-borne pathogens. Infection control and safety considerations are covered in more detail in Chapters 4 and 5, respectively. A daily bath or shower followed by the use of deodorant is also recommended.

Physical Fitness and Health

The role of a health care worker requires physical stamina. Good health improves the health care worker's appearance, attitude, job performance, and ability to cope with stress. Knowing oneself and being in tune with one's body—that is, recognizing the signs of illness or fatigue—can help recovery, reduce downtime from illness, and make one feel better about oneself. Good nutrition, appropriate eating habits (more fruits and vegetables), rest during lunch and break periods, regular exercising, and minimizing the risk of workplace injuries are essential to an individual's well-being. Practicing a healthy lifestyle while on and off duty will facilitate a return to work with a refreshed and more productive attitude. When people feel well, they tend to have a more positive outlook on life (**FIGURE 1–5**).

Back strain is an injury that contributes to unwanted illness and absences. However, it can easily be prevented by staying fit through regular exercise, use of back supports, and/or use of correct lifting techniques. In **FIGURE 1–6**, the health care worker is lifting a box of venipuncture supplies the wrong way by bending at her waist, which may trigger a back strain. **FIGURE 1–7** shows the correct way to lift, with the health care worker bending her knees to distribute the weight more evenly through her legs and body, and finally shown in the upright position.

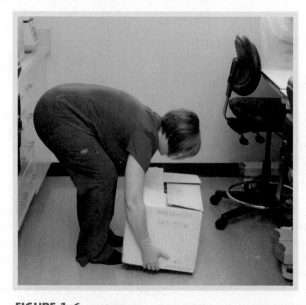

FIGURE 1–6

The Wrong Way to Lift

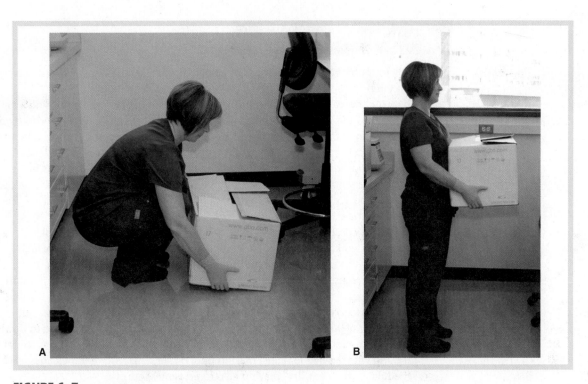

FIGURE 1–7
The Correct Way to Lift

A. Lift with your legs. B. Keep your back straight.

Stress in the Workplace

In most health care environments, the pace is hectic, there are many procedures and rules to follow, changes are common, worker relationships can be challenging, patients can get angry or agitated, and overtime work may be frequent. Also, life changes in one's personal life can add pressure to a career in the health care field. It takes a special effort to stay healthy and emotionally balanced, and to maintain a positive attitude. Aside from good nutrition and exercise, being prepared to deal with stress is a skill everyone needs. BOX 1–7 provides suggestions for relieving stress but the tips can be useful in preventing stress in the first place.

BOX 1–7

Ten Important Tips for Preventing or Relieving Stress

1. Find time to do your own thing. If you need privacy, structure some quiet time for yourself to meditate, pray, play an instrument, paint, or whatever activity you enjoy. Tai Chi or Qigong focuses on quieting the mind; and yoga has benefits such as improving sleep, mood, and quality of life. If you need an outlet, structure time for a hobby or a diversion outside of work to remove yourself from the stress, even if it is a brief period of time each day or week.

(continued)

BOX 1–7 (*continued*)

2. Look for humor in daily situations or associate with gentle people who can help you laugh or lighten up. Surround yourself with positive, energetic people.
3. Think of new ways to get exercise so that it does not get boring. Try adding a new exercise to your routine every few weeks. Try a new dance class or exercise form. If you cannot schedule an entire class, try short exercise sessions (10 minutes at three different times of the day is better than none at all). Even a short hike or walk can also reduce stress.
4. Eat nutritious low-fat foods and consider taking vitamins if your diet is not providing all the necessary nutrients. Think of your plate with at least 50 percent vegetables, 25 percent protein, and 25 percent carbohydrates. Also avoid candy—it is a short-lived "sugar high"; instead, eat a fruit snack.
5. Take more control over the sources of your stress. For example, if cooking meals after a hard day's work is stressful, cook multiple meals on your day off and freeze the rest so that they are easier to prepare during the busy workweek. If getting kids dressed and fed each morning is causing you to be late for work, lay out their clothes and breakfast foods the night before.
6. Establish adequate sleep habits. If you have insomnia, keep a sleep log about the quantity and quality of your sleep. If you have trouble sleeping, give yourself time to unwind before bedtime, use relaxation techniques, avoid stress-inducing activities prior to going to bed (arguing with family members, making phone calls, checking text messages, emails or your schedule for the next day, playing electronic games, etc).
7. Read interesting books, listen to new music, or watch interesting movies. Keep a life journal or a dream journal. If you forget to write in it, just skip a few days and pick it up again when you feel like it.
8. Go to a performance such as a concert, play, or dance program. Try to see an art exhibit or an art gallery open house.
9. Avoid harmful habits such as smoking, drinking excessively, or unnecessary drug use.
10. Do not be afraid to seek professional assistance (life coach, psychologist, therapist, etc.) when needed.

Quality Improvement and Assessment

PERCEPTIONS OF QUALITY

The concept of *quality* can be described in a variety of ways. The Clinical and Laboratory Standards Institute (CLSI), an organization that develops consensus standards for laboratory practice, defines **quality** as the "degree to which a set of inherent characteristics fulfills requirements"; other definitions include terms such as excellence, high standards, superiority, and the degree to which a service is performed correctly. The CLSI develops standards of practice for clinical laboratories. The standards are initially developed by a committee of experts in the field and go through a lengthy process of drafting, review, comment, and voting. During draft phases of the standards documents, CLSI seeks out comments from the public, and then the standards development committee addresses comments, errors, omissions, or other issues and finalizes the standards. All standards are available for purchase on the CLSI website, www.clsi.org/standards.

One can also consider quality in health care in two categories. First is the "scientific or technical" aspects of quality care; these entail how well clinical skills are applied to the situation—for example, whether the correct procedures/therapies are used for the patient. Second is the "nontechnical or interpersonal" aspects of quality care; these involve how well the personal needs of the patient are satisfied—for example, whether communication skills are adequate, the services are convenient and timely, or the patient is satisfied with the comfort and safety of the environment. Another way to describe quality in health care uses three major concepts:

■ **Efficacy**—The health care services provided have a positive impact on the patient's health; that is, the patient improves or gets well.

■ **Appropriateness**—The procedures performed on the patient are the correct ones for that particular condition or illness

■ **Caring Functions**—The services provided to the patient are available, timely, effective, safe, efficient, respectful, and sensitive to the patient's needs.

The quality of phlebotomy services focuses not only on meeting a *minimum* standard but also on the processes and assessments to constantly improve the services that are provided to stakeholders or customers.[4]

Stakeholders, or customers, are individuals, groups, organizations, or communities that have an interest in, or are influenced by, the quality of health care services. Internal stakeholders are individuals or groups within a health care organization itself; external stakeholders are individuals or groups outside the organization (**FIGURE 1–8**).

Phlebotomists have long been concerned about the quality of their work as evidenced by the following:

■ Standards of practice have been well established by organizations such as CLSI.

■ Educational programs have been established, and many are accredited (by the National Accrediting Agency for Clinical Laboratory Sciences [NAACLS]) to teach basic skills.

■ Certification and/or licensing examinations (ASCP, NPA, etc.) have been implemented to certify basic knowledge.

■ Associations have been established to voice and publicize the issues related to phlebotomy practice.

■ Codes of ethics have been designed.

■ Competencies have been identified by health care organizations.

■ Numerous resources are available for phlebotomists to improve their practices.

Therefore, it is imperative that phlebotomists assume some responsibility in **continuous quality improvement (CQI),** the concept of meeting and exceeding customer expectations by resolving immediate problems and finding opportunities for improvement where problems do not currently exist. These CQI efforts minimize cost, waste, and injury; enhance resources management; and improve stakeholder satisfaction.[1] Continuous quality improvement involves a constant and cohesive process of planning, teamwork, data monitoring, improvement, and reassessment.

Many health care organizations will adopt a specific quality improvement model or a framework for all to follow. One example of a quality framework is **Six Sigma,** a method designed to improve process performance by reducing variation, improving quality, enhancing financial performance, and improving customer satisfaction. Basically, it provides a data-driven, systematic approach to quality management through five phases, sometimes abbreviated as DMAIC:[5]

1. Define (the problem).
2. Measure (aspects of the current problem through data collection).
3. Analyze (the data to determine cause and effect issues).
4. Improve (by getting rid of places in the process where mistakes are made).
5. Control (the future processes by monitoring periodically).

Another quality management approach is the Lean process improvement methodology that focuses on improving quality by reducing delays, speeding up processes, eliminating waste, and taking immediate action. It is useful in determining which activities are "value-added" and which are not. Like other methods, the Lean process helps identify bottlenecks, identify best practices and measure progress toward set milestones

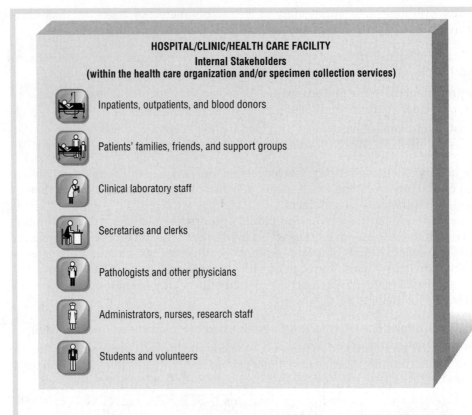

HOSPITAL/CLINIC/HEALTH CARE FACILITY
Internal Stakeholders
(within the health care organization and/or specimen collection services)

Inpatients, outpatients, and blood donors

Patients' families, friends, and support groups

Clinical laboratory staff

Secretaries and clerks

Pathologists and other physicians

Administrators, nurses, research staff

Students and volunteers

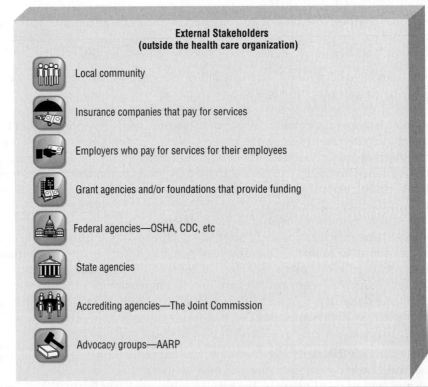

External Stakeholders
(outside the health care organization)

Local community

Insurance companies that pay for services

Employers who pay for services for their employees

Grant agencies and/or foundations that provide funding

Federal agencies—OSHA, CDC, etc

State agencies

Accrediting agencies—The Joint Commission

Advocacy groups—AARP

FIGURE 1–8

Examples of Stakeholders/Customers in Health Care

Globalization and Standardization: What's Up?

Did you know that the **International Organization for Standardization (ISO)** is a nongovernmental network of standards institutes from 155 countries that develops standards for manufacturing and service industries? According to its website, the ISO standards provide a "reference framework, or common technological language, between suppliers and their customers which facilitates trade and the transfer of technology." For applications in the clinical laboratory, ISO standards provide a quality management framework as well as standards for reporting laboratory test results. For more information, go to www.iso.org.

or goals. Some quality experts actually combine the two models into a "Lean Six Sigma," using components of both methods—the DMAIC framework and the principles of speed, efficiency, and quick action.[5] In addition, organizations such as the International Organization for Standardization (ISO), The Joint Commission, and the CLSI also provide guidelines for developing quality programs in health care facilities and laboratories (**BOX 1–8**).

The Clinical and Laboratory Standards Institute describes 12 Quality System Essentials (QSEs) for all workflow operations in the laboratory, from "preservice" through "service" to "postservice." They are summarized in **BOX 1–9**.

Summary of ISO's Quality Management Principles and CLSI's Twelve Quality System Essentials (QSEs)

The International Organization for Standardization (ISO) has developed 8 quality management principles that are to be used as a framework for organizations to improve performance. Basic topics are:

Principle 1: Customer focus
Principle 2: Leadership
Principle 3: Involvement of people
Principle 4: Process approach
Principle 5: System approach to management
Principle 6: Continual improvement
Principle 7: Factual approach to decision making
Principle 8: Mutually beneficial supplier relationships

For more details and information, see the vast resources and information available on the website: www.iso.org.

(continued)

BOX 1–9 (*continued*)

The QSEs include:

- Documents and records
- Organization and personnel
- Equipment, purchasing, and inventory
- Process control
- Information and occurance management
- Assessments—external and internal
- Process improvement
- Customer service
- Facilities and safety

Source: Adapted from Clinical and Laboratory Standards Institute (CLSI), *Quality Management System: A Model for Laboratory Services; Approved Guideline,* 4th ed., GP26-A4. CLSI, 940 West Valley Road, Suite 1400, Wayne, PA 19087-1898, www.clsi.org, 2011. For more information about acquiring this document, go to www.clsi.org.

Evaluating CQI is part of every health care worker's job, so knowing how to use tools and methods is essential. **Quality improvement** efforts for phlebotomy services usually focus on preexamination/preanalytical issues, for example:

- The health care worker's technique
- Patient identification procedures
- Waiting times
- Complications (e.g., excessive bleeding from the site)
- Recollection/repeat venipuncture rates
- Multiple sticks on the same patient
- Duplicate test orders for the same patient

These issues have the potential to result in negative outcomes for the patient. Thus, continuous improvement in minimizing these problems would be most beneficial to the patient and the health care worker. **TABLE 1–2** provides another way to consider components in a quality plan for phlebotomy.

TOOLS FOR QUALITY PERFORMANCE ASSESSMENT

Check sheets, run charts, and statistical tests can be used to review both the analytic and nonanalytic processes in the laboratory. Analytically, clinical laboratory scientists and technicians use data collection to ensure test sensitivity, specificity, precision, and accuracy. Nonanalytical data can be used to assess the timeliness of responses to requests, turnaround time for reporting test results, and effective communication. Tools for implementing continuous quality improvement include the following:

- **Brainstorming**—This is a method used to stimulate creative solutions in a group. Brainstorming is typically used at the beginning phases of assessing a quality issue. (See example in **BOX 1–10**.)
- **Cause-and-Effect (Ishikawa or Fish Bone) Diagrams**—These diagrams identify interactions among equipment, methods, people, supplies, and reagents (**FIGURE 1–9**).

TABLE 1–2

Components of a Quality Plan for Phlebotomy Services

Quality Aspect	Definition	Examples of Quality Monitoring in Phlebotomy
Structure	**Physical structure:** *Where are services provided?* Adequacy of supplies and equipment, safety devices, safety procedures, and availability and condition of equipment.	Expiration dates for supplies and reagents must be monitored because use of outdated blood collection tubes may cause faulty laboratory test results. When stocking collection tubes, place the tubes with a shelf life (expiration date) nearest the current date at the front of the shelf so that these tubes are used first. Perform **quality control (QC)** checks and preventive maintenance (PM) of laboratory instruments, including thermometers, sphygmomanometers (blood pressure cuffs), autoclaves, computers, and centrifuges.
	Personnel structure: *Are there adequate numbers of personnel and support staff?*	Ratio of staff to patients, qualifications of staff, and availability of the medical director or supervisors should be adequate.
	Management or administrative structure: *Are procedure manuals updated and readily available,* including security procedures for record keeping, and *can employees openly communicate with supervisors/administrators?*	Procedure manuals should be regularly updated and approved and available to those who need them. Employees should be able to contact a supervisor as needed. Phlebotomists and nursing staff should have access to an electronic or paper version of a manual that describes laboratory services, preparation of the patient, and special handling/processing of patients' specimens.
Processes	*Are procedures outlined and followed?* Steps are outlined and followed. This is usually accomplished through direct observation of practices, videorecording of health care interactions, patient interviews, and questionnaires.	Phlebotomists should perform the correct technical skills, and correct documentation procedures. Phlebotomy procedures that are commonly monitored are: ■ Patient identification: verbal, visual, handwritten, and/or automated ■ Isolation techniques ■ Precautions ■ Venipuncture or skin puncture procedures ■ Time required to complete venipuncture ■ Percentage of successful blood collection attempts on the first puncture ■ Percentage of 2nd attempts at collection ■ Appropriate use of collection devices ■ Appropriate transportation and handling ■ Completion of forms, documents, etc. ■ Specimen processing ■ Storage of specimens ■ Reporting results ■ Follow-up procedures when needed
Outcomes	*What is accomplished for the patient?* Poor patient outcomes have been described as the "5 Ds": death, disease, disability, discomfort, and dissatisfaction. Outcomes assessments often rely on information in the patient's medical record, laboratory reports, or what is self-reported.	Phlebotomists have a significant impact on patient outcomes so issues that are commonly monitored are: ■ Misidentified specimens ■ Hematoma formation: number and size ■ Infection rates ■ Contaminated or hemolyzed specimens ■ Excessive blood sampling ■ Repeat specimens or testing (redraws) ■ Response time ■ Volume of daily blood loss per patient ■ Number of patients who faint ■ Turnaround time for specimen collection ■ Turnaround time for lab test results ■ Correct timing of therapeutic drug monitoring ■ Patient satisfaction questionnaire results
Customer Satisfaction	*How satisfied are the stakeholders?* Determining satisfaction among patients and health care workers is usually accomplished by using questionnaires, mail-outs, and telephone or personal interviews. Although the information gathered using these techniques may be subjective, knowing why customers are dissatisfied and which customers are unhappy is extremely valuable.	Take the following into consideration: ■ Patient waiting time ■ Frequency and types of patient complaints ■ Frequency and types of MD/nurse complaints

Like brainstorming, this tool is useful in the early stages of quality assessment when figuring out the possible factors that affect a problem. It sorts ideas into key categories.

■ **Flowcharts**—This method is a visual representation of the steps or decision points in a process. A flowchart is useful for breaking a process into its components so that people can understand how it works (**FIGURE 1–10.**)

BOX 1–10

Brainstorming Exercise

This exercise can be performed by one individual or by groups of no more than three or four people. Groups are preferred because they tend to come up with a greater number and more creative ideas. Brainstorming sessions can be about any issue or problem as a first step in airing out ideas. As a start, use this quick exercise to practice using the brainstorming method.

One group should take the viewpoint of a new phlebotomist and the other group should take the viewpoint of the patient. (There are no "wrong" answers!)

Consider the idea of "excellence" or "perfection" in a phlebotomy encounter. What factors are important from your group's point of view? On a blackboard, whiteboard, or on paper that all group members can see, list as many and all ideas as you can in about 10 minutes. Get as many ideas as possible. Discussion of the ideas can take place in the next step. The important point for now is to get all possible ideas.

Next, in your group, come to a consensus about the order of importance of each idea. Make sure everyone in the group has a chance to participate and give his or her opinion about the order of importance.

Compare and discuss the lists from each group's viewpoint. Compare and contrast the order of priority for both groups. Come to a consensus about the order of priority of ideas for excellence in a phlebotomy encounter. Hopefully, participants will find that brainstorming is fun and can yield more ideas as a group process than as individuals.

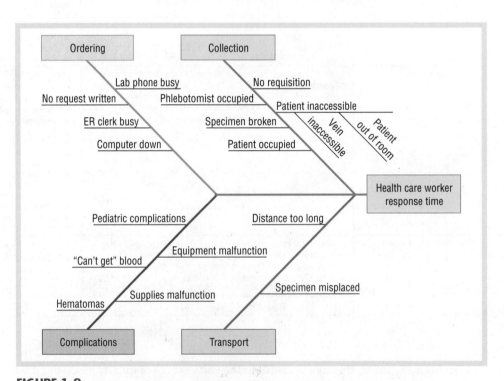

FIGURE 1–9

Cause-and-Effect Diagram

Cause-and-effect diagrams demonstrate interactions or factors that influence an outcome. For example, this cause-and-effect diagram demonstrates the issues affecting response time.

- **Pareto Charts**—Basically these are bar charts that show the frequency of problematic events; the Pareto principle says that "80 percent of the trouble comes from 20 percent of the problems" (**FIGURE 1–11**.) This is useful when there are many problems to address, but the team wants to focus on the most important or most frequent problem.

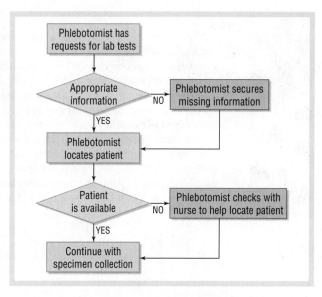

FIGURE 1–10
Flowchart

Flowcharts demonstrate steps in a process.

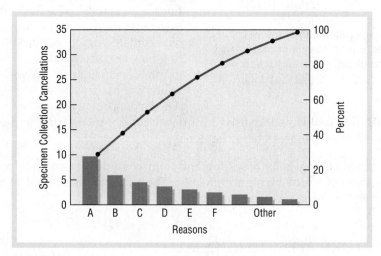

FIGURE 1–11
Pareto Chart

Pareto charts tally the number of times each specified problem occurs. Letters across the bottom indicate reasons for cancellations (e.g., the patient was unavailable, supplies were not accessible, duplicate orders, documentation was not complete, schedule conflict for patient, MD/nurse cancelled order).

- **Plan-Do-Check-Act Cycle (PDCA)**—This is a cycle for assessing and making positive changes, then reassessing.
- **Line Graphs, Histograms, and Scatter Diagrams**—These pictorial images represent performance trends. They are useful for charting numerical data distributions, and are usually used after the brainstorming and cause-and-effect diagrams have been explored.
- **Checkpoints and Tally Sheets**—These are structured, prepared forms for collecting and analyzing data for each attribute/reason (**TABLE 1–3**.)

TABLE 1–3

Example of a Tally Sheet

This table depicts a simple tally or check sheet used to collect data on "Interruptions to Morning Blood Draws on Unit 5."

Interruptions to Morning Blood Draws for Hospital Inpatients in Unit 5

Reason	Monday	Tuesday	Wednesday	Thursday	Friday	Saturday	Sunday	Total
Wrong patient in room	0	0	0	0	1	1	1	3
Additional information needed	1	0	1	0	0	1	1	4
Nurse requests assistance	4	0	1	0	2	3	2	12
Other	2	0	0	0	0	0	0	2
Total	7	0	2	0	3	5	4	21

Clinical Alert! Most of the time phlebotomists have a positive impact on health care, but always remember that they can have a negative impact on quality too. Unfortunately, they can cause pre-examination/preanalytical errors that can adversely affect patients. For example, misidentification of a patient can result in an erroneous cross-match and blood transfusion, which could be fatal to a patient (death). Inappropriate cleansing techniques or hand washing could result in transmitting **hospital- or health care-acquired infections (HAIs)**. Poor venipuncture techniques, such as improper needle insertion or excessive probing, could result in nerve damage (disability) or severe pain (discomfort). And lengthy waiting times, rude behavior, or messy work sites can contribute to an overall feeling of patient dissatisfaction.

- **Control Charts**—Control charts are graphs used to plot data over time (time of day, hours, minutes, days, months, etc.). They always have three important lines: upper control limit, lower control limit, and average control limit. These three lines are established based on historical data and standards of acceptable practice. By plotting new or current data on this graph, conclusions about variations are made—for example, Are the data out of control limits or are they in control? This tool is widely used for quality control monitoring in the laboratory and will be discussed more in later chapters.

There are many varied strategies for assessing and improving quality and performance of laboratories, most of which are highly effective. The phlebotomist should be a regular part of quality and performance assessments.

IMPORTANT FACTORS AFFECTING QUALITY IN SPECIMEN COLLECTION SERVICES

As mentioned earlier in this chapter, phlebotomists can consider the clinical laboratory testing process in several phases, with the primary goal of specimen collection being to obtain an accurate sample for analysis. The variables that are key to phlebotomists occur mostly before the specimen is actually analyzed (preexamination). Preexamination, examination, and postexamination (preanalytic, analytic, and postanalytic) phases in specimen collection, processing, and testing are part of every laboratory's operation. For purposes of this text, the quality discussion focuses on the preexamination phases, when the phlebotomist has the most impact. Examination and postexamination phases involve rigorous quality control procedures and other types of quality assessment procedures, including proficiency testing using specimens from outside approved sources and periodic inspections from authorized agencies. **FIGURE 1–12** summarizes the laboratory testing cycle, including examples of preexamination/preanalytic processes that are subject to quality reviews and monitoring. And Table 1–2 summarizes a Quality Plan for Phlebotomy Services that is in a framework that includes structures, processes, outcomes, and customer satisfaction.

In summary, the basic requirements for a *quality* specimen include the following:

1. Using standard precautions, the patient is identified, assessed, and prepared properly, and medication interference is avoided if possible.

Clinical Alert!

BLOOD LOSS DUE TO PHLEBOTOMY

For adults, blood loss due to venipuncture is usually well tolerated physiologically because the blood specimen constitutes only a small percentage of the total blood volume in the body. However, in some cases, patients are very ill and need to be closely monitored, so the frequency of blood collection and blood volume needed for testing may increase to a clinically significant level. Patients in intensive care units, those with arterial lines, and those with poor prognoses tend to have more total blood collected because of more frequent collections. The same is true for neonates and infants for whom even a small volume of blood may represent a large portion of the total blood volume. In these cases, phlebotomists must realize that blood conservation is a priority to avoid anemia and other complications. If too much blood is withdrawn from a patient in a short period of time, he or she may require a blood transfusion. Therefore, it is important to monitor blood loss daily if patients are neonates, have poor prognoses, or are being tested frequently. In these cases, the use of smaller test tubes and/or microcollection techniques might be warranted. This is discussed again in later chapters. Also refer to **BOX 1–11**.

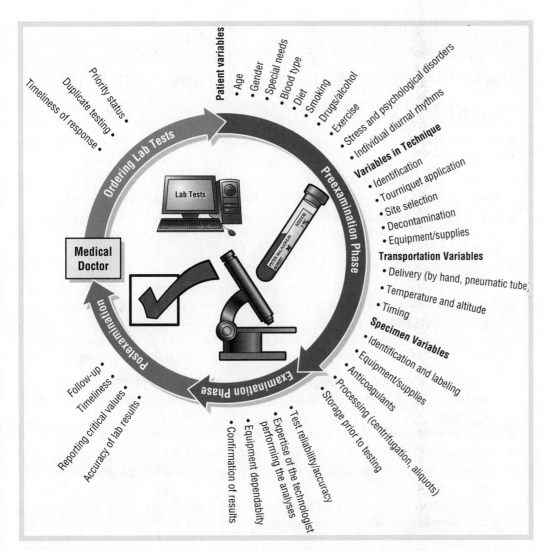

FIGURE 1–12

Laboratory Testing Cycle: Preexamination to Examination to Postexamination

The laboratory testing cycle begins with a physician's request for specific tests. After the laboratory is notified, the phlebotomist continues the preexamination phase by obtaining a specimen, which is then transported, processed, and prepared for the examination or analytic phase, when the specimen is tested/analyzed. The cycle ends with a test result going back to the MD who will make clinical decisions based on these results. Note the many variables that affect the entire process.

2. Specimens should be collected from the correct patients, using correct techniques, and labeled appropriately. Because the policy of most clinical laboratories is to discard specimens that are unlabeled or labeled incorrectly, the health care worker must abide by the laboratory policy describing acceptable identification of specimens. Potential errors in after-the-fact reidentification of a specimen by floor personnel can be extremely detrimental to the patient in question and are not acceptable. (See Chapter 10 for identification and labeling procedures.)
3. Correct anticoagulants and preservatives should be used with a sufficient amount of blood collected. Safety devices that minimize accidental needle-sticks should be used.
4. Specimens should be handled carefully so as not to cause damage and/or hemolysis.
5. Fasting specimens should be collected in a timely fashion and should actually be fasting samples. If they are not, the condition and follow-up actions should be documented.

BOX 1–11

Why Does the Laboratory Need So Much Blood for Testing?

In the laboratory, analytical variables that influence minimum blood volume requirements include the following:

- Analytical instruments require a minimum volume for testing.
- Analytical instruments may require a standard test tube size to function automatically.
- Special handling procedures are needed for separating plasma or serum into **aliquots** (smaller portions) for testing in different laboratory areas or for sending to a reference laboratory.
- Repeat testing is needed after a quality control failure.
- "Add-on" testing is ordered by a physician after the initial specimen is drawn.
- Tube manufacturers have volume requirements to ensure adequate dilution with an antico-agulant or other additive.

Strategies to reduce phlebotomy volume losses usually focus on organizing and coordinating blood draws. More specifically, phlebotomists can have an impact by assisting with the following:

- Coordinating all requests into a single phlebotomy event daily or by shift
- Scheduling blood draws on a regular and frequent basis to eliminate the need for random STAT requests
- Asking for a review of duplicate requests for tests that are already pending
- Maintaining a daily tally of blood loss when it is clinically indicated and for neonates
- Suggesting a review of standing orders that may no longer be needed because the patient has improved
- Assisting the laboratory in reducing turnaround time for test results through efficient, accurate, and timely preanalytical processes

6. Timed specimens should be correctly timed and documented.
7. Specimens without anticoagulants should be allowed to stand a minimum of 30 minutes so that clot formation can be completed. (Gel separator tubes, depending on the manufacturer, may shorten the time of clot formation.)

8. Specimens should be transported to the clinical laboratory in a timely fashion (within 45 minutes) to maintain freshness. A list of the specimens that are delivered after the designated time limits should be documented so as to help detect the source of the problem if needed.

All phlebotomists should aspire to provide the highest-quality patient specimens in a professional and safe environment 100 percent of the time.

ALERT

Clinical Alert!

INABILITY TO COLLECT A BLOOD SPECIMEN

Clinical laboratories should have a written procedure about what to do when a blood specimen cannot be collected. The procedure should describe the steps that should be taken by the phlebotomist when (1) collection attempts are unsuccessful (no more than two sticks by one phlebotomist), (2) the patient is unavailable, or (3) the patient refuses to have blood drawn.

Future Trends in Phlebotomy Practice

STANDARDIZATION AND GLOBALIZATION

As technology evolves and standardization and globalization of industries take place, so goes the health care industry. Through the efforts of ISO, CLSI, and many other professional organizations, phlebotomy practices have become more standardized along with credentialing criteria and educational requirements. In fact, several of the professional organizations mentioned in Box 1–3 now work collaboratively with many countries to provide international certification for phlebotomists. With the availability of online educational programs, opportunities are provided to people in many parts of the world. In addition, many countries (for example, Japan and the European Union) have adopted regulations similar to those in the United States that relate to privacy and confidentiality of health records. Universal signage symbols (**FIGURE 1–13**) and barcode technology (covered in Chapter 2) are now more accessible for use in health care settings throughout the world.

SMALLER AND FASTER THROUGH NANOTECHNOLOGY

Research efforts in clinical laboratory testing are toward smaller and faster. **Nanotechnology** (the manipulation of matter, including blood samples, on an atomic or molecular scale) and improved molecular sequencing, coupled with microfabrication of plastics, sophisticated biometrics, and electronic data processing, is opening many new avenues for testing blood specimens. These technologies have the potential to reduce blood sample sizes, reagent use, and costs, and increase instrument portability, ease of use, efficiency, and accuracy of some clinical testing processes.

DIRECT ACCESS TESTING (DAT) OR DIRECT TO CUSTOMER (DTC)

Since the general public has greater access to health information, patients are now more knowledgeable about health care decisions and more demanding of their own laboratory results. Many health care companies and organizations now offer direct testing results to consumers in a variety of nontraditional health settings—for example, health clubs, grocery stores, local pharmacies, religious facilities, and community centers. It is anticipated that this trend will continue to expand and open job opportunities for all health care workers who perform phlebotomy.

EDUCATION/CERTIFICATION

Technology has become a vital tool in education through the use of electronic books, virtual classrooms, and choices in how to complete courses. Internet access has enabled individuals to enroll in online CE courses, podcasts, webinars, etc., to get mandatory credit almost instantaneously, and/or take online certification examinations. However, in some cases, poor quality teaching, lack of standardization, or poor oversight may be lacking in phlebotomy programs, so phlebotomists should carefully evaluate all online options before investing time or money in a program. Well-established organizations, colleges, and universities exist that are reputable and legitimate and often offer better educational services at a lower cost.

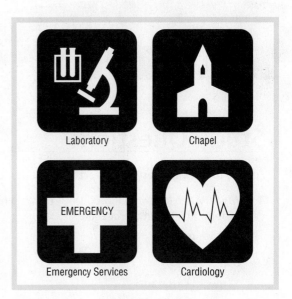

FIGURE 1–13
Universal symbols help patients and employees find their way in a health care facility without the need for text-based signs.

Courtesy of www.hablamosjuntos.org

Study Questions

For the following questions, select the one best answer.

1 Which of the following individuals is most likely to perform phlebotomy procedures?

a. office manager
b. pathologist
c. pharmacist
d. medical assistant

2 An example of how clinical laboratory test results are used is

a. body mass index
b. cataract screening
c. monitoring cholesterol levels
d. measuring heart rate

3 Specimen collection procedures are part of which phase of a laboratory workflow cycle?

a. preexamination
b. examination
c. postexamination
d. follow-up

4 Which of the following is a characteristic of a pathologist's responsibilities?

a. daily rounds with patients
b. treatment of conditions related to the respiratory system
c. oversight of a clinical laboratory
d. performance of point-of-care procedures

5 Which of the following is the main area of responsibility for every phlebotomist?

a. analytic testing
b. data collection
c. reporting results
d. preanalytic processes

6 Part of being a responsible member of a health care team involves

a. being confident at all times
b. understanding the mission, goals, objectives
c. always avoiding conflict
d. sticking to a decision regardless of advice from others

7 In order to protect themselves on the job, phlebotomists should have which character trait?

a. propensity for cleanliness
b. fear of infectious diseases
c. expressing themselves loudly
d. being suspicious of peers

8 Clinical laboratory standards of practice in the United States have been established by which of the following organizations?

a. FDA
b. CLSI
c. NRA
d. CMS

9 Which of the following tools is most useful for demonstrating steps in laboratory procedures.

a. Fish bone diagram
b. Brainstorming
c. Flowchart
d. Six Sigma

10 An example of an unfavorable patient outcome during or after a phlebotomy procedure would be if the patient

a. states that he is fearful of the procedure
b. faints after the venipuncture
c. has a loud radio going in the room
d. has several family members in the room

Case Study 1

Missing Laboratory Results A patient has been admitted to a hospital for a routine procedure that should require only a 24-hour hospitalization. The patient had laboratory tests performed the day before the scheduled admission. When the patient came to be admitted for the procedure, she was told that laboratory tests results were not yet available and she would have to have all tests repeated and return the following day for the procedure.

Questions

1 What are some possible causes for the missing laboratory results?

2 Describe the effects this scenario could have on the patient.

3 Describe the effects this scenario could have on stakeholder satisfaction.

Case Study 2

Morning Blood Draws Return to Table 1–3, "Interruptions to Morning Blood Draws on Unit 5." Review the data in this table and consider the following questions. Keep in mind that this is a hypothetical example and that you are an outsider making judgments so there are no real right/wrong answers in this scenario.

Questions

1 Describe the two most important trends you observe from the data in this table.

2 List some possible causes of these trends.

3 What should the quality team do next about this information?

Action in Practice 1

Building Character A new student in the clinical laboratory should begin using and/or developing character traits that are beneficial to the clinical environment. Oftentimes, these character traits are also helpful in daily life outside the workplace. Consider the following nonclinical encounter to help you envision and use positive character traits in daily life and at work. This can be done as an individual exercise, role-play exercise, or as a group discussion.

A close friend states that her house is full of clutter and debris and she feels overwhelmed. She states that she cannot get her family members to help her clean it up. She has asked you for advice with this problem.

Question

Analyze your friend's problem and consider the following character traits in justifying your advice to her:

- Sincerity and compassion
- Propensity for cleanliness
- Emotional stability and maturity

- Pride or satisfaction with a job
- Dedication to a higher standard
- Doing things right
- Respect for dignity and privacy
- Working as a team member
- Communicating with others

The Bakery Using an easy analogy is helpful to visualize the laboratory workflow. In a simplistic way, the laboratory works like a bakery making a special-order wedding cake. The process includes these steps:

a. Getting the order for the cake—selecting size, flavors, icing, decorations, etc.
b. Making the cake—measuring and mixing ingredients, pouring it into baking pans, setting baking time and temperature, etc.
c. Delivering the cake to the customer—maintaining the cake at the right temperature, transporting the cake, delivering it to the correct location, etc.

Questions

1. Think about this analogy and consider that the three processes are done by different people—for example, the telephone clerk, the baker, and the delivery person.

    ■ What kinds of errors can occur in each of the processes?
    ■ Which errors affect the customer the most?
    ■ Why is teamwork important in the baking example?
    ■ What happens if one step is incorrect and the other two are done perfectly?

2. Describe how this is similar to and different from the phases of laboratory testing.

COMPETENCY ASSESSMENT

Check Yourself

1 Describe the phases of laboratory testing and which phase is most important for the phlebotomist.

2 Phlebotomists can work in a variety of health care settings. Name at least 10 potential job sites for phlebotomists. Think about which work settings may appeal to you the most and why.

Competency Checklist: Basics of Phlebotomy Practice and the Clinical Laboratory

The health care worker should be able to identify common areas or departments of health care organizations, including clinical laboratories and various members of the health care team and their roles/responsibilities. The health care worker should do the following:

(1) Completed (2) Needs to improve

_____ 1. List at least five service areas/departments that are commonly found in large health care facilities.
_____ 2. List three ways in which laboratory test results are used.
_____ 3. Name at least five departments/sections common in clinical laboratory/clinical pathology.

_____ 4. List at least three types of laboratory personnel other than phlebotomists.
_____ 5. Name 10 types of locations where phlebotomy services can be performed.
_____ 6. Describe at least three clinical duties of a phlebotomist.
_____ 7. Describe at least three technical duties of a phlebotomist.
_____ 8. Describe at least three clerical duties of a phlebotomist.
_____ 9. Describe at least five character traits of a phlebotomist.
_____ 10. Name at least three professional organizations for phlebotomists and other laboratory personnel.

Competency Checklist: Quality Basics

The health care worker should have an understanding of fundamental factors related to providing quality services. The health care worker should do the following:

(1) Completed (2) Needs to improve

_____ 1. Provide three examples of external stakeholders (customers).
_____ 2. Provide eight examples of internal stakeholders (customers).
_____ 3. List five examples of how a phlebotomist may have a negative effect on quality and/or patient outcomes.
_____ 4. List 10 examples of quality improvement assessments that could be monitored for phlebotomy services.
_____ 5. Describe at least eight examples of preexamination/preanalytical factors that affect phlebotomy services.
_____ 6. Describe the difference between a flowchart and a cause-and-effect diagram.

REFERENCES

1. Clinical and Laboratory Standards Institute (CLSI). *Procedures for the handling and processing of blood specimens for common laboratory tests: Approved guideline,* 4th ed. Document H18-A4. Wayne, PA: Author.

2. American Hospital Association. (2014). Fast facts on U.S. hospitals. www.aha.org/research/rc/stat-studies/fast-facts.shmtl, accessed 2/25/2014.

3. Bailey, M. K. (2005, July). The telltale signs of a consummate lab professional. *Med Lab Observer,* 30–33.

4. Graham, N. O. *Quality in health care: Theory, applications, and evolution.* Gaithersberg, MD: Aspen, 1995.

5. Jacobson, J. M., & Johnson, M. E. (2006, March). Lean and Six Sigma: Not for amateurs. *Lab Med, 37*(3), 140–145.

RESOURCES

www.aama-ntl.org American Association of Medical Assistants (AAMA) provides a certification/recertification program and resources for medical assistants.

www.aha.org American Hospital Association "leads, represents and serves hospitals, health systems and other related organizations that are accountable to the community and committed to health improvement" and provides information about hospital statistics.

www.asq.org American Society for Quality (ASQ) is an organization devoted to quality. Basic resources about quality are available for numerous industries, including health care.

www.accessdata.fda.gov/scripts/cdrh/cfdocs/cfCLIA/clia.cfm This easy-to-use website is part of the U.S. Food and Drug Administration (FDA) and provides a database of all types of laboratory testing methods and CLIA categorization.

www.bexcellence.org Definitions, resources, and products for quality management systems are provided.

www.clsi.org Clinical and Laboratory Standards Institute (CLSI) provides information about standards for clinical laboratories and manufacturers of clinical laboratory supplies and equipment.

www.dhs.ca.gov/ps/ls/lfsb/html/phlebotomy.htm The California Department of Health Services provides information about state licensing and certification for phlebotomists in California.

www.isixsigma.com This website provides resources for achieving Six Sigma results, including live discussion groups, blogs, articles, and daily tips.

http://healthcare.utah.edu/careers/DressCodePolicy.pdf The University of Utah, Hospitals and Clinics, Human Resources, publishes a dress code policy for its employees.

www.iso.org The International Organization for Standardization is the largest developer of global standards for products and services in many industries, including health care, technology, and agriculture.

www.jointcommission.org The Joint Commission website provides information about accreditation services, standards, and performance measurement.

www.labtestsonline.org This website provides public information on clinical laboratory testing and professional requirements.

www2.medicine.wisc.edu/home/hr/dresscode The University of Wisconsin, Department of Medicine, also publishes its UW Health Dress Code and Appearance Policy.

www.naacls.org The National Accrediting Agency for Clinical Laboratory Sciences (NAACLS) is an accrediting agency for educational programs in phlebotomy and related health professions. The website includes valuable resources for educators.

www.phlebotomy.com The Center for Phlebotomy Education provides free practice tips, and markets numerous other phlebotomy products.

www.skymark.com/resources Skymark markets software for quality management tools and a free quality management resource center.

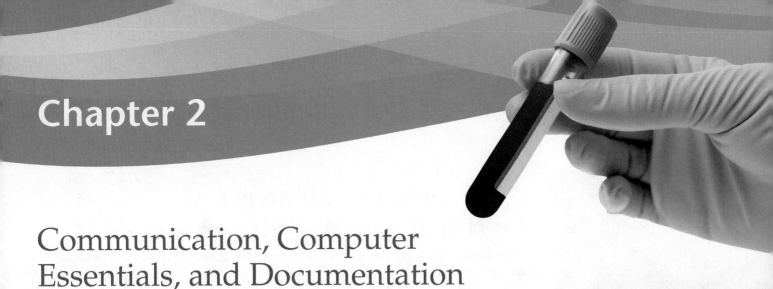

Chapter 2

Communication, Computer Essentials, and Documentation

Chapter Objectives

Upon completion of Chapter 2, the learner is responsible for doing the following:

1. Outline the basic communication loop.

2. Describe methods for effective verbal and nonverbal communication, active listening, and written communication.

3. List examples of positive and negative body language.

4. Describe methods to achieve cultural competence and sensitivity in the workplace.

5. Describe basic components of the medical record and provide examples of how to maintain confidentiality and privacy related to patient information.

6. Describe essential elements of laboratory test requisitions, specimen labels, and test results.

7. Identify potential clerical or technical errors that may occur during labeling or documentation of phlebotomy procedures.

8. Identify essential components and functions of computers in health care and list ways that health care workers use them to accomplish job functions.

KEY TERMS

active listening
bar codes
beliefs
blind
Braille
central processing unit (CPU)
clinical (or medical) record
cloud computing
computerized patient record (CPR)
confidentiality
critical value
culture
date of birth (DOB)
delta checks
electronic medical or health record
    (EMR or EHR)
e-mail
health literacy
laboratory information system (LIS)
pace (of voice)
quick response (QR) codes
radio frequency identification (RFID)
read-back
requisition
security password
specimen collection manual
STAT
tone (of voice)
traditions and practices
universal serial bus (USB)
values
zone of comfort

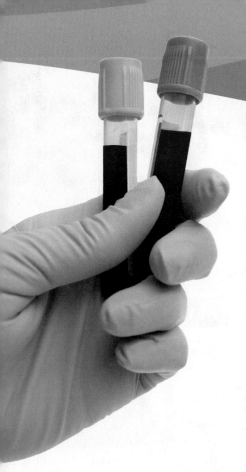

Communication Strategies for Health Care Workers

Communication using verbal and nonverbal skills, active listening, and electronic text or handwritten language is essential for everyday success. Nobody communicates alone; rather, it occurs when one person delivers a message so that the sender gets the desired response or reaction from the receiver. Effective interpersonal interactions can be depicted as a communication loop, as depicted in **FIGURE 2–1**. The verbal message must leave the sender (who encodes the message through the use of voice, tone, facial expression, etc.); it then travels through extraneous filters (noise, language barriers, hearing ability, etc.); it reaches the receiver (who must decode the message); and finally, the receiver provides a response or reaction (feedback) to the sender that the message has been received and understood. Without feedback, the sender has no way of knowing whether the message was accurately received or if the message was somehow blocked or

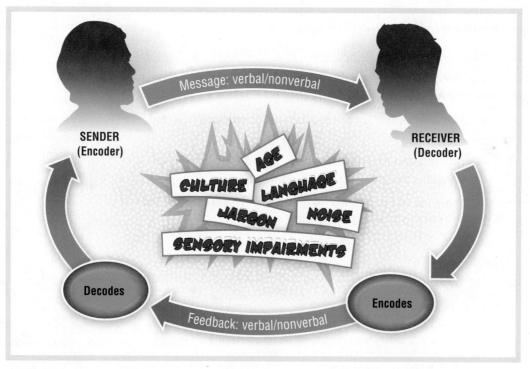

FIGURE 2–1

Communication Loop

The sender is at one end of the loop with a message to communicate. He converts the message using verbal and/or nonverbal codes. The sender (or encoder) carefully chooses the appropriate codes for his message using knowledge of the receiver, and the urgency and importance of the message. He can use any type of medium to encode the message (verbal, body language, writing, etc.). The receiver decodes the message correctly if s/he is familiar with the codes (verbal language, body language). The receiver's response or reaction is the feedback to the sender. Feedback provides evidence that either the message was correctly received or that is was misinterpreted. Many factors interfere with encoding and decoding messages.

changed by extraneous factors that filter out meaning from a message. Filters that affect the accuracy of the message include:

- Medical terminology or jargon
- Language differences
- Sensory ability (speech or hearing impairments)
- Pace, tone, and volume of one's voice
- Urgency of the situation
- Cultural meaning
- Environmental noise
- Age

FIGURE 2–2 shows that face-to-face communication is the single-most effective form of communication; health care workers must practice it every day so as to be sure that their message is the one they intended patients or coworkers to receive. In reality, people use multiple methods to enhance communication. In health care settings, so-called **read-back** policies are used between coworkers to assure that communication is accurate. After one worker has communicated a message to another, the read-back procedure consists of repeating the orders, instructions, or results back to the originating person. This ensures that the verbal orders, instructions, or results were interpreted correctly. For health care workers, the read-back practice is a valuable tool to use for patients, too. For example, if a health care worker is giving instructions to a patient about how to collect a urine sample, he or she can ask the patient, "Mrs. Jones, would you mind repeating the steps so we can ensure that you understand it all?"

In the following sections, communication is broken down into its four more detailed components, all of which are equally important:

1. **Verbal Communication**—Actual words are spoken.
2. **Nonverbal Communication**—Body language is used.
3. **Active Listening**—Verbal and nonverbal information is used to assess the situation.
4. **Written Communication**—Text-based language is used electronically or in printed format.

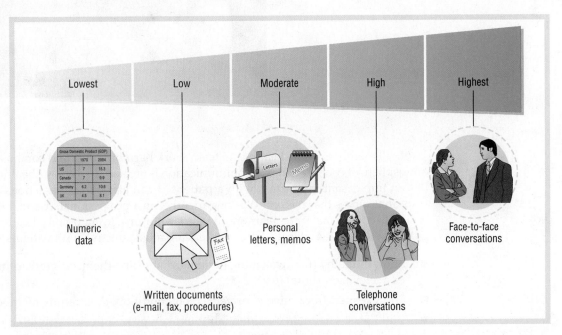

FIGURE 2–2

Degree of Communication Effectiveness

It is best to talk to patients one-on-one with minimal distractions and in a private environment. This provides the fastest and most effective communication method in phlebotomy situations.

VERBAL COMMUNICATION

Keep in mind that talking with patients about personal things such as their bodies is never easy. It may be particularly difficult with teenage patients, patients from cultural backgrounds that are different from that of the health care worker, and patients who are of the opposite gender. Likewise, communication with coworkers often involves different cultural issues, age differences, and variations in work habits (**FIGURE 2–3**).

FIGURE 2–3

Communicating with Patients and Team Members

Health care workers must be skilled in communicating with patients and team members. In these photos, note which components of communication are being utilized.

A. Patient and family member interaction with a medical assistant.
B. Health care team meeting.

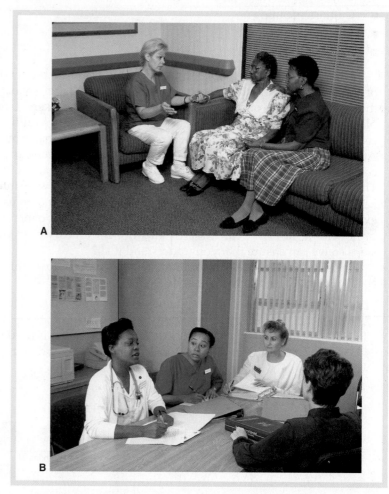

If all members of the health care team work harmoniously and compassionately, an atmosphere of cooperation and communication is created. If even one health care worker has an unpleasant interaction with a patient, it can affect the interactions of the entire team that serves that patient. Working together in a professional, friendly environment will collectively make the team more effective in providing quality health care for the patient (**FIGURE 2–4**). Health care workers are most effective with patients when they:

- Show empathy (for awakening patients, disturbing them, or interrupting their meal or a television show) (**BOX 2–1**).
- Show respect (for patients' privacy, their condition, their family members).
- Build trust (maintain confidentiality, explain procedures clearly, tell the truth).
- Establish rapport (show common courtesy, express interest).
- Listen actively (face the patient, maintain nonauthoritative posture, lean toward the patient, establish eye contact, relax and listen intently).
- Provide specific feedback (about their behavior, about a procedure)

Language and Age

Health care workers should use simple, straightforward vocabulary, with proper pronunciation and grammar, particularly with children or patients from other countries whose first language is not English. Using complex jargon or medical terminology can be confusing to laypeople. Nearly half of all adults in the United States struggle with **health literacy**—that is, they do not have adequate knowledge of health issues based on their written, spoken, or conceptual knowledge. Many also have trouble understanding physicians' instructions, reading medical directions, or making informed health care decisions.[1,2] In addition, the meaning of words varies with context and the age of the speaker. Generational differences can have a positive effect on communication with some basic insight, as indicated in 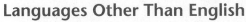TABLE 2–1. More detailed information will be presented for age-specific competencies with patients in the pediatric and geriatric sections of Chapter 13 because the language and gestures used for a pediatric patient are different from those used with a geriatric patient.

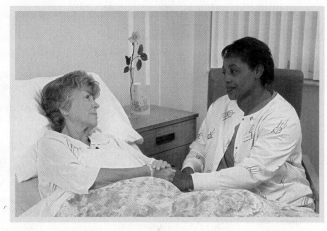

FIGURE 2–4

On occasion, a health care worker may need to sit down near the patient to spend extra time explaining the procedure or to answer questions. This health care worker is actively listening to the patient's concerns in a compassionate manner.

Languages Other Than English

In the United States, it is common to hear languages other than English spoken. As a sign of increasing globalization, in large metropolitan areas of the United States one sees signage in multiple languages and schools now teaching a variety of language courses that were not offered even five years ago. Patients who do not speak English can understand some basics from nonverbal cues, but to be sure the patient has been informed, the health care worker must know how to access the translation services that are now available in many forms—that is, health care workers who speak other languages, audiotapes or written information in various languages, language services available by phone or Internet, etc. In the absence of an interpreter, printed cards in different languages can be effective in transmitting information about the venipuncture procedures if the patient is literate.

Clinical Alert! In some states, children are not permitted to serve as translators for their parents when health care issues are discussed. Health care workers should check with their supervisors about the applicable laws in their states.

ALERT

BOX 2–1

Environmental Noise

A busy hallway, visitors, a television, a smartphone, a radio, or electronic music with headphones can prevent the patient from hearing accurately. In these cases, take steps, in a polite and professional manner, to reduce the sound level so the patient can hear necessary instructions. Examples might include phrases such as the following:

To visitors—"Excuse me please, it's important for me to explain this procedure to Mr. Smith. Would you mind if we have a quiet moment together for a few minutes? Thank you for your cooperation."

For the television, radio, music—"Mr. Smith, I'm sorry to interrupt your television show, but would you mind if we lower the volume for a few minutes so we can go over the procedure for collecting your blood sample? Thank you—this shouldn't take very long."

For headphones—"Mr. Smith, it's important that we discuss this procedure before beginning. Would you mind taking off your headphones for a few minutes? I'll be brief. Thank you for your cooperation."

TABLE 2–1

Communication across Generations: Know the Person You're Talking To

The workforce in the United States, which generally includes individuals older than age 18, can be categorized into four basic groups depending on their age or birth year. Collaboration among workers from different generations or between a patient and workers from different generations can be challenging but necessary to promote an effective health care team and quality patient care. Keep in mind that terms can change meaning across generations. Therefore, one should bridge the generational gap by learning the perspectives and motivations of others, by discussing expectations early on, and keeping up with new and changing technology.[3,4]

	Veterans/ Traditionalists/ Matures/Builders (born prior to mid-1940s)	Boomers (born mid-1940s–1964)	Generation Xers (born 1965–1981)	Millenials/Internet Generation Y/ Nexters (born 1982–2000)
Population	More than 44 million	More than 76 million	More than 54 million	More than 77 million
Important Aspects of Their Lives	WWII and Pearl Harbor bombing The Great Depression Korean War *Music:* Big Band Era, Frank Sinatra, Nat King Cole *Politics:* Bob Dole, Ronald Reagan, Jimmy Carter, George Bush, Sr.	Assassinations of John F. Kennedy and Martin Luther King Civil rights Women's liberation First moon landing *Music:* The Beatles, Elvis Presley, Beach Boys, Rolling Stones, Supremes, Jimi Hendrix, Motown, Woodstock *Politics:* Bill and Hillary Clinton, George W. Bush	John Lennon's murder *Challenger* disaster Fall of Berlin Wall Operation Desert Storm Personal computers Latchkey kids of boomers Music videos *Music:* U2, Madonna, Nirvana, Guns and Roses, Michael Jackson *Politics:* Barack Obama	Oklahoma City bombing and 9/11 O. J. Simpson trial Columbine school murders Gang violence War in Iraq Clinton-Lewinsky scandal Body piercing and tattoos Internet Video games Cell phones Kids with schedules and over-protective, supportive parents *Music:* Fall Out Boy, Jonas Brothers, Alicia Keys, Puff Daddy, Lady Gaga, Dave Matthews
Occupation Characteristics and Strengths	Practical, dedicated, disciplined, stable, and quiet Not comfortable with technology Prefer face-to-face meetings	Service oriented Seek personal gratification Optimistic and idealistic Team players Entered workforce with expectations of career-long loyalty to one organization Good mentors Don't like heavy workload demands; prefer flexible work shifts	Computer literate Adaptable, entrepreneurial, skeptical of large organizations Free agents in job market Need mentoring and frequent feedback Like multitasking and don't mind juggling work with home life Like to work independently	Technologically advanced, global and networked Value speed over detail Like group activities Self-confident, goal oriented, and compliant Inclusive Multitaskers, street smart Hopeful Polite Loyal to peers Entrepreneurial
View of Authority	Respectful	Love/hate	Unimpressed and not intimidated	Polite May seek guidance from authority Tests authority
Leadership Expectations	Accustomed to hierarchies	Prefer consensus management	Demand leadership competence	Pulling together for results Dislikes authoritarian types
Feedback Preferences	No news is good news	Annual performance evaluation is enough	Want frequent feedback on how they are doing	Want instant feedback

Because of the proximity of the United States to Central and South America, many patients from these countries travel to the United States for their health care. Also, according to the 2010 U.S. census, the Hispanic population grew by 43 percent since 2000, and now represents 16 percent of the total U.S. population.[5] Thus, a growing percentage of the population is Spanish speaking (BOX 2–2). It is beneficial for health care workers to develop some skill in Spanish; however, it is recommended that the health care worker practice the phrases with someone who can speak the language before attempting to communicate with a patient, because mispronounced words may lead to more confusion. (Basic requests in Spanish/English are listed in Appendix 12.)

BOX 2–2

Using a Second Language

Employees who can translate from one language to another and have proficiency in the medical terminology of that language (including those proficient in sign language) are valuable to their organizations because their translation services for patients are convenient and effective. However, sometimes using another language with coworkers has caused uncomfortable situations. Some employers prefer to have an "English-only" policy, rather than having groups of employees speaking other languages at work. These policies are hard to enforce and are often challenged legally because they may be perceived as discriminatory. Therefore, out of respect for all members of the health care team, use English at all times while communicating with coworkers. Social divisions and breaks in interpersonal relationships occur when one group of employees intentionally speaks a language that excludes peers or supervisors. This can be perceived as discourteous behavior.[6]

Regardless of the patient's language, the health care worker is responsible for communicating essential information. Always speak respectfully, in a highly professional manner, and with phrases that are clearly articulated. If a health care worker feels frustrated by an inability to communicate with a patient, he or she should seek assistance from a supervisor, translator, family member, or physician. Each patient should be treated compassionately, fairly, and with the utmost of dignity, regardless of language abilities.

Sensory Impairments

Health care workers must be knowledgeable about and sensitive to patients who have impaired hearing or sight (deafness or blindness). A question such as, "Is there a step you would like me to repeat before we begin?" yields better clues that the patient has heard and understood than saying, "Do you understand?" If it is obvious that the patient did not hear, try speaking slightly louder (not shouting) and slower and repeat statements if needed. Keep in mind that there are many technological advances (hearing aids, audible aids, smartphone, tablet applications, etc.) that enable individuals with impairments to communicate, live independently, and perform tasks of daily living. If the patient does not understand, provide written instructions or write down instructions for the patient, or if the patient can read sign language, use sign language to provide instructions. If the health care worker does not know sign language, arrangements should be made to find a coworker who can serve as an interpreter. The health care worker must be sure that the patient can understand the instructions or the procedure. Writing tools should be readily available.

It is estimated that only 20 percent of vision or sight-impaired people are totally blind; most have some remaining vision because they lost their sight gradually, often as they grew older. According to the National Federation of the Blind (NFB), people who are blind see about 10 percent of what a sighted person can see. There are several terms that can be used instead of *blind*, such as *visually impaired, low vision,* or *sightless,* however NFB uses the term **blind** for all people who need alternative techniques to do the same tasks that a sighted person can do normally. **Braille,** which is the traditional writing system for sightless individuals, consists of patterns of raised dots read by touch.

The ability for blind persons to live and work independently has become more commonplace due to many technological advances such as audible or talking watches and clocks, measuring devices and thermometers, and reading/scanning devices that convert text into verbal language. These assist in activities of daily life, and health care workers should be familiar with and respectful of patients who use them. In the health care setting, several simple commonsense facts and tips can make both the health care worker and the blind patient feel more at ease during an interaction:[7,8]

- When addressing a blind patient, speak directly to the patient. Do not raise your voice or speak to a companion if there is one. Remember that the patient cannot see a welcoming smile so introduce yourself as you shake hands and do not be afraid to say "Nice to see you." Blind people use this phrase also.

- Patients who are blind are entitled by law to use a long white cane or guide dog to walk independently. The white cane is specifically designed for each individual's height and the length should be about two steps in front of the individual. In all states, the law requires drivers to yield the right of way when they see an extended white cane. In health care, if the work spaces are small, you may caution them about a desk or countertop that may be in their way. Do not grab the patient's arm to steer them; instead, offer your arm and let the patient decide if he or she needs assistance. If so, the blind patient will take your arm and stay a half-step behind you to anticipate corners or steps. Describe steps or turns as you approach them. Remember that open cabinet doors and drawers can be hazards for a blind patient.

- If you are in a hospital room, and you need to move furniture or medications out of the way prior to a venipuncture procedure, be sure to put things back where they were before you entered.

- Let the patient know who is in the room if there are others present. If appropriate, describe and show the patient where the bathroom is, and where the light switch is. Blind patients like to know whether the lights are on.

- Describe all the procedures thoroughly and offer to answer any questions. Do not use phrases such as "Take a seat over there"; instead, offer your arm to direct the patient to the chair. Place his or her arm on the chair back so that he or she can sit down on his or her own.

- Do not ask questions just because you are curious about blindness. Do your research on your own time. Blind patients have many interests, as do others.

- Do not make small talk about the patient's other senses (e.g., smell, touch, or hearing). Remember that these senses did not change or get better due to blindness, but blind individuals simply rely on those senses more often to get information about their environment.

- Most people who are blind do not want to be fussed over. Think of the patient as a regular person who happens to be blind, *not* as a blind patient. The important thing is to communicate who you are and what you are doing.[7,8]

PROCEDURE 2–1 describes initial interactions with hearing or sight-impaired patients.

PROCEDURE 2-1

Initial Communication with a Patient Who Has a Hearing and/or Sight Impairment

Rationale   Patients with hearing or sight impairments (deafness or blindness) *must* understand health care procedures to ensure safe and effective treatment. Health care workers should use the most effective communication skills to inform the patient about specimen collection procedures. Adjustments should be made to accommodate various levels of hearing and/or patients that might have both hearing and sight impairments. In some cases, written instructions in English may be sufficient, but in other cases, a sign language interpreter may be needed or instructions in large print or Braille may be required. The health care worker should use good judgment and advice from supervisors or nursing staff on the best way to communicate with each patient.

Equipment/Supplies

- Written instructions and/or instructions in large print
- Braille or audiotaped instructions
- Pen/pencil/paper

Preparation

1 Reduce external noise as much as possible (e.g., turn off music or TV, pull privacy curtain, close hallway door). Refer to the additional tips mentioned above for assisting blind patients in ambulatory settings.

Procedure

2 When entering the hospital room, smile and establish eye contact while identifying yourself and stating the reason for your visit. If the patient is blind, he or she will not see your smile but will appreciate knowing who you are and why you are there. Be keenly aware of the verbal and nonverbal cues from the patient. If the patient does not respond, it is a sign that he or she has not heard or may not understand what you have said thus far. If the patient turns his or her head to one side, it may mean that he or she can hear better on that side. If it appears that the patient is following your opening conversation, then you may proceed with the description of the procedure and the identification process (covered in more detail later).

3 Face the patient and speak slowly and do not shout.

4 Describe the procedure fully.

5 Offer pencil and paper for the patient to use when necessary.

6 Use a written explanation to reinforce your message with patients who have hearing impairments. For patients who are blind, consider offering an audio version of the explanation.

7 For patients who have hearing impairments, give directions using actions as well as words.

8 Ask the patient "Is there a step you would like me to repeat before we begin?"

9 If there is still doubt that he or she understands, have the patient summarize what is to be done by stating "Okay, Mrs. Jones/ Mr. Smith, to be sure that you understand, can you summarize what we are going to do next?" The patient may verbalize or write down that he or she understands everything or may request a sign language interpreter. Before proceeding with the procedure, ask yourself, "Does this patient really understand this procedure?" If the answer is no, seek assistance from a supervisor or nurse. Do not proceed until you are sure the patient understands.

10 Show the utmost empathy and respect.

11 Notify a supervisor, the nurse, or a physician of any patient concerns.

Pace, Tone, and Volume of Voice

Pace refers to the rate of speed and urgency of the voice; **tone**, or intonation, refers to the pitch of the voice ranging from high (e.g., soprano or high keys of a piano) to low (e.g., baritone or low end of the piano); and *volume* refers to the "loudness" range (e.g., from a whisper to a shout). The pace, tone, and volume of one's voice can change a positive sentence into a negative-sounding statement and an understanding into a misunderstanding. The pace, tone, and volume of voice should match the words that are spoken. In urgent situations, words are usually spoken rapidly and loudly, at a higher pitch. Sarcasm is usually communicated just by changing the tone of voice and can even be detected on a telephone call. Health care workers can avoid sending mixed messages to patients by practicing a calm, soothing, and confident tone of voice, at a moderate pace and volume. **BOX 2–3** is a practice exercise for health care professionals to use in observing and controlling their own voices and facial expressions. Refer to **TABLE 2–2** for more tips about telephone etiquette.

Emergency Situations

Emergency, or **STAT**, blood collections are common in emergency rooms and in some complicated surgical or medical cases. These phlebotomy procedures require extra speed and accuracy without jeopardizing the "personal touch." Patients in emergency rooms may not have identification information with them and/or may be unconscious. All facilities, however, should have documented procedures for the identification process with which health care workers should be familiar. Individual patients should be considered in terms of their privacy, dignity, and individual needs, *not* by nicknames such as "Mr. L down the hall" or "the broken leg in 3C." Each individual is entitled to professional, respectful care in all circumstances.

BOX 2–3

Control Your Voice and Facial Expression

The following exercise is fun and useful for improving verbal and nonverbal communication skills. Practice it in front of a mirror or with a coworker.

Step 1. Using a pleasant voice (i.e., calm, compassionate, clear, professional tone), with a smile on your face, practice saying the following phrases:

- "Please ... "
- "Good morning, Mrs. Jones. How was your breakfast?"
- "Are you enjoying your television program this morning?"
- "Have you had lunch?"
- "May I please check your identification bracelet?"
- "Thank you."

Step 2. Next, repeat the phrases at a fast rate, high pitched, and more urgent voice (as if you are in a hurry) and with a worried look on your face.

Step 3. Now, using a slower, deeper tone of voice, with a frustrated, disdainful look on your face, repeat the phrases listed in step 1.

Step 4. List the specific features you liked about the first method with those features you disliked about the second and third methods. Try to contrast details of facial features (wrinkled eyebrows or smiling face), how the voice lowers or raises at the end of the statements, and how you feel when speaking in the three ways.

Step 5. Keep a mental impression (or take a video or photo) of the way you look and sound during the first step. Remember: A simple smile can often force a positive change in voice tone.

TABLE 2–2

Telephone and E-Mail Etiquette

Telephone Etiquette

On the telephone, your tone of voice reveals the message, no matter how carefully you choose your words.

Incoming calls

1. Try to answer on the first or second ring. Before answering, mentally focus on the caller and finish your prior conversations. It is uncomfortable for a caller to hear the end of your discussion while you are picking up the phone.

2. Smile as you answer the phone because it changes your tone. Keep a mirror near the phone to check your smile.

3. Identify the department/office/lab after the greeting: "Good morning, Dr. Barrett's office." Your voice can range from a whisper to extra loud (volume) and from slow to quick/excited (pace). Keep your voice at a moderate volume and pace. If the speaker asks you to repeat something, it is an indication that he or she cannot hear or does not understand, so take the clue and slow down using pauses between points and or increase your volume slightly.

4. Enunciate words and statements carefully.

5. Identify yourself using name and title: "This is James, the phlebotomist."

6. Ask how you may help the caller: "How may I help you?" (Use *may* instead of *can*.)

7. Seek information from the caller using proper etiquette and record the date and time: "May I have your name please?" "Could you spell that please?" "Could you repeat that please?"

8. Do not immediately place the caller on hold or cut the caller off with "Hold please"; allow the caller to state a reason for the call and give them the option to leave a message: "May I put you on hold for a few moments while I get information or would you prefer to leave a message?"

9. Do not leave the caller on hold for more than 30 seconds; check back to see if he or she wants to continue holding or leave a message.

10. Read the message back to the caller to ensure that it is correct. Double-check spellings, identification or phone numbers, and other pertinent information.

11. End the call with a professional closure, such as "Thank you" and "Good-bye." Allow the caller to hang up first, just in case he or she needs to add something at the last minute. Don't start talking to someone else until you are disconnected; otherwise the person on the other end may still hear you unintentionally.

Outgoing calls

1. Be prepared: Have pencils/pens, message pads, and the telephone in an accessible area near the computer screen if necessary.

2. Do not call to socialize while working and use discretion with confidential information (especially in a crowded work area).

3. State your name, your department and/or title, and the purpose of your call.

4. Leave preferred times and phone numbers where you can be reached if a follow-up call is necessary.

5. Double-check that the receiver has the correct information and/or ask for a "read-back" since most health care professionals will know what that means.

6. Thank the receiver for taking your message.

Other tips

1. Actors use gestures and mannerisms to help them change their tone of voice, so try to change your body language to a positive position—for example, erect posture, shoulders back, and head held high.

2. If you are upset by a caller, take a short walk and breathe deeply before answering other calls.

3. High-pitched voices are associated with panic, urgency, and excitement, so try to keep the pitch of your voice at a moderate level for most communications. If the situation is an emergency, a higher pitch of your voice can reinforce the critical message.

E-Mail Etiquette

E-mail documents are legal documents and are admissible evidence in court cases, so always be truthful and cautious about what you write.[9,10]

Incoming e-mail

1. Try to respond within 24 hours or at your earliest convenience, and if you are not able to, use a comment such as "Thank you for your patience," or "I apologize for the delay, but . . . ."

2. Use auto-reply messages when you are unavailable for more than a day.

3. If you need more time to respond, at least use a short reply such as "Thanks, I'll work on it." or "Thanks, but I need more time to work on it."

4. Save important e-mails (not junk).

5. When you open your e-mail, scan for priority messages.

Outgoing e-mail

1. Be factual and professional.

2. E-mail is forever. Think about the consequences of your message before you send it.

(continued)

TABLE 2–2

Telephone and E-Mail Etiquette (*continued*)

E-Mail Etiquette

3. E-mail is not anonymous. *Do not* send highly sensitive messages; proprietary information; messages that could be breaches of patient confidentiality; or offensive, obscene, discriminatory, or potentially embarrassing messages.

4. Draft important e-mails offline so they can be thoroughly prepared before sending.

5. Be short and concise, but thorough in responses.

6. E-mails are harder on the eyes than written documents, so make it visually easier to read by using bullet points and a meaningful subject line.

7. As a courtesy, call the recipient prior to sending a large file to make sure he or she wants to or can receive it.

8. Use of all capital letters/upper case, bolded letters, or underlined words can be INTERPRETED AS SHOUTING AND OFFENSIVE.

9. Avoid use of excessive symbols such as ????, !!!!!!!!!!!, or %$#&!!! Their meaning is unclear and may be construed as offensive.

Other tips

1. Always follow your health care facility's protocol for use of e-mail related to transmission of patient information, departmental data, etc.

2. Use of personal digital assistants (PDAs) is common, convenient, and acceptable; however, they present other e-mail issues primarily due to their size. Follow your organization's practices on the use of PDAs.

Bedside Manner

The climate established by a health care worker when entering a patient's room will affect the entire patient encounter. The feeling of confidence that comes from the knowledge that the collection tray is clean and well stocked is the first step in a good bedside manner. A pleasant facial expression, neat appearance, and professional manner set the stage for a positive interaction with the patient. The first 30 seconds after the health care worker enters the patient's room determines how that patient perceives the quality of patient care offered by that hospital. Most patients admit that the procedure they dread most is being "stuck" for blood collection, so make every effort to minimize the negative effects of the situation.

NONVERBAL COMMUNICATION

Some theories suggest that communication consists of 10 to 20 percent verbal and 80 to 90 percent nonverbal messages. Nonverbal cues, or body language, can be positive (i.e., facilitate understanding) or negative (i.e., hinder effective communication). Learning the meaning of nonverbal cues, which are summarized in **TABLE 2–3**, will be valuable to health care workers.

Smiling

A simple, compassionate smile can set the stage for opening lines of communication. It can make each patient feel that he or she is the most important person at that moment. In addition, most people look better with smiles on their faces than they do with frowns. It takes fewer muscle movements to smile than it does to frown.

ALERT

Clinical Alert! Health care providers are legally required to provide effective communication to patients who have hearing or sight impairments about their health care. Remember that English may be considered a second language for deaf or deaf-blind patients (with American Sign Language as their first language). Sometimes even written notes in English are not effective in communicating medical procedures. If a deaf patient requests a sign language interpreter, the health care provider must make efforts to comply with this request prior to initiating any procedure. If unable to do so, a supervisor should be consulted.

TABLE 2–3

Nonverbal Communication/Body Language

Positive Body Language	Examples
Aids communication Can make interactions more professional	Face-to-Face positioning Relaxed hands, arms, and shoulders Erect posture Eye contact, eye level (avoid looking down on someone) Smiling Appropriate "zone of comfort"
Negative Body Language	**Examples**
Is distracting Prevents effective communication Causes discomfort and uneasiness	Slouching, shrugged shoulders Rolling eyes or wandering eyes Staring blankly or at ceiling Rubbing eyes or excessive blinking Squirming or tapping foot or pencil Deep sighing or groaning Crossing arms or clenching fists Wrinkling forehead Thumbing through books or papers Stretching or yawning Peering over eyeglasses Pointing finger at someone

Eye Contact and Eye Level

The most expressive parts of the human face are the eyes. Therefore, eye contact is important in effective communication. For many patients and health care workers, eye contact promotes a sense of trust and honesty between them.

Eye level is also a consideration. Individuals are most comfortable if they are communicating at the same eye level. However, bedridden patients must always look up to those in the room, including the health care worker. This can create a feeling of intimidation, of being "looked down on," or of weakness (BOX 2–4). Knowing that this feeling exists can help the health care worker be more compassionate by making appropriate adjustments when needed—for example, raising the patient's bed or adjusting pillows. Most of the time, health care workers do not have the extra time to find a chair to sit in so that they are at eye level; however, if health care workers must explain a lengthy procedure or if it is noted that the patient is particularly anxious, the extra effort should be taken to explain the procedure while seated at eye level with the patient.

A word of caution about eye contact is needed when dealing with patients of certain cultures. For the most part, the general public in the United States views eye contact as a positive aspect of human nature, and avoidance of eye contact might mean that someone is not being truthful. However, some Asian and Native American cultures believe that prolonged eye contact is rude and an invasion of privacy. Muslim women may avoid eye contact also. Patients may not appreciate direct eye contact with a health care provider because it may make them feel self-conscious; or it may be unacceptable in their culture or may not be acceptable with the opposite gender. Take cues from the patient. If the patient does not look at the health care worker when she is speaking, perhaps the patient would feel more comfortable with more space between them or with less direct eye contact, or even another health care worker of the same gender as the patient. The health care worker can take the interaction at a slower pace to understand and monitor the patient's comfort level. The more secure and comfortable the patient feels, the easier the procedure will become.

BOX 2–4

Role Reversal Exercise: Too Close for Comfort

Having respect for an individual's personal space is part of being a compassionate health care worker. Each person's comfort zone varies with gender, culture, and situation. However, most people feel uneasy when strangers are touching them or are "too close for comfort." An example of this uncomfortable sensation is standing in a crowded elevator. People take great measures to move so that they are not touching strangers, and as people exit the elevator, the remaining people move and shift to provide more space around them. This same sense of uneasiness is felt by patients who are approached by unfamiliar health care workers.

To simulate a real patient–health care worker interaction, practice the following exercise with a coworker who is not a close friend. Eye contact should be made during this exercise.

1. Lie on a bed or sit in a chair as if you are a patient.
2. Have the coworker slowly approach you. He or she should begin 10 feet away and pause between steps.
3. Note at what distance you begin to feel awkward or uncomfortable. (Usually, this distance is about 2 to 4 feet.) This distance is the boundary of your zone of comfort.
4. Repeat the exercise with the same coworker. You will probably require a smaller zone of comfort because a person becomes a little more at ease after initial contact with an unfamiliar person.

Zone of Comfort

Most individuals begin to feel uncomfortable when strangers get too close to them physically. A **zone of comfort** is the area of space around a patient that is private territory, so to speak, where they feel comfortable with an interaction. If that zone is crossed, feelings of uneasiness may occur. Refer to Box 2–4.

For most Western cultures, there are four zones of interpersonal space:

- **Intimate space (direct contact up to 18 inches)**—for close relationships and health care workers who bathe, feed, dress, and perform venipunctures.

- **Personal space (18 inches to 4 feet)**—for interactions among friends and for many patient encounters.

- **Social space (4 feet to 12 feet)**—for most interactions of everyday life.

- **Public space (more than 12 feet)**—for lectures, speeches, etc.

A stranger who gets too close can cause the patient to feel nervous, fearful, or anxious. Health care workers must be understanding and approach nervous patients slowly and gently to avoid causing feelings of being threatened. This is particularly true with children, many of whom have a wide zone of comfort; that is, they do not like anyone to approach them except close relatives or friends. A skilled health care worker must be aware of his or her threat to a patient and use a calm, professional, and confident manner. It is helpful to approach the patient slowly while crossing the zone of comfort, not to be too hasty, and to talk to patients during the process (**BOX 2–5**).

BOX 2–5

Developing Sensitivity to Bedridden Patients

Health care workers should strive to be as compassionate as possible. Bedridden patients often feel intimidated because health care workers must repeatedly "look down" on them to provide care. Sometimes patients are also depressed because of their condition or prognosis. This exercise will help you imagine yourself in the patient's condition and can make you a more compassionate member of the health care team. Practice the exercise with a coworker whom you do not know very well.

1. Lie on a bed or blood donor chair while your coworker stands directly over you, looking down.
2. Have the coworker "go through the motions" of a venipuncture procedure by introducing him or herself, asking your name, and touching your arm, pretending to tie a tourniquet, and pretending to draw a blood specimen. Try to imagine the anticipation of the needlestick. Have the coworker maintain eye contact with you during parts of the procedure while conversing.
3. Repeat step 2, without any eye contact and mentally note the positive or negative aspects of this procedure.

Cultural Sensitivity

Culture is a system of values, beliefs, and practices that stem from one's concept of reality (**BOX 2–6**). Culture influences decisions and behaviors in many aspects of life. Learning about various ethnic groups and cultures is important for health care professionals so as to understand the reasons for patients' behaviors during times of health and illness.

Specific traits that vary among cultures were addressed earlier in this chapter (e.g., eye contact and zone of comfort). However, with the changing demographics of the U.S. population, it is vital for all health care workers to become more sensitive and compassionate about accepting cultural practices that vary from their own. When a health care

BOX 2–6

What Is Culture?

Culture is variable among groups of individuals, but it usually encompasses the following traits:

■ **Values**—the accepted principles of a group (individualism versus socialism, importance of education and financial security, competition versus cooperation, sanctity of life, etc.).
■ **Beliefs**—doctrine or faith of a person or group (spiritual orientation, family bonds, etc.).
■ **Traditions and practices**—customs and behaviors associated with groups (holidays, foods, music, dance, health care practices, etc.).

worker is unsure or unaware of acceptable patterns of behavior for a patient, the recommended action is to "follow the patient's lead." For example, if a patient speaks softly and slowly, speak in a similar manner. If the patient turns to a family member when speaking to you, include the family member in the conversation. If a patient moves closer to you during the conversation, try not to back away from the patient's zone of comfort. Since travel abroad is expensive, health care workers must educate themselves about cultural diversity in other ways. The best way to become more culturally competent is to allow patients to teach us, to become active observers of how culturally diverse patients interact with each other and with health professionals. Becoming keen observers of mannerisms, gestures, and facial expressions of group members, reading about cultural groups, watching films and videos, reading novels that depict different cultures, and reading newspapers published by cultural groups will make health care workers better and more informed at what they do.

In some cultures, the zone of comfort may be wide; in others, people naturally stand closer to each other. How much at ease a person feels with physical closeness can also vary with gender. Some women feel very uncomfortable having a male health care worker standing over them preparing to draw a blood specimen, and vice versa. It is particularly considerate to recognize this and respond accordingly. Again, respect for the patient's needs and dignity must be considered (**FIGURE 2–5**).

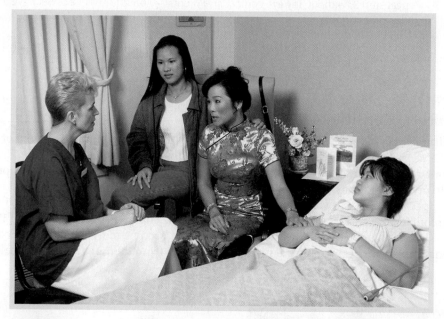

FIGURE 2–5
This health care worker is discussing a procedure with a patient and her family.

Negative Body Language and Distracting Behaviors

This section of text highlights some of the body language signs presented earlier in Table 2-3.

Wandering eyes   When people roll their eyes upward, they convey the sense of being bored, inattentive, or unwilling to perform a duty. Because this behavior is distracting, it should be avoided when communicating with, listening to, or observing patients, coworkers, or supervisors.

The same can be said about gazing out the window or looking up at the ceiling. If a health care worker enters a patient's room and begins addressing the patient while looking out the window, the patient will feel neglected, and the health care worker will appear unconcerned. If the window is too tempting to avoid a glance at, the health care worker can include the patient in his or her observations. A friendly comment about the weather might be appropriate; then the phlebotomy procedure can be continued when full attention can be given to the patient. The objective is to make the patient feel at ease through good communication techniques so that the procedure can be successful.

Nervous behaviors Behaviors such as squirming or tapping a pencil or a foot can be distracting. They can make a patient feel nervous, hurried, or anxious about the venipuncture. A calm and confident image maximizes the patient's comfort and trust. It is also helpful to recognize these behaviors in patients, especially children, so that efforts can be made to reduce fear. Allowing a few extra moments of conversation or preparation may help.

Breathing pattern A deep sigh can convey a feeling of being bored or a reluctance to do the job. Avoid sighing, especially when communicating with an angry, uncooperative patient. Likewise, if a patient sighs deeply or moans at the mere sight of the health care worker, this should be a cue that a little extra attention, conversation, or a smile might ease the patient's reluctance for the procedure.

Other distracting behaviors Many other actions can convey negative or defensive emotions. Among these are crossed arms, a wrinkled forehead, frequent glances at a clock or watch, rapid thumbing through papers, chewing gum, yawning, or stretching. Health care workers should realize that these behaviors can detract from their professional image when they are communicating with patients, families, visitors, coworkers, and supervisors (**FIGURE 2–6**). It is also important to realize what these cues mean if a patient exhibits them. Regular in-services or continuing education programs can be directed at reminding health care workers to be aware of positive and negative body language, both in their own behavior and that of patients.

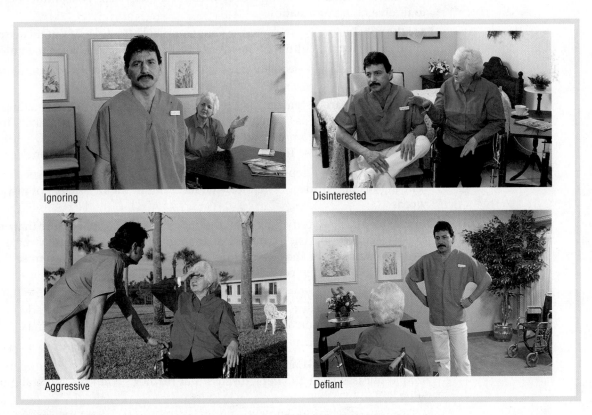

FIGURE 2–6
Examples of Negative Body Language

Nonverbal communication can have a negative effect on communication.

Active Listening

Listening to a patient or coworker involves verbal and nonverbal aspects. Active listening helps close the communication loop by ensuring that the message sent can indeed be repeated and understood. Listening skills do not depend on intellect or educational background; they can be learned and practiced. Listening carefully to the patient can have important ramifications in test results. For example, the nursing staff may have instructed the inpatient that he or she will be fasting, or will have "nothing by mouth," until after the early-morning blood collections, but the health care worker might hear comments such as, "I didn't have breakfast yet, but I drank some juice" or "They won't feed me." The first indicates that the patient broke the fast and had juice, which could affect some test results, and the second statement indicates that the patient probably has been fasting overnight. When in doubt, confirm that the patient has been fasting by simply asking the patient if he or she has eaten or had anything to drink other than water.

Active listening is paying undivided, complete attention to the speaker by concentrating on the verbal message, observing his or her nonverbal language, and offering appropriate feedback. It engages the mind more fully. *Passive listening* is listening without replying, like listening to the television or a lecturer.[1]

Steps for active listening The following list is presented as a starting point for the development of listening skills by health care workers. Because individuals can mentally process words faster than they can speak them, a good listener must concentrate and focus on the speaker. Development of these skills can help individuals in their professional as well as personal lives. It takes a conscious effort and practice.

Get ready—Concentrate on the speaker by "getting ready" to listen. Take a moment to clear your mind of distracting thoughts. Begin the interaction with an open, objective mind. Sometimes taking a deep breath can help clear your mind and prepare it to receive more information.

Face the speaker—Give the speaker your complete attention. Maintain eye contact as appropriate for the culture of the speaker. Also maintain the zone of comfort.

Pause occasionally—Use silent pauses in the conversation wisely to mentally summarize what has been said. Note the nonverbal cues.

Verify that you are listening—Let the speaker know that you are listening by using simple phrases such as "I see," "Oh," "Isn't that interesting," and so on, to reassure the speaker and to communicate understanding and acceptance. Do not interrupt unless you need to ask for an explanation about something that is unclear.

Avoid judgments—Keep personal judgments to yourself until the speaker finishes relaying his or her idea. Listen for true meaning in the message, not just the literal words.

Provide feedback—Verify the conversation with feedback. Make sure that everything said is clear to you. Ask for more explanation if necessary. Mentally review the key words to summarize the overall idea being communicated. Paraphrase the idea or conversation to ensure complete understanding.

Notice body language—Pay attention to body language and ask for clarification. A simple prompt such as "You look sad" or "You seem nervous" can add more meaning to the conversation and encourage the speaker to verbalize feelings.

Maintain eye contact—Eye contact communicates interest or concern.

Use encouragement—Encourage the listener to expand his or her thoughts by using simple phrases such as "Let's discuss that further," "Tell me more about it," and "Really?"

Practice, practice, practice—Practice active listening at work and at home.

WRITTEN AND ELECTRONIC COMMUNICATION

Written communication for health care workers varies with job responsibilities. If clerical duties are a part of the job description, the health care worker may fill out or develop many types of documents—for example, letters, appointment or employee schedules, quality control records, laboratory reports, medical records, and inventory records. Regardless of the function, concise and correct word usage, pronunciation, and grammar are essential. Documents should be proofread prior to use. When using handwritten communication, the writing must be legible and in permanent ink. Other essentials of documentation are described further in a later section of this chapter. Review Table 2–2 for information about e-mailing.

Health care workers should know that their computer interactions can be recorded and monitored. Most employers have policies about the use of social media during work hours. Some employers ban use completely, whereas others use filtering systems to allow employees to use media with restricted access, such as time limits, or certain hours of the day (i.e., lunch or dinner hours). Whatever the case, it is prudent to avoid disparaging remarks about work. Even though individuals have a right to free speech and whistleblower laws protect employees, there are also standards of practice and policies that protect supervisors and the health care organization.

ROLE OF FAMILY, VISITORS, AND SIGNIFICANT OTHERS

Family members and friends or partners of patients are often present when health care workers need to collect specimens. It is important to realize that their presence can make the patient feel more secure and comfortable. Sometimes, however, families and visitors are much more difficult to deal with than the patients. For instance, they might make requests that are beyond the health care worker's scope of acceptable or authorized responsibilities, and so it is best to inform the appropriate health care team member of the family's request. If several visitors are in the hospital room with the patient, they may be asked to step into the hall while the venipuncture is performed. If the health care worker believes that assistance is required (e.g., to give emotional support) and the patient agrees, a family member may be asked to stay during the procedure. This can make the family members feel helpful and provide reassurance to patients. Children should be accompanied by a parent or guardian.

Physicians, priests, and chaplains have the right to visit privately with patients. Unless the blood specimen is timed, the health care worker should respect that privacy and return to the patient after completing the other collections in the area. If the procedure is timed or STAT, the health care worker should apologize for the interruption, explain the nature of the request, and ask permission to collect the specimen.

With the exception of parents of pediatric patients, families and visitors should not be permitted in the clinical laboratory or provided with patient information, except by prior arrangement and permission of the patient. The patient's privacy and safety and the **confidentiality** of patient records must be considered.

PATIENT–HEALTH CARE WORKER COMMUNICATION

When encountering a patient for the first time, there are some essential steps to follow:

- After knocking (not pounding) on the hospital room door or after calling a patient from a clinic waiting room, the health care worker should introduce him- or herself and state that he or she is part of the hospital unit or laboratory staff, whichever is the case (**BOX 2–7**).

BOX 2–7

Greeting a Patient

The following scenario is a typical one that might occur at the opening greeting between a health care worker and a hospitalized patient. Imagine both the verbal and nonverbal factors involved. The *wrong responses* are suggested in italics. They can be used as a discussion tool of how the health care worker can have a negative impact.

Health care worker: Good morning, my name is Lauren. I work in the laboratory, and I am here to collect a blood sample for your laboratory tests. Could you state your name and spell it for me please?

Wrong response: Hi, are you Mrs. Betty Nelson? I have to get your blood for a test.

Patient (softly): My name is Betty Nelson.

Health care worker: Could you repeat that and spell it for me please?

Wrong response: Huh? What did you say? Speak up next time.

Patient: My name is Betty Nelson. B-E-T-T-Y N-E-L-S-O-N

Health care worker: Thank you, I think I have it now but I also need to check your identification bracelet with the laboratory requisitions. I will be taking a blood sample from your arm so that the laboratory can perform tests that your doctor ordered. Have you had breakfast yet?

Wrong response: Okay, let's get on with it because I have lots of patients to stick.

Patient: No breakfast yet; I just woke up.

Health care worker: OK, I need to look at your arms. Would you prefer your right side or left side?

Wrong response: Stick out your arm so I can take a look.

Patient: Nobody ever gets blood on the left side, so we'd better try the right side.

Health care worker: Thanks for that information; we can check the right side. Please hold out your arm so that I can feel for your veins.

Wrong response: Oh, don't worry about a thing. I'm pretty good at drawing from tough veins.

Patient: Okay, but will it hurt?

Health care worker: It will hurt a little, but I'll do my best to have it done quickly. Do you have any other questions?

Wrong response: No, I would never hurt anyone. I'm in a hurry so do you have any more questions?

Patient: Not really, just get it over with.

Health care worker: Thanks for your cooperation, Mrs. Nelson.

Wrong response: Well, I'm just doing what I was told! Let's get on with it.

■ The patient should be informed that a blood specimen is being collected for a test ordered by the physician. A statement indicating that this is a routine hospital protocol often reassures the patient. A lengthy discussion of why a certain test was ordered or what tests were ordered is inappropriate. These questions should be referred to the patient's physician. Health care workers must be truthful and thorough about explaining procedures.

- Health care workers should be calm, compassionate, and highly professional and should limit conversations to essential information.

- Patients must *not* be told "This won't hurt." Most blood collection procedures are indeed slightly painful; therefore, it is important that the patient be forewarned and prepared. Saying something such as "This will hurt a little but it will be over soon" is better than giving a false statement about the pain.

- During the procedure, the patient should be informed about how it is going (e.g., "This is going well" or "I'm almost finished"). Care should be taken not to be distracted from the phlebotomy procedure by excessive talk of unrelated issues.

- After the procedure, but before leaving the room, always thank the patient for his or her cooperation. A simple "Thank you" will suffice.

Communication for Confirming Patient Identification

Health care organizations differ slightly in their guidelines for patient identification, but all agree that proper identification is essential. The Joint Commission has made accurate patient identification a priority in order to reduce and prevent medical errors. It recommends using "at least two ways to identify patients," (neither to be the patient's room number) whenever taking blood samples or administering medications or blood products.[11]

If the patient is hospitalized, identification should be accomplished by a match between the test requisition (or requisition labels) and the armband, and by verbal confirmation from the patient. If a hospitalized patient does not have an armband, a positive confirmation must be made by a unit nurse who knows the patient. This process should be well documented by the health care worker. Patient identification is covered more thoroughly in later chapters.

Communication in Ambulatory Settings or in the Home

Special identification procedures should also be well documented for ambulatory patients, especially in cases of homebound patients, mobile vans, and other off-site locations. Armbands may not be used in all ambulatory settings; however, some form of an identification card is usually standard. It may include some demographic data and other identifying information, such as the patient's identification number, date of birth (DOB), address, or a combination of these. This information should be confirmed by the patient prior to blood collection (**FIGURE 2–7**).

It usually takes more time in an ambulatory setting or in a home health care setting to identify a patient because of the following factors:

- The health care worker must introduce him- or herself and clearly explain the purpose of the interaction.

- The patient should be directed to an appropriate place to sit or recline during the procedure. This may involve walking to a private area, blood collection booth, or special recliner.

- If the phlebotomy procedure is taking place in an unfamiliar setting, such as the patient's home, the health care worker must take extra time to find the nearest bathroom (for handwashing, blood spillage, etc.) and the nearest bed in case there are complications (e.g., fainting) during the phlebotomy procedure.

- In a patient's home, the health care worker may need to find a phone or carry a cell phone, tablet or laptop to clarify laboratory orders or inquire about patient information.

Clinical Alert ! The patient should always be asked "What is your name?" not "Are you Mr. Smith?" The first question is a more reliable and direct way of confirming identity. The second question is inappropriate and less reliable because a patient who is heavily medicated will often agree with anything that he or she is asked.

ALERT

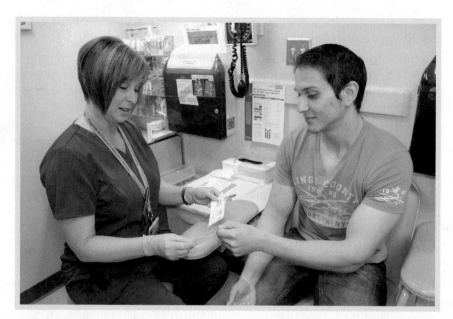

FIGURE 2–7
Identifying an Ambulatory Patient

- Information about the procedure should be fully explained (especially if it is a first-time blood collection for the patient or if it has been a long time since the last blood collection).

- Identifying the home-bound or ambulatory patient should be done meticulously and cautiously, using various methods to identify the patient positively (e.g., driver's license or identification card, confirmation of birthday and home address, etc.).

- The puncture site must be appropriately cared for, and it should be clear that the patient is physically fit to leave the area after the phlebotomy procedure. If the patient is homebound, the health care worker must be sure that the patient is no longer bleeding, the puncture site has been appropriately bandaged, and the patient is able to stay by him- or herself.

Some health care facilities insist that the health care worker ask for the ambulatory patient's full name and spelling, as well as birthdate, whereas others also require the mention of the patient's complete address and hometown to reinforce and confirm identity. This portion of the specimen collection procedure ensures that the remainder of the diagnostic testing protocol provides information on the correct person.

Computer and Documentation Basics

COMPUTERIZATION IN THE CLINICAL LABORATORY

Computers enhance quality patient care through efficient data collection and tabulation, elimination of duplicate work, and a decrease in transcription errors. A health care worker may play a role in data entry, medical records management, appointments and scheduling, electronic requisitioning and results reporting, bookkeeping, billing, supply and equipment inventory, quality control, and many other functions. In some cases, computerization has become so sophisticated that a health care worker may perform a bedside, point-of-care (POC), CLIA-waived laboratory test on a computer, and test results will be reported without any other human intervention or oversight (CLIA is the Clinical Laboratory Improvement Amendments of 1988). In a similar scenario, the health care worker could load a specimen from the patient directly onto an automated clinical analyzer where it is tested and results are reported electronically—again, without any direct oversight.

Thus, it is vital that health care workers understand the scope of work and uses of computers throughout the preexamination, examination, and postexamination processes. Health care workers can expect to find computers in every type of health care setting imaginable, from hospitals to doctors' offices, from mobile health units to ambulances, from battlefields to the space station (**FIGURES 2–8** and **2–9** and **TABLE 2–4**; also refer to **BOX 2–8**).

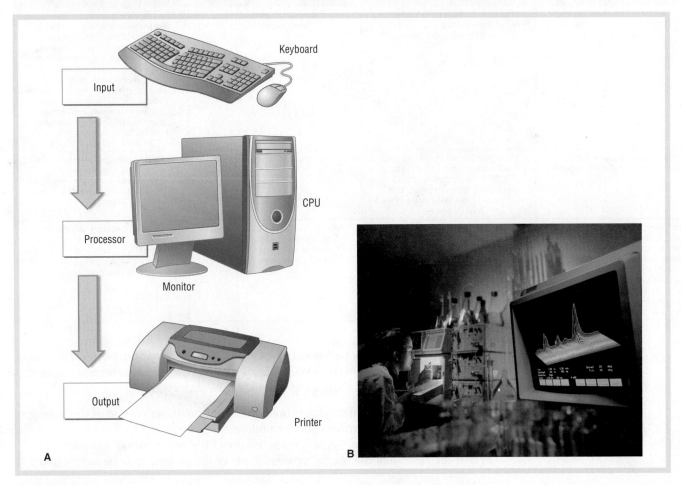

FIGURE 2–8

A. Components of a computer system. B. Monitor for a computer system.

Courtesy of William Tautic/Corbis/Stock Market

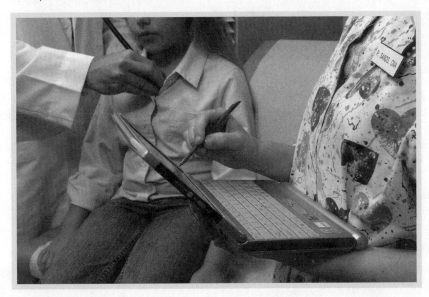

FIGURE 2–9

This medical assistant is using a laptop computer for bedside data entry.

TABLE 2–4

Computer Hardware, Software, Storage, and Internet Fundamentals

Hardware	Software	Storage	Internet
The programmable machine; the brain of the machine that executes activities	The instructions for the hardware that are written in a computer-programming language	Retains large amounts of information/data	The *Internet* is a system of thousands of worldwide interfacing networks. Access to the Internet occurs through a commercial Internet service provider (ISP) and allows for a wide variety of services (electronic mail, file transfers, information resources, interest groups, interactive collaborations, social networking, instant messaging, multimedia displays, real-time broadcasting, ordering supplies/equipment from vendors, and much more).
Central processing unit (CPU)—the main controller of the computer	Hospital information systems (HIS) and laboratory information systems (LIS); most laboratory analytic instruments have software that enables linkages to LIS or other health care computers.	Hard disk, magnetic tapes	Web 1—originally developed in 1960s as a military project; Web 2—evolved web of many layers of information not owned by any one organization
Peripherals: computer monitor/display, keyboard, printer, modem, scanner, bar code reader, other handheld devices, external hard drive, fax machine, cables, and **universal serial bus (USB)**, which refers to a range of devices from a standardized interface device to storage devices and other equipment	Applications: word processing, presentation software, statistical software, laboratory algorithms, firewall software, antivirus protection, Internet provider software	Disks, compact discs (CDs), CD-ROM (read only memory), USB (also known as flash, jump, or thumb drive), DVDs and DVD-ROMs	**Cloud computing**—a computer network that can be a wide area network (WAN) for numerous groups of users or local area network (LAN) within an organization

In the clinical laboratory pathway (preexamination, examination, postexamination), one may encounter a range of computerization from none to highly integrated, complex computer systems. Generally speaking there are three categories:

1. **Manual systems**—These require human intervention at each phase of the testing process (sample preparation, specimen integrity, testing).
2. **Semiautomated systems**—A specimen requires little or no human intervention at each phase of the testing process. Parts of the process may be automated

BOX 2–8

The Ergonomic Workspace

Prolonged and repeated use of computers is prevalent in our society and at work. However, desktop computer use can cause physical discomfort if one is not positioned properly.

Chair Push your hips as far back as they can go in the chair; adjust the seat height so that your feet are flat on the floor and your knees are equal to or slightly lower than your hips; support your upper and lower back; change positions frequently; adjust the armrests (if any) so that your shoulders are relaxed.

Keyboard Position the keyboard directly in front of your body and adjust the height so that your shoulders remain relaxed with your elbows in a slightly opened position and your wrists and hands straight.

Monitor Adjust the monitor directly in front of you so that your neck and shoulders are relaxed, and the top of the monitor should be about two to three inches above your seated eye level; adjust blinds or the monitor position so that there is no glare on the monitor (**FIGURE 2–10**).

Your body Take a 1- to 2-minute break after each 30 minutes of computer use; after each hour, take a 5- to 10- minute break; rest or refocus your eyes periodically to avoid fatigue; use correct posture and change positions slightly and frequently.

BOX 2–8 (*continued*)

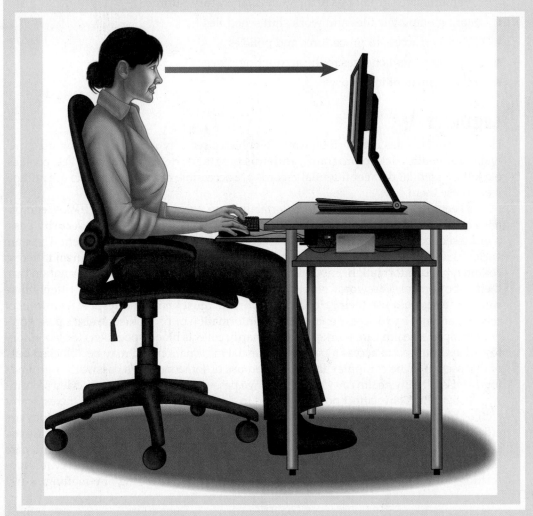

FIGURE 2–10

An Ergonomic Workspace

The health care worker should be positioned with feet flat, wrists, hands, and forearms parallel to the ground, and eyes about 20 inches away from the top of the monitor. Adjustable chairs can accommodate various heights and back positions so that muscle strain is relieved.

(sample processing, mixing reagents with the sample, quality control checks, loading specimen tubes onto the instrument, etc.).
3. **Automated systems**—Little or no human intervention is needed during the testing process; the entire process is automatically performed; human intervention occurs only when instrument error occurs or results are flagged because they are outside the defined limits.

Personal, tablet or laptop computers, **laboratory information systems (LIS)** (dedicated hardware and software for clinical laboratories and/or anatomical pathology), and/or mainframe computers and networks have become essential instruments in the clinical laboratory by carrying out functions such as

■ Providing lists of test requisitions for a patient

■ Generating patients' labels, specimen collection lists, and schedules

■ Updating the laboratory specimen accession records

■ Printing lists that identify which test procedures need to be performed on a patient's specimens

- Reporting test results
- Storing test results
- Sending laboratory test results to the nursing stations either as individual test reports or cumulative summaries of a patient's laboratory records
- Storing employee files and work shift schedules
- Providing access to procedures and policies
- Sending patient charges to the accounting office
- Management of inventory

SECURITY

Health care facilities use various ways to enhance security measures (passwords, firewalls, automatic backup programs, antivirus programs, deleting Internet files, cookies, etc.). It is essential that confidential records are accessible only to those who are authorized to use them.

In keeping with Health Insurance Portability and Accountability Act (HIPAA) compliance to protect patient records, most health care workers will be issued a **security password**, a sequence of characters that enable access to part(s) of a computer system. There are various levels of security that enable only those who are authorized to use them to access certain types of information. Supervisors typically have greater access to information than their subordinates. Passwords should *never* be shared with coworkers or written where someone else could use them. Health care workers must know and respect their level of security and not try to access unauthorized information or use someone else's password. For example, a health care worker who primarily collects blood specimens for laboratory tests does not need to access a patient's financial information and may be "blocked out" of that section in the computer. Unauthorized use of someone else's password is grounds for dismissal. Many health care facilities change passwords periodically for added security.

Also, HIPAA laws affect policies related to electronic transmission (e.g., faxes, scans, etc.) of laboratory information. Scans and faxes are useful sometimes because they are efficient, timely, and cost effective, especially when offsite services are offered. However, since the patient's permission is needed to disclose any information, each health care facility or laboratory should have clear policies related to the use of laboratory test requisitions or test results that are sent or received by faxing, scanning or e-mailing.

Laboratory Test Requisitions, Specimen Labels, and Blood Collection Lists

Laboratory tests are requested (at the beginning of the preexamination phase) by means of a laboratory **requisition**, which may be a handwritten form; a computer-generated, electronic order (semiautomated or automated method); or, in special circumstances, by a STAT verbal request (which is later followed by an official written or computerized requisition). Specimens should never be collected without an authorized requisition. The health care system is rapidly integrating paperless electronic methods for health care information management rather than paper-based systems. However, there are many sites and applications that still use and require manual methods (e.g., handwritten form). Health care workers should be open-minded and adaptable to new technologies used by their health care facilities.

MANUAL METHOD

Multipart requisition forms that can serve as both request and report forms are more subject to human error (e.g., transcription mistakes, lost requisitions, duplicate orders). Some of these problems can be minimized by instituting a centralized location for all requisition forms, using a sorting system once the requisition reaches the laboratory, and using a blood collection log. These forms may also be handy in the event of major computer failures (during power outages, or severe weather conditions, etc.). The forms are usually of a convenient size and can be easily attached to paper, as is used in older-type medical records files. Such forms are manufactured to provide clear copies and easy detachment (perforated edges). Color-coding can be used for different request forms for ease of identification, both in the ordering of tests and in the charting of results. The name of the facility or medical office is usually printed on each request form (**FIGURE 2–11**).

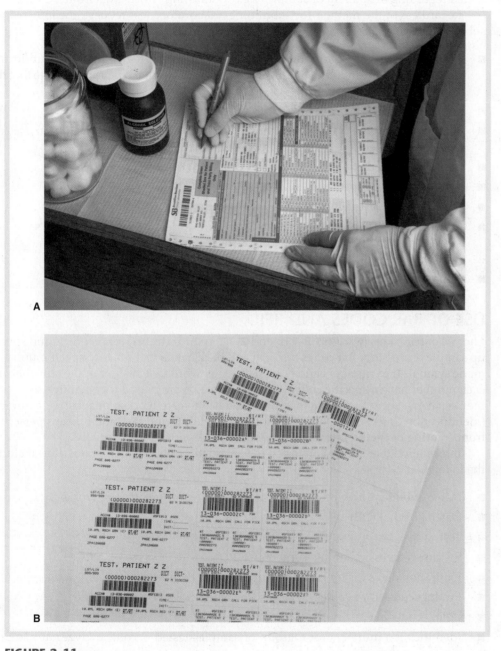

FIGURE 2–11

Example of a Multipart Laboratory Test Requisition

A. Use of multipart requisition forms is helpful in a manual system or as a temporary request until the formal request can be entered into a computer system. **B.** Bar coded, electronically generated test requisitions also serve as specimen labels. Note that various sizes of labels are printed on one sheet and can be peeled off as needed for each collection tube, aliquot, or microscopic slide.

SEMIAUTOMATED OR AUTOMATED METHOD

Electronic input of information is the most error-free means of initiating a laboratory test request. Because a computer system can perform automatic checks on the input, it may not accept a request for any test that is not in its test-information database or that is from an unauthorized person. Likewise, it may not accept a sample of urine for a test restricted to serum. It also allows the person entering the test request to obtain accurate and up-to-date information about specific determinations, such as revised specimen collection requirements, delivery instructions, assay techniques, reference ranges, and fees. Even with handheld computers that are used for bar code scanning, special comments may be added regarding the patient or sample (e.g., "nonfasting" or "drawn from a CVC line").

Regardless of the method for submitting a laboratory test request, the information submitted must include the following:

- Patient identification information (full name and unique registration or identification number, location, and/or a unique identification confidential specimen code that has an audit trail to the patient)

- Patient's gender and **date of birth (DOB)** or age

- Name of physician or legally authorized person ordering the test (the physician's address is needed if it is different from the laboratory's address)

- Test(s) requested

- Time and date of specimen collection

- Source of specimen when appropriate

- Other pertinent clinical information when appropriate (special comments; sampling site if it is other than the arm; or, for genetic testing, race/ethnicity may be necessary information for detection rates for specific diseases)

- Billing information, if applicable

USE OF BAR CODES AND RFID

The use of bar codes (**FIGURES 2–11B** and **2–12**) reduces transcription errors and speeds up sample processing. **Bar codes** are light and dark bands that relate to specific alphanumeric symbols (i.e., numbers and letters). In other words, each letter of the alphabet and each number have a specific code. When these bands are placed together in a sequence, they can correspond to a name (of a patient, a health care worker, or a test) or a number (identification or test code). This technology is accurate and fast, and it keeps personnel from entering or typing information, which reduces errors substantially.

Information that can be converted to bar coded symbols for laboratory use includes the following:

- Name and identification number (of patient and/or health care worker)

- Date of birth (DOB)

- Test codes

- Specimen accession or log numbers

- Expiration dates for inventory of supplies and equipment

- Product codes for needles, syringes, specimen collection tubes, etc.

- Billing codes

- Identification numbers for a group of samples tested on one analyzer at one time (i.e., a "batch-run")

Bar code labels can be commercially produced to be used on samples in extreme temperatures, cryogenic freezer storage, liquid nitrogen, multifreeze thaw cycles, alcohol immersion, autoclaving, steam sterilization centrifugation processes, water baths, humidity and moisture, chemical solvents, or diagnostic reagents. They can be produced in any size, shape, color, design, or with special adhesives. (Refer to Figure 2–12.)

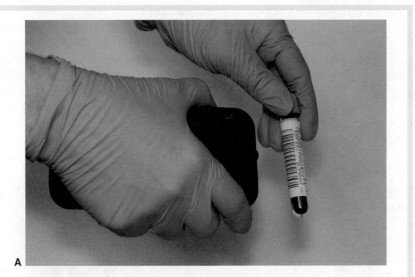

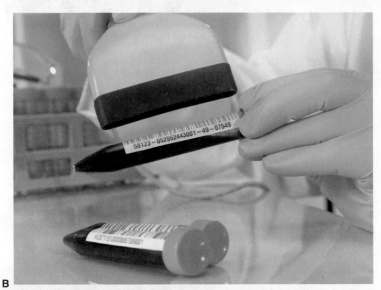

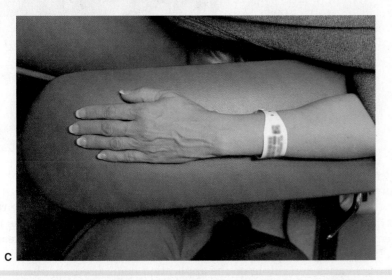

FIGURE 2–12

A. Bar codes can be read easily using a handheld scanner. **B.** Bar codes can be commercially produced in any format or language, and to withstand many environmental or laboratory conditions. **C.** Example of an identification wristband on a patient. Note that this wristband has 2 types of bar codes.

Quick response (QR) codes are two-dimensional bar codes first used in the auto industry but now often seen in commercial, marketing, and advertising applications because of their ease of use with smartphone reader apps. Scanning a QR code can direct the smartphone's browser to the website of an organization (health care facility), a product, a store, etc. The amount of data stored in the QR code relates to the size of symbol and character set version used (higher versions allow more storage capacity). Applications in health care settings are not yet fully developed. However, due to the ease of use with most smartphones, security risks may pose problems. (See **FIGURE 2–13** for examples of quick response codes.)

FIGURE 2–13

Example of QR Codes

A. Commercial QR codes. **B.** QR labels for a blood specimen tube.

© *angellodeco/Fotolia.*

Another form of electronic identification tag used in health care for identifying and tracking records, equipment and supplies, specimens, and patients is the **radio frequency identification (RFID)**. These ID tags are silicon chips that transmit data to a wireless receiver. In contrast to a bar code, RFID does not require "line-of-sight" reading with a scanner. It is possible to identify and/or track many items simultaneously. The frequency (and cost) varies depending on the application being used and the distance that the RFID tag needs to be from the wireless receiver. Lower frequencies can be used when the range of distance is relatively short. Each health care facility must evaluate key issues prior to implementation of RFID, including cost, standardization, and privacy protection measures.

A **STAT verbal request**, often called a *STAT request*, via the telephone is occasionally used in cases of emergency. The request should be documented either electronically or on a standardized form in the laboratory prior to the specimen collection, as shown in **FIGURE 2–14**. After the blood is collected, the official requisition must be submitted to correspond to that specimen.

EMERGENCY REQUEST FOR LABORATORY TESTS

Requesting Nurse:

Requesting Physician:

Patient name: Patient ID (if available):

Location:

    Room #: _____ ICU: _____ ER: _____ Other location: _____

Laboratory requisitions to follow: _____ Pick up on unit _____ Computer entry

List tests ordered:

Requested by:

Order taken by:

Date: _____ Time: _____ am / pm

FIGURE 2–14

Sample Documentation Form for Emergency (STAT) Verbal Request

Verbal emergency, or STAT, laboratory requests can be accepted only from authorized personnel and must later be followed by an appropriate laboratory requisition.

Specimen Labels

Clear and accurate specimen identification is essential and must begin immediately after the specimen is collected and continue through disposal of the specimen. Identification methods vary from manually copying all patient identification information directly onto the container to using prenumbered bar code labels as shown in Figure 2–12. Manually labeling specimens can be time consuming and prone to transcription errors, so use of preprinted labels, which are available from many commercial sources, is preferred. Based on laboratory requests from the physicians, the correct number of labels can be generated electronically containing the following information:

- Patient identification for each tube required to be drawn
- Specific tests requested
- Types of specimen collection tubes required for the requested tests
- Unique identification/accession numbers or sample numbers to be used for that particular collection time
- Smaller transfer labels for aliquot tubes, collection tubes, cuvettes, and microscope slides
- Blood drawing lists by floor or unit

This type of system eliminates the manually written entry log used at smaller facilities for recording the tests and accession number requested for each patient. Additional test requests ordered later in the day are entered into the computer, which assigns a specific time and number to the tests so that they can be easily separated from those requested in the morning. Labels for later collection can be electronically printed or made with an Addressograph machine. For even greater accuracy, speed, and convenience, handheld scanners and/or printers can be used at or near the patient's bedside.

USE OF A BLOOD DRAWING LIST

A blood drawing list (usually generated electronically each morning) is useful in a hospital setting for each floor or nursing unit. When the health care worker finishes on a particular floor, he or she can document its completion so that caregivers attending the patient can see which specimens have already been collected. Any additional specimens collected later in the day are documented also. In this way, the personnel on the health care team have a complete list of the specimen collections taken from each patient throughout the day.

Reporting Laboratory Results

WRITTEN REPORTS

After the examination/analytical phase, reporting laboratory test results constitutes the final phase (postexamination) of the clinical laboratory work pathway. It is estimated that between 60 and 70 percent of *all* clinical data originates in the laboratory. Both the Joint Commission and the College of American Pathologists (CAP) state that laboratory results should be confirmed, dated, and accompanied by permanent reports that are available in the laboratory, as well as on the patient's medical record via an electronic transmission or a hard copy. The CAP also states that each report should contain adequate patient identification, contain the date and hour when the procedures were completed, and be signed and initialed (manually or electronically) by the laboratory personnel performing the procedure. When electronic reports are used, laboratory documentation on instrument-generated worksheets by personnel performing the procedures is sufficient. It is suggested that health care personnel consider the following when designing a report form:[12]

- Identification of patient, patient location, and physician
- Date and time of specimen collection
- Description, source of specimen, and labeled precautions
- Compactness and ease of preparing the package for shipment
- Consistency in format
- Clear understandability of instructions or orders
- Logical location in patient's chart for reference laboratory reports
- Sequential order of multiple results on single specimens
- Listing of reference ranges or normal and abnormal/critical values
- Assurance of accuracy of request transcription
- Administrative and record-keeping value

Any unique institutional requirements for an acceptable report should be stated in the laboratory procedure manual and may include criteria such as quality control (QC) limits and/or **delta checks** (QC that allows for detection of clinically significant changes in laboratory results). Results can be documented in one of the following three ways: manual recording of test results, laboratory-instrument-printed reports, and electronic reports.

VERBAL REPORTS

The use of verbal and telephone reports has declined because of easier, more reliable computer access and the concern for privacy. Verbal reports tend to be more error prone but are useful for reporting STAT results and/or a **critical value**, a test result that may be life threatening and must be reported immediately to the patient's physician. Verbal reports should be accompanied by documentation with the following information: patient name and hospital number, name of person receiving the report, date and time, information given, and name of person issuing the report, as shown in **FIGURE 2–15**.

```
┌─────────────────────────────────────────────────────────────┐
│  ┌──────────────────────────────────────────────────────┐   │
│  │ PATIENT NAME:               PATIENT ID #:            │   │
│  │ PHYSICIAN:                                           │   │
│  │ PERSON REQUESTING INFORMATION:                       │   │
│  │ DATE OF TEST RESULTS:                                │   │
│  │                                                      │   │
│  │ INFORMATION GIVEN:                                   │   │
│  │                                                      │   │
│  │                                                      │   │
│  │ DATE & TIME OF INQUIRY:                              │   │
│  │                                                      │   │
│  │ REPORTED BY:                                         │   │
│  └──────────────────────────────────────────────────────┘   │
└─────────────────────────────────────────────────────────────┘
```

FIGURE 2–15

Sample Form Used for Reporting Verbal Laboratory Results

Reporting laboratory results is a serious responsibility, and each health care facility has policies for who is authorized to do so and under which conditions. Compliance with HIPAA regulations assures that patients' privacy and confidentiality wishes are maintained. Only employees who are authorized to do so should complete the required documentation when appropriate.

ELECTRONIC REPORTS

Various electronic devices can provide a rapid reporting system and are more reliable than verbal reports. Hospitals usually have multiple computers located in each unit. After the tests have been completed and verified in the laboratory, the results can be immediately displayed in each patient unit. A printer can be attached to each terminal to generate a temporary hard-copy report to authorized personnel. However, steps must be taken to ensure security, privacy, and confidentiality of patient results if reports are printed.

A health care facility's computer system can easily provide daily laboratory reports and cumulative reports for direct access into the patient's medical record. All reports should be available at times that are convenient for making clinical decisions by the medical staff.

The business office of the health care facility also receives data regarding laboratory procedures. This office must be notified of all laboratory charges, according to date requested and procedural code for patient billing. It is financially advantageous to send reports promptly.

Documentation Essentials and the Medical or Health Record

Documentation in all health care delivery organizations provides a legal record of the patient's visit and progress. Health care workers document progress in a **clinical (or medical) record** (MR) for each patient (**BOX 2–9**). Everything that is done to the patient should be documented, including orders, all clinical discussions, all test results, etc. All organizations must shift paper-based clinical records to electronic formats—that is, **electronic medical or health record (EMR or HMR)** or **computerized patient record (CPR)**, but implementation varies widely among health care settings.

Clinical Alert ! Authorized health care workers must report critical values to physicians in a timely manner. This often means paging or telephoning a physician at home and/or during off-hours. Although this can be an unwelcome task, it is important for the patient's welfare as well as to avoid liability risks. All laboratories should have policies about what should be done when results are in a critical range.

BOX 2–9

Components of a Medical Record

Each health care delivery organization's medical record will differ somewhat in its format. However, the following components are common to most. In a paper-based system, these may be in separate sections. In an EMR, there may be electronic tabs to categorize various sections.

Personal information—Patient's name, date of birth, identification number, address, marital status, closest relative, known allergies, physician's name, and diagnosis

Personal and family medical history—Initial assessment completed by the physician (MD or DO) and the registered nurse (RN)

Ordering documentation—Includes MD's and/or other qualified providers' (nurse practitioner [NP], clinical nurse specialist [CNS], physician assistant [PA]) orders for laboratory, radiology, pharmacy, and so on

Consent and release forms—Consent forms, authorization forms for release of medical information, and other forms for patient's preferences (e.g., advanced directives, do-not-resuscitate [DNR] orders, etc.)

Patient's plan of care—MD and nursing care diagnoses, interventions, and patient outcomes; can include flowcharts or checklists indicating recordings of the patient's temperature, pulse rate, respiratory rate, blood pressure, glucose screening levels, weight, and other assessments

Diagnostic test results—Results from all tests performed on the patient: laboratory, radiology, and so on

Medication administration record—Medication dosage and timing, route of administration, site, and date

Progress notes—Notes from qualified health providers (MD, NP, CNS, PA) about the patient's progress, interventions used, and treatment effectiveness

Consultations—Evaluation summaries by clinical specialists: infectious disease specialists, endocrinologists, and so on

Health care team notes—Progress notes from other departments such as nutrition, physical therapy, occupational therapy, counseling, and so on

Discharge plan or summary—Plans for after discharge from a hospital, including special diets, medications, home health visits, and follow-up appointments

Using an EMR eliminates or reduces paper, consolidates data so that they can be accessed from multiple sites, and allows the timely import of information from many ancillary sites (laboratory, pharmacy, etc.). The EMR is an important source of legal information and is admissible in a court of law. Any clinically significant information should be included in the medical record, including laboratory results. Since the laboratory generates a large proportion of the medical record, there is greater potential for delays and errors if the data are delivered in a paper format. Delays in reporting results can have serious patient health consequences—for example, the patient might have already left the hospital yet can have an abnormal test result. The format of the medical record varies by setting—a hospital versus a doctor's office—or by the amount of documentation that is required—from open-ended forms to checklists to fully automated results entry.

Documentation of all clinical events in the MR is important for the following reasons:[11]

■ **Monitoring the quality of care**—Documentation describes what has been done and how the patient responds. Accreditation guidelines and Joint Commission regulations mandate quality assessment activities such as infection rates, use of unnecessary procedures, repeated tests, turnaround times for laboratory results, etc. Refer to Chapter 1 for more information.

- **Coordination of care**—Collaboration occurs among health care providers to plan interventions, evaluate progress, and assist the health care team in making effective decisions. It provides for communication among all health care providers involved with the patient.

- **Accrediting and licensing**—The Joint Commission and other such agencies require standards for documentation in each medical record. Guidelines usually include an assessment, a plan of care, medical orders (e.g., laboratory, radiology), progress notes, and a discharge summary.

- **Legal protection**—Clinical records provide "proof" that the action was performed. They serve as supporting evidence in disability, personal injury, malpractice, and mental competency cases. Appropriate documentation is the key to winning or losing a case for individuals or employees of the health care facility. If a health care worker does not record what occurred, it is assumed that it was not done (**BOX 2–10**; also refer to Chapter 3 for more information about legal issues.)

- **Research**—In teaching institutions, documentation provides important data for research on new therapies, procedures, or drugs.

POLICIES AND PROCEDURES

All health care facilities have policy and procedure manuals (printed and/or electronic) that document and guide practices within the organization. Employees usually spend time during their orientation/training period learning the policies. Health care workers commonly utilize the manuals that are summarized in **TABLE 2–5** in a variety of settings. In particular the College of American Pathologists, an accrediting agency for clinical laboratories, requires that a **specimen collection manual** (printed or electronic) be available to health care workers at all sites where specimens are collected.

BOX 2–10

Important Tips for Documenting Clinical Information

- **Be accurate, objective, short, and legible.** Follow the facility's protocol for entering data. Record only the facts in short phrases, not opinions or assumptions; on hard copies (paper) write in ink and print the words. Comments should not assign blame (e.g., "Blood was not collected from Mr. Juarez because nurse Daly did not complete the proper requisition"). Likewise, comments about staffing shortages or working overtime are discouraged because they may not have a direct influence on the patient's medical condition.

- **Errors should not be erased.** Paper-based records should never be changed, deleted, or falsified to cover a mistake. Errors should be noted by marking a single line through it and writing the word *Error* next to it with one's initials next to the correction.

- **Electronic errors should be corrected by authorized individuals.** Again, follow the facility's protocol for error documentation.

- **Include all relevant information in a timely manner.** Notes should be entered about each event, procedure, or problem that occurs *as soon as possible* with the exact time and date. For example, if a health care worker is unable to identify a patient because of a missing armband, the notation should include the time, the date, the name of the nurse who positively identified the patient, and the health care worker's name. Electronic notations should be done by authorized personnel and according to the organization's policies.

TABLE 2–5

Procedures Important to Health Care Workers

The following topics are generally covered in Standard Operating Procedures and are particularly important for health care workers performing specimen collections.

Topic	Procedures
Specimen collection manual	■ Patient preparation ■ Type of collection container and amount of specimen required ■ Timing requirements (e.g., creatinine clearance, therapeutic drug monitoring) ■ Type and amount of preservative or anticoagulant needed ■ Special handling or transportation needs (e.g., refrigeration, immediate delivery) ■ Proper labeling requirements ■ Need for additional clinical data when indicated (e.g., fasting versus nonfasting).[11]
Administrative procedure manual	■ Performance evaluation procedures and job descriptions ■ Disciplinary policies and confidentiality/nondisclosure policies ■ Compensatory time, annual leave, and overtime policies ■ Attendance and punctuality policies ■ Holiday schedules ■ Handling of employee accidents ■ In-service requirements ■ Vaccination policies (e.g., hepatitis) ■ Telephone etiquette policies ■ Translation procedures for non–English-speaking patients ■ Release of information policies ■ Sexual harassment policies ■ Quality improvement plan ■ Patient billing methods ■ Dress code
Safety manuals	■ Fire safety ■ Internal and external disaster plan ■ Radiation safety ■ Exposure control plan, Material Safety Data Sheets ■ Hazard communication manual
Infection control manual	■ Handling specimens ■ Precautions ■ Isolation procedures ■ Disposal policies ■ Decontamination procedures ■ Hand hygiene procedures ■ Accidental percutaneous needlesticks ■ Postexposure procedures
Quality control (QC) manual	■ Maintaining appropriate supplies ■ Monitoring reagents and equipment ■ Proper use, storage, and handling of supplies ■ Stability of reagents and expiration dates ■ Measuring precision and accuracy
Other procedures important to health care workers	■ Reporting of critical values ■ Maintaining confidentiality and privacy ■ Laboratory test or billing codes ■ Inventory procedures for equipment and supplies ■ Acceptable symbols, abbreviations, and units of measure (refer to the appendices for examples) ■ Interdepartmental loans of supplies and equipment ■ Use of library resources ■ Handling specimens going to or coming from outside organizations ■ Instrument and maintenance manuals

LABORATORY SERVICES INFORMATION BOOK

Communication with other health care providers working outside the laboratory is enhanced by using an electronic information bulletin, or "floor book," of laboratory services (**BOX 2–11**). This should contain a directory of the laboratory departments and staff members, the location of the laboratory, contact numbers, operating hours, reference ranges, instructions, and pertinent standard laboratory procedures. The methods used for collection of all specimens—as well as the proper identification, storage, preservation, and transportation mechanisms to be used—are clearly specified. In addition, an alphabetical listing of all laboratory determinations, specimen requirements, special

> **BOX 2-11**
>
> # Ideas for Sharing Laboratory Information
>
> There are many ways to communicate laboratory information with coworkers and staff members outside the laboratory department. Here are some common methods to share or seek out information:
>
> - Task force meetings
> - Committees for patient safety or quality improvement
> - Quarterly, monthly, or weekly reports, tips for success
> - Newsletters, bulletin boards, blogs
> - Regional conferences, video conferences, webinars,
> - Onsite training programs
> - Advice from consultants

instructions, and tables with reference ranges for each measurement are often included. This is particularly helpful to phlebotomists, medical students, residents, fellows, and trainees.

CONFIDENTIALITY AND PRIVACY

Clinical information such as laboratory and radiology test results must be kept confidential and private. Health care workers who have access to this information must be careful not to disclose patient information in a casual, unnecessary fashion. Discussion that does not directly relate to the health care worker's role in caring for the patient should be avoided.

A health care worker might occasionally overhear communication between a physician and the patient. This communication is considered privileged and must not be shared with others without the prior consent of the patient. This assures compliance with HIPAA, which prohibits disclosure of any health information unless a written consent has been obtained from a patient. Health care providers are required to create "privacy-conscious" practices, which include informing patients about the use and disclosure of their health information and require that only the minimum amount of health information necessary be disclosed. Furthermore, providers and insurance companies must ensure internal protection of medical records, employee privacy training and education, proper handling of privacy complaints, and designation of a privacy officer.

Study Questions

For the following questions, select the one best answer.

1 Which is an example of a barrier to communication with a patient?

a. sender
b. decoder
c. television
d. supervisor

2 "DOB" stands for

a. don't offer beverages
b. date of breakfast
c. date of birth
d. department of blood work

3 Which of the following statements is appropriate during a phlebotomy procedure?

a. "This won't hurt a bit!"
b. "Your name is Mrs. O'Brien, isn't it?"
c. "You are required to cooperate with this."
d. "Could you please spell your last name for me?"

4 Which of the following is a key element in effective communication?

a. active listening
b. critical values
c. eye color distinctions
d. point-of-care procedures

5 Slouching posture, a nonverbal behavior, conveys what message?

a. confidence
b. pride
c. laziness
d. attention to detail

6 What feelings does one experience when a stranger gets "too close for comfort"?

a. anxiety
b. joy
c. confidence
d. security

7 The definition of *culture* includes which one of the following aspects?

a. anatomy and physiology
b. hair and eye color
c. traditions and values
d. combined family salary

8 EMR stands for which term?

a. effectiveness of medical reagents
b. electronic medical record
c. efficient monitoring of results
d. electronic medical research

9 Which of the following data should be considered confidential?

a. laboratory test results
b. patient's bill of rights
c. nonprofit status of the health facility
d. universal precautions

10 What method for requesting a laboratory test is the most "error-free"?

a. handwritten requisition
b. electronic method
c. verbal method
d. verbal STAT method

Case Study 1

One Patient, Two Health Care Professionals A 50-year-old woman is scheduled to have a hysterectomy later in the week. She is at the hospital for preoperative laboratory work and a chest x-ray. The nurse and phlebotomist are both in the room with the patient. The nurse is conducting a nursing assessment and reveals to the patient that the chest x-ray is abnormal. At the same time, the phlebotomist is ready to collect a blood specimen. Both health care workers can use a computerized handheld data-entry system to access information and to enter information about the patient in an electronic format.

Questions

1 If the patient's results are entered into the handheld device, who would be able to legally access that medical information?

2 Is it okay for the phlebotomist to collect a blood specimen while the nurse is conducting a health assessment?

3 Does the patient have to sign a consent form with regard to her electronic medical record?

4 Is this situation acceptable? If not, give some suggestions about how to improve it.

Case Study 2

The Patient and the Family Mrs. Rodriguez is pregnant and has come to see her obstetrician for a routine prenatal visit. She is accompanied by her 8-year-old daughter, her mother, and her two sisters. None of them speaks English very well, except the 8-year-old daughter. Mrs. Rodriguez's examination includes laboratory tests and urinalysis. She also needs to be screened for gestational diabetes. Elizabeth, an experienced health care worker who cannot speak Spanish, is assigned to collect the specimens from Mrs. Rodriguez.

Questions

1 Describe possible barriers to the effective communication between Mrs. Rodriguez and Elizabeth.

2 Even though there is limited information presented here, what factors seem important to Mrs. Rodriguez?

3 Describe at least five communication strategies that Elizabeth might use during her encounter with Mrs. Rodriquez.

4 What role(s) can the family members play in this situation?

5 Describe career development strategies that Elizabeth might consider to improve her ability to communicate effectively with patients such as Mrs. Rodriquez.

Action in Practice

Cultural Competency—Keep an Open Mind All health care workers should be culturally sensitive by helping to provide an environment that supports cultural differences. A health care worker who considers a patient's personal values, beliefs, and customs will be a more effective employee than one who does not.

Questions

Answer the following questions yourself, then discuss them either in a group or with a friend. Without being judgmental, listen carefully and learn about how others answer the same questions. You do not have to agree with another belief, but you should respect the right of others to have beliefs different from your own. There are no right or wrong answers to these questions.

1 How do you define social activities?

2 What are some of the activities you enjoy?

3 Do you believe in a Supreme Being?

4 What is your role in your family unit (father, mother, child, advisor, caregiver)?

5 Who is/are the primary decision maker(s) in your family?

6 When you were a child, what or who influenced you the most?

7 What is/was your relationship with your siblings and parents?

8 What does work mean to you?

9 What is your attitude toward health and illness?

10 How do you react to pain?

11 Who helps you cope during difficult times?

12 What foods are family favorites or considered traditional?

13 What types of foods did you eat as a child?

14 Would you consider yourself past oriented, present oriented, or future oriented?

Verbal Communication People sound differently from how they think they sound because the voice inside one's head is not the "real" voice. The true voice is what comes out of one's mouth and is heard by others. The words may indicate something pleasant, but a "mean" tone of voice changes the message entirely.

Questions

The only way to improve the way your voice sounds is to hear yourself as others hear you. (Also consider doing this exercise with a peer to get his or her impressions and feedback.)

1 Make a recording of your voice. Select a paragraph in this chapter and read it out loud while recording it.

2 Wait 5 to 10 minutes, relax, go to a mirror and smile at yourself a few times, then listen to yourself to get an impression of how you sound to others. You will notice whether your spoken message sounds as you want it to sound.

3 Ask yourself:

   ■ Do you sound tired or bored?
   ■ Do you sound angry or impatient or stressed?
   ■ At what volume (loud/soft) and pace (fast/slow) were you speaking?

   ■ Do you have an accent that might interfere with transitions between words or sentences?
   ■ Do you remember how you were sitting or standing during the reading? Was it comfortable?

4 Next try to put your favorite picture, photo, or favorite object near you. Sit in a comfortable chair with good posture, smile, and take a few deep breaths. Now read and record another paragraph in the chapter. Listen to it again to see if your voice improved.

5 Keep improving your tone of voice and communication skills until you believe that you can have a positive impact on how you come across to customers and peers.

Check Yourself

1 Describe adjustments you should make in your communication skills when you collect a specimen from a patient who cannot hear well and a patient who is legally blind.

2 Describe some courtesy tips that can help a sighted person become more at ease with a blind person.

Competency Checklist: Cultural Competency

Sometimes it is difficult to be introspective about your own biases, attitudes, and behaviors toward people or groups that are different from your own. Most adults do not perceive themselves as prejudiced. As a professional, it is important to treat all individuals with unbiased respect and compassion. To assess your own attitudes, rate yourself on the following criteria. Be honest with yourself when completing the checklist. Make a list of areas you think need improvement. For more information and more detailed assessment tools, refer to www.adl.org.

(1) Completed (2) Needs to improve

_____ 1. I have enough knowledge about the cultures of other racial, religious, and ethnic groups.

_____ 2. I periodically attend multicultural events, social events, and classes or seminars about generational or cultural diversity.

_____ 3. I never use degrading language or terms.

_____ 4. I do not use stereotypes about people based on their group, gender, etc.

_____ 5. I value cultural differences.

_____ 6. I give equal attention to all coworkers and patients regardless of race, age, religion, economic status, and physical ability.

_____ 7. I am not afraid to ask people who use biased language or behaviors to refrain from doing so.

Competency Checklist: Telephone Communication

All health care workers should ensure that correct information is communicated or received when on the telephone.

(1) Completed (2) Needs to improve

_____ 1. The telephone is answered on the first or second ring.

_____ 2. The correct greeting is used ("Good morning," give name and/or department, "How may I help you?").

_____ 3. Words and statements are enunciated and easy to understand.

_____ 4. A professional tone of voice is used.

_____ 5. A moderate volume is used for talking.

_____ 6. A moderate pace is used with appropriate pauses.

_____ 7. The caller is placed on hold after he or she states the reason for the call.

_____ 8. The caller is not left on hold for more than 30 seconds.

_____ 9. Messages are clearly and accurately written.

_____ 10. Spellings and phone numbers are repeated for accuracy.

_____ 11. There is a polite ending to the conversation ("Good-bye," "Thank you," etc.).

_____ 12. The caller is allowed to hang up first.

Competency Checklist: Handwritten Communication

Health care workers need to write legibly and articulately. Practice the following exercises and have them read and edited by another person to get feedback.

(1) Completed (2) Needs to improve

_____   1.   Write a short paragraph (5 to 10 sentences) about the last time you had a blood test. The reader should evaluate:

the clarity of the message

the readability of the handwriting

how well the description of the scene was understood

_____   2.   Practice writing your full name and initials 10 times very quickly. The reader should evaluate the

legibility of each letter in each of the 10 names

legibility of each letter in each of the 10 initials

Competency Checklist: Computer Components

Using computer equipment in the clinical laboratory, student laboratory, or an office, identify and define each of the following computer components and peripherals.

(1) Completed (2) Needs to improve

_____   1.   Computer monitor

_____   2.   Keyboard

_____   3.   Printer

_____   4.   Bar code reader (if available)

_____   5.   Scanner

_____   6.   Fax/Scan

_____   7.   Modem

_____   8.   CPU

_____   9.   Data storage units

_____ 10.   Software used on that computer

REFERENCES

1. Beaman, N., & Fleming-McPhillips, L. (2007). *Pearson's administrative medical assisting. Volume 1: Administrative competencies.* Upper Saddle River, NJ: Pearson Prentice Hall.

2. Gibbons, M. (2006, Feb). Reading, writing, life, death: Lack of health literacy threatens patients' lives, costs billions. *Advance for Administrators of the Laboratory,* http://laboratory-manager.advanceweb.com, accessed Feb 25, 2014.

3. Frerichs, J. (2007, March). Front-line supervisory skills: Generational differences in the workplace. Presented at the 2007 Leadership Exchange, American Society for clinical Pathology, Chicago.

4. www.wmfc.org/uploads/GenerationalDifferencesChart.pdf, accessed Feb 25, 2014.

5. United States 2010 Census Briefs, www.census.gov/2010census/, accessed Feb 25, 2014.

6. Harty-Golder, B. (2004, August). Liability and the lab: Lost in translation, foreign languages in the lab. *Medical Lab Observer,* p. 41.

7. National Federation of the Blind: Straightforward answers about blindness. www.nfb.org, accessed Feb 25, 2014.

8. Hall, L. (1981). Blind patients. *Brit Med J., 282*(714).

9. Penno, K. (2007, July 2). The eternal e-mail. *Advance for Medical Laboratory Professionals, 19,* p. 33 (accessed in archives March 19, 2013).

10. Patton, Matthew T. Woeful workplace etiquette. *Advance Healthcare Network for Nurses,* www.nursing.advanceweb.com, accessed January 13, 2014.

11. The Joint Commission: 2014 National Patient Safety Goals. (2014). http://www.jointcommission.org/, accessed Feb 25, 2014.

12. Clinical Laboratory and Standards Institute (CLSI). (2010). *Procedures for the handling and processing of blood specimens for common laboratory tests, approved guideline,* 4th ed., H18-A4. Wayne, PA: Author.

RESOURCES

www.adl.org The Anti-Defamation League (ADL) combats bigotry of all kinds by providing information and antibias educational resources.

www.cap.org This is the official website for the College of American Pathologists, an accrediting organization for clinical and anatomical laboratories.

www.xculture.org This website is part of the Cross Cultural Health Care Program, which provides educational materials and training opportunities for culturally and linguistically appropriate health care. The organization also provides training for medical interpreters.

www.diversityrx.org Diversity Rx promotes language and cultural competence to improve the quality of health care for minority, immigrant, and ethnically diverse communities. Educational resources are available.

www.ethnomed.org EthnoMed provides information about cultural beliefs and medical issues (such as fasting during religious holidays) pertinent to the health care of recent immigrants to the United States, many of whom are refugees fleeing war-torn nations.

www.ncihc.org The National Council on Interpreting in Health Care (NCIHC) provides standards and information to promote competent health care interpreting for individuals with limited English proficiency.

www.nfb.org The National Federation of the Blind provides advocacy, education, research, technology, and programs that encourage independence and self-confidence.

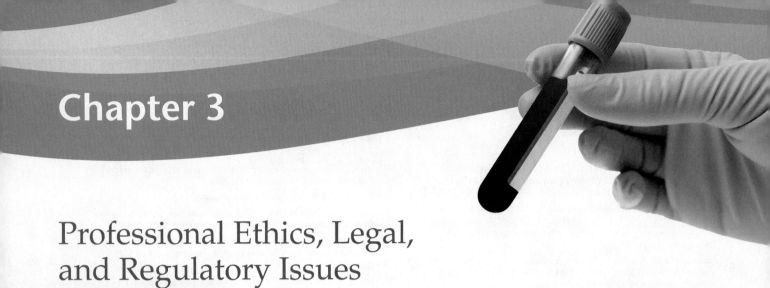

Chapter 3

Professional Ethics, Legal, and Regulatory Issues

Chapter Objectives

Upon completion of Chapter 3, the learner is responsible for doing the following:

1. Define basic ethical and legal terms and explain how they differ.

2. Describe types of consent used in health care settings, including *informed consent* and *implied consent.*

3. Describe how to avoid litigation as it relates to blood collection.

4. Define *standard of care* from a legal and a health care provider's perspective.

5. Identify key elements of the *Health Insurance Portability and Accountability Act (HIPAA).*

6. List key factors common to health professional liability insurance policies.

7. List common issues in lawsuits against health care providers and prevention tips to avoid lawsuits in phlebotomy.

The topics of law, ethics, and bioethics are all interrelated and difficult to discuss without referring to one another:

- "Laws are societal rules or regulations that are advisable or obligatory to observe. Laws protect the welfare and safety of society, resolve conflicts in an orderly and nonviolent manner, and constantly evolve in accordance with an increasingly pluralistic society."[1]

- **Ethics** refers to the moral standards of behavior or conduct that govern an individual's actions. Moral standards are developed throughout life, beginning with the childhood learning process of differentiating between right and wrong. All health care providers are confronted daily with professional choices. Choosing one type of needle instead of another and using a cleaning agent that creates an allergy in a patient are procedures that can be harmful and can impact both the patient and health care worker. When a health care provider makes an error, he or she must try to remedy the error and learn from it. The health care worker must be knowledgeable and recognize what can be harmful to a patient to avoid a wrong patient outcome.

- **Bioethics** (*bio* refers to "life") refers to the moral issues or problems that have resulted because of modern medicine, clinical research, and/or technology. Usually, bioethics refers to "life-and-death" issues such as abortion, when a patient should be allowed to die, and who receives organ donations.

Ethics Overview

All health care workers are faced with ethical decisions at one time or another (**BOX 3–1**). As health care situations become more complex, ethical decision making requires using a health care team approach as well as an individual approach. Each individual should reflect on his or her own standards of behavior and those of his or her professional affiliations. The simple set of questions that follow can serve as an "ethics check" for people facing an ethical dilemma or decision. To evaluate a difficult situation, simply ask yourself:[1]

- Is this legal and does it comply with institutional policy?
- Does it foster a "win-win" situation with the patient/supervisor or other individuals?
- How would I feel about myself if I read about this decision in the newspaper? How would my family feel?
- Can I live with myself after making this decision?
- Is it right?

Patients' Rights

All members of the health care team recognize that their first responsibility is to the patient's health, safety, and personal dignity. Many organizations, such as the **American Hospital Association (AHA)**, have recognized rights for patients in health care organizations. The AHA originally adopted a **Patient's Bill of Rights** in 1973, with the

> **BOX 3–1**
>
> # Example of Ethical Behavior for a Health Care Worker
>
> If a health care worker realizes that she or he has made a mistake in identifying a patient and specimens, the health care worker faces an ethical decision about whether to report her or his own mistake. Reporting it may result in disciplinary action. Consider the following points:
>
> - Each health care worker should go through the ethics check questions to conclude that the right ethical decision would be to report his or her mistake as soon as possible in order to avoid any clinical and/or treatment decisions based on the wrong test results.
>
> - This is the right decision because it complies with policy, it's ethically the right thing to do, and it fosters a win-win situation for the patient and the doctor. The alternative would be embarrassing, dishonest, and grounds for dismissal. In addition, legal risk is minimized for the health care worker and the health care facility if the error is appropriately corrected and documented. Reporting that an error has occurred and seeking corrective action are critical factors in health care professionalism.

latest revision in 2003, titled the **Patient Care Partnership**. The key elements involve a patient's rights to the following:[2]

- Quality health care
- Provision of a clean health care environment
- The patient's role in his/her own care
- Privacy rights
- Availability of assistance when leaving the hospital or with billing issues

NATIONAL PATIENT SAFETY GOALS (NPSGs)

The Joint Commission is an independent, nongovernmental agency that provides standards for the objective evaluation process that guides health care facilities to measure, assess, and improve performance for patient care and safety. This regulatory agency has existed longer than other health care policy-setting organizations in the United States. To be accredited through the Joint Commission, a health care institution must undergo an onsite evaluation by a survey team every three years and two years for the clinical laboratories. Today, this regulatory agency has developed into an international authority.

The Joint Commission has stated that the delivery of health care to patients should be done in a manner that is respectful and appropriate to an individual's language and culture as well as a factor in the safety and quality of patient care.[3] The Joint Commission's National Patient Safety Goals (NPSGs) were established to help health care organizations address specific areas of concern with regard to patient safety in health care facilities. For the clinical laboratory, the 2012 NPSGs are:

- **Identify patients correctly.** Use at least two ways to identify patients when providing laboratory preanalytical, analytical, and postanalytical procedures.
- **Improve staff communication.** Provide test results to the right person in a timely manner. For critical test results, the results need to be expedited for the physician to diagnose and treat the patient promptly.

■ **Prevent infection.** Use the hand-cleaning guidelines designated by the Centers for Disease Control and Prevention (CDC) or the World Health Organization (WHO).

Overall, the health care worker, as a major part of the health care team, should appreciate the rights and needs of patients as he or she assists in providing health care in hospitals, ambulatory care facilities, and other health care sites.

Governmental Laws

The legislative, executive, and judicial branches of government control laws. The legislative written laws are called *statutes* and are made at the federal, state, and county levels. The executive branch makes administrative laws, and the judicial branch establishes case law that is based on legal cases from lower-level judicial branches. The federal and state governments each have separate judicial court systems.

Basic Legal Principles

The laws governing medicine and medical ethics complement and overlap each other. For many years, even centuries, the decision of the physician or health care professional was unquestioned. This has changed, however. Health care consumers and patients have become more aware, more critical, and much more willing to sue anyone that their lawyer believes has been at fault, including health care workers who are collecting blood specimens.

LEGAL TERMINOLOGY

An understanding of basic legal concepts can help a health care worker define how personnel involved in the specimen collection process can be liable for their activities. Such understanding can also reduce the conflicts between the health care worker and the law.

Liability for the lack of a proper standard of health care may be imposed on any health care worker, including physicians, nurses, laboratorians, patient care technicians, and phlebotomists. The number of substantial awards against health care workers as a result of improper care has grown in recent years as patients have become more sensitive to treatment complications.

To grasp the legal implication of health care, the health care provider must have some knowledge of basic legal terminology. A few major definitions with health care examples can be found in **BOX 3–2**.

NEGLIGENCE

The word *negligence* is very important to health care providers. In the past decade, the number of legal cases in which a laboratory has been directly or indirectly involved has increased noticeably. *Negligence* is "a violation of a duty to exercise reasonable skill and care in performing a task."[4] *Torts* are civil wrongs that include negligence and malpractice. Most civil lawsuits in the clinical laboratory are due to negligence that falls under the category of tort law—a private action between individuals.

The following factors must be considered in alleged negligence cases:

■ **Duty**—Relates to those duties or responsibilities the hospital or health care provider has toward the patient; it also includes all the individuals who had a duty toward the patient to use the appropriate standard of care.

■ **Breach of duty**—Relates to whether the duty was breached and if the breach was avoidable. The plaintiff must be able to show what actually happened and that the defendant acted unreasonably.

BOX 3–2

Legal Terminology

- **Assault**—The unjustifiable attempt to touch another person or the threat to do so in such circumstances as to cause the other to believe that it will be carried out or to cause fear. An assault may be permissible if proper consent has been given (e.g., consent to obtain a blood specimen).

- **Battery**—The intentional touching of another person without consent; also, the unlawful beating of another or carrying out of threatened physical harm. Because battery always includes an assault, the two are commonly combined in the phrase *assault and battery*. Liability of hospitals, physicians, and other health care workers for acts of battery is most common in situations involving lack of or improper consent to medical procedures, such as blood collecting. Three examples follow:

  1. A small boy who refused to have his blood collected was locked in the blood collection room by the health care worker and was forced to have his blood drawn by the health care worker without the parents' consent. Attempting a blood collection on a child without the parents' consent can lead to the health care worker being charged with assault and battery.

  2. If a patient is feeling stressed because of pain and does not know which medical procedures will be performed and a health care professional displays threatening behavior, this can lead to legal intervention. The health care worker must obviously avoid using threatening language (e.g., "If you don't let me collect your blood, your illness will probably become critical").

  3. Sometimes with elderly patients or patients with specific mental disorders (i.e., Alzheimer's disease, dementia, Parkinson's disease), it is difficult to determine if the patient is competent to give consent for blood collection. In these situations, if the health care worker is uncertain whether the patient is refusing to have blood collection due to his or her mental state, the health care worker should contact the supervisor and/or physician so that the blood collection procedure does not lead to a charge of assault and battery.

- **Breach of duty**—(Also referred to as *neglect of* duty) An infraction, violation, or failure to perform. For example, something was performed when it should not have been performed or nothing was done when it should have been done. With medical privacy as a major issue in today's society, a health care provider must avoid a **breach of confidentiality** in releasing a patient's laboratory test results without authorization to do so.

- **Civil law**—Not a criminal action; the plaintiff sues for monetary damages. A **tort** is a civil wrong committed against a person or a person's property. The person or persons claimed to be responsible for the tort are sued for damages. Civil lawsuits involve the government or an individual versus another individual or entity (i.e., business).

- **Criminal actions**—Legal recourse for acts or offenses against the public welfare; these actions can lead to imprisonment of the offender. Criminal cases involve the government versus an individual or entity.

- **Defendant**—The health care worker or institution against whom the action or lawsuit is filed.

- **False imprisonment**—The unjustifiable detention of a person without a legal warrant.

- **Felony**—Varies by state but generally is defined as public offense; if the defendant is convicted, he or she will spend time in jail.

- **Fraud**—Deliberate deception or cheating either by conduct or words, frequently performed to obtain money—for example, billing for Medicare health care services that have not been provided.

BOX 3–2 (continued)

- **Invasion of privacy**—The unauthorized release of information about a patient. The law does not allow any personal information on a patient, such as HIV test results, to become public without the patient's permission.
- **Liable**—Under legal obligation, as far as damages are concerned.
- **Litigation process**—The process of legal action to determine a decision in court. Many malpractice cases are negotiated and settled out of court.
- **Malice**—Knowing that a statement is false or making a statement with reckless disregard of the truth.
- **Malpractice**—Professional negligence. Improper or unskillful care of a patient by a member of the health care team, or any professional misconduct or unreasonable lack of skill.
- **Misdemeanor**—The general term for all sorts of criminal offenses not serious enough to be classified as felonies; usually punishable by fines, prison penalties, or forfeiture.
- **Misrepresentation**—Use of misleading information or omission of important facts.
- **Negligence**—Failure to act or to perform duties according to the standards of the profession.
- **Plaintiff**—The claimant who brings a lawsuit or an action.
- **Res ipsa loquitur**—The doctrine or principle that "the thing speaks for itself." It is a rule of evidence that occurs when the plaintiff is injured in such a way that he or she cannot prove how the injury occurred or who was responsible for its occurrence. This doctrine is usually applied in medical malpractice cases in which the injured party was in surgery, is unconscious, or was an infant. An example is an infection that resulted from an unsterile instrument.
- **Respondeat superior**—Under this concept, supervisors and directors may be held liable for the negligent actions of their employees.
- **Subpoena**—Court order for a person and documents (e.g., health care worker and phlebotomy technical procedures) to be brought to court proceedings.
- **Tort**—A civil wrong committed against a person or a person's property. The person or persons claimed to be responsible for the tort are sued for damages. Tort law is based on fault. The accountable person either did not meet his or her responsibility or performed a task below the allowable standard of care. Torts are civil wrongs and *not* based on contracts.

- **Foreseeability**—Relates to the concept that certain events may reasonably be expected to cause specific results. For example, using a long, large needle to collect blood from an elderly patient with frail veins will foreseeably lead to vein damage and accumulation of blood in the skin around the venipuncture.
- **Proximate causation**—Relates to whether the breach of duty actually contributed to or caused injury; also concerns all the parties involved in contributing to the alleged injury. There must be a direct line from the conduct to the injury.
- **Injury or harm**—The demonstration that an actual physical injury occurred. As an example, as a health care worker collected blood from a patient, the needle went through the vein into the median nerve and the patient subsequently lost the use of three fingers of his hand due to nerve damage.
- **Damages**—The actual injury and the amount of money awarded to the plaintiff (injured client) that is based on compensating for the resultant injuries, pain, suffering, and permanent disability.

Many circumstances could be considered negligence if health care providers are not extremely careful. For example, there have been legal cases in which the confusion of patient samples led to a patient's death.[5]

MALPRACTICE

Malpractice, or professional negligence, is defined as improper or unskillful care of a patient by a member of the health care team, or any professional misconduct or unreasonable lack of skill.

If the physician is the medical director overseeing clinical laboratory testing, in most cases he or she is responsible under the law for the standard of care and the performance of all aspects of laboratory testing. Therefore, a breach of standard on the part of the health care worker collecting blood for laboratory assays could place both the physician and the health care worker at risk.

HIPAA

The use of electronic transfer of patient's medical information is regulated by the federal **Health Insurance Portability and Accountability Act (HIPAA) (FIGURE 3–1).**[6] This law created legal requirements for the protection, security, and appropriate sharing of a patient's personal health information. The information is referred to as **protected health information (PHI)**. HIPAA requires that health care providers obtain a patient's written consent before disclosing medical information for the routine uses of diagnosis, treatment, payment, or health care operations (e.g., laboratory data collection for quality assurance). Thus, each laboratory must give patients information on their rights and on the ways their laboratory test results will be used.[7] Health care workers must review and sign a confidentiality and nondisclosure agreement that describes the sensitivity of patient information. This signature verifies that the health care worker will

- Maintain the confidentiality of all patients' information, including laboratory tests to be performed.
- Keep the computer password for entering the laboratory patients' database secure from others' knowledge.
- Maintain the confidentiality of patients' information when looking at the computer database of patients' medical record information.[8]

Some examples of seemingly innocent activities that can lead to lawsuits include:

- Discussing patient information with a patient's family member without the patient's permission
- Throwing laboratory test requests into the regular trash
- Not logging off the computer after entering blood collection updates
- Sending a patient's laboratory test requests to be printed and forgetting to take it off the printer
- Forgetting to clear phone numbers from fax machines, copiers, etc.

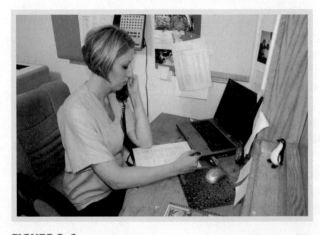

FIGURE 3–1

Blood collection involves entry of specimens collected on patients in a confidential manner.

PATIENT CONFIDENTIALITY

Negligence cases can arise out of violation of the right to privacy or of **patient confidentiality**: "No one except the patient may release patient results without a clinical need to know." Patient or employee laboratory test results must be considered strictly confidential. Negligence can be claimed, for example, if employees' or patients' drug abuse test results are released to anyone other than the attending physician or other authorized individuals. This is particularly true regarding employee or athlete drug or alcohol abuse screening and human immunodeficiency virus (HIV) testing. Confidential materials include communications between the physician and the patient; the patient's verbal statements; medical computer entries on patients; and nonverbal communications, such as laboratory test results.

CONFIDENTIALITY AND HIV EXPOSURE

An increasing concern for health care workers collecting blood from patients who are homebound is the health care worker's rights in relation to accidental exposure to blood or body fluids, whether by a needlestick or some other means. In some states, laws allow health care workers to know the identity of a patient who has acquired immunodeficiency syndrome (AIDS) or who is HIV positive. Many states, however, do not provide for the easy acquisition of this sensitive patient information. A home health care worker who routinely collects blood specimens from homebound patients should obtain information on the state's law regarding confidentiality and HIV status.[9] It can be obtained from the health care worker's employer, from legal counsel, or from a national or state health professional organization.

It is important to use the proper blood collection techniques with safety precautions and required infection control procedures for homebound patients. If exposure to the blood occurs through a needlestick, a lancet, or another means, the home health care worker needs to be certain of obtaining the patient's HIV status and other potential infectious diseases (e.g., Hepatitis C) to ensure that the proper immediate and long-term self-protective procedural steps can be taken.

If employed by a health care facility, the health care worker should follow the guidelines established by the facility. It is important for a self-employed health care worker to monitor his or her own HIV status. Also, counseling should be sought to obtain emotional support during this stressful time.

STANDARD OF CARE

If a patient has suffered injury resulting from blood collection for laboratory testing, the patient must show that the health care worker who collected the blood failed to meet the prevailing **standard of care**. All health care workers must conform to a specific standard of care to protect patients. It is a measuring stick representing the conduct of the average health care worker in the community. The community has become a national community as a result of national laboratory standards and requirements. The standard of care is set by statutes; licensing requirements; rules and regulations of regulatory or professional organizations (e.g., American Hospital Association, The Joint Commission); internal health care facility policies, procedures, rules, and regulations; and professional publications. Some of these agencies are mentioned in Chapter 1.

> **ALERT**
>
> # Clinical Alert!
>
> - Minors must have the informed consent of their parents or legal guardians for medical care, including blood collections.
> - Persons who are unconscious or injured in such a way that they are unable to give consent must have consent provided from the closest adult relative if existing laws permit. Health care delivery organizations should have explicit procedures for these circumstances.
> - An adult who has the mental capacity of a child and who has an appointed guardian must have consent provided by the guardian.
> - Since language can be a barrier to informed consent, an interpreter may be necessary so that information for consent may be given in the patient's native tongue.
> - States have enacted legislation requiring that informed consent be obtained before most HIV specimen collection and testing are performed. The statutes indicate the type of information that must be given for the patient to be considered "informed." This information includes
>   1. An explanation of the test
>   2. Potential uses of the HIV test
>   3. Testing limitations and the meaning of its results

INFORMED CONSENT

Informed consent is the voluntary permission given by a patient to allow touching, examination, and/or treatment by health care providers. It allows patients to determine what will be performed on or to their bodies. Without informed consent, intentional touching can be considered a criminal offense. In the health care environment, patients must be informed of the possible consequences of having or not having particular medical treatments. An informed consent form is then signed by the patient for approval of medical treatment(s), including blood collection (**FIGURE 3–2**).

Integral to consent is the patient's belief that the health care worker to whom the consent is given has the knowledge, skills, and technical ability to perform such tasks. Thus, the patient can expect the blood collector to know the proper blood collection techniques and procedures. The patient may also give consent for a venipuncture procedure through the actions of holding out his or her arm, rolling up a sleeve, or simply turning the arm in the correct position for the blood collection procedure.

INFORMED CONSENT FOR RESEARCH PURPOSES

As a result of unethical treatment of humans in the past for research purposes, the United States passed a law in 1974, the National Research Act, that established Institutional Research Boards (IRBs) at institutions (e.g., hospitals, universities) that perform

---

MEMORIAL HEALTH

COMPLETE ORIGINAL IN INK FOR HOSPITAL CHART
PATIENT MUST BE AWAKE, ALERT AND ORIENTED WHEN SIGNING

DATE: _____   TIME: _____   ✳ AM ✳ PM

I AUTHORIZE THE PERFORMANCE UPON_____
OF THE FOLLOWING OPERATION (state nature and extent):_____
_____
_____

TO BE PERFORMED UNDER THE DIRECTION OF DR. _____

1. I HAVE BEEN ADVISED THAT THERE IS A FAVORABLE LIKELIHOOD OF SUCCESS, BUT I UNDERSTAND THAT A COMPLETELY SUCCESSFUL OUTCOME MAY NOT BE ACHIEVABLE, AND THERE ARE NO GUARANTEES REGARDING THE OUTCOME. I ALSO UNDERSTAND THAT CERTAIN ADVERSE EVENTS COULD OCCUR AS A RESULT OF THE PERFORMANCE OF THE PROCEDURE OR TREATMENT, INCLUDING PAIN, INFECTION, LACERATION OR PUNCTURE OF INTERNAL ORGANS, BLEEDING, NERVE DAMAGE OR EVEN IN RARE CASES, DEATH. I UNDERSTAND THAT HOSPITALIZATION OR OTHER INSTITUTIONAL CARE, HOME CARE OR CARE BY HEALTH PROFESSIONALS MAY BE NEEDED FOLLOWING THE PROCEDURE OR TREATMENT, RELATED TO FULL RECOVERY, RECUPERATION OR CONVALESCENCE. I UNDERSTAND THE ALTERNATIVES TO THIS PROCEDURE, INCLUDING MY RIGHT TO REFUSE TO CONSENT TO IT, AND I NEVERTHELESS HAVE DECIDED TO CONSENT TO PERFORMANCE OF THE PROCEDURE OR TREATMENT.

2. I CONSENT TO THE PERFORMANCE OF OPERATIONS AND PROCEDURES IN ADDITION TO OR DIFFERENT FROM THOSE NOW CONTEMPLATED, WHETHER OR NOT ARISING FROM PRESENTLY UNFORESEEN CONDITIONS WHICH THE ABOVE NAMED DOCTOR OR HIS/HER ASSOCIATES OR ASSISTANTS MAY CONSIDER NECESSARY OR ADVISABLE IN THE COURSE OF THE OPERATION.

3. I CONSENT TO THE DISPOSAL BY HOSPITAL AUTHORITIES OF ANY TISSUES OR PARTS WHICH MAY BE REMOVED.

4. THE NATURE AND PURPOSE OF THE OPERATION/PROCEDURE, POSSIBLE ALTERNATIVE METHODS OF TREATMENT, THE RISK AND BENEFITS INVOLVED, AND THE COURSE OF RECUPERATION HAVE BEEN FULLY EXPLAINED TO ME. NO GUARANTEE OR ASSURANCE HAS BEEN GIVEN BY ANYONE AS TO THE RESULTS THAT MAY BE OBTAINED.

5. I UNDERSTAND AND AGREE WITH THE ABOVE INFORMATION. I HAVE NO QUESTIONS WHICH HAVE NOT BEEN ANSWERED TO MY FULL SATISFACTION. I UNDERSTAND THAT I HAVE THE RIGHT TO ASK FOR FURTHER INFORMATION BEFORE SIGNING THIS CONSENT.

I have crossed out any paragraph above which does not apply or to which I do not give consent.

PATIENT SIGNATURE: _____   WITNESS SIGNATURE: _____
(OR PARENT OR GUARDIAN IF PATIENT IS UNDER 18 YEARS OF AGE)   *(OF PATIENT, PARENT OR GUARDIAN SIGNATURE)*

RELATIONSHIP: _____   WITNESS SIGNATURE: _____
                                          ● **TELEPHONE CONSENT** *(2ND WITNESS NEEDED FOR TELEPHONE CONSENT)*

FIGURE 3–2

Sample of an informed consent document to perform surgery, sedation, and other medical procedures such as blood collection.

research. These IRBs were established to review and approve only those research proposals that included protocols that would protect the human subjects involved. The IRB ensures that human subjects do not bear any inappropriate risk and have properly consented to their involvement.

Frequently, in hospitals, health care facilities, and health science universities, health care workers become involved in collecting blood from research participants for research projects. The National Research Act states that any research project utilizing human subjects requires the informed consent of those individuals. In order to collect blood for a research project, the participants must understand the nature of the research study and the risks and benefits involved if they are to make an informed decision about their participation.

Informed consent for research requires a "consent document" that includes the following:

- **Full disclosure**, which explains the full nature of the research and any risks (e.g., blood collection problems) and benefits to the participant.
- Describes the level of confidentiality of the research data. If at all possible, the patient should never be capable of being identified through the research study.
- Describes the measures that the researcher will take to ensure that confidentiality is maintained.

This information must be presented to and signed by the participant in the research before any blood collection can occur for the research activities. In addition, working as a blood collector in the research project requires attending a course on the protection of human subjects in research projects (**FIGURE 3–3**).

IMPLIED CONSENT

Implied consent occurs when the patient's nonverbal behavior indicates agreement. Implied consent exists when immediate action is required to save a patient's life or to prevent permanent impairment of the patient's health. In other words, an emergency removes the need for informed consent. The essence behind implied consent is that if the person was able to do so, they would have agreed to treatment by signing an informed consent form. By being rushed to the hospital, it is implied that the person wants to be treated and gives their consent to treatment—even though the person is unable to do so. The requirements for implied consent differ legally from one state to another. Health care providers need to know the legal boundaries of implied consent because someday they may need to decide whether to perform a vital emergency procedure (e.g., cardiopulmonary resuscitation).

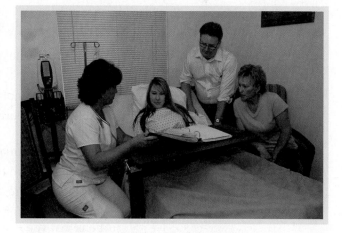

FIGURE 3–3
It is important for a patient to be informed and to sign the appropriate informed consent forms before he or she participates in a research study.

STATUTE OF LIMITATIONS

The **statute of limitations** is a law that defines how soon after an injury (e.g., due to malpractice) a plaintiff must file the lawsuit or be forever barred from doing so. The purpose of this law is to prevent the threat of a lawsuit from hanging over a possible defendant's (e.g., health care provider's) head forever and to force legal action while memories are fresh, records are available, and witnesses are still living.

The statute of limitations for professional negligence in most states is two years. A complete and accurate medical record with laboratory testing results is the best defense in these cases because the attending physician and health care workers for the patient may have little recollection of the events in question.

Legal Claims and Defense

In a malpractice lawsuit, the first statement of a case by the plaintiff(s) against the defendant(s) is the complaint. It states a cause of action, notifying the defendant(s) of the reason for the lawsuit (**FIGURE 3–4**).

Several steps are followed at the beginning of a malpractice lawsuit:

- If the case is not dismissed before trial, the parties to a lawsuit have the right to **discovery**, which means to examine the witnesses before the trial. Examination before trial is a method used to enable the plaintiff(s) and defendant(s) to learn more regarding the nature and substance of each other's case.

- This discovery process consists of oral testimony under oath and includes cross-examination by the lawyers.

- The **deposition** is the testimony of a witness that has been recorded in a written legal format. Either party in the lawsuit—plaintiff or defendant—may obtain a court order permitting examination and copying of laboratory reports, incident reports from personnel files, **medical records**, phlebotomy and laboratory policies and procedures, training manuals, and so forth, as well as other facts and information that may help in the discovery.

- In addition to the deposition, the parties may undergo cross-examination at the time of the trial. They will provide testimony regarding the cause for the case that will be recorded and filed with the court.

A health care worker who receives a summons to provide a deposition before a trial and/or testimony during a trial for a lawsuit will find the following guidelines helpful:

- Answer only the questions asked.
- Be organized in your recollection of the facts regarding the incident.
- Do not be antagonistic in answering the questions.
- Explain the laboratory and/or blood collection procedures and policies in simple terminology for the jury.
- Do not overdramatize the facts that you are presenting.
- Dress neatly and be groomed appropriately.
- Be polite, sincere, and courteous.
- Be sure to ask for clarification of questions that you did not clearly hear and questions that you did not understand.
- If you are not sure of an answer, indicate that you do not know the answer or that you are not sure.
- Above all, be truthful.

EXPERT WITNESS

Expert testimony, as well as scientific or medical data, is sometimes used to assist in establishing the standard of care required in any given situation. An **expert witness** may assist a plaintiff in proving the wrongful act of a defendant or may assist a defendant in refuting such evidence. At the time of testifying, each expert's training, experience, and special qualifications will be explained during the deposition and later to the jury during the trial.

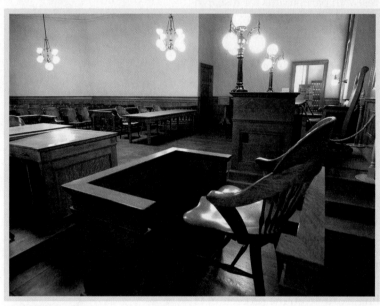

FIGURE 3–4
Being in the interior of a court of law can be very unsettling for both the plaintiff and defendant in a malpractice lawsuit.

EVIDENCE

Evidence during the trial is used to prove or disprove the lawsuit. Evidence must be complete, relevant, and important to the outcome. It may include items such as vacuum tubes and tube holders, needles, safety apparatuses such as biohazardous waste containers, infection control logs and reports, The Joint Commission standards, educational and training records for the involved health care workers, board certification standards for health care workers, and laboratory policies and procedures.

ADVICE TO AVOID LAWSUITS

Justice is expensive in the United States. Lawyers' fees typically range from $400 to $700 per hour, and associated costs can lead to thousands of dollars in legal fees. Also, legal proceedings are time consuming, expensive, and most of all, emotionally devastating to both the plaintiff(s) and the defendant(s). Thus, to avoid a malpractice lawsuit, the health care provider should heed the advice given in **TABLE 3–1**.

RESPONDEAT SUPERIOR

Respondeat superior (a Latin term meaning "let the master answer") is a legal doctrine that holds employers responsible for acts of their employees within the scope of the employment relationship. Not only may the injured party sue the employee directly, but

TABLE 3–1

Lawsuit Prevention Tips for Minimizing Risks

Common Issues in Lawsuits against Health Care Providers	Prevention Tips for Health Care Workers Involved in Blood Collection
Documentation	Always document the time and date and include the blood collector's initials on the blood collection containers.
Reporting of incidents	Document the information legibly and spell correctly. If an adverse incident occurs to the patient and/or the blood collector before, during, or after blood collection, report the incident to your immediate supervisor and complete the appropriate documentation in a legible manner.
Failure to follow health care facility's procedure	Be knowledgeable of the policies and procedures of the health care facility and the clinical laboratory. If you must deviate from a policy or a procedure, discuss the incident with your immediate supervisor and decide on the appropriate action.
Failure to ensure patient's safety	Monitor the patient in an appropriate, timely manner during and after blood collection. Return bed rails to the raised position if the bed rails were raised prior to blood collection. Lock the patient in the blood collection chair for the duration of the blood collection procedure. Ask each patient if he or she has a tendency to faint at the sight of blood. If an outpatient says that he or she might faint or does faint during blood collection, place the patient in a supine position to collect blood, and monitor the patient for at least 20 minutes after collection before allowing him or her to stand up and leave the facility. Remove all supplies and equipment after the procedure.
Improper treatment and performance treatment	Use proper technique and equipment (e.g., gloves) when performing procedures. When performing treatments, follow the procedures of the health care facility and the clinical laboratory. Update your collection skills and techniques through continuing education classes; maintain up-to-date performance evaluations that are well documented by the supervisor with any corrective action.
Failure to monitor and to report	Report any significant changes in a patient's condition (e.g., patient continues to bleed from puncture site after blood collection).
Equipment use	Learn how to use blood collection equipment as designed. Use biohazardous waste containers as indicated in procedures. If involved in offsite blood collections, carry biohazardous waste containers and hand cleanser as well as extra blood collection supplies and equipment. If involved in offsite collections, have the correct types and amounts of insurance coverage to address liability exposures with respect to transporting biohazardous specimens.
Patients with HIV	Be conscious of actions that could result in a lawsuit: Discrimination in treatment; Nosocomial transmission of infections; Breach of confidentiality. Follow health care facility's procedures for blood collection and disposal of biohazardous waste.

the employer, if sued, may also seek indemnification from the employee. *Indemnification* is compensation for the financial loss suffered from the employee's act.

Legal Cases Related to Clinical Laboratory Activities

Most phlebotomy cases are settled after a lawsuit is filed but before the court renders a judgment. It is important to remember that many cases are not cited in the literature because often health care institutions or health care workers negotiate, arbitrate, and settle out of court. The following sections discuss cases that are of interest to health care workers involved in blood collection.

CASES RESULTING FROM IMPROPER TECHNIQUE AND NEGLIGENCE

Health care workers who collect blood by venipuncture must be thoroughly trained and skilled in proper technique, safety, and the use of collection equipment. Problems that can arise and have led to phlebotomy lawsuits are listed here:

1. Patient falling
2. Hematoma/Hemorrhage from inadequate pressure to the vein
3. Abscess or other infections at the venipuncture site
4. Injuries from fainting before, during, or after blood collection
5. Nerve damage due to poor venipuncture technique
6. Complications from collecting blood from the same side as a mastectomy (removal of breast)
7. Wristband or identification error leading to wrong diagnosis and treatment and death in some cases
8. Three attempts to take blood from the same venipuncture site with three failures in blood collection, leading to a hematoma and nerve damage in the patient's arm.
9. Forgetting about a tourniquet on the patient's arm, leading to loss of blood circulation and nerve damage in the patient's arm.
10. Attempted blood collection in the lower radial area (i.e., wrist) of the arm, leading to radial nerve damage in the patient's arm and hand.

For help with avoiding the first six problems, review Chapter 9. For the remaining problems, review Chapter 10. For detailed information about identification processes, refer to Chapters 2 and 10.

EXAMPLES OF PAST PHLEBOTOMY LAWSUITS

In one case settled out of court, a health care worker had not received proper blood collection training. She performed a venipuncture by inserting the needle approximately two inches above the antecubital fold. The needle went through the vein, through muscle, and into the nerve, severely injuring the patient's arm, which remained permanently damaged even after three surgeries to repair the damage resulting from the hematoma and nerve injury.

Another case involved a medical technologist under pressure to collect specimens from ambulatory patients as quickly as possible. One of the patients stated prior to blood collection that she had fainted during blood collection at a previous time. The health care worker, however, took no precautions to avoid the possibility of the patient's syncope (fainting), collected the patient's blood, and allowed the patient to leave immediately. The patient fainted at the elevator and suffered permanent loss of smell and a permanent "ringing sound" in her ears.

In another case, a health care worker collecting bedside glucose results misread the glucometer and caused the deaths of three patients with diabetes. The errors might have been avoided with better training, supervision, and quality monitoring.

In yet another case, a phlebotomist collected blood at an excessive angle of needle insertion from the patient's basilic vein when the median cubital vein was clearly an option for collection. The blood collection resulted in injury to the patient's median nerve and a malpractice lawsuit. In addition, documentation errors were evident for the collection. In all, the patient was awarded thousands of dollars for the health care worker's violations regarding proper standard of care.[10]

Another case involved a phlebotomist who had often collected blood from an elderly patient who had monthly blood coagulation testing to monitor her Coumadin (anticoagulant medication) levels. The phlebotomist had used butterfly needles (e.g., small needles) in the past blood collections since the elderly patient had fragile, small veins. However, this time the phlebotomist collected the blood with a large needle, even after the patient requested that the phlebotomist use a small needle since the patient knew how fragile her veins were with so many venipunctures. This venipuncture led to the patient having a hematoma (area around the puncture swells, usually due to blood leakage into the tissues). The hematoma covered the entire arm of the patient within a few minutes after the blood collection. However, the phlebotomist ignored it and sent the patient home. The hematoma led to nerve damage in the patient's arm and hand and the patient was awarded compensation in a case settled out of court for the resultant surgeries and suffering incurred through this poorly performed venipuncture.

HIV-Related Issues

If a health care worker becomes infected with HIV during employment at a health care facility, worker's compensation benefits are usually available. The health care worker must, however, demonstrate a causal connection between his or her HIV infection and his or her employment. This causal connection includes having a documented incident report at the health care facility involving a needlestick injury, a puncture wound, or other exposure to HIV-contaminated blood or body fluids. In addition, the worker's lifestyle will be investigated to determine whether the exposure occurred elsewhere. Preemployment health evaluations may prove useful later should the health care worker allege contraction of infection during the time of employment. Employers are legally responsible for monitoring postexposure follow-up.

If a health care worker resigns because of contracting AIDS, unemployment benefits may be available if the worker can show that he or she believed in good faith that continued employment would jeopardize his or her health.

Professional Liability Insurance

Because hospitals are places where seriously ill patients are admitted and treated with highly sophisticated medical technology, the likelihood for problems is greater in them than in other health care settings. Often, the health care staff in the hospital or clinical laboratory is on a blanket professional liability insurance policy. If, however, the health care worker is employed by a pathologist who has a contract with an institution or owns a clinic, he or she may be protected by the pathologist's professional liability insurance policy.

The health care worker, with less money than a hospital or no malpractice insurance, has not been a target for lawsuits in the past. The advances in technology and increased complexity of health care, however, have increased legal exposure for allied health and nursing professionals. The health care worker who routinely deals with the public in patient–health care worker relationships is indeed liable. Therefore, each individual should examine the possibility of malpractice suits and the need for professional liability insurance from a personal standpoint.[11] (**BOX 3–3**.)

BOX 3–3

Purchasing Professional Liability Insurance

If the health care worker decides to purchase professional liability insurance, the following factors should be carefully considered:[12]

1. Does the employer carry liability insurance?
2. Is adequate dollar value coverage provided? In recent lawsuits, total damages of $1 million or more have been awarded against physicians.
3. What are the coverage limitations? How much does one have to lose if sued?
4. What are the procedures that must be followed for the policy to provide coverage? Some policies state that divulging the amount of coverage or the fact of coverage voids the policy.
5. The health care worker should not assume that the lawyers representing the hospital, laboratory, or clinic will have his or her best interests at heart. The attorney's first obligation is to serve those who have hired him or her. There have been cases in which the hospital was cleared of all charges, but the health care professional was held liable for damages.
6. Is a job change expected soon?
7. Are specimen collecting services provided offsite or in patients' homes?

With the purchase of professional liability insurance, the attorney's fee and court costs are usually covered. Some professional organizations offer professional liability insurance at a reasonable or reduced rate. A genuine concern for others and careful attention to technique are good investments of the health care worker's time. A record of continuing education courses, seminars, workshops, performance evaluations, and academic credits should be a part of each health care worker's personal file.

Clinical Laboratory Regulations

The federal government has several agencies that regulate and oversee all clinical laboratories; they include the U.S. **Food and Drug Administration (FDA)**, the **Centers for Medicare & Medicaid Services (CMS)** in the federal Department of Health and Human Services, the Occupational Safety and Health Administration (OSHA), and the Department of Transportation (DOT). Some of these will be discussed more extensively in later chapters. The CMS regulates all clinical laboratories through the **Clinical Laboratory Improvement Amendments of 1988 (CLIA 1988)**, which are periodically revised.[13,14] Regulations apply to *any* site that tests human specimens whether the tests are simple to perform or technologically complex, and they include all testing sites from small **physician's office laboratories (POLs)** to large hospital laboratories. The regulations include establishing qualifications for health care personnel who perform the tests, periodic inspections, proficiency assessments, and the investigation of complaints. (**BOX 3–4** provides more information about CLIA requirements.)

Other regulatory agencies also oversee clinical laboratories, depending on the health care setting, the type and complexity of the testing they do, and employee certification. Among these are the American Association of Blood Banks (AABB), the American Red Cross, the American Society for Clinical Pathology (ASCP), the College of American Pathologists (CAP), and The Joint Commission.

BOX 3–4

CLIA Approval for Laboratories

The Clinical Laboratory Improvement Amendments of 1988 categorizes laboratory tests according to the level of complexity of the testing procedure and the risk involved for the patient if errors are made in performing or interpreting the test. The tests may also be reclassified from one category to another as technology advances. For more detailed information, see http://www.fda.gov/medicaldevices/deviceregulationandguidance/ivdregulatoryassistance/ ucm124208.htm. All laboratories are subject to CLIA 88 regulations and are required to obtain a certificate from the CMS. The certificate is based on the level of complexity of the tests performed. For the moderately complex or highly complex testing, the inspection considers all procedural steps in laboratory testing—preanalytic, analytic, and postanalytic. Thus, the blood collection procedures area is a major part of CLIA inspections.

Waived tests are those tests that are the easiest to perform, the least susceptible to error, and the least risky to patients. Examples include urinalysis, urine pregnancy tests, blood glucose screening tests, rheumatoid factor tests or mononucleosis tests using blood agglutination, occult blood detection from stool samples, spun microhematocrits, and erythrocyte sedimentation rates. These tests are commonly done in ambulatory settings, on hospital units near the bedside, and in other remote locations. The list of approved waived laboratory tests performed frequently by phlebotomists has expanded over the years. These waived tests can be found at http://www .cms.gov/Regulations-and-Guidance/Legislation/CLIA/downloads/cr4136.waivetbl.pdf.

Tests of moderate complexity are those tests that are simple to perform but may involve more risk to the patient if results are inaccurate. Examples include white and red blood cell counts, hemoglobin, hematocrit, blood chemistries, and urine cultures.

Tests of high complexity are those tests that are complex to perform and may allow for reasonable risk of harm to the patient if results are inaccurate. These include tests that require sophisticated instrumentation and oversight by a pathologist or Ph.D.-level scientist. Examples include molecular analyses, bone marrow evaluations, immunoassays, flow cytometry, cytogenetics analysis, and electrophoresis.

Also, some states (including California, New York, and Florida) have licensure regulations and/or testing requirements that vary according to the technical responsibilities for laboratory personnel. Phlebotomists should be knowledgeable about the licensure requirements when applicable because they may be allowed to perform certain procedures in one state, but not in another. For example, many phlebotomists are allowed to perform basic point-of-care tests in most states, but they are not allowed to do so in California.

Study Questions

For the following questions, select the one best answer.

1 The standard of care currently used in malpractice legal cases involving health care providers is based on the conduct of the average health care provider in which area?

a. state
b. city
c. national community
d. local community

2 What are factors or key points that must be considered in *all* alleged negligence cases?

a. duty, damages
b. breach of duty, battery
c. proximate causation, invasion of privacy
d. res ipsa loquitur

3 Which of the following legal branches makes administrative laws?

a. legislative branch
b. judicial branch
c. U.S. Supreme Court
d. executive branch

4 A federal regulatory agency that has oversight of all clinical laboratories is:

a. FDA
b. CMS
c. CLIA
d. ASCP

5 The statute of limitations for professional negligence in most states is:

a. 6 months
b. 1 year
c. 2 years
d. 5 years

6 Which legal concept refers to the voluntary permission by a patient to allow touching, examination, and/or treatment by health care providers?

a. implied consent
b. assault and battery
c. battery
d. res ipsa loquitur

7 When should incident reports involving accidental HIV exposures be reported?

a. at the end of the work shift
b. immediately
c. after 24 hours
d. after seeing the employee health physician

8 Informed consent refers to

a. the patient's right to look at her or his medical records
b. the sign-off by the patient for the health care worker to provide the patient with the results of his or her laboratory results
c. a health care worker's right to perform blood collection on the patient since the patient has signed hospital documents for having medical procedures
d. a physician who informs the patient that he or she removed the patient's appendix even though the patient was not aware before the surgery that this would happen

9 A national organization that develops guidelines and sets national standards for laboratory procedures is the

a. Joint Commission
b. American Physical Therapy Association
c. American Diabetes Association
d. American Cancer Society

10 Informed consent for research requires a "consent document" that includes which of the following?

a. provides the level of confidentiality of the research data
b. full disclosure of the research
c. describes measures that the researcher will take to ensure confidentiality
d. all of the above

Case Study

A health care worker in the ambulatory outpatient clinic was checking in an elderly outpatient for blood collection who indicated that she has been on Coumadin (a blood thinner) therapy for the past seven months.

Question

What precautions should the health care worker take for this patient when collecting her blood?

Action in Practice

Mr. Johnson, a health care worker who recently completed his training program at San Saba Community College, acquired a position at University Hospital on the early morning shift. He must enroll in the various insurance programs for employees at the University Hospital.

Questions

1 What is the first question that Mr. Johnson should ask about professional liability insurance at University Hospital?

2 Provide three other questions that he should ask about the enrollment.

COMPETENCY ASSESSMENT

Check Yourself

1 What are the steps that are followed at the beginning of a malpractice lawsuit?

2 What is the difference between *implied consent* and *informed consent*?

Competency Checklist: Ethical, Legal, and Regulatory Issues

This checklist may be completed as a group or individually.

(1) Completed (2) Needs to improve

_____ 1. Describe four methods for protecting health information.

_____ 2. List six lawsuit prevention tips for minimizing risks.

REFERENCES

1. Lewis, M. A., & Tamparo, C. D. (1998). *Medical law, ethics, and bioethics for ambulatory care,* 4th ed. Philadelphia: F. A. Davis.

2. American Hospital Association. www.aha.org/aha/issues/Communicating-with-Patients/pt-care-partnership.html, accessed June 1, 2013.

3. The Joint Commission. www.jointcommission.org/PatientSafety/hlc/, accessed June 1, 2013.

4. Rakich, J. S., Longest, B. B., & Darr, K. (1992). *Managing health services organizations.* Baltimore: Health Professions Press.

5. *Parker v. Port Huron Hospital,* 105, N.W. 2d 854 (1981).

6. Health Insurance Portability and Accountability Act of 1996, 18 USC S264.

7. Travis, J. (2003, February 10). Complying with HIPAA: Are you ready? *ADVANCE for Med Lab Prof, 15*(4): 16–18, 25.

8. Understanding HIPAA Privacy—U.S. Department of Health and Human Services. www.hhs.gov/ocr/privacy/hipaa/understanding/coveredentities/index.html, accessed May 22, 2013.

9. Brent, N. J. (1990). Confidentiality and HIV status: The nurse's right to know. *Home Healthcare Nurse, 8*(3): 6–8.

10. Ernst, D. (1999, April). Phlebotomy on trial. *Med Lab Obser,* 46–50.

11. Pozgar, G. D. (2002). *Legal aspects of health care administration.* Gaithersburg, MD: Aspen.

12. Guido, G. W. (2006). *Legal & ethical issues in nursing,* 4th ed. Upper Saddle River, NJ: Pearson Prentice Hall.

13. Department of Health and Human Services (DHHS), Health Care Financing Administration (HCFA), Public Health Service: 42 CFR 405 et seq, 57 FR 7002–7186, February 28, 1992.

14. Centers for Disease Control and Prevention: Current CLIA Regulations. www.phppo.cdc.gov/clia/regs/toc.aspx.

RESOURCES

Howanitz, P. (2005). Errors in laboratory medicine. *Arch Pathol Lab Med, 129,* 1259–1264.

Loewy, E. H. & Loewy, R. S. (2004). *Textbook of healthcare ethics.* Boston: Kluwer Academic Publishers.

Thompson, J. B., & Thompson, H. O. (1985). *Biomedical decision-making for nurses.* Norwalk, CT: Appleton-Century-Croft.

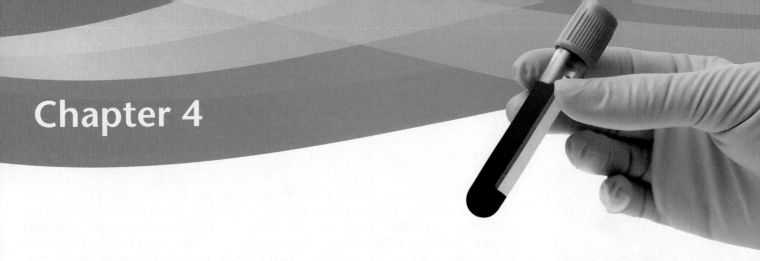

Chapter 4

Infection Control

Chapter Objectives

Upon completion of Chapter 4, the learner is responsible
for doing the following:

1. Explain the infection control policies and procedures that must be followed in specimen collection and transportation.

2. Define the terms *health care–associated, health care–acquired,* and *nosocomial infections.*

3. Identify the basic programs for infection control and isolation procedures.

4. Explain the proper techniques for handwashing, gowning, gloving, masking, double bagging, and entering and exiting the various isolation areas.

5. Identify steps to avoid transmission of blood-borne pathogens.

6. Identify ways to reduce risks for infections and accidental needlesticks.

7. Describe measures that can break each link in the chain of infection.

8. Identify the steps to take in the case of blood-borne pathogen exposure.

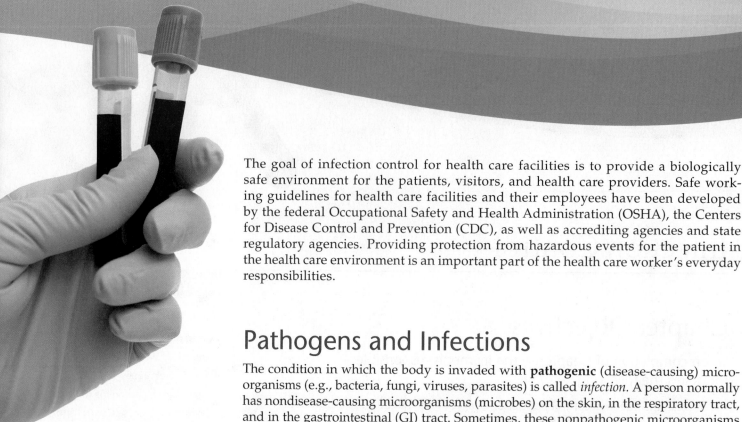

The goal of infection control for health care facilities is to provide a biologically safe environment for the patients, visitors, and health care providers. Safe working guidelines for health care facilities and their employees have been developed by the federal Occupational Safety and Health Administration (OSHA), the Centers for Disease Control and Prevention (CDC), as well as accrediting agencies and state regulatory agencies. Providing protection from hazardous events for the patient in the health care environment is an important part of the health care worker's everyday responsibilities.

Pathogens and Infections

The condition in which the body is invaded with **pathogenic** (disease-causing) microorganisms (e.g., bacteria, fungi, viruses, parasites) is called *infection.* A person normally has nondisease-causing microorganisms (microbes) on the skin, in the respiratory tract, and in the gastrointestinal (GI) tract. Sometimes, these nonpathogenic microorganisms enter parts of the body where they normally do not belong and cause disease. For example, *Escherichia coli (E. coli),* normally found in the GI tract, can cause a bladder infection from poor hygiene. If the infectious microorganism can be transmitted to an individual by direct or indirect contact or as an airborne infection, the result is a **communicable disease**.

In health care institutions, the patients are usually ill because of infection or injury. Health care settings continuously have pathogenic and nonpathogenic microorganisms carried by patients, visitors, and health care providers. The term **blood-borne pathogens (BBPs)** describes any infectious microorganism present in blood and other body fluids and tissues that can cause infectious diseases, including:

- Hepatitis A, B, C, D, and E
- HIV (AIDS)
- Syphilis
- Malaria
- Human T-cell lymphotrophic virus (HTLV) types I and II

HEALTH CARE–ASSOCIATED (NOSOCOMIAL) INFECTIONS

Health care-associated (nosocomial) infections (HAIs) are those that are acquired by a patient after admission to a health care facility, such as a hospital, clinic, nursing home, or psychiatric institution. Of the 35 million patients admitted to hospitals annually in the United States, about 1.7 to 3 million acquire a nosocomial infection. In the United States, the Centers for Disease Control and Prevention reports that health care–associated infections have caused approximately 99,000 deaths per year. Approximately 1 out of every 20 hospitalized patients will contract an HAI.[1] The CDC provides research on the types of HAIs in the nationwide health care facilities to determine methods to decrease and hopefully avoid these infections. (**BOX 4–1** provides a list of infectious diseases identified by the CDC that may lead to HAIs.)

BOX 4–1

Diseases and Organisms in Health Care Settings Leading to Health Care-Associated Infections

- *Acinetobacter*
- *Burkholderia cepacia*
- Blood-borne pathogens
- *Clostridium difficile*
- *Clostridium sordellii*
- Enterobacteriaceae (carbapenem-resistance)
- Hepatitis
- Human Immunodeficiency Virus (HIV)
- Influenza
- *Klebsiella*
- Methicillin-resistant *Staphylococcus aureus*
- Mycobacterium abscessus
- Norovirus
- *Staphylococcus aureus*
- Tuberculosis (TB)
- Vancomycin-intermediate *Staphylococcus aureus* and Vancomycin-resistant *Staphylococcus aureus*
- Vancomycin-resistant Enterococci (VRE)*

*Reprinted from U.S. Department of Health and Human Services, Centers for Disease Control and Prevention. Obtained from CDC's HAIs Diseases and Organisms in Health-Care Settings. www.cdc.gov/HAI/organisms/organisms.html#b, accessed February 18, 2013.

In an attempt to control them, **infection control programs** have been developed, using guidelines established by the CDC, The Joint Commission, and state regulatory agencies. Managers of each health care institution are responsible for developing and implementing an infection control program. These programs address the issues of proper **asepsis, isolation procedures,** education, and management of community-acquired infections, as well as health care–associated infections. An infection control preventionist or nurse usually works closely with or in the clinical microbiology laboratory and communicates with personnel in the health care facility and with home health care providers to make the necessary assessments.

The **Centers for Disease Control and Prevention (CDC),** as part of the U.S. Public Health Service, oversees the investigation and control of various diseases, especially those that are communicable and threaten the U.S. population. The CDC provides infection control and safety guidelines to protect health care workers and patients from infection. The cornerstones for infection protection of patients and health care

TABLE 4–1

Microorganisms Causing Health Care–Associated (Nosocomial) Infections in Hospital Areas

Hospital Areas	Commonly Identified Pathogenic Agents
Burn unit	All gram-negative bacilli (especially *E. coli*) Gram-positive rods *Staphylococcus aureus* (MRSA*) predominant *Pseudomonas aeruginosa* predominant Fungi
Dialysis unit	Hepatitis and other viruses Bacteria; especially microbes resistant to drugs (i.e., MRSA) Fungi
Intensive care or postoperative care unit	Any microorganisms
Nursery unit	*S. aureus* (This pathogen is of increasing concern in the Nursery due to it being instant *Staphylococcus aureus* [MRSA].) Group B *Streptococcus* *E. coli* *S. pneumoniae* Other Gram-negative bacilli Viruses (i.e., Rotavirus)

*MRSA is an abbreviation for methicillin-resistant *Staphylococcus aureus*.

workers, particularly when collecting blood, are **aseptic techniques,** which include the following:

- Frequent hand hygiene (handwashing or alcohol-based hand rubs)
- Use of barrier garments and personal protective equipment
- Waste management of contaminated materials
- Use of proper cleaning solutions
- Use of standard precautions
- Use of sterile procedures when necessary

These protective measures must become part of a health care worker's routine procedures and standards for practice. Because each health care facility has its own infection control program and policy manual, the health care worker should read and be familiar with both.

If the health care worker works for a home health care agency, it is imperative that he or she has knowledge of infection control protocols for home health care, because the home is an uncontrolled, unpredictable setting in which to provide care. Infections can be transmitted in a variety of ways, and each health care worker should realize that she or he can be infected and can transmit infectious agents. TABLES 4–1 and 4–2 list causative agents for nosocomial infections.

ALERT

Clinical Alert!

Antibiotic-Resistant Pathogens: MRSA and VRE

The abbreviation MRSA represents methicillin-resistant *Staphylococcus aureus;* VRE is an abbreviation for vancomycin-resistant enterococci. Both of these pathogens are antibiotic resistant and create serious medical problems in the United States and worldwide since these bacteria are highly infectious and are virtually impossible to treat due to their drug resistance.

TABLE 4–2

Microorganisms Causing Health Care-Associated (Nosocomial) Infections in Patients

Body Areas	Commonly Identified Pathogenic Agents
Blood and cerebrospinal fluid	Any microorganisms
Ear	*Pseudomonas aeruginosa*
	Streptococcus pneumoniae
	Gram-negative bacilli
Eye	*Staphylococcus aureus*
	Neisseria gonorrhoeae
	Gram-negative bacilli
	Moraxella lacunata
	Haemophilus influenzae
	S. pneumoniae
	P. aeruginosa
Gastrointestinal tract	*Shigella*
	Clostridium difficile
	Enteropathogenic *Escherichia coli*
	Vibrio cholerae
	Campylobacter
	Helicobacter pylori
	Salmonella
	Parasitic protozoans
	Candida albicans
	Some viruses (i.e., Noravirus, Rotavirus)
	N. gonorrhoeae
Genital tract	*Haemophilus vaginalis*
	C. albicans (yeast)
	Streptococcus pyogenes
Respiratory tract	*Corynebacterium diphtheriae*
	Bordatella pertussis
	Staphylococcus epidermidis
	Campylobacter
	S. aureus
	S. pneumoniae
	H. influenzae
	Any Gram-negative bacilli
	Fungi
	Certain viruses (i.e., Influenza A2 and B, Parainfluenza, Rhinovirus)
	S. aureus
	S. pyogenes
Skin	*C. albicans*
	Smallpox
	Herpes virus
	Enterovirus
	Measles
Urinary tract	Any microorganism in sufficient numbers
Wounds and abscesses	Any microorganisms

Personal Safety from Infection During Specimen Handling

All patients' specimens should be handled with caution to prevent the possibility of acquiring blood-borne pathogen infections from infectious organisms found in blood and other body fluids (i.e., Hepatitis A, B, C, D, and E viruses; human immunodeficiency virus [HIV]; syphilis; malaria); (**BOX 4–2**).

This preventive approach, called **universal precautions,** was established through the **Occupational Safety and Health Administration (OSHA),** an agency of the U.S. Department of Labor. The precautions established by OSHA require employers to provide measures that will protect workers exposed to biological hazards, including training to avoid exposure to blood-borne pathogens. Health care workers who are routinely exposed to blood (i.e., possible needlestick injuries) and body fluids must take the precautions of wearing gloves to protect themselves from infection as well. These requirements have occurred as a result of the 1991 OSHA standards for occupational exposure to blood-borne pathogens (29 CFR 1930.1030) and the Needlestick Safety and Prevention Act that took effect April 18, 2001, which updated the 1991 OSHA standards.[2,3] These federal regulations include several requirements for prevention, such as needlestick protection

BOX 4–2

Blood-Borne Pathogens

Examples of body fluids that can potentially carry the HIV and Hepatitis B virus as well as other blood-borne pathogens include the following:

- Blood
- Saliva involved in dental procedures
- Cerebrospinal fluid
- Cell cultures
- Human tissue
- Semen and vaginal secretions
- All body fluids containing blood

Transmission Routes

- Exposure to broken skin
- Increased risk if contact involves a large area of skin or BBP contact is prolonged
- Increased risk with increased BBP levels
- Misuse of sharps (e.g., eyes, nose, and/or mouth splashed by infected body fluid)

Engineering Controls

- Leak-proof containers
- Sharps containers
- Needleless devices (e.g., retractable syringes, self-sheathing needles)

Personal Protective Equipment

- Gloves
- Lab coats, scrub suits, gowns
- Goggles, safety glasses

devices (see Chapter 8) and the placing of warning labels on containers (refrigerators, freezers, infectious waste, etc.) that contain blood or other potentially infectious materials. The labels required are fluorescent orange or orange-red and feature the biohazard alerts shown in **FIGURES 4–1** and **4–2**.

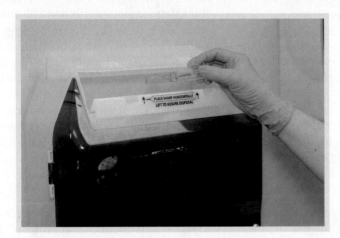

FIGURE 4–1
Health Care Worker Discarding Needle Apparatus into Biohazard
Waste Container

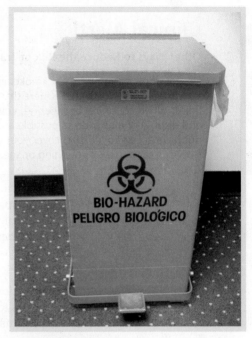

FIGURE 4–2
Biohazard Label in English and Spanish
Courtesy of Centers for Disease Control and Prevention (CDC)

SHARPS/NEEDLESTICK INJURY PREVENTION

Accidental needlesticks are another risk for health care workers because of their potential to transmit infections. Sharps injuries can be caused by

- Failure to activate the safety device after using a needle
- Attempting to recap a needle
- Transferring blood specimens from a syringe into collection tubes
- Use of needles without safety devices
- Overfilling the biohazard sharps container
- Use of nonretractable puncture devices for fingersticks

It is obvious that these causes are preventable by the use of sound practices (according to procedures), the correct use of safety devices, and adequate training. This will be discussed in greater detail as phlebotomy procedures are presented.

EXPOSURE CONTROL

Any incident of exposure to potentially harmful blood-borne pathogens or other infectious body fluids should be reported

ALERT

Clinical Alert! The Occupational Safety and Health Administration requires managers at health care facilities to provide—at no cost to the worker—confidential medical evaluation, treatment, and follow-up for any employee who has had a blood-borne exposure incident (e.g., needlestick). Immediately after an exposure incident, the employee must:

- Decontaminate the needlestick site or other sharps injury (i.e., shards of glass) with soap and water or an appropriate antiseptic (e.g., iodine) for 30 seconds.
- Flush the exposed mucous membrane site (e.g., eyes, nose, or mouth) with water or sterile saline for 10 to 15 minutes. Use an eyewash station if available to flush the site. Contact lenses must be removed immediately and disinfected before reuse or discarded.
- Report the incident to the supervisor, who will direct the employee to the appropriate clinic for medical evaluation, treatment, and counseling.

The medical evaluation involves the following steps:

1. The exposed health care worker (HCW) is identified in a confidential manner and tested for HIV, Hepatitis B virus (HBV), and Hepatitis C virus (HCV) with permission from the health care worker. Hopefully, the HCW has previously received the Hepatitis B virus vaccine, as required for working in a health care environment.
2. The exposed health care worker should receive counseling, medical evaluation, possible antiviral treatment and postexposure testing at 4 weeks, 12 weeks, and 4 months later.
3. The exposed health care worker is counseled to be alert for acute viral symptoms within 12 weeks of exposure. This entire medical evaluation must be completely confidential.

Clinical Alert!

Other Ways to Reduce the Risk of Transmitting Infections

Do not drink, eat, chew gum, smoke, apply cosmetics, or handle contact lenses in work areas where there is exposure to blood or body fluids. When coughing or sneezing, cover your mouth with a tissue and dispose of it as soon as possible and wash your hands. If you do not have access to a tissue, cover your cough with your upper arm or sleeve. Wear a mask if coughing or sneezing is frequent.

immediately to the supervisor and the employer's personnel health department. Each health care worker should know who to contact, where to go, and what to do if possibly exposed to harmful pathogens.[4,5] The report must include the safety-engineered blood collection device that did not work effectively to protect the health care worker during blood collection as well as details of the exposure (i.e., date, time, location, volume of blood or other body substance exposed to, duration of contact). If exposures are not reported, it is difficult to prove retrospectively that an exposure to an infectious agent was work related. These exposure-control written incidents must also be maintained for legal documentation if lawsuits arise because of an ineffective safety-engineered blood collection device.

EMPLOYEE HEALTH

Infection control programs also monitor employee health programs. The primary objective is to minimize the risk of infection and hazardous circumstances for employees and patients. Most employees are screened for the following diseases prior to employment:

- Measles
- Mumps
- Tuberculosis
- Hepatitis
- Diarrheal disease
- Syphilis
- Skin diseases

Immunization for a variety of diseases is often made available initially and throughout employment, free of charge, such as those listed in **BOX 4–3**. The information in the box updates the previously published summary of recommendations for vaccinating health care personnel in the U.S. Centers for Disease Control and Prevention.

BOX 4–3

Summary of Main Changes* from 1997 Advisory Committee on Immunization Practices/Hospital (now Health Care) Infection Control Practices Advisory Committee Recommendations for Immunization of Health Care Personnel (HCP)

Hepatitis B

- HCP and trainees in certain populations at high risk for chronic hepatitis B (e.g., those born in countries with high and intermediate endemicity) should be tested for HBsAg and anti-HBc/anti-HBs to determine infection status.

BOX 4–3 (continued)

Influenza

- Emphasis that all HCP, not just those with direct patient care duties, should receive an annual influenza vaccination.

- Comprehensive programs to increase vaccine coverage among HCP are needed; influenza vaccination rates among HCP within facilities should be measured and reported regularly.

Measles, Mumps, and Rubella (MMR)

- History of disease is no longer considered adequate presumptive evidence of measles or mumps immunity for HCP; laboratory confirmation of disease was added as acceptable presumptive evidence of immunity. History of disease has never been considered adequate evidence of immunity for rubella.

- The footnotes have been changed regarding the recommendations for personnel born before 1957 in routine and outbreak contexts. Specifically, guidance is provided for 2 doses of MMR for measles and mumps protection and 1 dose of MMR for rubella protection.

Pertussis

- HCP, regardless of age, should receive a single dose of Tdap as soon as feasible if they have not previously received Tdap.

- The minimal interval was removed, and Tdap can now be administered regardless of interval since the last tetanus or diphtheria-containing vaccine.

- Hospitals and ambulatory-care facilities should provide Tdap for HCP and use approaches that maximize vaccination rates.

Varicella

- Criteria for evidence of immunity to varicella were established. For HCP they include

  1. Written documentation with 2 doses of vaccine,
  2. Laboratory evidence of immunity or laboratory confirmation of disease,
  3. Diagnosis of history of varicella disease by health-care provider, or diagnosis of history of herpes zoster by health-care provider.

Meningococcal

- HCP with anatomic or functional asplenia or persistent complement component deficiencies should now receive a 2-dose series of meningococcal conjugate vaccine. HCP with HIV infection who are vaccinated should also receive a 2 dose series.

- Those HCP who remain in groups at high risk are recommended to be revaccinated every 5 years.

---

* Updated recommendations made since publication of the 1997 summary of recommendations (CDC Immunization of Health-Care Workers: Recommendations of the Advisory Committee on Immunization Practices [ACIP] and the Hospital Infection Control Practices Advisory Committee [HICPAC]. *MMWR, 46,* 1997, No. RR-18).

Abbreviations: HBsAg = hepatitis B surface antigen; anti-HBc = hepatitis B core antibody; anti-HBs = hepatitis B surface antibody; Tdap = tetanus toxoid, reduced diptheria toxoid and acellular pertussis vaccine; HIV = human immunodeficiency virus.

Source: From: CDC Immunization of Health-Care Personnel Recommendations of the Advisory Committee on Immunization Practices (ACIP). *MMWR* / November 25, 2011 / Vol. 60 / No. 71.

Chain of Infection

Nosocomial (health care–associated) infections result when the **chain of infection** is complete (**BOX 4–4**). The components that make up the chain are the (1) pathogen (e.g., *Streptococci*); (2) reservoir (e.g., infected patient); (3) portal of exit (e.g., respiratory droplets); (4) mode of transmission (e.g., health care worker clothing); (5) portal of entry (e.g., nasal cavity); and (6) susceptible host (e.g., another health care worker or a hospital patient).

PATHOGEN

The microorganisms that cause infectious disease include bacteria, fungi, viruses, prions, protozoa, and worms. Some of these were listed earlier in the chapter.

RESERVOIR

In a normal environment, relatively few things are sterile; therefore, potential reservoirs of infection cover a wide range. Inanimate objects, as well as people, have various microorganisms, many of which help carry out normal body functions. Some of these microorganisms, however, are more pathogenic than others. Pathogenic infections are numerous in the health care environment. For instance, human hands provide a warm, moist environment for microorganisms. Therefore, a physician, phlebotomist, nurse, other health care providers, and hospital visitors can transmit organisms from themselves or an infected patient to another potential host. Laboratory coats, scrub suits, and other clothing that comes in contact with infectious agents and is then worn around other patients is another potential source of infection. Since tourniquets come in contact with intact skin, a tourniquet should be used on only one patient and discarded (single-use).

BOX 4–4

Chain of Infection

- A *pathogen* must be present.
- A *reservoir* is frequently the patient who has or is carrying the pathogen (e.g., *Streptococcus*, which causes strep throat).
- *Portal of exit* describes how the pathogen is released from the reservoir (e.g., the patient's respiratory droplets are expelled on the health care worker's coat when the patient sneezes).
- **Mode of transmission** is the trail the pathogen takes to pass directly from the **source** to the new host (e.g., touching infected individuals, individuals spreading infection through coughing or sneezing, inadequate ventilation, invasive medical instruments, etc.).
- *Portal of entry* is the means by which a pathogen enters the new host (e.g., nasal cavity, wounds, etc.).
- A **susceptible host** (e.g., hospital patient) who cannot fight off the pathogen (e.g., elderly patient, cancer patient)

PORTAL OF EXIT

The pathogen can exit from an infected person (the reservoir) by body fluids (e.g., blood, debris of an infected wound, urine, etc.) that are excreted; or by respiratory droplets that are released into the air by sneezing and coughing.

MODE OF TRANSMISSION

The fourth link in the chain of infection involves transmission from the reservoir to the next host. Pathogenic agents may be transmitted by five modes:

1. Direct contact
2. Air
3. Medical instruments
4. Other objects
5. Other vectors

Direct contact involves close or intimate contact with an infected person. For example, some patients acquire staphylococcal infections, chicken pox, hepatitis, or diarrhea after touching other infected individuals. During contact, the infective microorganism rubs off one person onto another. Handwashing is the best means of preventing infections transmitted by this route.

Microscopic airborne droplets may carry infectious agents, such as the causative agent of tuberculosis and Legionnaire's disease. Droplets may become airborne when an individual coughs or sneezes, when linens are shaken, when dust is stirred by sweeping, or when ventilation is inadequate. Preventive measures include covering the mouth when coughing or sneezing, wearing a mask, isolating specific patients, and ensuring good ventilation.

As mentioned previously, invasive medical instruments may expose a susceptible patient to pathogenic agents. To prevent instrument-induced infections, health care personnel should discard instruments, such as tourniquets and catheters, after each use. Safety needles and holders should be used only once, and then disposed of in appropriate containers. Other inanimate objects, such as toys in the pediatric areas, common toilets and sinks, linens, and water fountains are all potential modes of transmission. Some microbes can survive on surfaces for days. Objects that can harbor infectious agents and transmit infection are called **fomites**. **BOX 4–5** lists fomites found in health care settings.

BOX 4–5

Where Fomites Are Found in Health Care Facilities

- Computer keyboards
- Doorknobs
- Telephones
- Countertops
- Scrub suits
- Phlebotomy trays
- Eyeglasses

- Pens and pencils
- Water-faucet handles
- Laboratory coats
- Manuals and books
- Phlebotomy supplies and equipment
- IV equipment

Preventing transmission by fomites can be accomplished by

- Following isolation techniques
- Using sterile technique for injections or venipuncture
- Wearing gloves during equipment handling
- Restricting the use of common toys or facilities

Many insects (mosquitoes, ticks, fleas, mites, etc.) and rodents act as vectors or vehicles in transmitting infectious diseases, such as plague, rabies, and malaria. Patients may be exposed to these vectors in unsanitary conditions in a home setting or in areas where the diseases are prevalent. As examples, vectors can transmit infectious microbes through animal or insect bites via saliva into the susceptible host.

PORTAL OF ENTRY

The pathogen must have an entrance pathway into the "susceptible host." An example is the bacteria *Staphylococcus aureus* that enters through the mouth or nasal passage of the susceptible host.

SUSCEPTIBLE HOST

The sixth and final link in the chain of infection is the susceptible host. Factors that affect a host's susceptibility are age (e.g., very young and very old), drug use, the degree and nature of the illness, and the status of the immune system. The patient's progress in the hospital significantly affects his or her chances of acquiring an infection. Underlying diseases, such as diabetes, HIV, acquired immune deficiency syndrome (AIDS), and cancer, as well as therapeutic measures (chemotherapy, radiation therapy, antibiotics), all change the status of the body and make it a potential host for infection.

BREAKING THE CHAIN

Infection control programs aim at breaking the infection chain (**FIGURE 4–3**) at one or more links. Handwashing procedures for sterile technique, proper waste disposal, appropriate laundry services, and housekeeping are ways of controlling the sources. Isolation techniques, control of insects and rodents, and use of disposable protective equipment and supplies help interrupt the modes of transmission. Host susceptibility is controlled by speeding the patient's recovery. Immunizations, transfusions, proper nutrition, medication, and adequate exercise all help the patient regain health.

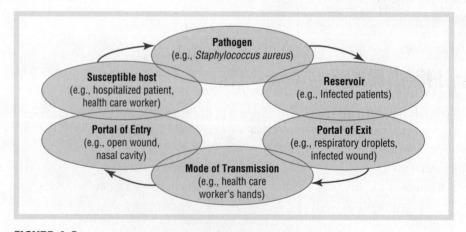

FIGURE 4–3

The Chain of Infection

Health care-associated infection can be interrupted by infection control procedures.

Standard Precautions

Isolation procedures, methods of removing individuals with contagious diseases from society, date to antiquity. Although the supplies for and methods of isolation have been updated, the fear of being contaminated and the stigma associated with a patient in isolation are still present. The psychological effects of being a patient in isolation are profound. Therefore, the health care provider should make an effort to reduce the patient's anxiety by communicating in a calm, professional, and reassuring manner.

Standard precautions (**FIGURE 4–4**) have been designed through the CDC to decrease the risk of transmission of microorganisms from both recognized and unrecognized sources of infection in hospitals. Standard precautions include *universal precautions* that are designed to prevent transmission of all infectious agents in the health care setting. They provide protection from contact with blood, all body fluids, mucous membranes, and nonintact skin.

FIGURE 4–4
Infection Control
Courtesy of BREVIS Corp.

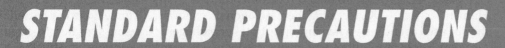

FOR INFECTION CONTROL

Hand Hygiene
Wash after touching **body fluids**, after **removing gloves**, and between **patient contacts**. If hands are not visibly soiled, use an alcohol-based hand rub for routinely decontaminating hands.

Gloves
Wear **Gloves** before touching **body fluids**, **mucous membranes**, and **nonintact skin**.

Mask & Eye Protection or Face Shield
Protect eyes, nose, mouth during procedures that cause **splashes** or **sprays** of **body fluids**.

Gown
Wear **Gown** during procedures that may cause **splashes** or **sprays** of **body fluids**.

Patient-Care Equipment
Handle soiled equipment so as to prevent personal contamination and transfer to other patients.

Environmental Control
Follow hospital procedures for cleaning beds, equipment, and frequently touched surfaces.

Linen
Handle linen soiled with **body fluids** so as to prevent personal contamination and transfer to other patients.

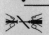
Occupational Health & Bloodborne Pathogens
Prevent injuries from needles, scalpels, and other sharp devices.
Never recap needles using both hands.
Place sharps in puncture-proof sharps containers.
Use **Resuscitation Devices** as an alternative to mouth-to-mouth resuscitation.

Patient Placement
Use a Private Room for a patient who contaminates the environment.

"Body Fluids" include **blood**, **secretions**, and **excretions**.

Form No. **SPR-C**   BREVIS CORP., 225 West 2855 South, SLC, Utah 84115 www.brevis.com   © 2004 Brevis Corp.

Transmission-based precautions are used in addition to standard precautions for patients with known or suspected infections that are spread in one of three ways: (1) airborne transmission, (2) droplet transmission, or (3) contact transmission.[6,7,8]

- **Airborne precautions** reduce the spread of airborne droplet transmission of infectious agents such as rubeola, varicella, and *Mycobacterium tuberculosis*.

- **Droplet precautions** are used to reduce the transmission of diseases such as pertussis, meningitis, pneumonia, and rubella. These diseases can be transmitted through contact of the mucous membranes of the eye, mouth, or nose with large-particle droplets that occur through sneezing, coughing, or talking.

- **Contact precautions** reduce the risk of transmission of serious diseases such as respiratory syncytial virus (RSV), herpes simplex, wound infections, and others through direct or indirect contact.

TABLE 4–3 provides detailed recommendations by the Department of Health and Human Services, CDC, for using these isolation precautions. All three types of precautions may be used at one time when multiple routes of pathogenic transmission are suspected in a patient. These precautions are always used with standard precautions. In **FIGURES 4–5**, **4–6**, and **4–7**, the precautions are provided as signage to health care workers.

TABLE 4–3

HICPAC* Recommendations for Transmission-Based Precautions

	Contact	Droplet	Airborne
Purpose	■ Prevent transmission of known or suspected infected or colonized microorganisms by direct or indirect hand or skin-to-skin contact that occurs when providing direct or indirect patient care. Conditions in which contact precautions are required: diphtheria, herpes simplex, scabies, *Staphylococcus* infection, Hepatitis A, and respiratory syncytial virus wound or skin infection	■ Prevent transmission of large-particle droplets, larger than 5 microns (μm) (e.g., diphtheria, pertussis, streptococcal pharyngitis, pneumonia, scarlet fever, meningitis, rubella)	■ Prevent transmission of small-particle residue of 5 microns (μm) or smaller droplets (e.g., measles, varicella, tuberculosis)
Patient	■ Private room	■ Private room	■ Private room
Placement	■ Can be placed in room of patient with same microorganism	■ Can be placed in room of patient with same diagnosis	■ Can be placed in room of patient with same diagnosis ■ Monitoring of negative air pressure ■ Keep door closed ■ Keep patient in room
Respiratory Protection	■ Mask not necessary (Respiratory hygiene/cough etiquette) Instruct symptomatic persons (e.g., patients, visitors, health care workers) to cover their mouth and nose when sneezing/coughing; use tissues and dispose in no-touch receptable.	■ Use mask when working within 3 feet of patient.	■ Use respiratory protective equipment. ■ Do not enter room of patients with rubeola or varicella if susceptible to these infections. Follow health care institution's policy for possible cases of multidrug-resistant TB, SARS, influenza, and other highly contagious respiratory diseases.
Gloves and Gown	■ Wear gloves when entering room. ■ Change gloves after contact with infective material, such as wound drainage or fecal material. ■ Wash hands immediately after removing gloves. ■ Wear gown when working with patients with diarrhea, ostomies, or wound drainage not contained in dressing. ■ Wear gown if contact with patient or environment will occur.	■ Follow standard precautions.	■ Follow standard precautions.
Patient Transport	■ Transport only if essential. ■ Ensure precautions are maintained to minimize risk of transmission.	■ Transport only if essential. ■ Place mask on patient when outside room.	■ Transport only if essential. ■ Place mask on patient when outside room.
Patient Care Items	■ Patient care items and environmental surfaces are cleaned daily. ■ Dedicate equipment to single patient use (e.g., stethoscope, thermometer).		

*Hospital Infection Control Practices Advisory Committee.

Source: Adapted from Department of Health and Human Services: CDC, *Federal Register* "Guidelines for Isolation Precautions in Hospitals"; and CDC Guideline for Isolation Precautions: Preventing Transmission of Infectious Agents in Healthcare Settings 2007, authored by J. D. Siegel, E. Rhinehart, M. Jackson, L. Chiarello, and the Healthcare Infection Control Practices Advisory Committee. www.cdc.gov/ncidod/dhqp/pdf/isolation2007.pdf

FIGURE 4–5

Airborne Precautions

Courtesy of BREVIS Corp.

AIRBORNE PRECAUTIONS
(in addition to Standard Precautions)

STOP VISITORS: Report to nurse before entering.

Use Airborne Precautions as recommended for patients known or suspected to be infected with infectious agents transmitted person-to-person by the airborne route.

Patient Placement

Place in an **AIIR** (**A**irborne **I**nfection **I**solation **R**oom). **Monitor air pressure** daily with visual indicators.

Keep door closed when not required for entry and exit.

In ambulatory settings instruct patients with a known or suspected airborne infection to wear a surgical mask and observe Respiratory Hygiene/Cough Etiquette. Once in an AIIR, the mask may be removed.

Patient Transport

Limit transport to **medically necessary purposes.**

If transport outside an AIIR is necessary, instruct patients to **wear a surgical mask**, and observe Respiratory Hygiene/Cough Etiquette.

Hand Hygiene

Hand Hygiene according to Standard Precautions.

Personal Protective Equipment (PPE)

Wear a fit-tested, NIOSH-approved **N95** or higher level respirator for respiratory protection when entering the room of a patient when listed diseases are suspected or confirmed.

APR7.LA ©2008 Brevis Corporation www.brevis.com

FIGURE 4–6

Droplet Precautions

Courtesy of BREVIS Corp.

DROPLET PRECAUTIONS
(in addition to Standard Precautions)

STOP VISITORS: Report to nurse before entering.

Use Droplet Precautions for patients known or suspected to be infected with pathogens transmitted by respiratory droplets generated by a patient who is coughing, sneezing or talking.

Personal Protective Equipment (PPE)

Don mask upon entry into the patient room or cubicle.

Hand Hygiene

Hand Hygiene according to Standard Precautions.

Patient Placement

Private room, if possible. Cohort or maintain spatial separation of 3 feet from other patients or visitors if private room is not available.

Patient Transport

Limit transport to **medically necessary purposes.**

If transport or movement in any healthcare setting is necessary, instruct patient to **wear a mask** and follow Respiratory Hygiene/Cough Etiquette.

No mask is required for persons transporting patients on Droplet Precautions.

DPR7.LA ©2008 Brevis Corporation www.brevis.com

FIGURE 4–7
Contact Precautions

Courtesy of BREVIS Corp.

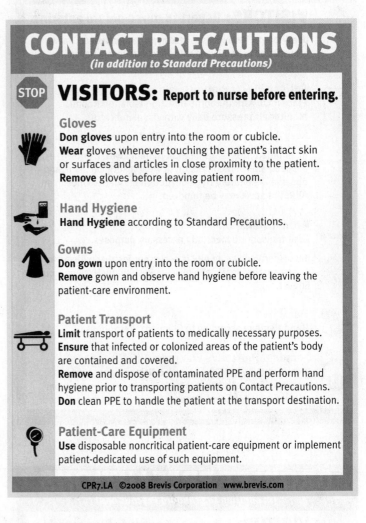

USE OF STANDARD PRECAUTIONS

Health care providers should follow these guidelines when collecting blood from a patient in order to avoid contracting an infectious microorganism:

1. Use **personal protective equipment (PPE)** (i.e., gloves, facial masks, respirators, gowns, shields) to prevent **percutaneous** (through the skin) and **permucosal** (through mucous membranes of the mouth, eye, and nose) exposure when contact with blood or other body fluids of any patient is anticipated. This will prevent transmission by fomites.

   ■ Gloves should be worn for
     ● Handling objects or surfaces soiled with blood or body fluids
     ● Performing venipunctures, skin punctures, and intravenous (IV) line collections

   ■ Gloves should be changed after contact with each patient and hands washed or alcohol hand sanitizers used after glove removal and before donning (putting on) new gloves.

   ■ Masks and protective eyewear or face shields should be worn to prevent exposure of mucous membranes of the mouth, nose, and eyes during procedures that are likely to cause droplets or splashes of blood or other body fluids.

- A personal respirator should be used if the risk of tuberculosis is present.
- Footwear (i.e., covers the entire foot) that protects against broken glass possibly contaminated with blood or other body fluids should be worn (i.e., flip flops, sandals, and clogs are *not* recommended).

2. Hands and other skin surfaces should be washed immediately and thoroughly if contaminated with blood or other body fluids. Hands should be washed immediately after gloves are removed! Proper handwashing technique is shown in **PROCEDURE 4–1**. Although alcohol-based hand antiseptics are not appropriate for use when hands are visibly dirty or contaminated, alcohols are more effective than plain or antimicrobial soap for standard handwashing or hand antisepsis by health care providers.[1] It is handy to keep a plastic bottle of alcohol-based hand antiseptic in the pocket of the laboratory coat just in case the alcohol-based (waterless) antiseptic agent is not available at the patient's bedside (**FIGURE 4–8**). However, keep in mind that OSHA requires that hands be washed with soap and water every third time the hands are cleaned.

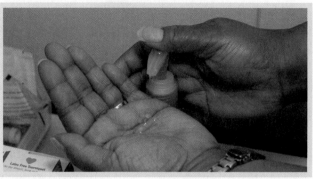

FIGURE 4–8
Alcohol-Based Antiseptic

Alcohol-based hand antiseptic kills 99.9 percent of the most common microorganisms in 15 seconds.

PROCEDURE 4–1

Handwashing Technique

Rationale   To perform proper handwashing technique.

Procedure

1 Remove jewelry (including rings, with the exception of watches, wedding bands, and bracelets) and stand at the sink without allowing clothing to touch the sink. Wet hands with water. Foot pedals are preferable for controlling the flow of water, but they are not available in all health care facilities (**FIGURE 4–9**).

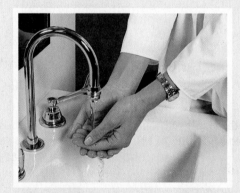

FIGURE 4–9

2 Dispense a small amount of soap to the hands (1 to 2 teaspoonfuls or the amount recommended by the manufacturer) (**FIGURE 4–10**). If using bar soap, keep the bar in your hands and use enough soap to form a lather by moving your hands over each other and between the fingers of each hand.

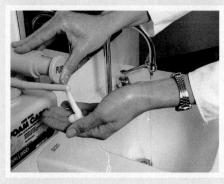

FIGURE 4–10

(continued)

PROCEDURE 4–1

Handwashing Technique (continued)

3 Rub hands together vigorously for at least 15 seconds, covering all surfaces of the hands and fingers (**FIGURE 4–11**).

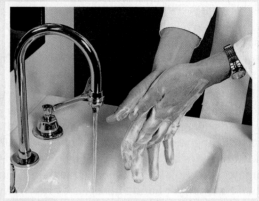

FIGURE 4–11

4 Rinse hands in a downward motion with water (**FIGURE 4–12**) and dry thoroughly with a clean disposable towel. Multiple-use cloth towels of the hanging or roll type are not acceptable for use in health care settings because they can transmit microorganisms.

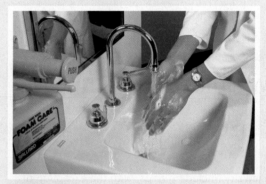

FIGURE 4–12

5 Turn off the faucet with a dry disposable towel if not using a foot pedal (**FIGURE 4–13**).

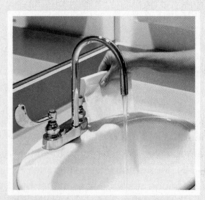

FIGURE 4–13

It is important to wash your hands after any contact with blood, body fluids, or contaminated objects, whether or not gloves are worn. Placing gloves on dirty hands can transfer microorganisms after the gloves are taken off. Proper donning and removing of gloves is shown in **PROCEDURE 4–2**.

PROCEDURE 4–2

Donning and Removing Gloves

Rationale   To place gloves on properly for blood collection and removal after procedure is performed.

Equipment

- Clean gloves (clean, nonsterile gloves are appropriate for most blood collection procedures)
- Trash container

Procedure

1 Complete handwashing prior to donning gloves (**FIGURE 4–14**).

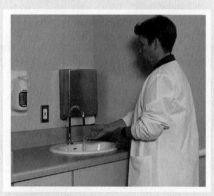

FIGURE 4–14

2 Remove gloves from glove dispenser (**FIGURE 4–15**).

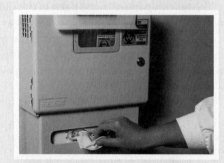

FIGURE 4–15

3 Slip your fingers into the openings of the glove as you hold the glove at the wrist edge with your other hand. Then pull the glove up to your wrist (**FIGURE 4–16**).

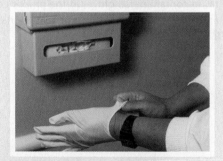

FIGURE 4–16

PROCEDURE 4–2

Donning and Removing Gloves (continued)

4 With your gloved hand, place your fingers under the wrist edge of the second glove and slip your fingers into the openings (**FIGURE 4–17**).

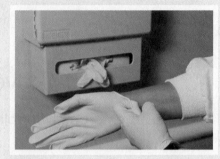

FIGURE 4–17

5 For glove removal, grasp the wrist of one glove at the cuff by the other gloved hand and pull it off of your hand as the glove turns inside out (**FIGURE 4–18**).

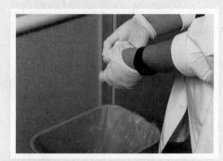

FIGURE 4–18

6 After placing the rolled-up glove in the palm of the gloved hand, remove the second glove by slipping one finger under the glove edge and pulling it inside out as the glove goes down the hand. This glove will roll over the other glove with no exterior glove exposure from either glove (**FIGURE 4–19**).

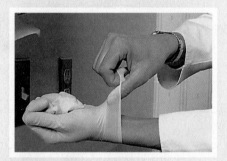

FIGURE 4–19

7 Dispose of these contaminated gloves in the proper container, not at the patient's bedside. Then complete hand hygiene (**FIGURE 4–20**).

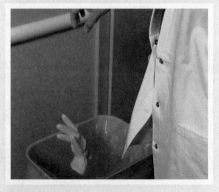

FIGURE 4–20

3. Take precautions to prevent skin injuries caused by needles and other sharp instruments or devices:

   - During blood collection procedures
   - During the disposal of used needles, lancets, etc.
   - When handling any sharp instruments after procedures

4. To prevent infections from blood-borne pathogens as a result of needlestick injuries, health care workers should:

   - Use only safety-engineered needle and sharps devices.
   - *Not* recap needles, purposely bend or break them by hand, remove them from disposable syringes or holders, or handle them for any reason.
   - Immediately dispose of the blood tube holder and safety needle as a single unit after blood collection.
   - Place disposable syringes and needles, lancets, and other sharp items, after they are used, in puncture-resistant containers for transport to the biohazardous waste center.

Clinical Alert!

- Standard precautions have been designed to be used for patients, health care providers, and visitors in health care facilities.
- Standard precautions reduce the risk of infections being transmitted from health care workers to patients, patients to patients, patients to health care workers, and health care workers to other health care workers or visitors.
- These precautions apply in the following situations:
  - Contact with blood
  - Contact with body fluids
  - Contact with mucous membranes and wounds

ISOLATION FOR HOSPITAL OUTBREAKS

Occasionally, outbreaks of particular infections occur in one or more hospital areas. For example, infection control surveillance may reveal that the nursery unit is having an excessive number of cases of staphylococcal infection. To control the outbreak, the infection control staff may dictate the need for special precautions, isolation procedures, or employee screening for staphylococcal carriers. With the increased possibility of respiratory infections (i.e., MRSA, multidrug-resistant tuberculosis, various influenza viruses), the CDC is requesting health care workers to instruct patients and accompanying individuals who have signs and symptoms of respiratory infection to cover their mouths and noses when coughing or sneezing, use and dispose of tissues, and perform hand hygiene after hands have been in contact with respiratory secretions. Any health care worker entering or exiting these areas should be made aware of the special circumstances.

Clinical Alert!

- Do not wear artificial fingernails or extenders when collecting blood from patients in high-risk hospital areas (e.g., intensive care unit, premature nursery). Many health care facilities prohibit the use of artificial nails or extenders due to the spread of pathogenic infections and fungus to immunosuppressed patients.
- Keep natural fingernails less than 1/4-inch long (**FIGURE 4–21**).
- Wear gloves when there is possible contact with blood or other potentially infectious materials.
- Remove gloves after collecting blood from a patient. *Do not* wear the same pair of gloves for the blood collection of more than one patient.
- Since gloves can possibly contain defects (holes), a quick visual inspection of each glove will avoid a potential breakage/leakage.
- Sweaty hands or other chemicals that may be present in a clinical laboratory environment can cause gloves to dissolve and/or become permeable. If working in a laboratory setting, change gloves frequently (about every 30 minutes).

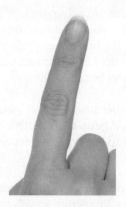

FIGURE 4–21

ALERT

PROTECTIVE, OR REVERSE, ISOLATION (PROTECTIVE ENVIRONMENT)

A few hospitals in the United States have large **protective (reverse) isolation** facilities for patients with combined immunodeficiencies who must live in an environment that is completely sterile. All food and articles are sterilized before they are taken into the patient's room. Some patients must live in these protected environments when they are recovering from cancer treatments (e.g., stem cell transplant).

INFECTION CONTROL IN SPECIAL HOSPITAL UNITS

Other areas where patients are at a high risk of infection are the nursery, the burn unit, the postoperative care unit, the **intensive care unit (ICU),** and the dialysis unit. The clinical laboratory plays an important role in infection control in these hospital units and is also subject to specific infection control procedures.

Infection Control in a Nursery Unit

Newborns are easy targets for infections of all sorts because their immune systems are not fully developed at birth. Neonates may pick up pathogens from their mothers, other babies, or hospital personnel. The best way to minimize infection is to use the special infection control procedures of the nursery and neonatal ICU. Special clothing may be worn by nursery personnel, changed daily, and limited to the unit. Often, a baby is assigned a single nurse to limit the possible sources of infection transmission. Many health care institutions have an anteroom (interior room) where the health care worker can perform the infection control procedures of hand hygiene, gowning, gloving, etc. prior to entering the nursery or neonatal ICU. Babies whose mothers have genital herpes must be isolated from other infants. Mothers with genital herpes must also be isolated. All individuals having contact with either the mothers or the children must be gowned and gloved, and double-bagging (as described later in this chapter) procedures must be used for disposal of contaminated articles in the patient's room.

Infection Control in a Burn Unit

Patients with burns are also highly susceptible to infection. Burn infections are one of the most serious complications that occur in the early period following burn injury. In some institutions, infection rates for burn patients are lower because of the availability of a completely isolated environment for each patient. Each bed is surrounded by a plastic curtain with sleeves. Hospital personnel use these sleeves to have contact with the patient. All supplies and equipment are kept outside the curtain. In hospitals lacking these facilities, burn patients are housed in private rooms. Gowning, gloving, double bagging, and strict hand hygiene procedures should be used. All articles in the room, as well as the room itself, should be disinfected or sterilized frequently.

Infection Control in an Intensive Care Unit or Postoperative Care Unit

Patients in ICUs are more critically ill, have numerous invasive devices (e.g., IV lines, urinary catheters) and, by nature, more susceptible to infections than other patients. In some hospitals, intensive care units are open areas, with numerous patients in one large room so as to be more easily monitored. Patients with known infections are isolated according to the types of infections they have, and strict handwashing and gloving policies are necessary in all ICUs.

Postoperative patients are susceptible to infection because surgical wounds or drains enable bacteria to gain easy access to deeper tissues. Again, each patient who becomes infected should be isolated and dealt with according to the type of infection acquired.

Infection Control in a Dialysis Unit

Patients needing dialysis are most often immunosuppressed, which makes them a high-risk group for contracting infection, especially hepatitis. Protective gowns and gloves may be worn in the unit, and strict hand hygiene and gloving techniques should be adhered to.

Specific Isolation Techniques and Procedural Steps

In most hospitals, all supplies required for isolation procedures (**PROCEDURES 4–3, 4–4, 4–5,** and **4–6**) are located in an area or on a cart just outside the patient's room (**FIGURE 4–22**). These include:

- Disposable gloves
- Gown
- Mask
- Protective eyewear

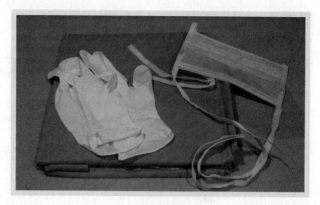

FIGURE 4–22
Supplies for Isolation Procedures

PROCEDURE 4–3

Gowning, Masking, and Gloving

Rationale   To prevent the transmission of microorganisms from health care workers to patients or from patients to health care workers.

Equipment

- Alcohol-based rub or soap and water
- Gown
- Mask
- Face shield or goggles
- Chemically clean disposable gloves or sterile disposable gloves

Procedure

Follow these isolation procedural steps:

1 Complete hand hygiene as described in Procedure 4–1 (**FIGURE 4–23**).

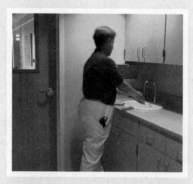

FIGURE 4–23

2 Use new gowns large enough to cover all clothing (**FIGURE 4–24**).

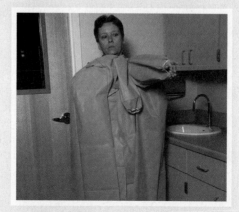

FIGURE 4–24

(continued)

PROCEDURE 4-3

Gowning, Masking, and Gloving (continued)

3 Touching only its inside surface, place one arm at a time through the gown's sleeves and wrap the gown completely around the body so that the opening is in back. Pull down the sleeves. Then the neck ties or Velcro should be secured around the neck; and the tie strings around the waist need to be tied. Gowns are generally made of cloth and paper (**FIGURE 4–25**).

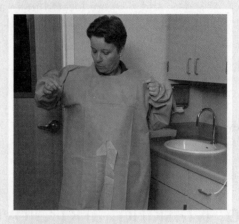

FIGURE 4–25

4 Don mask if required (**FIGURES 4–26** and **4–27**). Masks protect the health care worker from small-particle droplets that may carry pathogens. Often, a small metal band on the mask can be shaped to fit the nose. Two ties are usually made, the first around the upper portion of the head and the second around the upper portion of the neck.

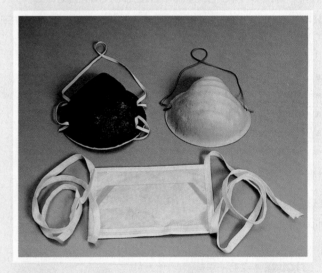

FIGURE 4–26
Sample Masks Used for Isolation Procedures

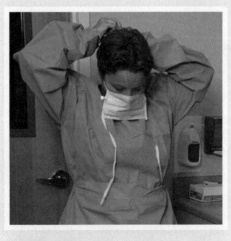

FIGURE 4–27

PROCEDURE 4-3

Gowning, Masking, and Gloving (continued)

5 Wear a face shield or goggles during procedures that may possibly generate blood or body fluid droplets (i.e., splashes or sprays), such as from severe patient coughing (**FIGURE 4-28**).

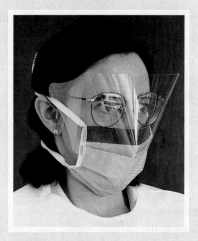

FIGURE 4-28

6 Pull gloves over the ends of the gown sleeves to prevent contamination of exposed skin (**FIGURE 4-29**). Chemically clean disposable gloves may be used for most isolation procedures. For isolation procedures in which the patient must be protected from any microorganisms, use sterile disposable gloves. Do not wear rings and other pieces of jewelry because they may puncture a glove during patient contact.

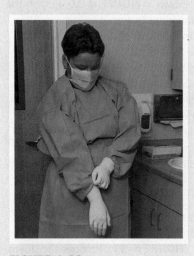

FIGURE 4-29

PROCEDURE 4–4

Removal of Isolation Gown, Mask, and Gloves

Rationale   To prevent the transmission of microorganisms, remove the personal protective equipment at the doorway or in the outer room (anteroom), except for the respirator. Remove the respirator after leaving the patient's room and closing the door.

Equipment

- Large red isolation bag
- Linen hamper
- Special container for disposing the masks

Procedure

After the completion of blood collection in an isolation room, follow these steps for removing the isolation gown, mask, and gloves:

1 Remove the gloves as shown in **FIGURE 4–30**. Pull off the first glove in such a manner as to turn it inside out. Place the rolled-up glove into the palm of the hand that is still gloved. Remove the second glove by slipping the index finger of the ungloved hand between the glove and the hand. Then pull the glove down and off as it turns inside out. Dispose of both gloves in a red garbage bag in the isolation room. After the removal of the gloves, remove the goggles or face shield by touching the head band or ear pieces. (*Do not touch the outside of goggles or face shield because of contamination.*)

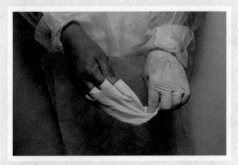

FIGURE 4–30

2 Unfasten the gown's ties. Take off the gown by pulling down from the neck and shoulders first and then pull the arms out of the gown (**FIGURE 4–31**). Remove the gown and fold it with the contaminated side turned in and with care taken not to touch the outer side.

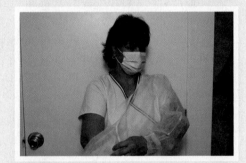

FIGURE 4–31

PROCEDURE 4–4

Removal of Isolation Gown, Mask, and Gloves (continued)

3 To prevent contamination, use the gowns only once. Dispose of the gown in the linen hamper or, if disposable, in a garbage bag in the isolation room (**FIGURE 4–32**).

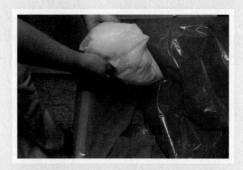

FIGURE 4–32

4 Remove the mask by carefully untying the lower tie first, then the upper one (**FIGURE 4–33**). Hold only the ends of the ties. Properly dispose of the mask inside the room. In some cases, a special container for masks is placed just outside the room to prevent exposure of hospital personnel to airborne pathogens while inside the isolation room.

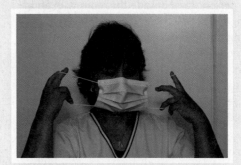

FIGURE 4–33

5 Wash hands in the room and again at the nearest sink after exiting the room (**FIGURE 4–34**). Use a clean paper towel to open the door. Hold the door open with one foot and discard the used paper towels in the wastebasket directly inside the patient's room.

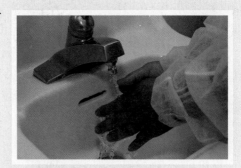

FIGURE 4–34

PROCEDURE 4–5

Disposing of Contaminated Items

Rationale   To properly dispose of contaminated items and prevent the transmission of microorganisms. Trash, linens, and other articles in an isolation room may be removed by using one sturdy biohazard bag or the **double bagging** procedure (explained here).

Equipment

- Two large red isolation bags

Procedure

1   Put contaminated material in one bag and seal the bag while inside the room, as shown in **FIGURE 4–35**.

2   Have another person stand outside the room with another opened, clean, impermeable bag (**FIGURE 4–36**). The person standing outside the room should have the ends of the bag folded over their hands to shield from possible contamination. Place the sealed bag from the room in the clean bag. The person outside the room can then fold over the edges, expel the air, and seal the outer bag. The bag must be labeled with biohazard warnings.

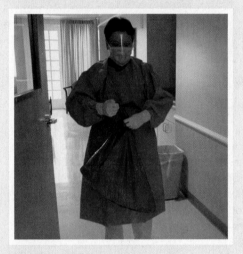

FIGURE 4–35

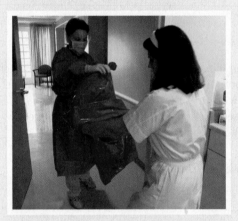

FIGURE 4–36

PROCEDURE 4–6

Removal of Patient's Specimen from Isolation Room

Rationale   To properly transport a blood specimen or other specimens from a patient in isolation to prevent transmission of microorganisms.

Equipment
- Blood tube(s)
- Clean biohazard bag

Procedure

1 Follow the required procedure for entering the isolation room.

2 Label blood tube(s) with the patient's name, hospital ID number, and other required identification criteria of the health care facility, and the word *isolation* before entering the isolation room.

3 Collect the blood and place the tube(s) in a clean plastic biohazard bag outside the room (**FIGURE 4–37**).

4 Complete hand hygiene.

5 Transport the blood specimen to the laboratory with the appropriate laboratory request form.

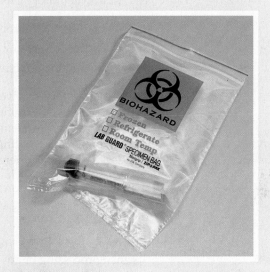

FIGURE 4–37
Biohazard Bag for Transport of Patient Specimens from Isolation Room

ISOLATION ITEM DISPOSAL

The supplies needed for isolation item disposal include:

- Garbage bag
- Linen hamper
- Large red isolation bag
- Specimen container
- Plastic bag with biohazard label
- Laundry bag
- Puncture-resistant disposal container for needles and sharps
- Gloves
- Antiseptic agent or antimicrobial agent

Isolation bags for transporting specimens should be turned halfway inside out and left near the door outside the room; someone may be available to hold the bag outside the door. Only the needed supplies should be taken into the room. Phlebotomy requisitions may be left outside the room on the isolation cart. If collecting a blood specimen, the health care provider may use a tourniquet in the room or use the one brought in. The specimen should be labeled at the bedside and the pen left in the room. Used needles, swabs, and other used objects should be put in appropriate containers inside the room. Any blood on the outside of the specimen container should be removed with a paper towel. While standing in the doorway, and touching only the inside of the isolation bag, the health care worker should place the specimen inside the bag. Gloved hands should be washed in the room. The faucet may be turned off with a paper towel.

Infection Control and Safety in the Clinical Laboratory

The clinical laboratory contributes to infection control programs in the following manner:

- Maintaining laboratory records for surveillance purposes
- Reporting on infectious agents, drug-resistant microorganisms, and outbreaks
- Evaluating the effectiveness of sterilization or decontamination procedures

The laboratory receives numerous patients' specimens for diagnostic procedures to be performed to determine causes of diseases and disorders. Health care workers in the laboratory must be extremely cautious because they often handle specimens with infectious agents. The following essentials of standard precautions and safe laboratory work practices should be adhered to when in the laboratory:

- Perform frequent hand hygiene.
- Assume all patients and specimens are infectious for HIV and other blood-borne pathogens.
- Use personal protection equipment, including a face shield, when performing specimen processing or any procedure that might initiate an aerosol or splash from blood or other body fluids.
- Use appropriate waste-disposal practices.
- Maintain good personal hygiene, including wearing clean clothes, keeping hair clean and tied back if necessary, keeping fingernails clean, and washing hands frequently.
- Do not eat, drink, smoke, or apply cosmetics (including lip balm).
- Avoid storing food and drinks in the laboratory refrigerator or freezer used for reagents and specimens.
- Avoid wearing a laboratory coat or other personal protective equipment outside of the designated area for use (i.e., no laboratory coats in lunchroom or at home).
- Do not insert or remove contact lenses.
- Avoid biting nails or chewing on pens.
- Cough or sneeze into a tissue and discard immediately. Wash hands afterwards. If no tissue is available, cough into one's upper arm or sleeve
- Avoid wearing loose bracelets, long necklaces, or long earrings.
- Carefully dispose of safety needles, lancets, and other blood collection supplies in appropriate biohazardous-labeled containers.
- Maintain good health by eating balanced meals, getting enough sleep, and getting enough exercise.
- Report personal illnesses to supervisors.
- Become familiar with and observe *all* isolation policies.
- Learn about the job-related aspects of infection control, and share this information with others.
- Caution all personnel working with known hazardous material (this can be done with proper warning labels).
- Report violations of the policies.

- Cover patients' specimens at all times during transportation and centrifugation.
- Centrifuge specimens within a biohazard safety hood.
- Clean phlebotomy trays at least once a week with a 1:10 bleach solution.
- Clean the specimen collection area with a decontaminating 1:10 bleach solution.

DISINFECTANTS AND ANTISEPTICS

Disinfectants are chemical compounds used to remove or kill pathogenic microorganisms. Chemical disinfectants are regulated by the **Environmental Protection Agency (EPA)**. A list of EPA-registered products may be obtained by contacting the EPA's Antimicrobial Division. **Antiseptics** are chemicals used to inhibit the growth and development of microorganisms, but they do not necessarily kill them. Antiseptics may be used on human skin, whereas disinfectants are generally used on surfaces and instruments because they are too corrosive for direct use on skin. Chlorhexidine gluconate (CHG) is used extensively in health care as an antiseptic for skin. The bactericidal action of CHG surpasses antiseptic preparations containing povidone-iodine. Thus, it is used in skin preparation for blood culture collections as well as blood transfusions.

A disinfectant with a product label claiming that the disinfectant is *HIVcidal* or *tuberculocidal* or a disinfectant having a chlorine bleach (5.25% sodium hypochlorite) dilution of 1:10 is recommended by CDC to be used to disinfect tourniquets and items contaminated with blood or other body fluids. A more dilute solution of chlorine bleach (1:100) can be used for routine cleaning of surfaces. Gloves and gowns should be worn when performing decontamination procedures. All dilute solutions of chlorine bleach need to be made weekly to prevent the loss of the germicidal activity.[5] The minimal contact time for disinfectants to be effective is 10 minutes.

TABLES 4–4, **4–5**, and **4–6** list some of the more common hospital disinfectants and antiseptics. Also refer to Appendix 6.

TABLE 4–4

Common Antiseptics and Disinfectants for the Health Care Setting

Compound	Uses and Restrictions
Alcohols	
Ethyl (70%)	Antiseptic for skin
Isopropyl (70%) (isopropanol)	Antiseptic for skin
Chlorhexidine gluconate	Antiseptic for skin
Chloramine	Disinfectant for wounds
Hypochlorite solutions (bleach)	Disinfectant
Ethylene oxide	Disinfectant (toxic)
Formaldehyde	Disinfectant (noxious fumes)
Glutaraldehyde	Disinfectant (toxic)
Hydrogen peroxide	Antiseptic for skin
Tincture of iodine	Antiseptic for skin (can be irritating)
Benzalkonium chloride	Antiseptic for skin
Iodophors	Antiseptic for skin (less stable)
Phenolic compounds	Disinfectant
1–2 percent phenols	Disinfectant
Chlorophenol	Disinfectant (toxic)
Hexylresorcinol	Antiseptic for skin
Triclosan	Antiseptic for skin
Quaternary ammonium compounds	Antiseptic for skin (ingredient in many soaps)

TABLE 4–5

Antimicrobial Spectrum and Characteristics of Hand-Hygiene Antiseptic Agents*

Group	Gram-Positive Bacteria	Gram-Negative Bacteria	Mycobacteria	Fungi	Viruses	Speed of Action	Comments
Alcohols	+++	+++	+++	+++	+++	Fast	Optimum concentration 40%–95%; no persistent activity
Chlorhexidine (2% and 4% aqueous)	+++	++	+	+	+++	Intermediate	Persistent activity; rare allergic reactions
Iodine compounds	+++	+++	+++	++	+++	Intermediate	Cause skin burns; usually too irritating for hand hygiene
Iodophors	+++	+++	+	++	++	Intermediate	Less irritating than iodine; acceptance varies
Phenol derivatives	+++	+	+	+	+	Intermediate	Activity neutralized by nonionic surfactants
Triclosan	+++	++	+	–	+++	Intermediate	Acceptability on hands varies
Quaternary ammonium compounds	+	++	–	–	+	Slow	Used only in combination with alcohols; ecologic concerns

*Hexachlorophene is not included because it is no longer an accepted ingredient of hand disinfectants.

Note: +++ = excellent; ++ = good, but does not include the entire bacterial spectrum; + = fair; – = no activity or not sufficient.

Source: Guideline for Hand Hygiene in Health-Care Settings. *MMWR,* October 25, 2002, Vol. 51, No. RR-16.

TABLE 4–6

Parameters and Applications of Selected Hand Hygiene Antiseptics

Antiseptics	Concentration, %	Speed of Action	Residual Activity	Use
Alcohols	60 to 70%	Fast	No	As component of gels and foams; hand-rubbing before and after patient contact
Chlorhexidine gluconate	0.5 to 4%	Intermediate	Yes	As component of disinfectant; 0.5 to 1% solutions for handwashing, 2 to 4% for surgical scrub
Iodophors	0.5 to 10%	Intermediate	+/-*	Handwashing and antiseptic for patient skin

*Evidence for iodophor residual activity is contradictory and depends on formulation, use, and concentrations.

Source: WHO Guidelines on Hand Hygiene in Healthcare, 2009. World Health Organization www.who.org.

Study Questions

The following may have one or more answers.

1 Which of the following is the most effective replacement for latex gloves?

a. low-powder latex gloves
b. hypoallergenic latex gloves
c. nitrile gloves
d. cotton gloves

2 What is/are the primary function(s) of isolation procedures?

a. keep the hospital clean
b. prevent transmission of communicable diseases
c. protect the general public from disease
d. provide protective environments

3 Which chemical is most effective as an antiseptic for cleaning the blood collection site?

a. iodine
b. povidone-iodine
c. chlorhexidine
d. ethyl alcohol

4 Nurses, physicians, and other health care workers are responsible for changing their gloves:

a. only if the patient has an infectious disease
b. after every third patient on the blood collection list
c. after every patient
d. after blood collection on the patients in the dialysis center

5 For health care workers, most occupational exposure to HIV occurs following:

a. blood contact with eyes
b. needlestick injuries
c. blood or body fluid contact with respiratory membranes
d. blood contact with skin

6 Airborne precautions may be required for patients with infections such as

a. tuberculosis
b. staphylococcus
c. Hepatitis A
d. Rocky Mountain spotted fever

7 According to the OSHA standards for occupational exposure to blood-borne pathogens, which of the following is NOT personal protective equipment?

a. 10% household bleach
b. fluid-resistant gown
c. goggles
d. respirator

8 Safe working conditions in the health care environment are federally regulated by

a. The Joint Commission
b. OSHA
c. ASCP
d. JCAHO

9 When collecting blood from a person with AIDS in his or her home, the best way to dispose of the contaminated needle and holder is to

a. detach the needle from the needle holder and dispose
b. place the needle and holder together as a unit in a puncture resistant container in the home
c. recap the needle and bring it back to the appropriate disposal area in the clinical laboratory
d. recap the needle and dispose of it in the closest available biohazard container

10 Gloves, gown, and mask are examples of

a. work practice controls
b. personal protective equipment (PPE)
c. engineering controls
d. administrative controls

Case Study

Accidental Injury Sally Landers had been on the job for only 8 months. She was a health care worker at a rural hospital in the Southwest where she had been hired to do early-morning blood collections and deliver specimens to the centralized laboratory. She was tired when she went to work one Friday morning. She drew blood from a frail middle-aged man, Mr. Gilmore. She had trouble with the collection procedure in that she had to stick him twice before she acquired the blood specimen. Sally was relieved when she finally finished the procedure. As she began to clean up and discard the used equipment, she noticed that the biohazard container was full. She decided, however, that it could probably hold the needles she had used on Mr. Gilmore. She used her fingers to push the used needles and needle holders into the container and she felt a sharp puncture. She realized that she had stuck herself with a contaminated sharp object. She gathered the specimens she had drawn and quickly left. She immediately reported the injury to her supervisor.

Questions

1 Describe what Sally did correctly and incorrectly.

2 Which procedures would need to be reviewed with Sally?

3 What additional education would you recommend for Sally?

Action in Practice

A *Staphylococcus* infection of the skin on the arm above the antecubital area started occurring in many of the elderly adults in the long-term care facility at Grand Oaks Health Care Center. Upon investigation it was discovered that the patients with the skin infections had recent venipunctures to collect blood. What was a major possibility for the skin infections in these patients?

Questions

1 Identify the links in this chain of infection:

Pathogen

Reservoir

Portal exit

Mode of transmission

Portal of entry

Susceptible host

2 Explain how you can break the chain of infection.

COMPETENCY ASSESSMENT

Check Yourself

1 You have collected blood from a patient in isolation for "droplet precautions." What steps should occur to exit this room?

2 When you have completed a phlebotomy procedure and taken off your gloves, what should you proceed to do prior to collecting blood from the next patient?

Competency Checklist: Infection Control

This checklist can be completed as a group or individually.

(1) Completed (2) Needs to improve

_____ 1. Describe or identify four pieces of personal protective equipment in the blood collection area.

_____ 2. List the personal protective equipment required to enter an isolation room for droplet precautions.

REFERENCES

1. CDC Health Care Associated Infections (HAI): www.cdc.gov/HAI/burden.html, accessed February 18, 2013.

2. U.S. Department of Labor and Occupational Safety and Health Administration (OSHA). (1991, December 4). Occupational exposure to blood-borne pathogens; final rule (29 CFR 1910.1030). *Federal Register,* 44004–44182.

3. OSHA Revised Bloodborne Pathogens Standard 1910.1030. Needlestick Safety and Prevention Act; April 18, 2001.

4. Updated U.S. Public Health Service Guidelines for the Management of Occupational Exposures to HBV, HCV, and HIV. Recommendations for postexposure prophylaxis. *MMWR,* June 29, 2001, 50(RR11).

5. Clinical and Laboratory Standards Institute. (2005). *M29-A3 protection of laboratory workers from occupationally acquired infections: Approved guideline.* 3rd ed.

6. Centers for Disease Control and Prevention. (1996). Guidelines for isolation precautions in hospitals, part 1: Evolution of isolation practices. *Am J Infect Control, 24*(1): 24–31.

7. Siegel, J. D., Rhinehart, E., Jackson, M., & Chiarello, L. (2007). Guideline for isolation precautions: Preventing transmission of infectious agents in health care settings. The Health Care Infection Control Practices Advisory Committee. *Infect Control Hosp Epidemiol, 35* (10), Supplement 2: S65–S164.

8. Molinari, J. A. (2003). Infection control: Its evolution to the current standard precautions. *J Am Dent Assoc, 134,* 549–574.

RESOURCES

www.apic.org Association for Professionals in Infection Control and Epidemiology.

www.cdc.gov Centers for Disease Control and Prevention.

www.cdc.gov/flu/pdf/protect/cdc_cough.pdf Centers for Disease Control and Prevention; Cover Your Cough Poster.

http://www.cdc.gov/mmwr/preview/mmwrhtml/rr5116a1.htm Guideline for hand hygiene in health-care setting. (2002). *MMWR, 51* (RR14).

www.jointcommission.org/assets/1/6/2013_LAB_NPSG_final_10-23.pdf, accessed February 21, 2013. The Joint Commission. (2013). 2013 National patient safety goals.

www.niosh.gov National Institute for Occupational Safety and Health.

www.who.org World Health Organization. WHO Guidelines on Hand Hygiene in Healthcare, 2009.

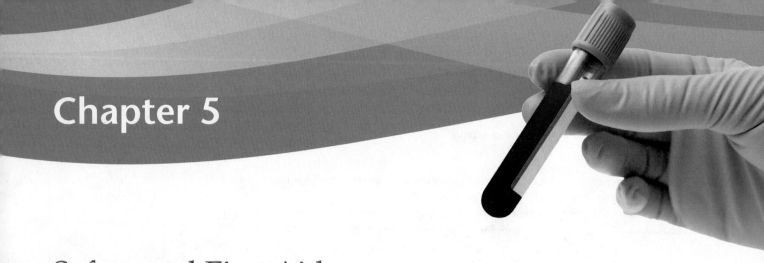

Chapter 5

Safety and First Aid

KEY TERMS

cardiopulmonary resuscitation (CPR)
global harmonization
Global Harmonization System (GHS)
HazCom
Material Safety Data Sheets (MSDSs)
RACE: Rescue Alert Confine Extinguish

Chapter Objectives

Upon completion of Chapter 5, the learner is responsible for doing the following:

1. Discuss safety awareness for health care workers.

2. Explain the measures that should be taken for fire, electrical, radiation, mechanical, and chemical safety in a health care facility.

3. Describe the essential elements of a disaster emergency plan for a health care facility.

4. Explain the safety policies and procedures that must be followed in specimen collection and transportation.

5. Describe the safe use of equipment in health care facilities.

6. List three precautions that can reduce the risk of injury to patients.

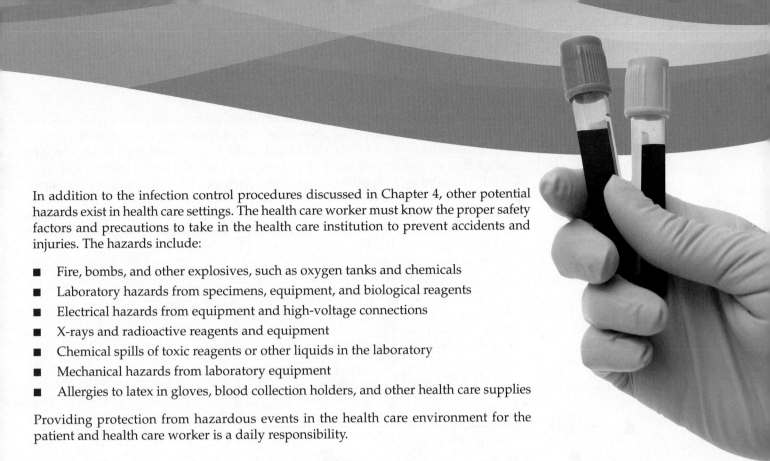

In addition to the infection control procedures discussed in Chapter 4, other potential hazards exist in health care settings. The health care worker must know the proper safety factors and precautions to take in the health care institution to prevent accidents and injuries. The hazards include:

- Fire, bombs, and other explosives, such as oxygen tanks and chemicals
- Laboratory hazards from specimens, equipment, and biological reagents
- Electrical hazards from equipment and high-voltage connections
- X-rays and radioactive reagents and equipment
- Chemical spills of toxic reagents or other liquids in the laboratory
- Mechanical hazards from laboratory equipment
- Allergies to latex in gloves, blood collection holders, and other health care supplies

Providing protection from hazardous events in the health care environment for the patient and health care worker is a daily responsibility.

Fire Safety

Fire safety is the responsibility of all employees in the health care institution. Fire or explosive hazards may occur in the laboratory or other areas of the health care facility. Health care workers should be familiar with not only the use and location of the fire extinguishers but also the procedures to follow during a fire. They should also be knowledgeable of the exact locations of fire extinguishers and fire blankets. The blankets should be available to smother burning clothes or to use as a fire shield if fire is blocking the exit. Health care institutions usually conduct periodic safety education programs in which the health care worker can participate to become skillful in and knowledgeable about the use of fire safety equipment (**FIGURE 5–1**).

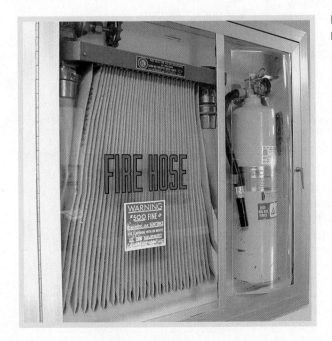

FIGURE 5–1
Fire Extinguisher and Fire Hose

CLASSIFICATION OF FIRES

The components of fire are fuel, oxygen, and heat, plus the necessary chain reaction. Three general classifications of fires have been adopted by the National Fire Protection Association (NFPA).[1] As shown in **FIGURE 5–2**, Class A fires require an ABC extinguisher or pressurized water extinguisher for wood, paper, clothing, and trash. Class B fires need an ABC extinguisher or carbon dioxide (CO_2) extinguisher for liquid, grease, and chemical fires. Class C fires are electrical fires and a CO_2, halon, or ABC extinguisher can be used. The ABC extinguisher is the one found in most health care facilities, so health care workers need not worry about which extinguisher to use in case of fire.

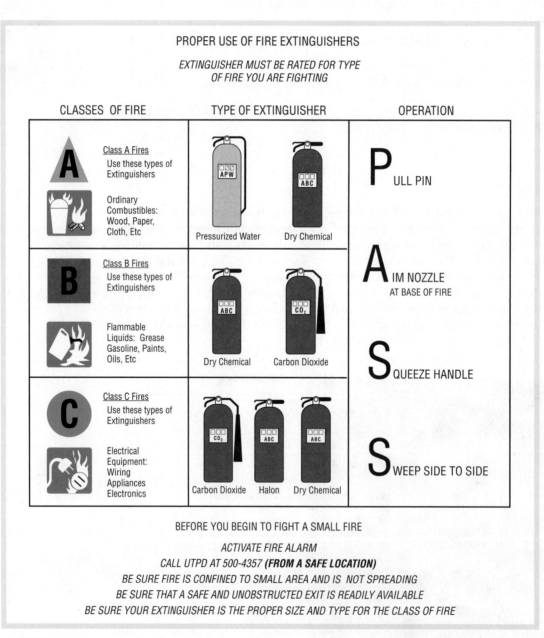

FIGURE 5–2

Proper Use of Fire Extinguishers

Courtesy of Health and Environmental Safety, The University of Texas Health Science Center at Houston.

EMERGENCY RESPONSE TO POSSIBLE FIRE

If a fire or explosion occurs in the workplace, the health care worker should *not* do the following:

- Block entrances
- Reenter the building
- Panic
- Run

Instead, the health care worker *should* **RACE: <u>R</u>escue <u>A</u>lert <u>C</u>onfine <u>E</u>xtinguish** by doing the following (**FIGURE 5–3**):

- Pull the nearest fire alarm.
- Call 911 or the hospital's fire emergency number, which should be posted on or near the phone.
- Remove patients from danger if the fire is on a patient floor.
- Close windows and doors to prevent spreading of the fire.
- If the fire is small and isolated from other possible fuel sources, use an ABC extinguisher to fight it:

  1. Pull pin off extinguisher (**FIGURE 5–4**).
  2. Aim extinguisher at the base of fire and squeeze the handle.
  3. Spray the solution toward base of fire, but do not point directly at an individual.

- If the fire threatens to block exits or is not small, leave the area immediately. Take the stairs, not the elevator.
- If clothing is on fire, drop to the ground and roll, preferably in a fire blanket.
- If caught in a fire, crawl to the exit. Because smoke rises, breathing is easier at floor level. Breathing through a wet towel is also helpful.

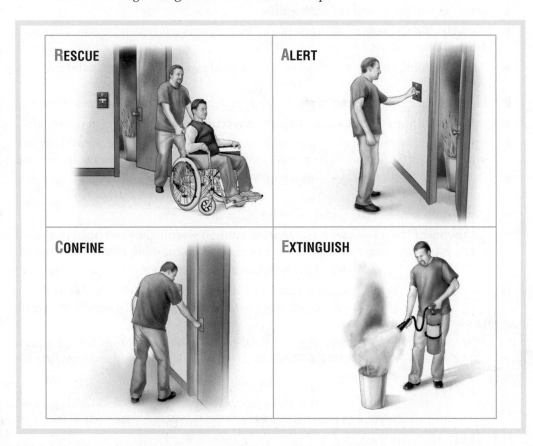

FIGURE 5–3
Using RACE in Fire Emergencies

RESCUE

ALERT

CONFINE

EXTINGUISH

FIGURE 5–4
Pulling Pin Off Fire Extinguisher

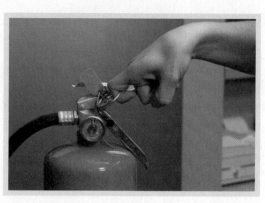

FIGURE 5–4
Pulling Pin Off Fire Extinguisher

Remember that every time a new environment is entered (i.e., health care facility, home health visit), the health care worker needs to become familiar with the locations of fire exits and other safety equipment.

Electrical Safety

A major hazard in any area of a health care institution is the possibility of electrical current passing through a person. For example, in the clinical laboratory or physician office laboratory, the health care worker sometimes operates electrical equipment, such as a centrifuge. He or she should be aware of the location of the circuit-breaker boxes in order to assure a fast response in the event of an electrical fire or an electrical shock. The health care worker using electrical equipment should consider the following:

- Do not use power cords that are frayed.
- Do not use control switches and thermostats that are not in good working order.
- Know where the closest fire extinguisher is located.
- Avoid handling electrical equipment and instruments when standing on a wet floor or having wet hands.
- Always unplug the centrifuge or other electrical equipment before maintenance is performed.
- Electrical equipment in need of repair needs to be performed by those trained to do so.
- Avoid using any electrical cords that are frayed or show other signs of damage.
- Any electrical instrument that liquid has been spilled on or in, or whose wiring has come in contact with liquid, should be immediately unplugged and dried prior to further use.
- If liquid is spilled on equipment in a patient's room, notify the floor nurse immediately.
- Do not overload electric outlets with lots of plugs.
- If equipment has a label with an electrical caution warning, do not open it, since it may contain batteries that store electricity even when the equipment is unplugged.
    - Avoid using extension cords.
    - While collecting blood, avoid contact with any electrical equipment, since the electricity may pass through you and the needle and shock the patient.
    - Use three-prong "hospital-grade" electrical plugs for all equipment (**FIGURE 5–5**), since they have a long prong for grounding the equipment.

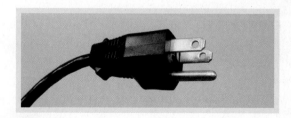

FIGURE 5–5
Three-Prong Grounded Plug

If an electrical accident occurs involving electrical shock to an employee or a patient, be aware of the two points described in **BOX 5–1**.

What to Do in Case of an Electrical Accident

1. The electrical power source must be shut off. If this is impossible, carefully remove the electrical contact from the victim, using something that does not conduct electricity, such as placing your hand in a glass beaker and pushing the power supply away from the victim. The rescuer should not attempt to touch the victim without heeding these precautions.

2. Medical assistance should be called and **cardiopulmonary resuscitation (CPR)** started immediately. The victim should not be moved prior to the arrival of medical assistance. A fire blanket or other warm clothing should be put over the victim to keep him or her warm until medical help arrives.

Radiation Safety

The three cardinal principles of self-protection from radiation exposure are time, shielding, and distance. Radiation exposure is cumulative; thus, limiting the length of exposure at any one time is a major factor in minimizing the hazard.

Areas where radioactive materials are in use and stored must have warning signs (**FIGURE 5-6**) posted on the entrance doors. All radioactive specimens and reagents must also be properly labeled with the radioactive sign.

The health care worker may encounter potential hazards from radiation exposure only if he or she must collect specimens from patients in the nuclear medicine or x-ray department or must take specimens to the radioimmunoassay section in a research or a clinical chemistry laboratory. Thus, the health care worker should be cautious when entering an area posted with the radiation hazard sign and should be knowledgeable of the institution's procedures pertaining to radiation safety. Limit the time of exposure to

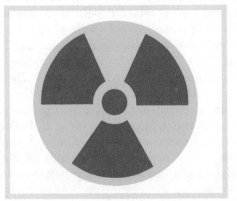

FIGURE 5-6
Radiation Hazard Sign

patients who have received radioactive implants. A person must have limited exposure to radioactivity since high exposures can lead to leukemia and various types of cancer. If the health care worker must collect specimens in areas where high levels of radioactivity may occur (i.e., nuclear medicine), he or she must wear a dosimeter badge to determine the amount of radioactivity received (**FIGURE 5–7**).

FIGURE 5–7
Dosimeter

A dosimeter can measure dose rates of radiation and is useful in determining health care personnel exposure levels.

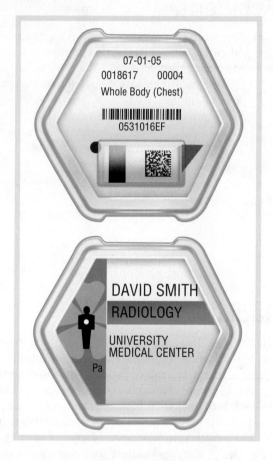

These badges *must* be turned into the health care facility's Safety Department according to the facility's scheduled intervals to check the radioactivity exposure level. The health care worker must abide by these periodic radioactive badge readings for his or her protection. Health care workers who are pregnant should be aware of the potential hazard of radiation to the fetus.

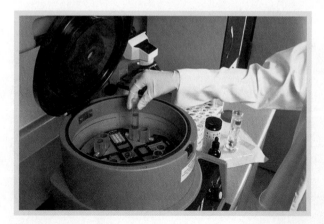

FIGURE 5–8

Example of a Centrifuge

Mechanical Safety

The centrifuge is a frequently used instrument for blood specimen preparation and testing (**FIGURE 5–8**). Thus, a health care provider who collects and prepares blood specimens for testing should learn how to maintain this instrument and become familiar with its parts. For example, he or she should know if the carriers are in the correct position prior to use. If the carriers are not in the correct position, they can swing out of the holding disks into the side of the centrifuge. Also, the wrong head, the wrong cups, or imbalanced tubes can lead to the same dangerous problem. If this particular type of accident occurs, tubes containing patients' specimens or spinning chemicals may be propelled onto the side of the centrifuge and broken, and a dangerous, hazardous problem created. Thus, it is of utmost importance to abide by the preventive maintenance schedule and procedures for the centrifuge.

Chemical Safety

Because a health care worker must sometimes pour preservatives, such as hydrochloric acid (HCl), into containers for 24-hour urine collections and transport these specimens to the patients' floor, she or he should be knowledgeable of chemical safety (**FIGURE 5–9**). Mixing chemicals (e.g., bleach with other cleaning agents) can lead to dangerous gases and possible harm to health care workers. Labeling may be the single-most important step in the proper handling of chemicals. Laboratory workers should be able to ascertain from appropriate labels not only the contents of the container but also the nature and extent of hazards posed by the chemicals (**TABLE 5–1**). Carefully read the label before using any reagents (**BOX 5–2** for requirements of labeling). Regulations for hazardous materials and reagents are being modified due to worldwide classifications of such materials.

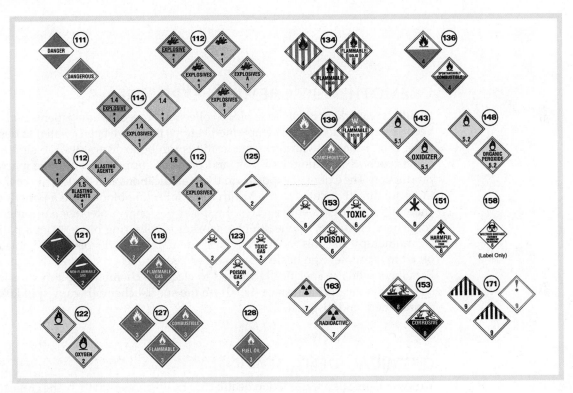

FIGURE 5–9
Department of Transportation (DOT) Hazardous Materials Warning Signs

TABLE 5–1

Hazard Classes and Placard Colors

Hazard Class	Hazard Type	Color Code
1	Explosives	Orange
2	Gases	Red or green
3	Liquids	Red
4	Solids	Red and white
5	Oxidizers and organic peroxides	Yellow
6	Poisonous and etiologic agents	White
7	Radioactive materials	Yellow and white
8	Corrosives	Black and white
9	Miscellaneous	Black and white

BOX 5–2

Chemical Labels

Labels for hazardous chemicals must

- Provide a warning (e.g., corrosive) (Figure 5–9).
- Explain the nature of the hazard (e.g., flammable, combustible) (Figure 5–9).
- State special precautions to eliminate risks.
- Explain first-aid treatment in the event of a chemical leak, a chemical spill, or other exposure to the chemical.

CHEMOTHERAPY CHEMICAL EXPOSURE

Health care workers involved in blood collection procedures on patients with cancer may become exposed to chemotherapy medications that have been created to destroy cancer cells. Direct contact with these medications can be toxic and lead to significant health effects such as vomiting, hair loss, and possible suppression of bone marrow cellular production. The extent of exposure to these medications and the toxicity of these medications are directly related to the health risk. Collecting blood from a patient undergoing chemotherapy treatment requires the usual personal protective equipment for blood collection. However, if a health care worker is collecting blood from a patient having chemotherapy and this medication is accidentally spilled from the IV pole or knocked off from a counter, the health care worker needs to leave the area as soon as possible. Personnel who are specifically trained to clean up chemotherapy medications need to be immediately notified, since they have the special chemotherapy spill kits for proper containment and disposal.[2]

CHEMICAL IDENTIFICATION

Various chemicals are needed in health care facilities, especially in the clinical laboratory department. Because chemicals may pose health or physical hazards, OSHA amended the Hazard Communication Standard (29 CFR 1910.1200, Right to Know/HCS Standard) to include health care facilities.[3]

In addition to mandating labels, the Right to Know law, also known as the OSHA **HazCom** standard, requires chemical manufacturers to supply **Material Safety Data Sheets (MSDSs)** for their chemicals. The MSDS is required for any chemical with a hazard warning label (**FIGURE 5–10**). An MSDS lists general information, precautionary measures, and emergency information (**BOX 5–3**).

Regulations for hazardous materials and reagents are being modified due to **global harmonization.** This new term refers to the worldwide development of hazardous materials classification and transportation regulations that are consistent among all countries (**FIGURE 5–11**). The change to the **Global Harmonization System (GHS)** requires the use of the GHS-sanctioned safety data sheets (SDS) format for the hazard communication sheets. Safety data sheets contain virtually all of the identical information as Material Safety Data Sheets, but the order and format have been standardized.

The National Fire Protection Association developed an "NFPA 704 marking system" for hazardous chemicals that is frequently used in health care facilities (**FIGURE 5–12**). The system uses a diamond-shaped symbol, four colored quadrants, and a hazard rating

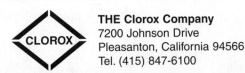

THE Clorox Company
7200 Johnson Drive
Pleasanton, California 94566
Tel. (415) 847-6100

Material Safety
Data Sheets

Health	2+
Flammability	0
Reactivity	1
Personal Protection	B

I – CHEMICAL IDENTIFICATION

Name	regular Clorox Bleach	CAS No.	N/A
Description	clear, light yellow liquid with chlorine odor	RTECs No.	N/A

Other Designations	Manufacturer	Emergency Procedure
EPA Reg. No. 5813-1 Sodium hypochlorite solution Liquid chlorine bleach Clorox Liquid Bleach	The Clorox Company 1221 Broadway Oakland, CA 94612	• Notify your supervisor • Call your local poison control center OR • Rocky Mountain Poison Center (303)573-1014

II – HEALTH HAZARD DATA

• Causes severe but temporary eye injury. May irritate skin. May cause nausea and vomiting if ingested. Exposure to vapor or mist may irritate nose, throat and lungs. The following medical conditions may be aggravated by exposure to high concentrations of vapor or mist: heart conditions or chronic respiratory problems such as asthma, chronic bronchitis or obstructive lung disease. Under normal consumer use conditions the likelihood of any adverse health effects are low. FIRST AID: EYE CONTACT: Immediately flush eyes with plenty of water. If irritation persists, see a doctor. SKIN CONTACT: Remove contaminated clothing. Wash area with water. INGESTION: Drink a glassful of water and call a physician. INHALATION: If breathing problems develop remove to fresh air.

III – HAZARDOUS INGREDIENTS

Ingredients	Concentration	Worker Exposure Limit
Sodium hypochlorite CAS# 7681-52-9	5.25%	not established

None of the ingredients in this product are on the IARC, NTP or OSHA carcinogen list. Occasional clinical reports suggest a low potential for sensitization upon exaggerated exposure to sodium hypochlorite if skin damage (e.g., irritation) occurs during exposure. Routine clinical tests conducted on intact skin with Clorox Liquid Bleach found no sensitization in the test subjects.

IV – SPECIAL PROTECTION INFORMATION

Hygienic Practices: Wear safety glasses. With repeated or prolonged use, wear gloves.

Engineering Controls: Use general ventilation to minimize exposure to vapor or mist.

Work Practices: Avoid eye and skin contact and inhalation of vapor or mist.

V – SPECIAL PRECAUTIONS

Keep out of reach of children. Do not get in eyes or on skin. Wash thoroughly with soap and water after handling. Do not mix with other household chemicals such as toilet bowl cleaners, rust removers, vinegar, acid or ammonia containing products. Store in a cool, dry place. Do not reuse empty container; rinse container and put in trash container.

VI – SPILL OR LEAK PROCEDURES

Small quantities of less than 5 gallons may be flushed down drain. For larger quantities wipe up with an absorbent material or mop and dispose of in accordance with local, state and federal regulations. Dilute with water to minimize oxidizing effect on spilled surface.

VII – REACTIVITY DATA

Stable under normal use and storage conditions. Strong oxidizing agent. Reacts with other household chemicals such as toilet bowl cleaners, rust removers, vinegar, acids or ammonia containing products to produce hazardous gases, such as chlorine and other chlorinated species. Prolonged contact with metal may cause pitting or discoloration.

VIII – FIRE AND EXPLOSION DATA

Not flammable or explosive. In a fire, cool containers to prevent rupture and release of sodium chlorate.

IX – PHYSICAL DATA

Boiling point.................................212°F/100°C (decomposes)
Specific Gravity (H_2O = 1)............1.085
Solubility in Water.........................complete
pH..11.4

FIGURE 5–10

Example of a Material Safety Data Sheet (MSDS)

BOX 5–3

Important Protective Measures for Chemical Use

- The proper personal protective equipment and clothing must be worn when a health care worker is working with chemicals.
- A buttoned laboratory coat, safety glasses, face shield, and gloves provide protection and prevent skin contact. The laboratory coat must provide optimal protection against chemicals and infectious agents. Aprons may be used to provide additional protection.
- When transporting acids or alkalis, an acid carrier—a specially designed container for carrying large quantities of hazardous solutions—should be used.
- The entrance of any room in which hazardous chemicals are in use or in storage must be posted with a caution sign specifying the types of chemicals present.
- No chemicals should be stored above eye level because of the danger of breakage or spillage involved in reaching for them.
- No chemicals should be stored in unlabeled containers.
- No chemicals should be poured into previously used containers or dirty containers.
- All explosives should be stored in an explosion-proof or a fire-proof room that is separate from other flammable materials.

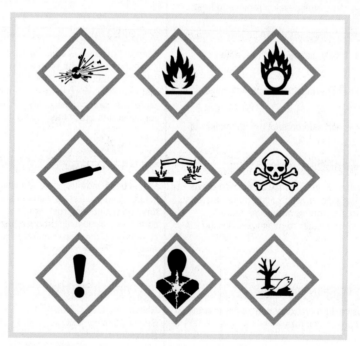

FIGURE 5–11

Labels Used to Identify Hazardous Materials in the Global Harmonization System (GHS).

These labels will become used more often as the GHS becomes worldwide as intended.

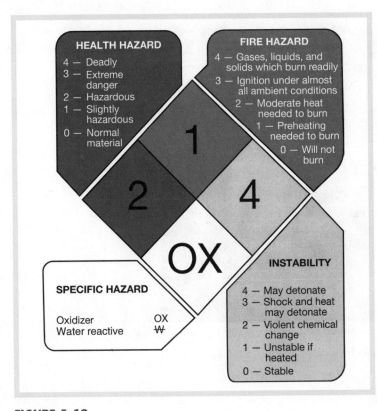

HEALTH HAZARD
4 — Deadly
3 — Extreme danger
2 — Hazardous
1 — Slightly hazardous
0 — Normal material

FIRE HAZARD
4 — Gases, liquids, and solids which burn readily
3 — Ignition under almost all ambient conditions
2 — Moderate heat needed to burn
1 — Preheating needed to burn
0 — Will not burn

SPECIFIC HAZARD

Oxidizer   OX
Water reactive   W̶

INSTABILITY
4 — May detonate
3 — Shock and heat may detonate
2 — Violent chemical change
1 — Unstable if heated
0 — Stable

FIGURE 5–12
NFPA 704 Marking System

Sodium Hypochlorite
(Bleach)

FIGURE 5–13
Example of OSHA-Mandated Labeling

scale of 0 to 4. The health hazard is shown in the blue quadrant, the flammability hazard is shown in the red quadrant, the instability hazard is indicated in the yellow quadrant, and the specific hazard is shown in the white quadrant. The red, blue, and yellow quadrants will each contain a number from 0 to 4. The number 4 indicates a high degree of hazard, and 0 indicates a low degree of hazard. The white quadrant will contain markings referring to a specific type of hazard such as an oxidizer (OX) or water reactivity (W). The W symbol indicates not to use water to suppress a fire in that marked area. Common laboratory chemicals such as isopropyl alcohol or diluted bleach (sodium hypochlorite) in squirt bottles require regulatory labels (**FIGURE 5–13**).

SAFETY SHOWERS AND THE EYEWASH STATION

Safety showers should be nearby for use if an accidental chemical spill occurs. Because permanent damage to the skin can result from chemical burns, the victim of a chemical accident must immediately rinse for at least 15 minutes after removing contaminated clothing.

In case of a chemical spill in the eye, the victim should rinse his or her eyes at the eyewash station for a minimum of 15 minutes (**FIGURE 5–14**). Contact lenses must be removed prior to the rinsing in

Clinical Alert ! A rule of thumb for chemicals is to ALWAYS add acid to water or other liquids. NEVER add water to acid! It can lead to a sudden chemical reaction that causes hazardous spatters and splashing.

ALERT

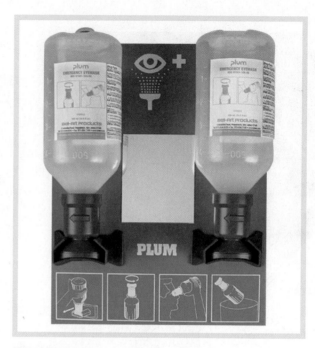

FIGURE 5–14
Eye Wash Station

Courtesy of Bel-Art Products

order to thoroughly cleanse the eyes. The victim should not rub his or her eyes because doing so may cause further injury. It is preferable to take the victim to the emergency department for treatment after his or her eyes have been rinsed for 15 minutes.

CHEMICAL SPILL CLEAN-UP

If a chemical spill occurs, the health care worker should immediately obtain a spill clean-up kit from the clinical chemistry section and contact the appropriate safety department for assistance. The kit includes absorbents and neutralizers to clean up acid, alkali, mercury, and other spills (**FIGURE 5–15**).

The absorbent and neutralizer used depend on the type of chemical spill; they have an indicator system that identifies when the spill has been neutralized and can be considered safe for sweep up and disposal. Avoid breathing vapors from the spill. In addition, rubber gloves and other appropriate personal protective equipment should be immediately available for the clean-up. The health care worker should become familiar with the procedures for cleaning up chemical spills in his or her place of employment and emergency contact phone numbers at the health care facility.

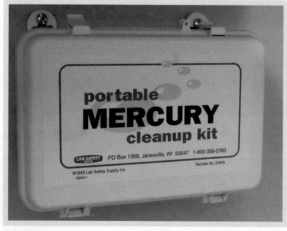

FIGURE 5–15
A Spill Clean-Up Kit

DISPOSAL OF CHEMICALS

Chemical disposal procedures must comply with all local and state regulations. Certain chemicals can be disposed of in sanitary sewer systems in accordance with the regulations. Thus, the health care worker must be familiar with the laboratory procedures for chemical waste disposal.

Equipment and Safety in Patients' Rooms

Each member of the health care team is responsible for the safety of the patient.[4] All health care professionals are responsible for patient safety from the time the patient enters the health care setting until his or her departure. First, when collecting blood from a hospitalized patient, provide privacy for the patient during the procedure (**FIGURE 5–16**).

As a matter of general patient safety, do the following in the patient's room:

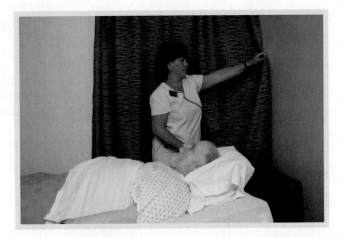

FIGURE 5–16
Patient Privacy

1. Make certain that all specimen collection supplies, needles, and equipment are either properly disposed of or returned to the specimen collection tray after blood collection.
2. Check to see whether the bed rails are up or down. If the bed rails were up when you entered the room, always be sure they are up before leaving the patient.
3. Check for food or liquid spilled on the floor, urine spills, or intravenous (IV) line leakage. Floors on which the patient and health care professionals walk must be dry. They should be free of obstacles and slipping hazards. Thus, in cases of spills, make certain that the area is cleaned and dried for the safety of the patients and hospital personnel.
4. During blood collection, be very cautious not to touch any electrical instrument located adjacent to the patient's bed, because if the instrument malfunctions, the health care worker may ground the patient and, as a result, a microshock could pass through the health care worker and into the patient. A serious problem could result from such a shock if the patient has an electrolyte imbalance or is wet with perspiration or other fluid. Furthermore, the needle inserted in the patient's arm could produce ventricular fibrillation and death if the patient has a pacemaker or an unstable heart ailment.
5. Report the following problem immediately to the nursing station: If the patient has an IV line and the site is swollen and red, the IV needle is probably no longer in the vein, which means that the IV solution is infiltrating into the surrounding tissues. Some chemicals in IV solutions are toxic to body tissue, so gangrene could result from such infiltration. Also, if blood is backing up the IV line from the needle insertion to the IV drip container, the IV solution container is empty. Report this problem immediately.
6. If the patient's alarm for the IV drip is sounding, report this problem to the nursing station immediately.
7. If the patient is in unusual pain or is unresponsive, notify the nursing station immediately.

Patient Safety Outside the Room

Health care workers should be aware of possible hazards to patients outside the patients' rooms. As a matter of general safety practice, the following guidelines should be followed:

1. Because trays, carts, and ladders may be placed around a hallway corner, the health care worker should be careful not to travel too quickly from one room to another and around corners.
2. Items lying on the floor, such as flower petals, may cause someone to slip and should be reported for clean-up.
3. Avoid running in a health care facility, because patients and visitors may become alarmed and begin to run as well. Also, someone may be hurt if the health care worker runs into him or her (e.g., a cardiac patient walking in the hall with an IV stand or another health care worker carrying a specimen collection tray).

Patient Safety Related to Latex Products

Patients, as well as health care workers, may be allergic to latex products (**FIGURE 5–17**). The signs and symptoms of an allergic reaction to latex may include a skin rash; hives; nasal, eye, or sinus irritation; and sometimes shock. **TABLE 5–2** provides examples of items frequently used in the health care environment that contain latex. **FIGURE 5–18** shows an example of a "Latex-Safe Environment" sign.

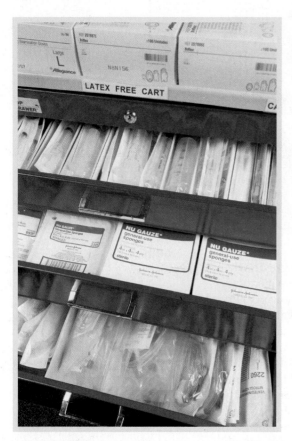

FIGURE 5–17
Latex-Free Cart

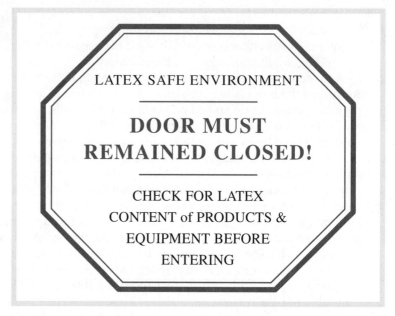

LATEX SAFE ENVIRONMENT

DOOR MUST REMAINED CLOSED!

CHECK FOR LATEX CONTENT of PRODUCTS & EQUIPMENT BEFORE ENTERING

FIGURE 5–18
Latex-Safe Environment Sign

Disaster Emergency Plan

Many health care institutions have developed procedures to be followed in case of a hurricane, flooding, earthquake, bomb threat, and other disasters. The health care worker should become familiar with these procedures because he or she must be prepared to take immediate action whenever conditions warrant (**FIGURE 5–19**).

TABLE 5–2

Products Containing Latex

Medical Equipment	Personal Protective Equipment	Office Supplies	Medical Supplies
Tourniquets	Gloves	Adhesive tape	Condom-style urinary collection device
Syringes	Goggles	Erasers	Enema tubing tips
Stethoscopes	Rubber aprons	Rubber bands	Injection ports
Oral and nasal airways	Surgical masks		Rubber tops of stoppers on multidose vials
IV tubing			Urinary catheter
Disposable gloves			Wound drains
Breathing circuits			
Blood pressure cuffs			

Source: Reprinted from *Preventing Allergic Reactions to Natural Rubber Latex in the Workplace,* The Centers for Disease Control and Prevention, National Institute for Occupational Safety and Health Alert, Atlanta, GA, June 1997.

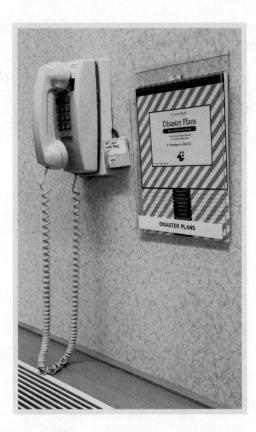

FIGURE 5–19
Disaster Plans and Phone

Emergency Procedures

The health care worker should become knowledgeable of emergency care procedures because accidents do occur even though precautionary measures are in place. He or she must be able to detach him- or herself from the emergency situation to some degree in order to perform well and deliver the best possible health care. In an emergency situation, the following objectives must be met for the victim: Prevent severe bleeding, maintain breathing, prevent shock and further injury, and send for medical assistance.

BLEEDING AID

Severe bleeding from an open wound can be controlled by applying pressure directly over the wound. The Occupational Safety and Health Administration requires adherence to "standard precautions" when health care workers respond to emergencies that provide potential exposure to blood and other potentially infectious materials. Health care workers responding to an emergency should be protected from exposure to blood and other potentially infectious materials through the use of personal protective equipment (gloves, mask, etc.). A clean handkerchief or other clean cloth (compress) should be placed over the wound before applying pressure with a gloved hand. In an emergency in which a clean cloth is not available, a gloved hand should be used until a cloth compress can

Clinical Alert ! Follow these procedures if someone telephones and threatens to bomb the health care facility:

- Listen to the person and keep him or her talking.
- Listen for background noises for caller's location.
- Listen for caller's accent, language, and so on.
- Ask the caller where the bomb is located and what time it will go off.
- Write down everything the caller says.
- Notify the health care facility's security officer.

If a bomb threat procedure is in place, it needs to be used by all health care workers.

ALERT

be located. Bleeding of a limb (i.e., an arm or a leg) can be decreased by elevation. The injured portion should be raised above the level of the victim's heart unless the injured portion is broken. Even with elevation, however, pressure should be maintained on the wound until medical assistance arrives. A tourniquet should not be used to control bleeding except in the case of an amputated, mangled, or crushed arm or leg or for profuse bleeding that cannot be stopped otherwise.

CIRCULATION AID

To maintain circulation in a victim, a health care provider must know the techniques of basic CPR (**PROCEDURE 5–1**). Thus, he or she should check with the supervisor about the availability of CPR classes at the health care institution, because this emergency technique must be demonstrated so that the employee can learn the proper skills.

PROCEDURE 5–1

Breathing Aid

Rationale   To apply immediate mouth-to-mouth resuscitation when a victim's breathing movements stop or her or his lips, tongue, or fingernails become blue

(*Note:* Any delay in using this technique may cost the victim's life.)

Equipment

- Mouth-to-mouth barrier device

Procedure

To perform mouth-to-mouth breathing, do the following:

1 See if the victim is conscious by gently tapping the shoulders of the victim and speaking loudly, "ARE YOU OKAY?" (**FIGURE 5–20**). If there is no response, call out for help and start aid immediately.

2 Place the victim on his or her back on a firm, flat surface. Exercise caution if the person has a spinal or neck injury. Avoid twisting the victim's body.

3 Open the airway passage by checking for obstructions: tongue, chewing gum, vomitus, and so on.

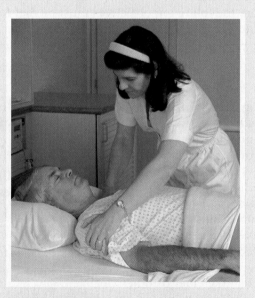

FIGURE 5–20

Breathing Aid (continued)

4 Place one hand on the victim's forehead and, applying firm, backward pressure with the palm, tilt the head back (**FIGURE 5–21**). Place the fingers of the other hand under the bony part of the victim's lower jaw, near the chin, and lift to bring the chin forward until the teeth are nearly closed. Support the jaw as the head is tilted back. This position is called the head-tilt/chin-lift.

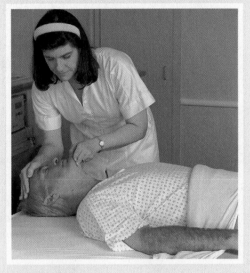

FIGURE 5–21

5 Listen and feel for return of air from the victim's mouth and nose for approximately 3 to 5 seconds (**FIGURE 5–22**). Also, simultaneously, look for the victim's chest to rise and fall.

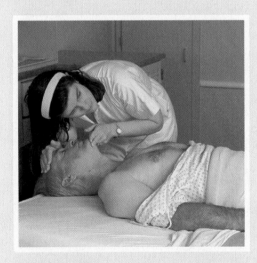

FIGURE 5–22

6 If there is no breathing, maintain the head-tilt/chin-lift and pinch the victim's nose shut with your fingers to prevent air from escaping. Open your mouth widely, take a deep breath, and seal your mouth over the victim's mouth with a barrier device (**FIGURE 5–23**). Blow into the victim's mouth by giving two rescue breaths, each over one second with enough volume to produce a visible chest rise. Watch for the victim's chest to rise.

7 Give two full ventilations. If this still does not start an air exchange, reposition the head and try again. Again, look, listen, and feel for breathing. Improper chin and head positioning is the most common cause of difficulty with ventilation.

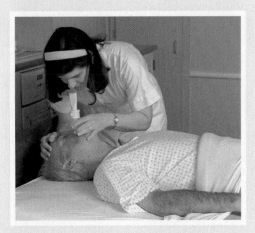

FIGURE 5–23

SHOCK PREVENTION

Shock usually accompanies severe injury. It may result from bleeding, extensive burns, an insufficient oxygen (O_2) supply, and other traumatic events. Early signs include pale, cold, clammy skin; weakness; a rapid pulse; an increased, shallow breathing rate; and frequently, nausea and vomiting. The main objectives in treating a shock victim are to improve circulation, to provide sufficient O_2, and to maintain normal body temperature.

The following six actions are recommended if first aid is given to a shock victim:

1. Correct the cause of shock if possible (e.g., control bleeding).
2. Keep the victim lying down.
3. Keep the victim's airway open. If he or she vomits, turn the head to the side so that the neck is arched.
4. In the absence of broken bones, elevate the victim's legs so that the head is lower than the trunk of the body.
5. Keep the victim warm.
6. Call for emergency assistance.

Actions that are *not* recommended include the following:

1. Giving fluids to a victim who has an abdominal injury (because the person is likely to require surgery or a general anesthetic)
2. Giving fluids to an unconscious or semiconscious person

Study Questions

The following may have one or more answers.

1 What organization developed a labeling system for hazardous chemicals that are frequently used in health care facilities?

a. CDC
b. FDA
c. NFPA
d. CLSI

2 If a chemical is spilled onto a health care worker, he or she should first

a. rinse the area with a neutral chemical to stop the possibility of a burn
b. rub the area affected by the chemical with one hand
c. rinse the area with water
d. wait to see whether it starts to burn the skin

3 Global Harmonization System includes which of the following?

a. hazardous materials classification
b. fire extinguisher types
c. electrical circuit safety standards
d. laboratory equipment maintenance

4 Which of the following is a main objective in treating a shock victim?

a. improve circulation
b. provide sufficient drinking water
c. provide sufficient food for maintaining energy
d. maintain a cold body temperature to suppress tissue damage

5 The first step in providing breathing aid to a victim in an emergency situation is to

a. place the victim on his or her back
b. see if the victim is conscious by gently tapping shoulders
c. place one hand on the victim's forehead to tilt backward
d. send for medical assistance

6 Which of the following should occur first if a fire breaks out in the health care facility?

a. run from the floor where the fire is located
b. call the assigned fire number
c. use the fastest elevator to escape from the floor where the fire is located
d. open all windows before leaving the area of the fire

7 Safety equipment in the chemical area of the health care facility will most likely include

a. a mouth-to-mouth barrier device
b. a dosimeter reader
c. a respirator mask
d. an emergency shower

8 The hazard labeling system developed by the National Fire Protection Association has a blue quadrant to indicate

a. flammability hazard
b. health hazard
c. instability hazard
d. specific hazard

9 If an electrical accident occurs that involves electrical shock to an employee or a patient, the first thing that the health care worker should do is

a. move the victim
b. shut off electrical power
c. start CPR
d. place a blanket over the victim

10 What are the major principles of self-protection from radiation exposure?

a. distance, using MSDS, shielding
b. time, reactivity, instability
c. combustibility, flash point, distance
d. shielding, time, distance

Case Study

The clinical laboratory supervisor needs an inventory of the Globalization Harmonization System's safety data sheets for the laboratory inspection process. She has asked you to look up the SDS for bleach that is diluted and used to disinfect the countertops and other items in the laboratory setting.

Questions

1 What is the chemical name for bleach?

2 Go to www.osha.gov/dsg/hazcom/ghs. html to find the safety data sheets for this chemical and then list

   a. the hazardous materials identification number for health and fire

   b. the first aid measures that should occur after skin contact

   c. handling and storage procedures for this chemical

3 Compare the SDS for this chemical to the previously used MSDS.

Action in Practice

Safety in Home Health Care Specimen Collections The home health aide, Maddie McGuy, works for Northshore Home Health Agency. Her job is multifaceted because she performs history and physical assessments, and when required, she collects blood for laboratory testing. One day she went to collect blood and urine samples from Ms. Hernandez, a 91-year-old woman who spoke very little English. She greeted Ms. Hernandez and found the bathroom and a suitable spot to collect blood from her. She felt confident that Ms. Hernandez had understood her communication. She was successful on the first attempt to collect the blood sample, and she helped Ms. Hernandez to the bathroom to collect the urine sample. Ms. Hernandez followed directions except she did not close the urine bottle tightly because she lacked the strength in her hands. Maddie did not notice that the lid was not on tightly. She placed all the specimens in the container she had brought. She decided to leave the container top open because she knew her next stop was just one block away. On the way to the next house, a car ran a stop sign so Maddie had to jam on the brakes of her car, and the container with specimens fell off the seat of the car. The urine specimen spilled all over the floor of her vehicle.

Questions

1 What could Maddie have done to avoid the situation?

2 What should Maddie do now?

Check Yourself

1 Locate at least two safety placards designated by the National Fire Protection Association 704 marking system in the area where you work.

2 What does the acronym PASS stand for as related to fire extinguishers?

Competency Checklist: Safety and First Aid

This checklist can be completed as a group or individually.

(1) Completed (2) Needs to improve

_____ 1. Describe the steps in providing "bleeding aid" to a victim.

_____ 2. Describe four protective measures for chemical use.

REFERENCES

1. National Fire Protection Association (NFPA). *National fire codes*. www.NFPA.org. (accessed March 2, 2008).

2. Centers for Disease Control and Prevention (CDC). *Preventing occupational exposure to antineoplastic and other hazardous drugs in health care settings*. www.cdc.gov/niosh/docs/2004-165/pdfs/2004-165.pdf (accessed December 31, 2012).

3. https://www.osha.gov/Publications/osha3021.pdf US Dept of Labor OSHA Workers' Rights 3021-09R 2011

4. The Joint Commission. (2012). *2012 national patient safety goals*. www.jointcommision.org/PatientSafety/NationalPatientSafetyGoals/012_lab_npsgs.htm (retrieved December 31, 2012).

RESOURCES

Department of Transportation (DOT). Materials, Transportation Bureau, Information Services Division, Washington, DC 20402. (202) 366–4000.

Dickinson, E. (Ed.) (2003). *First responder: A skills approach*, 6th ed. Upper Saddle River, NJ: Prentice Hall.

www.cap.org College of American Pathologists (CAP).

www.cdc.gov Centers for Disease Control and Prevention (CDC).

www.nfpa.org National Fire Protection Association (NFPA).

www.jointcommission.org The Joint Commission.

www.osha.gov/dsg/hazcom/ghs.html (OSHA).

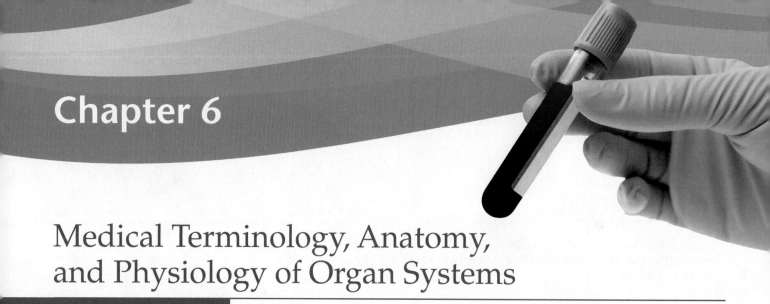

Chapter 6

Medical Terminology, Anatomy, and Physiology of Organ Systems

Chapter Objectives

Upon completion of Chapter 6, the learner is responsible
for doing the following:

1. Define medical terminology using word elements such as roots, prefixes, and suffixes.

2. Define words commonly used in the clinical laboratory.

3. Describe how laboratory testing is used to assess body functions and disease.

4. Define the differences among the terms *anatomy*, *physiology*, and *pathology*.

5. Describe the directional terms, anatomic surface regions, and cavities of the body.

6. Describe the role of homeostasis in normal body functioning.

7. Describe the purpose, function, and structural components of the major body systems.

8. Identify examples of pathologic conditions associated with each organ system.

9. Describe the types of specimens that are analyzed in the clinical laboratory.

10. List common diagnostic tests associated with each organ system.

Medical Terminology

Chapter 2 discussed communication using verbal and nonverbal methods, but the actual *definitions*, or literal meanings, of words refer to another essential aspect of professional communication. Health care workers must learn how to pronounce basic medical terms, know what they mean, and actually use the correct terms in practice to be productive and respected members of the team. Each field of medicine may have unique technical terms; however, there are fundamental tools that make learning and understanding the terms easier. Medical terminology becomes less awkward with practice and strategies to understand how words are formed.

Medical terms are different from everyday English language because they sound different, they come primarily from Greek or Latin origins, there can be more than one word element for a particular meaning, and changing a simple prefix can change the entire meaning of the word. Hippocrates, a Greek physician (460–377 BC), developed standards for medical practice and early terminology, but since technology rapidly changes, new terms are continuously developing. Many terms for the body's organs or structures originate from Latin—for instance, *vessel* comes from the Latin word *vascillum*, or "little vessel," and *capillary* originates from *capillus*, or "hairlike." Most of the terms that describe diseases originate from Greek—for example, *lipo-* means "fat" and *-oma* means tumor, so *lipoma* means a "fatty tumor"; *hepat-* means "liver" and *-itis* means "inflammation," so *hepatitis* means "inflammation of the liver."[1]

Medical terms consist of several parts:

- **Word root (R)**—The word root is the main part of the word that describes what the word is about—for example, *cardio-* is the word root for *heart*, so every time a medical term contains *cardio-*, it has something to do with the heart, and *phleb-* is a word root relating to *vein*.

- **Prefix (P)**—The prefix is added *before* the root, at the *beginning of the word*. It makes the word more specific—for example, *endo-* is the prefix meaning "inside."

- **Suffix (S)**—The suffix is added *after* the root, at the *end of the word*. It also adds to the meaning of the root—for example, *-itis* is the suffix for "inflammation," and *-tomy* is the suffix for "cut or incision."

- **Combining vowel (CV)**—Sometimes a vowel (usually *i, o, u,* or *y*) is added to make a word easier to pronounce. It does not add meaning. The combining vowel *o* is most often used in medical terminology—for example, *steth-* is the word root for *chest*, and *-scope* is the suffix for *instrument*; inserting an *o* between them makes the new word easier to say *(stethoscope)*.

Combining the examples just given results in the following words:

- **Endocarditis**—(endo/card/itis) is an inflammation of the inside lining of the heart. In this example, there was no need to add a CV because the prefix already has an *o*.

- **Microscope**—(micro/scope) is an instrument for examining small objects. In this example, again, there was no need to add a CV.

- **Phlebotomy**—(phleb/o/tomy) is a cut or incision into the vein. In this example, the *o* in the middle helps make the pronunciation easier.

When different prefixes or suffixes are added to the word root, the meaning changes. You can build a huge medical vocabulary by learning the meanings of Greek and Latin word parts and how to combine them (see **FIGURE 6–1** and **TABLES 6–1**, **6–2**, **6–3**, and **6–4**).[1]

KEY TERMS CONTINUED

nervous system
neurons
nucleolus
nucleus
occult blood
oliguria
organelles
organ systems
osteomyelitis
osteoporosis
ova and parasites (O&P)
pathogenesis
pathology
peristalsis
peritoneal fluid
physiology
pituitary gland
pleural fluid
posterior
proteinemia
proteinuria
proximal
pulse rate
red blood cells (RBCs)
reproductive system
respiration rate
respiratory acidosis
respiratory alkalosis
respiratory system
sensory neurons
skeletal (striated voluntary) muscles
skeletal system
steady state
superficial
synovial fluid
urinary system
ventral
visceral (nonstriated, smooth, involuntary) muscles

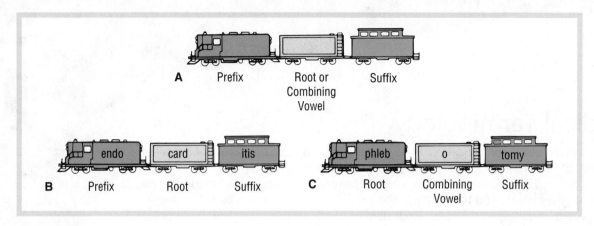

FIGURE 6–1
Word Elements in Medical Terminology

BASIC RULES FOR COMBINING WORD ELEMENTS

A few basic rules make medical terminology easier to learn and use and help in avoiding mistakes.[1] Remember that changing a simple prefix can change the entire meaning of a word. Always be cautious about correct spelling and pronunciation of terms, especially diagnostic laboratory tests and abbreviations. Health care workers involved in specimen collections must ensure accuracy in the terminology they use. (Refer to Appendices 6, 9, and 10 for additional information about common laboratory assays, units of measurement, symbols, abbreviations, and formulas commonly used in the clinical laboratory.)

TABLE 6–1

Primary Word Elements: Prefixes

Prefixes That Pertain to Position or Placement		
ab away from	**epi** upon, above	**meso** middle
ad toward	**ex** out, away from	**para** beside
ana up	**extra** outside, beyond	**peri** through
ante before	**hyper** above, excessive	**retro** backward
cata down	**hypo** below, deficient	**sub** below, under
circum, peri around	**infra** below	**super** above
ecto out, outer	**inter** between	**supra** above, beyond
endo within	**intra** within	
Prefixes That Pertain to Numbers and Amounts		
ambi both	**milli** one-thousandth	**quadri** four
bi two, double	**multi** many, much	**quint** five
centi a hundred	**nano** 10^{-9}, tiny	**semi, hemi** half
deca ten	**nulli** none	**tetra** four
dipl double	**poly** many	**tri** three
di (s) two	**primi** first	**uni** one
Prefixes That Are Descriptive and Are Used in General		
a, an without, lack of	**dys** bad, before, difficult	**oligo** scanty, little
ante, anti, contra against	**eu** good	**pan** all
auto self	**hetero** different	**pre** before, in front of
brachy short	**homeo** similar, same	**pro** before
brady slow	**hydro** water	**pseudo** false
cac, mal bad	**mega** large, great	**sym, syn** together
dia through	**micro** small	

Adapted from J. Rice, *Medical Terminology: A Word Building Approach.* Upper Saddle River, NJ: Prentice Hall, 2008, updated 2013.

TABLE 6–2

Primary Word Roots Related to the Cardiovascular System

Root	Meaning
ang/i, angi/o, vas/o	vessel
angin	to choke
arter	artery
arteri/o	artery
ather/o	fatty substance, porridge
capillus	hairlike
card	heart
card/i, cardi/o	heart
cubitum	elbow, forearm
cyte	cell
derm	skin
electr/o	electricity
embol	to cast, to throw
erg/o	work
erythr/o	red
hem/o	blood
infarct	infarct (necrosis of an area)
lipid	fat
log	study
man/o	thin
my/o	muscle
phleb	vein
phleb/o	vein
pulmonar	lung
rrhyth	rhythm
scler	hardening
sera	serum
sphygm/o	pulse
steth/o	chest
tens	tension
thromb	clot
ven/i	vein

Adapted from J. Rice, *Medical Terminology: A Word Building Approach.* Upper Saddle River, NJ: Prentice Hall, 2008, updated 2013.

- Practice using medical terminology with someone who is familiar with the correct pronunciation. A study partner can give you tips about the sound of the word so that confusion is avoided. It is even recommended that you read this section out loud. (Also remember the lessons from Chapter 2 about pace, volume, and tone of voice.) Following are some basic tips on pronunciation:
  - *ch* most often sounds like *k;* for example, *chronic* (kro-nic).
  - *ps* sounds like *s;* for example, *psychology* (si-kol-o-jee).
  - *pn* sounds like *n;* for example, *pneumonia* (nu-mo-ni-a).
  - *c* sounds like an *s* when it comes before *e, i,* and *y;* for example, *cytoplasm* (si-to-plazm), *centrifuge* (sen-tri-fuj).
  - *g* sounds like *j* when it comes before *e, i,* and *y;* for example, *generic* (jen-er-ik).
  - *i* sounds like *eye* when added to the end of a word to form a plural; for example, *bacilli* (ba-sil-li), *bronchi* (bron-ki).

TABLE 6–3

Primary Word Elements: Suffixes

Suffixes That Pertain to Pathologic Conditions		
-algia, dynia pain	**-oma** tumor	**-ptosis** drooping
-cele hernia, tumor, swelling	**-osis** condition of	**-ptysis** spitting
-emesis vomiting	**-pathy** disease	**-rrhage** bursting forth
-itis inflammation	**-penia** deficiency	**-rrhagia** bursting forth
-lysis destruction, separation	**-phobia** fear	**-rrhea** flow, discharge
-megaly enlargement, large	**-plegia** paralysis, stroke	**-rrhexis** rupture
-oid resemble		

Suffixes Used in Diagnostic and Surgical Procedures		
-centesis surgical puncture	**-opsy** to view	**-stasis** control, stopping
-desis binding	**-plasty** surgical repair	**-stomy** new opening
-ectomy surgical excision	**-plexy** surgical fixation	**-tome** instrument to cut
-gram a weight, mark, record	**-rrhaphy** suture	**-tomy** incision
-graph to write, record	**-scope** instrument	**-tripsy** crushing
-meter measure	**-scopy** to view	

Suffixes That Are Used in General		
-blast immature cell, germ cell	**-phasia** to speak	**-pnea** breathing
-cyte cell	**-philia** attraction	**-poiesis** formation
-ist one who specializes, agent	**-phraxis** to obstruct	**-therapy** treatment
-logy study of	**-physis** growth	**-trophy** nourishment, development
-phagia to eat	**-plasia** formation, produce	**-uria** urine

Adapted from J. Rice, *Medical Terminology: A Word Building Approach.* Upper Saddle River, NJ: Prentice Hall, 2008, updated 2013.

- The combining vowel is often an *o*. For example, **osteoporosis** (oste/o/por/osis) is a condition in which the bone becomes porous. It is easier to say with the addition of the *o* than to say "osteporosis."
  - When the suffix starts with a vowel, there is no need to use a combining vowel; for example, gastr/ (stomach) + *o*ma (tumor) = gastroma, a tumor of the stomach.
  - If there are two or more roots in a term, keep both combining vowels; for example, electr*o* (electricity) + cardi*o* (heart) + -gram (record) = electrocardiogram.
- When changing a word from the singular to plural, substitute the plural endings as follows:
  - *-a* as in *bursa* to *-ae* as in *bursae*
  - *-ax* as in *thorax* to *-aces* as in *thoraces*
  - *-nx* as in *phalanx* to *-nges* as in *phalanges*
  - *-en* as in *foramen* to *-ina* as in *foramina*
  - *-is* as in *crisis* to *-es* as in *crises*
  - *-ix* as in *appendix* to *-ices* as in *appendices*
  - *-on* as in *spermatozoon* to *-a* as in *spermatozoa*
  - *-um* as in *ovum* to *-a* as in *ova*
  - *-us* as in *nucleus* to *-i* as in *nuclei*
  - *-y* as in *artery* to *-i* and add *-es* as in *arteries* or phlebotomy to *phlebotomies*
- Some words of Greek origin are hard to spell because they may begin with a silent letter or have a silent letter within the word. Correct spelling is important because one mistake can change the meaning. The examples that follow demonstrate this:
  - *kn*, *mn*, and *pn* are pronounced as *n* as in *knuckle, mnemonic, pneumonia*
  - *ps* is pronounced as *s* as in *psychiatry*

TABLE 6–4

Using Common Suffixes

The suffix -*ology* is common in health care; it means "the study of." Here are some examples of specialty areas in health care.

Term	The study of . . .
Anesthesiology	Loss of sensation/pain management
Cardiology	Diseases of the heart, arteries, veins, and capillaries
Cytology	Cellular structure and functions
Dermatology	Skin
Endocrinology	Diseases of the endocrine (glands and hormones) system
Epidemiology	Epidemic diseases
Gastroenterology	Diseases of the stomach or intestinal or digestive system
Gynecology	Diseases of the female reproductive system
Hematology	Blood and blood-forming tissues
Histology	Microscopic structures of tissues
Immunology	Diseases of the immune system; allergic disorders
Microbiology	Microbes
Nanotechnology	Engineering devices of the smallest sizes
Nephrology	Diseases of the kidney and urinary systems
Neurology	Diseases of the nervous system
Oncology	Tumors
Ophthalmology	Diseases of the eye
Parasitology	Parasites
Pathology	Pathogens or disease-causing agents
Proctology	Diseases of the rectum, colon, anus
Psychiatry	Disorders of the mind
Radiology	Radioactive substances used in prevention, diagnosis, treatment
Serology	Antibodies in the serum
Urology	Urinary system

The suffix -*itis* is common in health care; it means "inflammation of." Here are some examples of disorders/diseases using this suffix.

Term	Inflammation of the . . .
Appendicitis	Appendix
Arthritis	Joints
Bursitis	Bursa
Cholecystitis	Gall bladder
Colitis	Colon
Cystitis	Bladder
Dermatitis	Skin
Diverticulitis	Colon wall
Encephalitis	Brain
Gastritis	Stomach wall
Gastroenteritis	Stomach and intestines
Hepatitis	Liver
Meningitis	Meninges
Nephritis	Kidney
Osteochondritis	Bone and cartilage
Osteomyelitis	Bone
Pancreatitis	Pancreas
Peritonitis	Abdominal wall
Rhinitis	Nasal membranes
Tendonitis	Tendons
Tonsillitis	Tonsils

- *pt* is pronounced as *t* as in *ptosis*
- *g* is silent in the word *phlegm* (pronounced flem)
- changing one letter, *b* to *d,* changes the word meaning, for example, *abduct,* meaning to lead away, changes to *adduct,* meaning toward the middle
- *anti-* means against; *ante-* means before or forward
- *hyper-* means above, beyond, or excessive; *hypo-* means below, under
- *peri-* means around; *per-,* means through

Anatomy and Physiology Overview

The design of the human body is elaborate and sophisticated. **Anatomy** is the study of its physical structure and **physiology** is the study of its functional processes. A human body can be divided into eight structural levels:

1. Atoms (carbon, hydrogen, oxygen, nitrogen, iron, etc.)
2. Molecules (chemical constituents)
3. **Organelles** or small structures within cells
4. Cells (the basic living units of all plants and animals)
5. Tissues (groups of similar cells)
6. Organs (two or more tissues)
7. **Organ systems** (groups of organs)
8. The organism (the human body) itself

Trillions of cells make up each individual (**TABLE 6–5**). Similar groups of cells are combined into tissues, such as muscles or nerves, and tissues are combined into systems,

TABLE 6–5

Terms and Definitions that Describe the Human Cell

Cell Structures/Terms	Definition or Primary Functions
Cell membrane	Protects the cell; provides for communication via receptor proteins; surface proteins serve as positive identification tags; allows some substances to pass into and out of the cell while denying passage to other substances; this selectivity allows cells to receive nutrition and dispose of waste.
Cytoplasm	Provides storage and work areas for the cell; the work and storage elements of the cell, called *organelles,* are the ribosomes, endoplasmic reticulum, Golgi apparatus, mitochondria, lysosomes, and centrioles.
Ribosomes	Make enzymes and other proteins; nicknamed "protein factories."
Endoplasmic reticulum (ER)	Carries proteins and other substances through the cytoplasm.
Golgi apparatus	Chemically processes the molecules from the endoplasmic reticulum and then packages them into vesicles; nicknamed "chemical processing and packaging center."
Mitochondria	Involved in cellular metabolism and respiration; provide the principal source of cellular energy and are the place where complex, energy-releasing chemical reactions occur continuously; nicknamed "power plants."
Lysosomes	Contain enzymes that can digest food compounds; nicknamed "digestive bags."
Centrioles	Play an important role in cell reproduction.
Cilia	Hairlike structure(s) that project from epithelial cells; help propel mucus, dust particles, and other foreign substance from the respiratory tract.
Flagellum	"Tail" of the sperm that enables the sperm to "swim" or move toward the ovum.
Nucleus (*nuclei* for two or more)	The control mechanism that governs the functions of the individual cell (i.e., growth, repair, reproduction, and metabolism). Inside the nucleus is a **nucleolus,** which also aids in cell metabolism and reproduction. The nucleus contains a genetic blueprint (**deoxyribonucleic acid, DNA**) with thousands of **genes** that code for an individual's characteristics, such as eye color, sex, and height. If the nucleus is damaged/destroyed, in most cases the cell will die; however, even though **red blood cells (RBCs)** lose their nuclei when they mature, the cells continue to carry O_2 for several months.
Chromosome	Threadlike array of nucleic acids and proteins found in the nucleus, that carries the genetic information in genes. There are 46 chromosomes in each nucleus of normal human cells. Each chromosome provides a code for different aspects of the body.

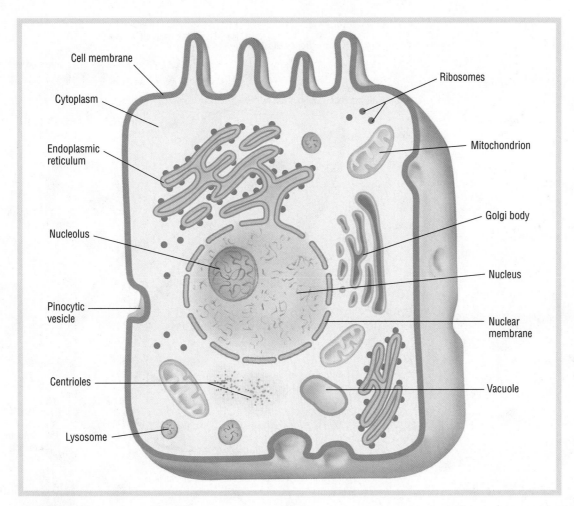

FIGURE 6–2

Cellular Structures

The size and shape of a cell depend on its function. Some cells fight disease-causing viruses and bacteria; some transport gases, such as oxygen (O_2) and carbon dioxide (CO_2); some produce movement, store nutrients, or manufacture proteins, chemicals, or liquids; and others, such as the egg and the sperm, can create a new life. Despite such diverse functions, most cells have basic structural elements in common.

such as the circulatory or reproductive system. These organ systems work simultaneously to serve the needs of the body. No one system works independently of the others (**FIGURES 6–2** and **6–3**).

Survival is the primary function of the human body, and many complex processes work independently and together to achieve this function. In human physiology, the body strives for a **steady state,** or **homeostasis.** Literally, *homeostasis* means "remaining the same." It is a condition in which a healthy body, although constantly changing and functioning, remains in a normal, healthy state of equilibrium. Homeostasis, or a steady-state condition, allows the normal body to stay in balance by compensating for changes. For example, if the body is taking in too much water, it responds to this imbalance by excreting water from the kidneys (urine), skin (perspiration), intestines (feces), and lungs (water in expiration). Another important concept for homeostasis is **metabolism,** which includes both the process of making necessary substances (**anabolism**—cells use energy to make complex compounds from simpler ones) or breaking down chemical substances in order to use energy (**catabolism**—chemical reactions to change complex substances into simpler ones while simultaneously *releasing* energy for the body to use).

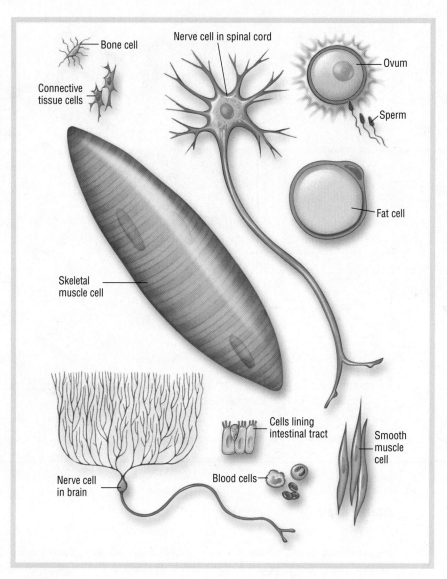

FIGURE 6–3
Examples of Human Cells

Both phases are required to maintain metabolic functions in a healthy individual. Body energy is always needed, whether for moving a chair, for allowing the heart to beat, for making tears, or for producing perspiration. A healthy body maintains constancy of its chemical components and processes in order to survive when environmental conditions are changing. Each organ system and body structure plays a part in maintaining homeostasis.

Health care workers can help assess homeostasis, or normal functioning, by taking "vital signs"—for example, temperature, **pulse rate,** and **respiration rate** (together known as *TPR*), and blood pressure. Methods for taking vital signs are described in Appendix 4.

In addition, clinical laboratory testing can provide a wealth of information about the individual organ systems and the integrated processes. Specimens, such as blood, bone marrow, urine, cerebrospinal fluid (CSF), **synovial** (joint) **fluid, pleural fluid** (from around the lungs), **ascites** or **peritoneal fluid** (from the abdominal cavity), pericardial fluid (from around the heart), biopsy tissue, semen, and others, can be microscopically

TABLE 6–6

Samples Collected from the Human Body

In a clinical or pathology laboratory, many types of samples are analyzed. Sometimes samples can be obtained easily in a clinic or at the patient's home; other times, minor surgery and anesthesia are required to remove the sample for analysis. Often the patient is somewhat embarrassed by the specimen collection process because it involves bodily wastes or fluids, or functions that are usually done in a private restroom. Health care workers should be sensitive to patients' privacy, especially when assistance is required in collecting the specimen.

Samples Eliminated Naturally	Examples
■ Can be collected by the patient ■ Usually painless ■ Can be collected at home or clinic ■ Printed instructions often suffice ■ May require verbal instructions ■ Elderly or children may need assistance	■ Urine: Patient urinates into a special container; instructions are given for cleansing prior to urinating; sometimes a catheter is inserted by a physician; sometimes 24-hour samples are collected in the hospital or at home. ■ Stool/Feces: Collected during toileting; instructions are given for food restrictions and to prevent contamination with urine. ■ Sputum: Patients will cough-up the specimen into a special container. ■ Semen: Male patients must ejaculate into a special container and instructions often include how to transport the specimen. ■ Saliva: Usually collected using a swab or expectorating into a special container.

Samples Collected Using a Swab	Examples
■ Can be collected in a clinic or hospital ■ Performed by a health professional ■ Painless or minor discomfort ■ Quick	■ Nose and Throat: Collected by moving a swab over the infected area; for throat, a quick gag reflex maybe uncomfortable but is brief; for nasal swab, the swab maybe inserted deep into the nasal passage and the discomfort is also brief. ■ Wounds: Swab is moved over the infected area to gather fluid or pus; since wounds or sores may be tender, it is likely that there will be brief pain. Sometimes a needle may be used to aspirate fluid or pus from the site. ■ Vaginal Secretions, Pap Smear: A swab or tiny brush is used to take sample; pain may be brief and position of the legs is uncomfortable for the patient.

Samples Requiring More Invasive Procedures	Examples
■ Range from minimally invasive fingerstick to venipuncture to minor surgery ■ Range from a few minutes (venipuncture) to longer procedures (biopsies) ■ All require specialized collection tubes, cleansing/sterilizing procedures, and appropriate training or certification to perform the procedures	■ Blood: Venipuncture, capillary punctures, or arterial punctures require penetrating the skin to access the blood vessel. Procedure is painful for a short duration. ■ Tissue Biopsy: Most commonly from breast, lung, or skin. Needle biopsies are performed by a physician, needle is inserted into the site and cells or fluid is withdrawn with a syringe. Tissue biopsies are done with surgical incision where a portion of the tissue is removed. ■ Cerebrospinal Fluid (CSF): Performed by a lumbar puncture (spinal tap) where needle is inserted between two vertebrae and into the spinal canal where CSF is withdrawn and placed into sterile vials. ■ Bone Marrow: Usually collected from the iliac crest of the hip bone; may require a sedative; requires a special needle for aspirating the marrow or collection of a core. Patient experiences brief discomfort and pain. ■ Other body fluids (synovial, peritoneal, pleural, pericardial) usually require aspiration using a needle and syringe and sterile container.

analyzed, assayed, and cultured to determine **pathogenesis** (the origin of the disease). Health care workers may have a part in the collection, processing, or testing of these specimens (**TABLE 6–6**).

Anatomic Regions and Positions

The human body has distinctive characteristics: a backbone, bisymmetry, body cavities, and 11 major organ systems. Anatomical terms provide a description of the body's landmarks. These terms are helpful during an assessment of a patient to make the patient's condition understandable to others. The following terms may be useful when evaluating a patient; describing a venipuncture complication, an interfering surgical wound site, or a burned area of the body; and searching for the location of a vein, artery, or potential venipuncture site (**FIGURES 6–4, 6–5, 6–6**, and **6–7**).

- **Anterior**: In front of (Example: I will collect a blood specimen from the *anterior* side of the arm.)
- **Posterior**: Toward the back (Example: There is a large bandage on the *posterior* side of the arm.)
- **Medial**: Toward the midline (Example: The heart is *medial* to the right shoulder.)

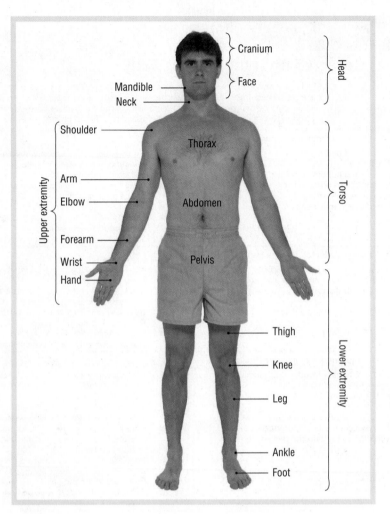

FIGURE 6–4
Body Regions

- **Lateral**: Toward the sides of the body (Example: The hip is *lateral* to the navel.)
- **Dorsal**: Back side (Example: The mole was on the *dorsal* side of her shoulder.)
- **Ventral**: Front side (Example: The scrape was on the *ventral* side of the knee.)
- **Proximal**: Near the point of attachment (Example: The leg broke on the *proximal* side of the knee.)
- **Distal**: Distant or away from the point of attachment (Example: The birthmark was *distal* to the wrist.)
- **Superficial**: Near the surface of the body (Example: *Superficial* veins show up easily on her skin.)
- **Deep**: Far from the surface of the body (Example: Major arteries are in the *deep* tissues.)

Terms that describe body positioning can also help communicate patient details prior to, during, or after a phlebotomy procedure including the following:

- **Normal Anatomic Position**—Erect, standing position with arms at rest and palms forward (Due to the risk of the patient fainting or falling, never perform a venipuncture on a patient who is standing.)

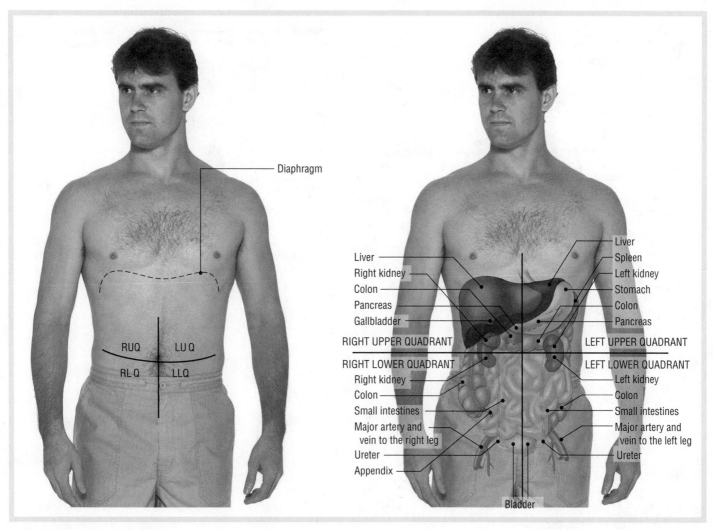

FIGURE 6–5
Abdominal Quadrants

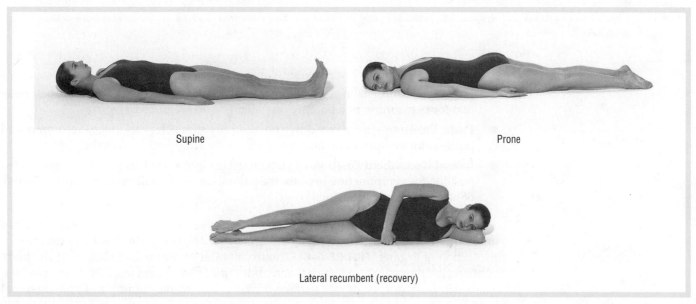

FIGURE 6–6
Anatomical Postures

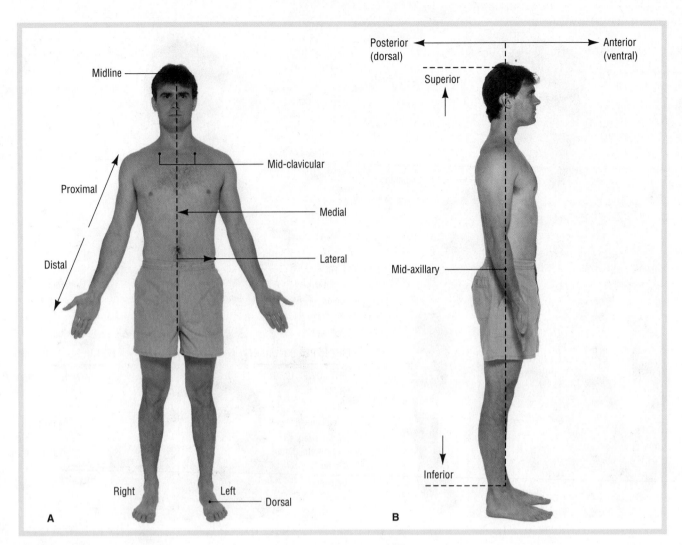

FIGURE 6–7

Terms Related to Body Orientation

Body movements and locations can be described in terms related to imaginary planes that divide the body. A. The sagittal plane (midline) divides the body into two halves. B. The plane that divides the body into front and back is referred to as the *superior/inferior plane* or the *cranial/caudal plane.*

- **Supine Position**—Lying or reclining face up on his or her back (This is the best position for performing phlebotomy on patients who are in bed.)

- **Prone Position**—Lying face down on his or her stomach (This is *not* a recommended position for venipuncture because of the awkward orientation of the arms.)

- **Lateral Recumbent Position**—Lying on left or right side (This is *not* a recommended position for venipuncture because the patient can easily roll over, increasing the risk of harmful needle insertion.)

Body regions can be categorized in various ways. One way is to begin at the top and work down in large regions, as in Figure 6–4. The body also has body cavities for protection of organs (**FIGURE 6–8**). The front, anterior, or ventral surface of the body contains the thoracic (lungs, heart) and abdominopelvic (stomach, intestines) cavities. The back, posterior, or dorsal surface contains the cranial (brain) and spinal (spinal

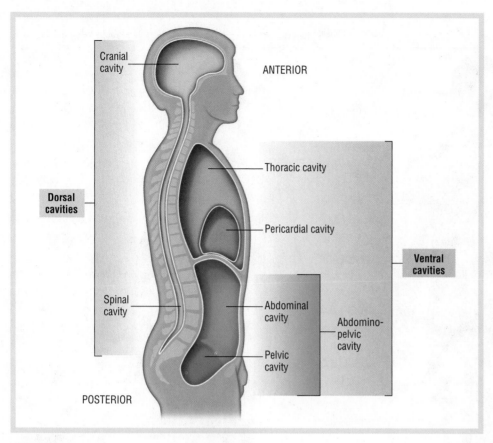

FIGURE 6–8
Body Cavities

cord) cavities. The human body can also be described according to imaginary planes or transecting lines, as in Figure 6–7. Areas and directions of the body can be described by their distance from or proximity to one of the **body planes** (**FIGURE 6–9**).

TABLES 6–7 and **6–8** offer further details about additional body regions that help locate areas and structures on the body. Develop mental imagery for anatomical structures, regions, and organs of the body. This becomes particularly important when dealing with the delicate anatomy of the arms, hands, and legs.

Clinical Alert ! When speaking with patients, health care workers should refer to the *patient's right* and the *patient's left* sides, not the health care worker's right or left side. This comes up when the health care worker asks to see a patient's right or left arm prior to vein selection for venipuncture. Even though the task seems easy, some health care workers confuse right and left arms when they are face to face with a patient. Practice using the terms by directly facing a friend and pointing to the friend's right and left side until it is done correctly each time. Do not confuse your own right and left side with the patient's right or left side. This task becomes important when there are specific instructions to collect blood from only one side of a patient because of a clinical condition.

ALERT

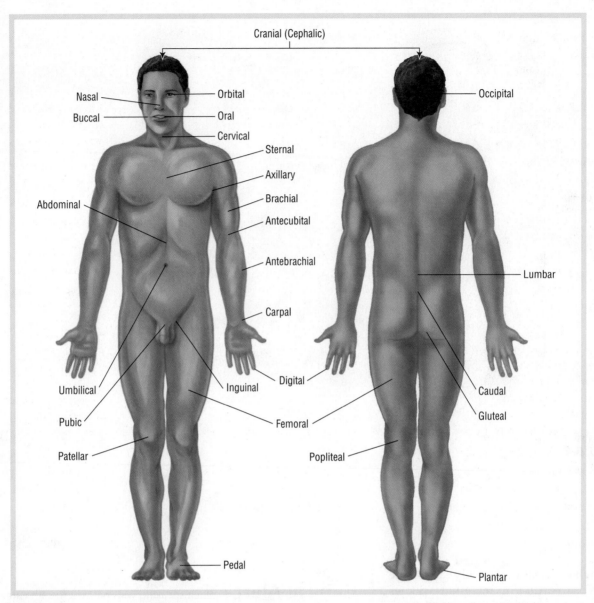

FIGURE 6–9
Anterior and Posterior Body Regions

TABLE 6–7

Directional Terminology

Directional Term	Meaning	Use in a Sentence
Proximal	Near point of reference	The wrist is *proximal* to the fingers.
Distal	Away from point of reference	The shoulder is *distal* to the fingers.
External	On the outside	The *external* defibrillator is used on the outside of the chest.
Internal	On the inside	He received *internal* injuries from the accident.
Superficial	At the body surface	The cut was only *superficial*.
Deep	Under the body surface	The patient had *deep* wounds from the chainsaw.
Central	Locations around center of body	The patient had *central* chest pain.
Peripheral	Surrounding or outer regions	The patient had *peripheral* swelling of the feet.

Adapted from B. Colbert, *Anatomy & Physiology for Health Professions.* Upper Saddle River, NJ: Prentice Hall, 2007.

TABLE 6–8

Terminology Examples of Body Regions and Their Location

Body Region	Location	Medical Example
Antebrachial	Forearm	This is located between the wrist and elbow.
Antecubital	Depressed area in front of elbow	Use this area to draw blood or start an IV.
Axillary	Armpit	The location can be used to take temperature.
Brachial	Upper arm	Take blood pressure.
Buccal	Cheek	Check buccal region for central cyanosis.
Carpal	Wrist	Carpal tunnel syndrome is painful here.
Cervical	Neck	Cervical collar needed for neck injuries.
Digital	Fingers	Place digital oxygen sensors here.
Femoral	Upper inner thigh	Check femoral pulse for effective CPR.
Gluteal	Buttocks	The injection site is in the gluteal area.
Lumbar	Lower back	Lumbar pain often occurs on long car trips.
Nasal	Nose	Medications can be given by nasal spray.
Oral	Mouth	Oral route is most common for medications.
Orbital	Eye area	Orbital injury can cause damage to sight.
Palmar	Wrist	Do not perform a venipuncture on the palmar side of the hand.
Patellar	Knee	Patellar injuries are common in sports.
Pedal	Foot	People with heart problems may have pedal edema (swelling).
Plantar	Sole of foot	Plantar warts can be painful.
Pubic	Genital region	The pubic region is often checked for body lice.
Sternal	Breastbone area	The sternal area is used for CPR.
Thoracic	Chest	The thoracic area is used to listen to heart and lung sounds.

Adapted from B. Colbert, *Anatomy & Physiology for Health Professions.* Upper Saddle River, NJ: Prentice Hall, 2007, Updated 2013.

Major Organ Systems

This portion of the chapter highlights the basic anatomy and physiology of each organ system except the lymphatic system and the circulatory, or cardiovascular, system, which are covered in Chapter 7. This section also identifies common disorders, diseases, or illnesses of the major organ systems and laboratory tests to detect abnormalities. The term **disorder** is a generic term referring to any pathologic condition of the mind or body; a **disease** is a specific, measurable condition characterized by specific clinical symptoms, patient history, and laboratory or radiology results; and **illness** is a more subjective, nonmeasurable term for any departure from wellness (pain, suffering, distress). For example, a person may have high blood pressure (a disorder known as *hypertension* and caused by arterial disease) but may not feel ill. Conversely, a person may have painful headaches (and feel ill) but may not have measurable clinical results to explain the headaches. The following sections provide a general understanding of organ systems, their role in bodily functioning, and common laboratory procedures useful in detecting abnormalities within the organ system.

TABLE 6–9 and **FIGURE 6–10** provide an overview of the major organ systems. For each system covered in more detail, there is a summary of the structure, function, disorders, and common laboratory tests.

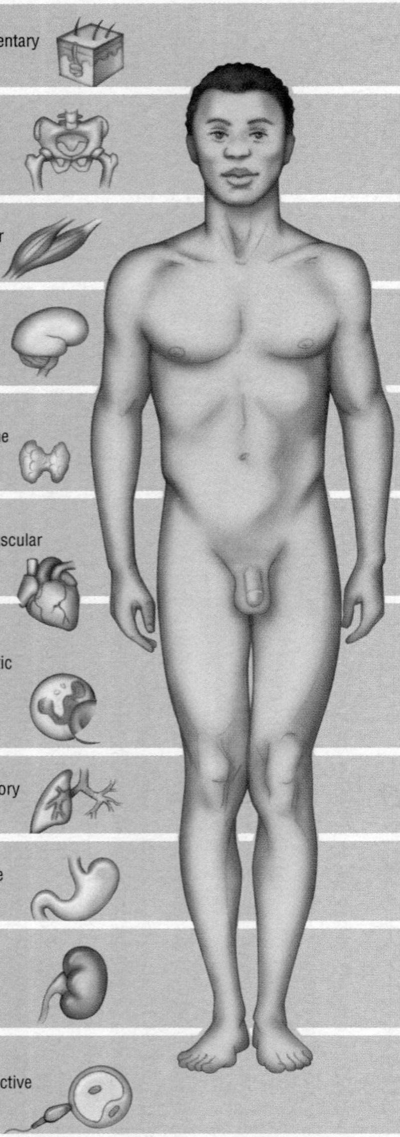

Organ System	Major Functions	Common Disorders*	Common Laboratory Tests*
Integumentary system	*Protection*: Temperature regulator, and sensory receptor.	Infections, cancers, wounds	Skin scrapings potassium hydroxide (KOH) preparation Biopsy staining procedures
Skeletal system	*Framework and Movement*: Shape, support, protection, and storage place for minerals. Movement is made possible through joints.	Arthritis, gout, tumors, infections, developmental conditions, eg., dwarfism	Calcium, phosphate, alkaline phosphatase uric acid, Vitamin D, blood cell counts, cultures, cytogenetic analysis
Muscular system	*Framework and Movement*: Muscles produce movement, maintain posture, and produce heat.	Muscular dystrophy, multiple sclerosis tendinitis, infections	Muscle enzymes, eg., creatine phosphokinase (CK), lactate dehydrogenase
Nervous system	*Communication and Control*: Transmits impulses, responds to change, responsible for communication and control over all parts of the body.	Infections, eg., meningitis, encephalitis, tumors, epilepsy, Parkinson's disease amyotrophic lateral sclerosis (ALS)	Hormone, protein, and enzyme analysis microbial cultures
Endocrine system	*Communication and Control*: The glands of the endocrine system produce hormones, chemical messengers, that provide for communication and control over various parts of the body.	Addison's disease, Cushing's Syndrome, diabetes, hyper or hypothyroidism, goiter	Hormone analysis, thyroid function tests
Cardiovascular system	*Transportation and Immunity*: Transports oxygen and carbon dioxide, delivers nutrients and hormones, regulates blood clotting and removes waste products.	Tumors, heart disease, hemophilia and other blood clotting disorders, infections	Heart enzymes, hemoglobin, hematocrit (H&H), cell counts, platelet function tests, coagulation factors, bone marrow analysis, cytogenetic analysis
Lymphatic system	*Transportation and Immunity*: The lymphatic system stimulates immune response, protects the body, and transports proteins and fluids.	Tumors, eg., lymphoma, Hodgkin's disease, immune disorders, infections	Bone marrow analysis, immune function tests
Respiratory system	*Distribution and Elimination*: Furnishes oxygen for use by individual tissue cells and removes their gaseous waste products, carbon dioxide.	Infections, eg., pneumonia, tuberculosis, sore throats, laryngitis, coughs, colds, influenza	Blood gases, eg., CO_2, & O_2, blood pH, electrolytes (sodium, chloride, potassium), bicarbonate, microbial cultures
Digestive system	*Distribution and Elimination*: Digestion, absorption, and elimination.	Peridontal disease, stomach disorders, eg., ulcers, acid reflux, hernias, intestinal disorders, eg., appendicitis	Occult blood test, microbial cultures, and parasitic analysis
Urinary system	*Distribution and Elimination*: Produces urine, transports urine, and eliminates urine. The kidneys help maintain electrolyte, water, and acid—base balance of the body.	Acidosis and alkalosis	Protein, glucose, ammonia, creatinine, blood urea nitrogen, electrolytes
Reproductive system	*Cycle of Life*: Responsible for sexual characteristics of the male and/or female. Proper functioning ensures survival of the human race.	Tumors, infertility, cysts, cancer, sexually transmitted diseases (STD) enlarged prostate	Cytogenetic analysis, semen analysis, biopsies, hormone analysis, prostatic specific antigen (PSA)

* Disorders and laboratory tests listed are only a few examples. The lists are not comprehensive.

FIGURE 6–10
Organ Systems of the Body

TABLE 6–9

Organ System Functions

Normal Body Functions	Organ Systems
Protection	Integumentary
Support	Skeletal
Movement	Muscular
Control	Nervous
Regulation	Endocrine
Fluid Regulation	Cardiovascular
Transport	Lymphatic
Environmental Control and Exchange	Respiratory
	Digestive
	Urinary
Birth	Reproductive

ROLE OF THE CLINICAL LABORATORY IN ASSESSING BODY FUNCTIONS

Clinical laboratory tests play a crucial role in four areas of health care:

1. Screening (e.g., diabetes, cholesterol)
2. Diagnosis (e.g., detecting viral or bacterial infections, sexually transmitted diseases [STDs], tumor markers)
3. Treatment (e.g., serum drug levels, cholesterol level follow-up)
4. Monitoring

Data that are generated from laboratory tests are combined with information from many other departments (e.g., x-rays, nutritional assessments, counseling) and analyzed by the medical team (doctor, physician's assistant, nurse, etc.) to make decisions about how to proceed with patient care. Laboratory test results help form an accurate clinical picture of the patient's internal condition. Thousands of substances can be detected by using laboratory methods, so knowledge about some of the more common laboratory tests is helpful. Examples of laboratory tests are noted under each body system discussed; however, the list does not include all tests currently available.

INTEGUMENTARY SYSTEM

Structure and Function

The **integumentary system** consists of:

- Skin, as depicted in **FIGURE 6–11**
- Hair
- Sweat glands (sudoriferous) and oil glands (sebaceous)
- Teeth
- Fingernails, as depicted in **FIGURE 6–12**

It serves for protection and regulatory functions such as insulation, thermal regulation, excretion, and the production of vitamin D. Skin is the largest organ of the body (covering about 3,000 square inches and weighing about 6 pounds), protecting the deeper tissues by providing a barrier to entering microorganisms and foreign

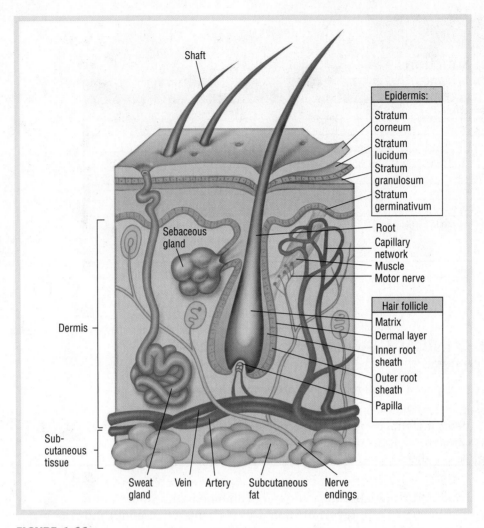

FIGURE 6–11

Cross-Section of Skin

The skin or integument consists of the epidermis, dermis, subcutaneous tissue, and its appendages (hair, nails, glands). These layers rest on top of muscle tissue. Note that the nerve endings and capillary network extend almost to the outer edges of the skin. This is the area that is punctured during a skin puncture procedure or "fingerstick."

FIGURE 6–12

The Fingernail

Note the close proximity of the bone (phalange) to the surface of the skin and the tip of the finger.

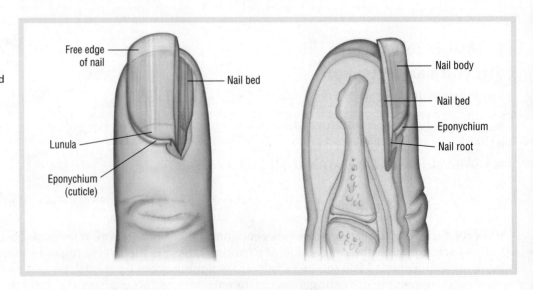

bodies and by protecting from hazardous exposures such as heat and cold. The skin also prevents water loss or allows for perspiration as needed by the body during exercise or fever or due to weather conditions. Sebaceous glands in the skin produce oils for hair and skin protection, and sweat glands produce perspiration, which helps cool the body as needed and eliminates some waste. **Melanin** in the skin provides skin color and protects underlying tissues from absorbing ultraviolet rays. Ultraviolet light stimulates production of inactive vitamin D in the skin. The liver and kidneys then activate vitamin D so that it is beneficial to the body. Other functions of the skin are to store fat in the layers next to the underlying tissues and to allow an individual to experience sensations such as touch, temperature, pain, and pressure. Hair on the head provides protection by acting as a heat insulator; eyebrows keep perspiration out of the eyes; eyelashes protect eyes from foreign objects; and hairs in the nasal passages filter out dust and harmful microorganisms. Likewise, fingernails protect the tips of the hands. Teeth aid in breaking up food to begin the digestive process.

Disorders of the Integumentary System

- Bacterial infections, such as acne and impetigo (caused by *Staphylococcus aureus*)
- Decubitis ulcers, also known as bedsores or pressure ulcers, are caused by partial blood flow obstruction to the soft tissue as a result of inactivity or constant pressure or friction to an area of the skin. Common in bedridden patients or those confined to a wheelchair; affected sites are the hips, coccyx, elbows, knees, ankles, etc.
- Viral infections, such as fever blisters or cold sores
- Rubeola, rubella, chickenpox, and herpes zoster (shingles)
- Fungal infections, such as ringworm and athlete's foot
- Allergic reactions, such as urticaria
- Dermatitis (inflammation of the dermal layers of skin), eczema (red, itchy, skin inflammations), and psoriasis (red, scaly patches on skin)
- Insect bites and burns
- Skin cancers, such as malignant melanoma (**FIGURE 6–13**)

Common Laboratory Tests for the Integumentary System

- For many of these conditions, skin scrapings and/or biopsy specimens are taken for analysis; tests can include bacteriologic, viral, or fungal tissue cultures; potassium hydroxide (KOH) preparations; or biopsy staining procedures.

SKELETAL SYSTEM

Structure and Function

The **skeletal system** consists of:

- **Bones**—Cells surrounded by calcified intercellular substances that allow for a rigid structure
- **Cartilage**—Similar to bone cells, but surrounded by a gelatinous material that allows for more flexibility
- **Joints**—Connective tissue that holds bones together, of various types (ball and socket, hinge, etc.)
- **Ligaments**—Tough connective tissue that connects one bone to another for flexibility and leverage
- **Tendons**—Cordlike structures that attach muscle to bone

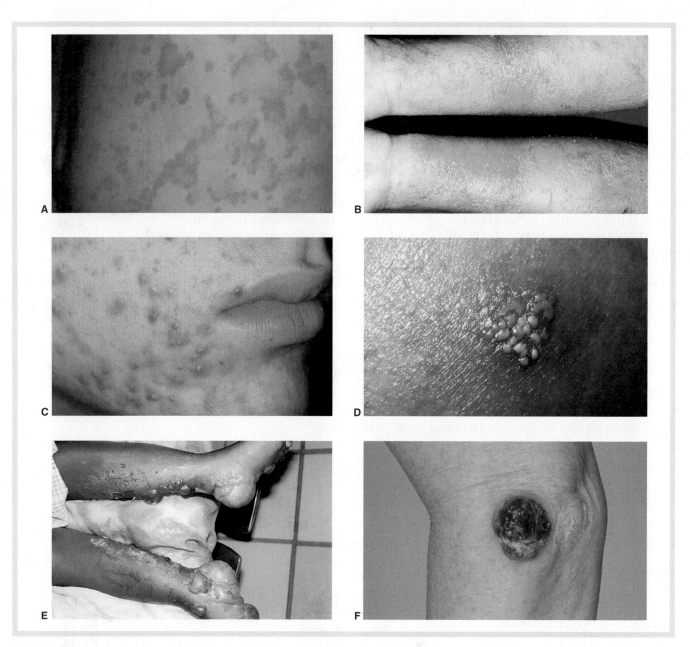

FIGURE 6–13

Disorders of the Integumentary System

A. Urticaria (hives). *(Courtesy of Jason L. Smith, M.D.)* B. Dermatitis (caused by poison ivy). *(Courtesy of Jason L. Smith, M.D.)* C. Acne. *(Courtesy of Jason L. Smith, M.D.)* D. Herpes simplex. *(Courtesy of Jason L. Smith, M.D.)* E. Burn, second degree. *(Courtesy of Jason L. Smith, M.D.)* F. Malignant melanoma. *(Biophoto Associates/Photo Researchers, Inc.)*

The skeletal system serves the body in five major ways: support, protection for softer tissues (brain and lungs), movement and leverage (**FIGURE 6–14**), **hematopoiesis** (blood cell formation) in the bone marrow, and mineral storage.

More than 200 bones are contained in the human body, and they are classified into four groups based on shape. *Long bones* include leg bones (e.g., femur, tibia, fibula) and arm and hand bones (e.g., humerus, radius, ulna, phalanges). *Short bones* include carpals and tarsals, or wrist and ankle bones, respectively. Among *flat bones* are several cranial bones, the ribs, and the scapulae (shoulder blades). Finally, *irregular bones* include

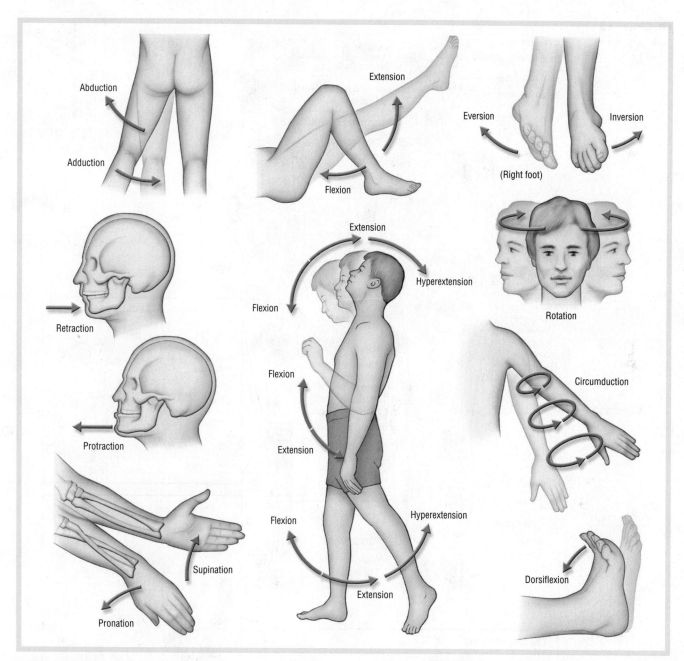

FIGURE 6–14
Terminology Related to Movement

cranial bones (e.g., sphenoid, ethmoid) and bones of the vertebral column (e.g., vertebrae, sacrum, coccyx) (**FIGURE 6–15**).

Bones are connected to each other by a variety of joints that permit many movements, as shown in Figure 6–14. Bone structure differs between male and female skeletons. Besides being somewhat larger and heavier, the male has a pelvis that is deeper, with a narrow pubic arch. In contrast, the female pelvis is shallow and broad and has a wider pubic arch to facilitate childbirth.

In general, bones consist of several layers covered by a membrane, the periosteum. The periosteum contains blood vessels that bring blood from inside the bone to the outer layer. Refer to Figure 6–15. The outer layer, or compact bone, is more rigid and heavier than the inner layer, which is like a honeycomb. The inner layer is spongy bone but is just as strong as compact bone. In the center of a bone is the marrow, which produces most

FIGURE 6–15
Skeletal System

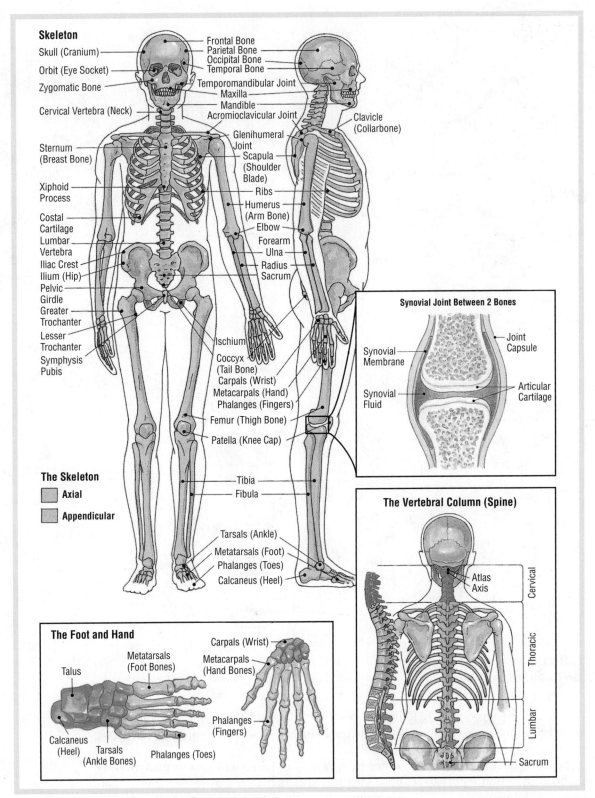

Skeleton

Skull (Cranium)
Orbit (Eye Socket)
Zygomatic Bone
Cervical Vertebra (Neck)
Sternum (Breast Bone)
Xiphoid Process
Costal Cartilage
Lumbar Vertebra
Iliac Crest
Ilium (Hip)
Pelvic Girdle
Greater Trochanter
Lesser Trochanter
Symphysis Pubis

Frontal Bone
Parietal Bone
Occipital Bone
Temporal Bone
Temporomandibular Joint
Maxilla
Mandible
Acromioclavicular Joint
Glenihumeral Joint
Scapula (Shoulder Blade)
Ribs
Humerus (Arm Bone)
Elbow
Forearm
Ulna
Radius
Sacrum

Clavicle (Collarbone)

Ischium
Coccyx (Tail Bone)
Carpals (Wrist)
Metacarpals (Hand)
Phalanges (Fingers)
Femur (Thigh Bone)
Patella (Knee Cap)

The Skeleton
Axial
Appendicular

Tibia
Fibula

Tarsals (Ankle)
Metatarsals (Foot)
Phalanges (Toes)
Calcaneus (Heel)

Synovial Joint Between 2 Bones
Synovial Membrane
Synovial Fluid
Joint Capsule
Articular Cartilage

The Vertebral Column (Spine)
Atlas
Axis
Cervical
Thoracic
Lumbar
Sacrum

The Foot and Hand
Metatarsals (Foot Bones)
Talus
Carpals (Wrist)
Metacarpals (Hand Bones)
Phalanges (Fingers)
Calcaneus (Heel)
Tarsals (Ankle Bones)
Phalanges (Toes)

blood cells. Approximately 5 billion red blood cells (RBCs) are produced daily by about half a pound (227 g) of bone marrow. Marrow is located in all the bones of an infant, but in adults it is in the skull, sternum (or breastbone), vertebrae, hipbones, and ends of the long bones.[1] Minerals stored in bones include calcium and phosphorus. When these minerals are needed in other parts of the body, they are released from the bone through the bloodstream.

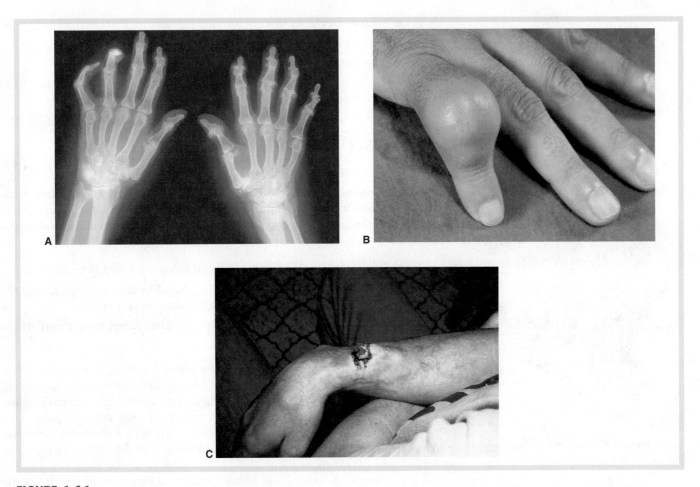

FIGURE 6–16

Conditions Affecting the Skeletal System

A. X-ray showing osteoarthritis joint changes. *(Getty Images/Stone Allstock.)* B. Gout of the finger joint. *(© Medical-on-Line / Alamy.)* C. Open fracture of the wrist.

Disorders of the Skeletal System

- Inflammatory conditions such as osteoarthritis, bursitis, and gout (**FIGURE 6–16**)
- Bacterial infections such as **osteomyelitis**
- Porous (containing holes, pores or cavities) bone conditions such as osteoporosis
- Bone fractures
- Developmental conditions such as gigantism (large stature or development due to excessive growth hormone production) or dwarfism (short stature due to insufficient production of growth hormone)
- Scoliosis (curvature of the spine), and rickets (soft or bent bones due to vitamin D deficiency), bone tumors

Common Laboratory Tests for the Skeletal System

- Serum calcium and phosphate levels
- Serum alkaline phosphatase (ALP) levels
- Uric acid
- Vitamin D
- Anti-nuclear antibodies (ANA)

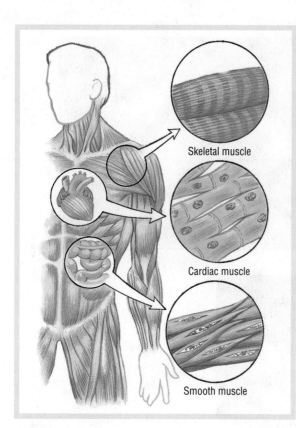

FIGURE 6–17

The Three Types of Muscle: Skeletal, Cardiac, and Smooth

- Erythrocyte sedimentation rate (ESR)
- Complete blood cell (CBC) counts
- Microscopic analysis
- Microbial cultures of the bone marrow and synovial fluid (fluid between joints and bones)

MUSCULAR SYSTEM

Structure and Function

The **muscular system** refers to all muscles of the body, including those attached to bones and those along the walls of internal structures, such as the heart. On the basis of location, microscopic structure, and neural control, muscles are classified as follows:

- **Skeletal (striated voluntary) muscles**: Attached to bones
- **Visceral or smooth (nonstriated, involuntary) muscles**: Lining the walls of internal structures, such as veins and arteries
- **Cardiac (striated involuntary) muscles**: Make up the wall of the heart (**FIGURE 6–17**)

Muscles provide movement, maintain posture, and produce heat. Movement takes place not only during locomotion but also during body movements, changes in the size of openings, and propulsion of substances (e.g., propulsion of blood through veins or passage of food through intestines). Posture is maintained during sitting and standing by continued partial contraction of specific muscles. Muscle cells that provide mechanical energy for movement also release energy in the form of heat. All three muscle types work by extending, contracting, and conducting and by being easily stimulated.

Skeletal muscles (more than 400 in humans) compose approximately 40 percent of a man's body. In contrast, women have less muscle and more fat than men. Muscles are strongest at about age 25, but with proper nutrition and exercise, they can remain strong throughout life. Without sufficient exercise, muscles become smaller and weaker. Glycogen is the form of stored glucose in muscles. Without stores of glycogen, muscles must wait for glucose, which is transported through the bloodstream. Exercise increases the amount of glycogen available for muscles, which in turn allows them to function more easily (**FIGURE 6–18**).

Disorders of the Muscular System

- Muscular dystrophy (MD) (gradual wasting and weakening of the skeletal muscles)
- Conditions that disrupt nerve stimulation (as in severe accidents and myasthenia gravis, which is muscular fatigue due to overuse)
- Muscle cramps and tendonitis (inflammation of the tendons)
- Muscle atrophy (muscles waste away from lack of use)
- Multiple sclerosis (MS) and amyotropic lateral sclerosis (ALS) (MS and ALS are nervous system diseases that involve destruction of the nerves. This results in impaired nerve impulses that can cause weak, numb, or atrophied muscles.)
- Viral infections, such as poliomyelitis (Poliomyelitis is a preventable nervous system disease that can cause atrophy and deformities of muscles in late stages. Vaccinations prevent the disease.)

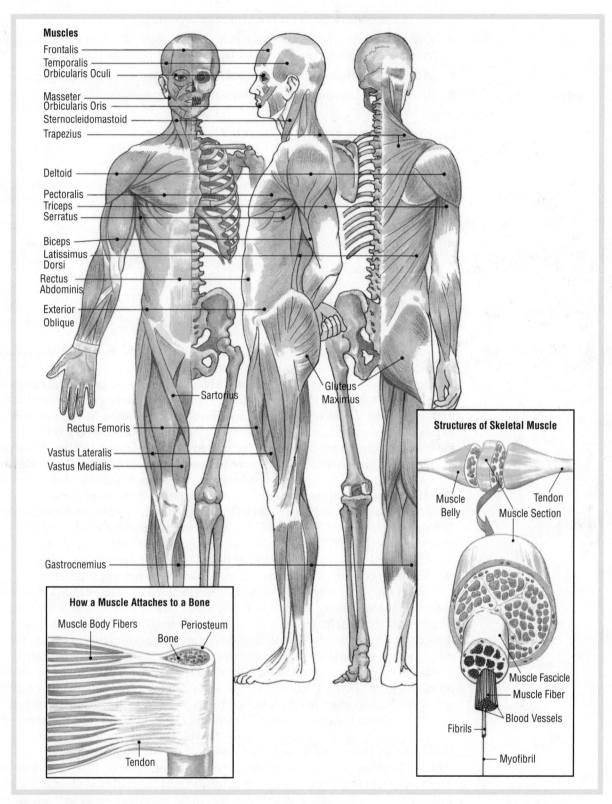

FIGURE 6–18
Muscular System

Common Laboratory Tests for the Muscular System

- Clinical assays of specific muscle enzymes, such as heart enzymes (troponins, creatine phosphokinase [CK], and lactate dehydrogenase [LDH])
- Analysis of autoimmune antibodies
- Microscopic examination, or culturing, of biopsy tissue

NERVOUS SYSTEM

Structure and Function

The **nervous system** provides communication in the body, sensations, thoughts, emotions, and memories. Nerve impulses and chemical substances regulate, control, integrate, and organize body functions. The nervous system consists of:

- **Neurons** (specialized nerve cells)
- Brain
- Spinal cord
- Brain and spinal cord coverings (meninges)
- Cerebrospinal fluid (CSF)

An estimated 10 billion neurons or more reside in the human body, most of which are in the brain. The nervous system can be thought of as two systems: The central nervous system (CNS) is made up of the brain and spinal cord, and the peripheral nervous system (PNS) is everything outside of the brain and spinal cord. **Sensory neurons** transmit nerve impulses to the spinal cord or the brain from muscle tissues. **Motor neurons** transmit impulses to muscles from the spinal cord or the brain (**FIGURE 6–19**). Both the brain and the spinal cord are covered by protective membranes (**meninges**). Between these protective membrane layers are spaces filled with **cerebrospinal fluid (CSF)** that provides a cushion for the brain and the spinal cord. Furthermore, the brain and spinal cord are protected by the skull and vertebral column respectively. The bony segments of the vertebral canal are divided into regions as shown in **FIGURE 6–20** (cervical, thoracic, and lumbar vertebrae). There are seven cervical vertebrae (C1–C7) that extend from the head to the thorax, 12 thoracic vertebrae (T1–T12) that extend from the chest to the back, and five lumbar vertebrae (L1–L5) that extend to the lower back. At the lower end of the vertebral column, the sacrum (S1–S5) and coccyx are fused elements of the sacral and coccygeal vertebrae.

The brain, along with the cranial nerves, functions in all mental processes and many essential motor, sensory, and visceral responses. The spinal cord and the spinal nerves control sensory (touch), motor (voluntary movement), and reflex (knee-jerk) functions. Reflexes are responses to stimuli that do not require communication with the brain. A simple reflex, such as moving a finger from something hot, occurs even before the brain realizes the pain. Specific cranial and spinal nerves control all complex or simple action processes in the body. There are 31 pairs of spinal nerves (nerves that branch off the spinal cord), each of which is identified by its location to the nearest vertebrae. Nerves that branch from the spinal cord (C5 through T1) and extend into the arm region (the brachial plexus) are the axillary, radial, musculocutaneous, median, and ulnar nerves. These nerves control all muscle movement of the shoulder, arm, and hand and also control sensations of the skin of the entire shoulder, arm, and hand. In summary, the nervous system is the primary communication and regulatory system in the body. The autonomic nervous system entails the functions that work without voluntary control of an individual, such as heartbeat, rate of breathing, tear and saliva production, and bladder constrictions.

Disorders of the Nervous System

- Infectious conditions (viral or bacterial) such as encephalitis (inflammation of the brain), meningitis (inflammation of the linings of the brain and spinal cord), tetanus, herpes, and poliomyelitis

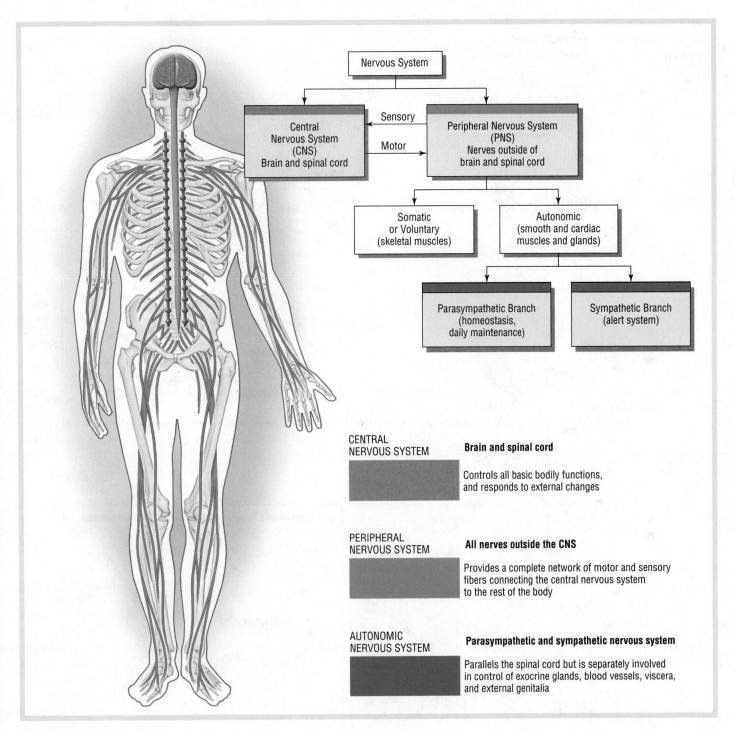

FIGURE 6–19
Organization of the Nervous System

- Conditions such as ALS, MS, Parkinson's disease (a degenerative disorder characterized by hand tremors, loss of facial expression, shuffling walk), cerebral palsy (CP; brain damage at birth that typically causes lack of muscle control) (**FIGURE 6–21**)
- Epilepsy (episodes of abnormal electrical discharges in the brain that may cause convulsions or loss of consciousness), hydrocephaly (excessive amounts of CSF in the brain that can lead to intracranial pressure and other complications), neuralgia (pain along a nerve), strokes, and headaches
- Injuries that can also result in paralysis or partial paralysis

FIGURE 6–20

Nervous System

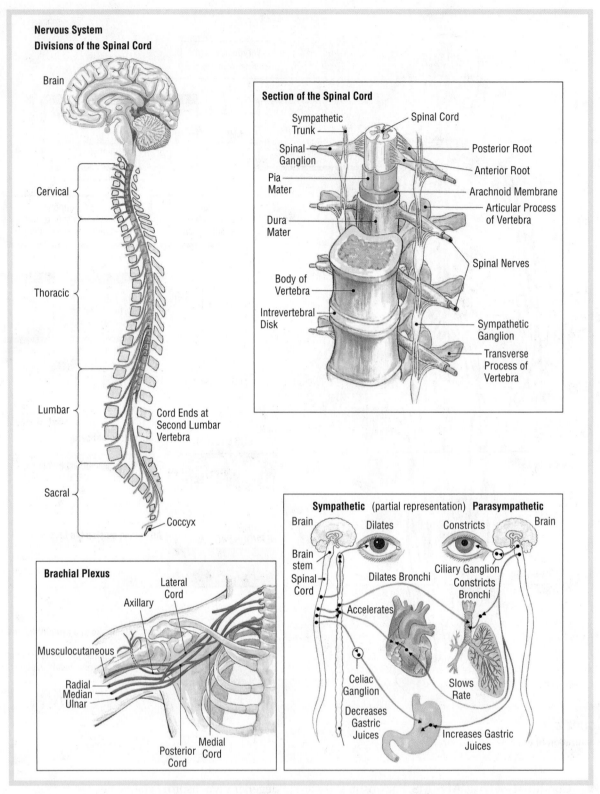

Nervous System
Divisions of the Spinal Cord

Brain

Cervical

Thoracic

Lumbar

Cord Ends at
Second Lumbar
Vertebra

Sacral

Coccyx

Section of the Spinal Cord

Sympathetic Trunk

Spinal Cord

Spinal Ganglion

Posterior Root

Anterior Root

Pia Mater

Arachnoid Membrane

Articular Process of Vertebra

Dura Mater

Body of Vertebra

Spinal Nerves

Intrevertebral Disk

Sympathetic Ganglion

Transverse Process of Vertebra

Brachial Plexus

Lateral Cord

Axillary

Musculocutaneous

Radial
Median
Ulnar

Posterior Cord

Medial Cord

Sympathetic (partial representation) **Parasympathetic**

Brain

Dilates

Constricts

Brain

Brain stem

Spinal Cord

Dilates Bronchi

Ciliary Ganglion

Constricts Bronchi

Accelerates

Celiac Ganglion

Slows Rate

Decreases Gastric Juices

Increases Gastric Juices

As a special note to health care workers performing blood collection, nerve damage, including partial paralysis, can also occur as a result of accidental injury during phlebotomy procedures. Injury may be the result of excessive probing with the needle, sticking the needle in a poor site for venipuncture, deep needle penetration all the way into the nerve, and/or if the patient suddenly jerks his or her arm during the venipuncture procedure, causing the needle to puncture a nerve. Choose venipuncture sites that are

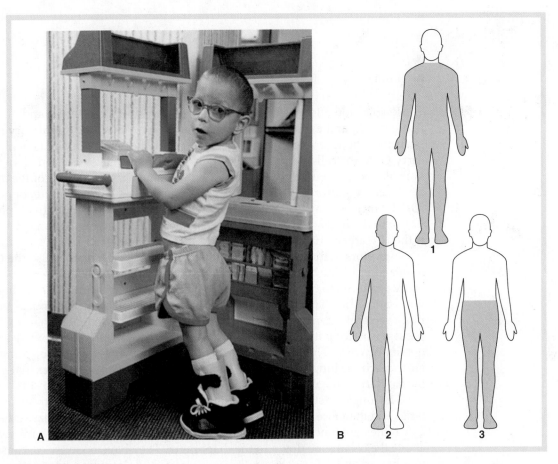

FIGURE 6–21

Conditions Affecting the Nervous System

A. A child with cerebral palsy has abnormal muscle tone and diminished physical coordination. B. Paralysis can be classified as follows: 1. Quadriplegia—complete or partial paralysis of the upper and/or lower extremities; 2. Hemiplegia—paralysis of one-half of the body when divided along the median sagittal plane; 3. Paraplegia— paralysis of the lower part of the body.

least likely to cause nerve damage and take precautions to have the patient's movements stabilized as much as possible. Under no circumstances should health care workers use the anterior or palmar side of the wrist to collect a blood specimen because the risk of hitting a nerve is high due to nerve locations close to the skin's surface. Details of venipuncture site selection are covered in Chapter 10.

Common Laboratory Tests for the Nervous System

■ Chemical assays can reveal drug interactions, as well as hormonal, protein, and enzyme alterations.

■ Infections can be detected by bacterial, viral, or fungal cultures or by the presence of specific antibodies in the CSF.

RESPIRATORY SYSTEM

Structure and Function

The main components of the **respiratory system** are in the head, the neck, and the thoracic cavity and consist of the

■ Nose
■ Pharynx

- Larynx
- Trachea
- Bronchi
- Lungs

Respiration allows for the exchange of gases between blood and air. When gases (oxygen [O_2] and carbon dioxide [CO_2]) enter the blood, the **circulatory system** transports them between lungs and tissues. Together, the respiratory and circulatory systems carry O_2 to the cells and remove CO_2 from the tissue cells. Oxygen allows the body to burn its fuel from ingested nutrients. It makes up about one-fifth of the air around us. The average person inhales and exhales about 15 times per minute, or approximately 20,000 times per day. As a person breathes in, the O_2 travels through air passages to the lungs. In the lungs, the exchange of gases occurs. Oxygen is exchanged for CO_2, which is then breathed out as the person exhales.

Receptors in the nose provide the sense of smell. The nose is also the primary filter for air entering the body. In the nose, the throat, and the bronchial tree, mucus is continuously produced to trap unwanted particles and prevent them from entering the lungs or vocal cords. Tiny hairlike cilia line the passageways and sweep the mucus to the nose and mouth so that it can be coughed up, sneezed, or swallowed. The pharynx is a tube-type passageway for both food and air. Along with the larynx (voice box), it determines the quality of voice. The trachea and the bronchial passages provide openings for outside air to reach the lungs. Within the bronchi are grapelike **alveolar sacs** that are enveloped by capillaries and allow diffusion between air and blood (**FIGURE 6–22**).

The lungs are structured into millions of branches of alveoli with surrounding capillaries and therefore can quickly take in large amounts of O_2 and release large amounts of CO_2 if they are functioning properly. The lungs are soft and spongy and reach from just above the collarbone down to the diaphragm. They have no muscles; consequently, the diaphragm and other surrounding muscles help enlarge and contract the chest cavity as respiration occurs. Humans have two lungs: the right lung has three lobes, and the left lung has only two, to allow room for the heart. An adult's lungs hold 3 to 4 quarts (approximately 3 to 4 liters) of air, depending on how vigorously the person is moving or exercising. In patients with pneumonia, the alveolar sacs become inflamed and fluid or waste products block the minute air spaces; thus, normal O_2 and CO_2 exchange is difficult.

Red blood cells (RBCs) transport O_2 and CO_2 as part of a molecule called **hemoglobin.** After O_2 crosses the respiratory membranes (in the lung) into the blood, about 97 percent of the O_2 combines with the iron-containing heme portion of hemoglobin inside the RBCs. The remaining 3 percent dissolves in plasma. Oxygen goes from the alveolar capillaries through the blood vessels to the tissue capillaries. Oxygen and CO_2 rapidly combine with hemoglobin in RBCs to form oxyhemoglobin and carbaminohemoglobin, respectively. Association (chemical combination) and dissociation (chemical release) with hemoglobin depend on the gaseous pressure. In lung capillaries, O_2 pressure (partial pressure of oxygen [PO_2]) increases and CO_2 (partial pressure of carbon dioxide [PCO_2]) decreases, which allows O_2 to rapidly associate, or combine chemically, with hemoglobin, and CO_2 to dissociate, or be released, from carbaminohemoglobin. Thus, humans inhale O_2 into the lungs and exhale CO_2 from the lungs. In tissue capillaries, the opposite occurs: O_2 pressure decreases and CO_2 pressure increases, which allows O_2 to dissociate from oxyhemoglobin and CO_2 to combine with hemoglobin. Thus, O_2 is released into tissues and muscles, and CO_2 is picked up, taken to the lungs, and exhaled.

Carbon dioxide has an important effect on the pH (acidity) of the blood. Normal body pH has a narrow range of between 7.35 and 7.45. Deviations from the normal or reference range can be dangerous and deadly. As CO_2 levels increase, the blood pH decreases (becomes more acidic), and chemoreceptors in the brain cause a faster rate of respiration (hyperventilation) in order to blow off excess CO_2 from the body (Figure 6–22). (The urinary system also plays a role in maintaining body pH, as described later in this chapter.)

FIGURE 6–22
Respiratory System

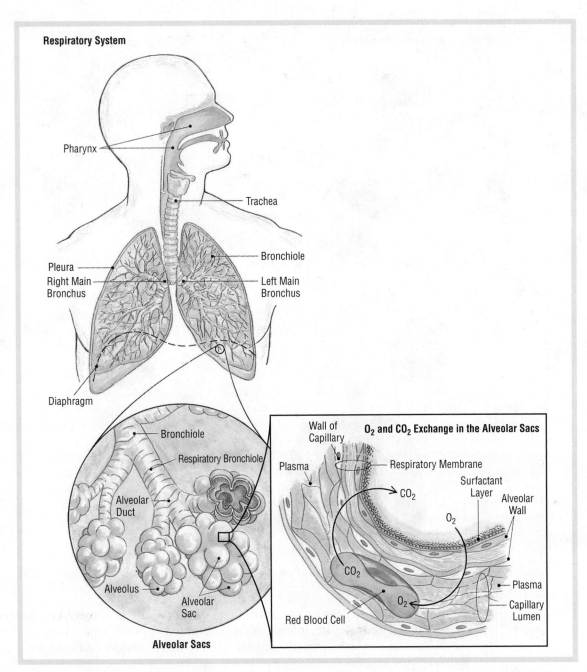

Disorders of the Respiratory System

■ Infectious conditions, including tuberculosis (TB), multidrug-resistant TB (MDR TB), laryngitis, bronchitis, colds, sore throat, whooping cough, tonsillitis, rhinitis, coughs, sneezing, runny noses, bronchitis, pneumonia, *Pneumocystis carinii* pneumonia, Legionnaires' disease, pleurisy, respiratory distress syndrome, respiratory syncytial virus and influenza, and severe acute respiratory syndrome (SARS) outbreaks

■ Conditions such as asthma (often caused by allergies and characterized by coughing, difficulty breathing or a tight feeling in the chest), emphysema (the lung sacs are enlarged and do not function properly; most commonly caused by smoking), and cystic fibrosis (hereditary disease that results in chronic obstructive pulmonary disease, frequent lung infections, and other related symptoms), and tumors **(FIGURE 6–23)**

FIGURE 6–23

Normal Bronchiole, Asthma, and Emphysema

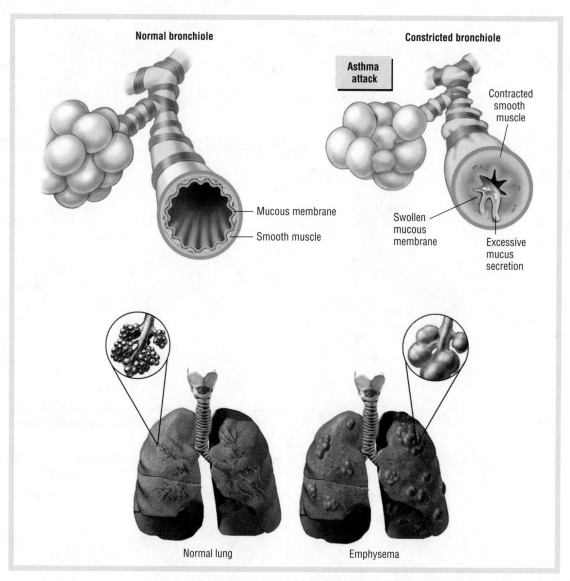

- In cases of pneumonia, the air sacs in the lungs fill with fluid, and gaseous exchanges cannot occur. Pneumocystis infections are considered opportunistic infections (i.e., they become pathogenic when the patient is immunosuppressed) and are associated with acquired immunodeficiency syndrome (AIDS).

Common Laboratory Tests for the Respiratory System

- Blood gases (CO_2 and O_2), blood pH
- Chemical constituents (sodium, chloride, bicarbonate, and potassium)
- Lung biopsies, throat swabs, sputum cultures, and bronchial washings can be examined microscopically or cultured for pathogenic microorganisms. Procedures for collecting specimens for a throat culture and a sputum specimen are included in Chapter 16.

DIGESTIVE SYSTEM

Structure and Function

The gastrointestinal (GI) tract is made up of the

- Mouth and teeth
- Pharynx

- Esophagus
- Stomach
- Intestines (small and large)
- Vital accessory organs (salivary glands, liver, gallbladder, pancreas, and appendix) (**FIGURE 6–24**)

Digestion (breaking down food), absorption (nutrients taken in and transported by the blood and lymph systems), and elimination (solid wastes excreted) are the main functions of this system. The **digestive system,** or **gastrointestinal system,** breaks down food chemically and physically into nutrients that can be absorbed and transported throughout the body to be used for energy by all body cells and to eliminate the waste products of digestion through the production of feces. Many proteins, enzymes, and juices are released by these components to facilitate digestion, absorption, and movement through the GI tract. The food passageway, or alimentary canal, which begins at the mouth and ends at the anus, has an average length of 27 feet in adults. (One meal can take 15 hours to 2 days to pass through.) Circular muscles surround the intestines to assist the movement of food through the body using wavelike contractions called **peristalsis.** (Peristalsis is such an effective process that a person can even swallow upside down!) If the process is reversed, vomiting enables the body to reject food.

Saliva produced in the mouth moistens food and contains an enzyme that helps begin the breakdown of carbohydrates into simple sugars such as glucose. (If a salt cracker is chewed a long time, saliva begins the breakdown process so it may taste sweet.) Also, the liver secretes bile, which aids in fat digestion and absorption. In addition, it is involved in carbohydrate metabolism, protein and fat catabolism, and synthesis of many vital blood proteins for clotting and regulatory purposes. Each component functions either mechanically or chemically to keep the body in homeostasis.

The digestive system helps regulate the intake and output of essential proteins, carbohydrates, fats, minerals, vitamins, and water. The body can then use these substances by catabolizing them for stored energy or by anabolizing them to build other complex compounds, such as hormones, other tissue proteins, and enzymes. Materials that are not digested in the alimentary canal are eliminated from the body as fecal material or urine.

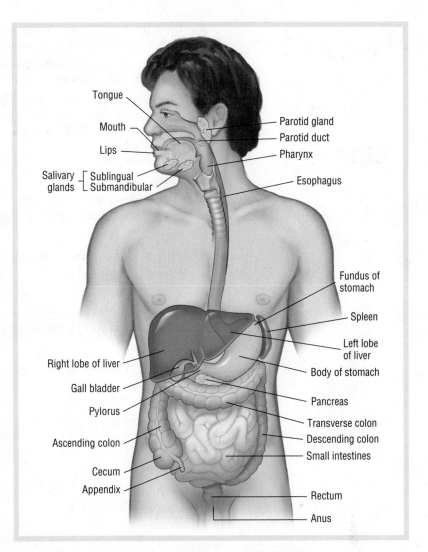

FIGURE 6–24
Digestive or Gastrointestinal System

Disorders of the Digestive System

- The oral cavity can contain dental caries, or tooth decay, and periodontal disease, which is an inflammation and degeneration of the gums, ligaments, and bone around the teeth.

- Stomach disorders can include gastroesophageal reflux disease (GERD) or acid reflux, hiatal hernias (protrusion through the diaphragm), irritable bowel syndrome (IBS), vomiting, infections with *Helicobacter pylori* (*H. pylori* is a bacterium causing ulcers and possibly cancers of the stomach and intestines), and peptic ulcer disease (PUD).

- Intestinal disorders (affecting small and large intestines) include polyps, maldigestion, malabsorption, cancer, appendicitis, colitis, diverticulitis, constipation, diarrhea, dysentery, and hemorrhoids.

- Pancreatitis is an inflammation of the pancreas.

- Liver inflammation is referred to as hepatitis and can be caused by various agents, such as excessive alcohol consumption and viral hepatitis.

- A common disorder of the gallbladder is gallstones, which can cause blockage of the bile duct, pain, and inflammation.

- Numerous bacterial and parasitic infections can also affect the digestive tract. Examples include staphylococcal food poisoning, salmonellosis, *H. pylori*, typhoid fever, cholera, giardiasis, tapeworms, pinworms, hookworms, and ascariasis (roundworm).

Common Laboratory Tests of the Digestive System

- Tissue biopsies
- **Occult blood** test (testing for blood in feces) and fecal occult blood test for fecal fat (procedures for performing a fecal occult blood test are included in Chapter 16)
- Bacterial cultures
- Analysis for **ova and parasites (O&P)**
- Gastric analysis
- Analysis of blood specimens for ammonia, amylase, bilirubin, carcinoembryonic antigen (CEA), carotene, cholesterol, complete blood count (CBC), glucose, glucose tolerance test (GTT), lipase, triglycerides

URINARY SYSTEM

Structure and Function

This system consists of the

- Two kidneys
- Two ureters
- Bladder
- Urethra (**FIGURE 6–25**)

The primary purpose of the **urinary system** is to produce and eliminate urine. The kidneys' main function is to regulate the amount of water and electrolytes (sodium, potassium, chloride, calcium, phosphate, magnesium) and to excrete nitrogenous waste products (urea) from protein metabolism. Between 1,000 and 5,000 milliliters of blood circulate through the kidneys every minute. Inside the kidneys' microscopic tubules, glomerular filtration, tubular reabsorption, and tubular secretion are basic processes by which the kidneys perform their functions. As the large volume of blood passes through the kidneys, it is first filtered, then nutrients are reabsorbed into the bloodstream while a concentrated solution containing the waste products is produced and excreted through the production of urine. A detailed graphic representation is shown in Figures 6–25 and **6–26**.

The proper concentration of these blood constituents is vital to maintaining homeostasis. Electrolytes function to maintain the body's acid-base balance. The normal ratio of acid (carbonic acid) to base (bicarbonate) is 1:20. Blood pH and blood gas determinations provide useful information about acid-base balance in the body. Normal blood pH is within a range of 7.35 to 7.45. The kidneys help correct the body's acid-base imbalances. As blood passes through specialized kidney cells, called *glomeruli*, water and solutes are filtered out. Only the necessary amounts of these substances are reabsorbed into the blood. The rest are excreted as waste products in the urine. Ureters collect urine as it forms and transport it to the bladder, which serves as a reservoir until the urine can be voided. The urethra is the terminal component of the urinary system. In women, it is merely a passageway from the bladder, whereas in men, it eliminates both urine and semen from the body.

Two-thirds of human body weight is water. About 60 percent of the body's water is inside cells, and the rest is in the bloodstream or tissue fluids. The salt content of the body's water is extremely important for survival. The kidneys eliminate excess salt and excess water from the tissues.

FIGURE 6–25
Urinary System

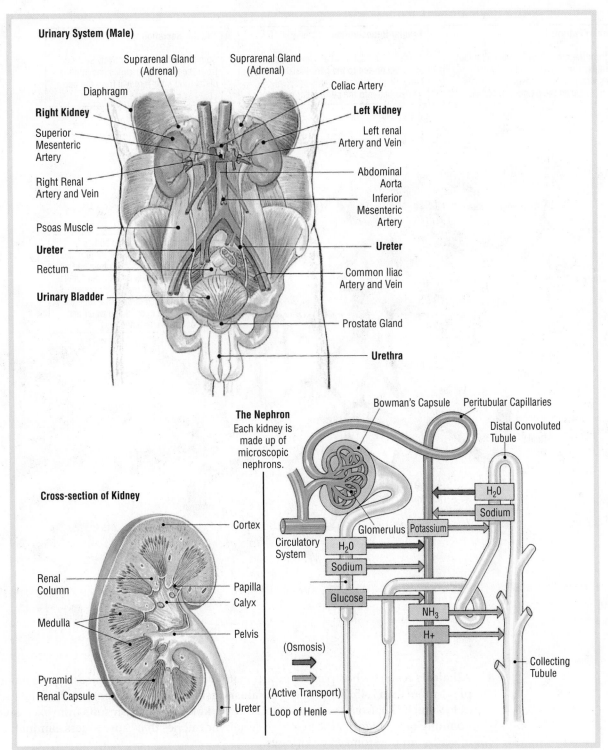

Disorders of the Urinary System

- **Acidosis** occurs when the blood pH decreases to less than 7.35, thus the bloodstream becomes acidic. If the condition worsens, the individual can become comatose. **Respiratory acidosis** is a serious condition that results when the respiratory system is unable to eliminate adequate amounts of CO_2 (in conditions such as a collapsed lung or blockage of respiratory passages). **Metabolic acidosis** results when the body retains acids or loses bicarbonate buffers or the kidneys eliminate acidic substances. There are several causes of metabolic acidosis, and they can result in kidney (renal) failure and/or death.

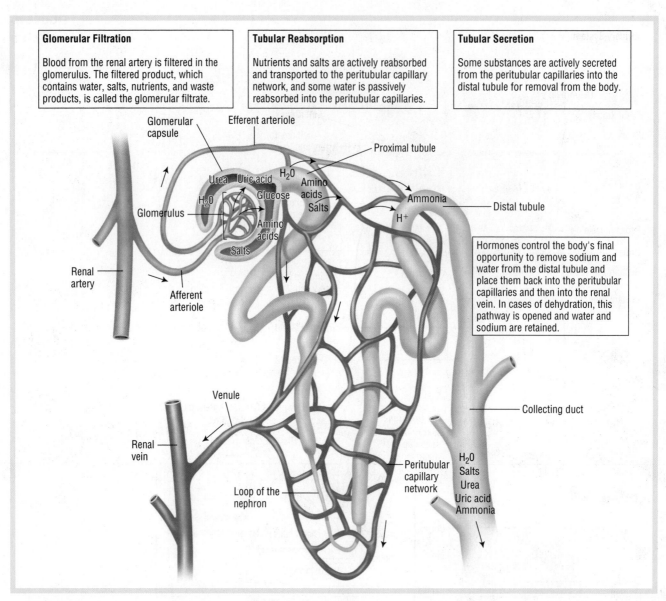

Glomerular Filtration

Blood from the renal artery is filtered in the glomerulus. The filtered product, which contains water, salts, nutrients, and waste products, is called the glomerular filtrate.

Tubular Reabsorption

Nutrients and salts are actively reabsorbed and transported to the peritubular capillary network, and some water is passively reabsorbed into the peritubular capillaries.

Tubular Secretion

Some substances are actively secreted from the peritubular capillaries into the distal tubule for removal from the body.

Hormones control the body's final opportunity to remove sodium and water from the distal tubule and place them back into the peritubular capillaries and then into the renal vein. In cases of dehydration, this pathway is opened and water and sodium are retained.

FIGURE 6–26

The Renal Tubule

- **Alkalosis** results when plasma bicarbonate increases, thereby increasing the blood pH to more than 7.45. **Respiratory alkalosis** results from hyperventilation or the loss of too much CO_2 from the lungs. **Metabolic alkalosis** usually results from excessive vomiting or an abnormal secretion of certain hormones that cause excess elimination of acid from the stomach or kidneys.

The kidneys are vitally important in compensating for respiratory acidosis or alkalosis. Conversely, the respiratory system is vitally important in compensating for metabolic and respiratory acidosis or alkalosis. If the kidneys are not functioning properly, a mechanical filtering process (dialysis) must be used or one of the kidneys must be replaced with a transplant.

Kidney diseases can be characterized in five major categories:

- Nephritic syndrome (caused by cancer, diabetes, renal vein thrombosis, pericarditis, malaria, syphilis, bee stings, transplant rejection, etc.) involves signs of blood in the urine (**hematuria**), protein in the urine (**proteinuria**), hypertension, uremia, and low urine output (**oliguria**). These signs are specifically associated with a thin glomerular basement membrane. Another term nephrotic syndrome is also a nonspecific description that is related to high levels of proteinuria and low levels of protein in the blood (**proteinemia**) or hypoproteinemia. Neither term, nephritic or nephrotic syndrome, represent a definitive diagnosis, but both terms are used to describe symptoms while a patient is being diagnosed.[2]

- Acute kidney disease (caused by hypovolemia-decreased blood volume possibly the result of internal bleeding, cardiac failure, acute tubular necrosis, shock, hemolytic uremic syndrome, vasculitis-inflammation of blood vessels, etc.)

- Chronic kidney disease (caused by systemic lupus erythematosus, polyarteritis rodosa, malignant hypertension, renal vein thrombosis, tuberculosis, pyelonephritis, diabetes, hypertension, urinary tract obstruction, etc.)

- Glomerulonephritis (caused by infections, immune diseases, hypertension, diabetes)

- End stage renal disease (ESRD) (caused by glomerulonephritis, tubular diseases, hypertension, polycystic disease, interstitial disease systemic lupus erythematosus)[2]

Common Laboratory Tests for the Urinary System

- Renal functions can be determined by evaluating circulating blood levels of substances, filtration capacity of the nephrons, excretion of compounds by the kidneys, and by the ability to maintain electrolyte and water balance. Thus, urinary substances are routinely analyzed using a dipstick method with urine and/or laboratory evaluations on blood specimens. Urinalysis is covered more thoroughly in Chapter 16.

- Laboratory tests include the measurement of osmolality, glomerular filtration rate (GFR), and chemical constituents, such as proteins, glucose blood, microorganisms, and cells in the urine, as well as chemical analysis of albumin, ammonia, creatinine, total protein, blood urea nitrogen (BUN), uric acid, blood pH, blood gases, and electrolytes in the blood.

- The creatinine clearance test evaluates the degree to which kidneys are filtering out waste products of metabolism.

ENDOCRINE SYSTEM

Structure and Function

The endocrine system consists of two types of glands:

- **Exocrine glands** secrete fluids, such as sweat, saliva, mucus, and digestive juices, which are transported through channels or ducts.

- **Endocrine glands,** or ductless glands, release their secretions (hormones) directly into the bloodstream and include the hypothalamus, pituitary, thyroid, parathyroid, thymus, and adrenal glands as well as the ovaries and testes.

This glandular system has the same functions as those of the nervous system: communication, control, and integration. **Hormones** play an important role in the metabolic regulation that influences growth and development, in fluid and electrolyte balance, in energy balance, and in acid-base balance. The **pituitary gland,** or master gland, as it is sometimes called, stimulates the other glands to produce hormones as needed. It controls and regulates hormone production through chemical feedback. The pituitary hormones also regulate retention of water by the kidneys, cause uterine contractions during childbirth, stimulate breast milk production, and produce growth hormone (GH). This hormone controls growth by regulating the nutrients that are taken into cells. It also works with insulin to control blood sugar levels. The thyroid gland produces a hormone that affects cell metabolism and growth rate. Parathyroid glands regulate calcium and phosphorus in the blood and the bones. The thymus gland affects the lymphoid system. The **adrenals** (two glands) produce hormones as a result of emotions such as fright or anger. This hormone production causes an increase in blood pressure, widened pupils,

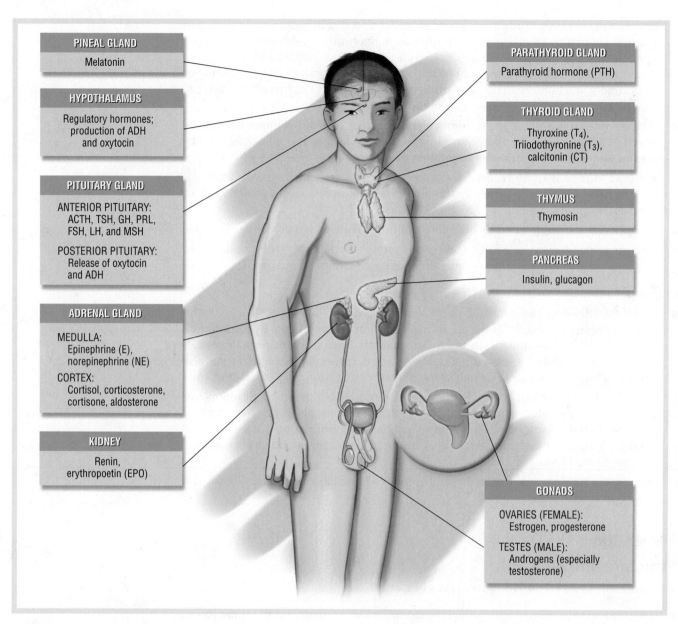

FIGURE 6–27

The Endocrine Glands and Their Hormones

and heart stimulation. The adrenals also produce hormones that regulate carbohydrate metabolism and electrolyte balance.[1] The gonads (ovaries and testes) produce estrogens and progesterone, and testosterone, respectively (**FIGURE 6–27**). The pineal gland secretes melatonin, a regulatory hormone. The pancreas contains exocrine tissue, which secretes pancreatic juice to aid in digestion, and endocrine tissue to secrete hormones, such as insulin and glucagon.

Disorders of the Endocrine System

- Many are inherited and result in excessive or insufficient hormone production.
- Disorders include Addison's disease, Graves' disease, Hashimoto's thyroiditis, Cushing's syndrome, dwarfism, acromegaly, gigantism, diabetes insipidus, diabetes mellitus, subacute thyroiditis, trophoblastic tumors, hypo- or hyperthyroidism, neonatal hypothyroidism, hyperinsulinism, hypoglycemia, goiter (enlarged thyroid gland)

Common Laboratory Tests for the Endocrine System

■ Since many hormones are transported by the bloodstream, abnormalities are easily detected by analyzing blood samples. Chemical assays are available for all types of constituents that are regulated by the endocrine system, including glucose, insulin, renin, serotonin, erythropoietin (EPO), antidiuretic hormone (ADH), adrenocorticotropic hormone (ACTH), growth hormone (GH), prolactin (PRL), follicle stimulating hormone (FSH), luteinizing hormone (LH), melanocyte-stimulating hormone (MSH), glucagon, cortisol, and others.

■ Specific thyroid function tests are available: antithyroglobulin antibodies, antithyroid peroxidase antibodies, free T_4 index (FT_4I), thyroxine-binding globulin (TBG), triiodothyronine (T_3), total T_3 (TT_3), thyroxine (T_4), free thyroxine (FT_4) and thyroid stimulating hormone (TSH), thyrotropin releasing hormone.[3,4]

REPRODUCTIVE SYSTEM
Structure and Function

The **reproductive system** is responsible for the production of offspring. Male and female structures are different even though they have similar roles (**FIGURE 6–28**).

Male reproductive structures include

■ Testes
■ Seminal vesicles
■ Prostate gland
■ Epididymis
■ Ejaculatory ducts
■ Urethra
■ Penis
■ Spermatic cords

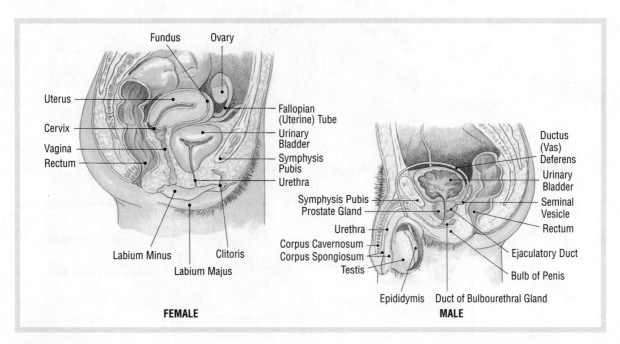

FIGURE 6–28
Reproductive System

The primary functions of this system are spermatogenesis (sperm production); storage, maintenance, and excretion of seminal fluid; and secretion of hormones (the most important of which is testosterone).

Female reproductive structures include

- Ovaries
- Fallopian tubes
- Uterus
- Vagina
- Labia
- Breasts, mammary glands

These structures play a role in ovulation, fertilization, menstruation, pregnancy, labor, lactation, and secretion of hormones (estrogens and progesterone) (**FIGURE 6–29**).

A sperm is one of the smallest cells in the body, whereas the mature egg is the largest. Each of these cells contains a nucleus with 23 chromosomes. Because a mother's egg and a father's sperm contain different sets of DNA, various genetic characteristics are paired. One of the pairs of chromosomes determines the sex of the fetus. The egg contains only an X chromosome; however, the sperm may contain an X or a Y chromosome. Therefore, if an X sperm fertilizes the egg, an XX pair of chromosomes forms, and the neonate will be a girl; if a Y sperm fertilizes the egg, an XY pair forms, and it will be a boy. The 46 combined chromosomes contain the DNA-coded blueprint, otherwise know as the **genome,** for the newborn (**FIGURE 6–30**).

FIGURE 6–29
Pregnant Female

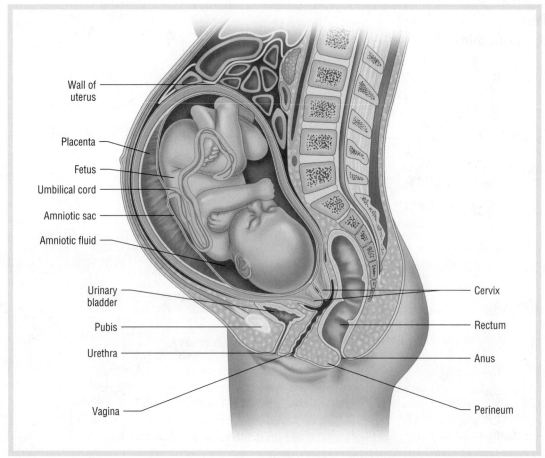

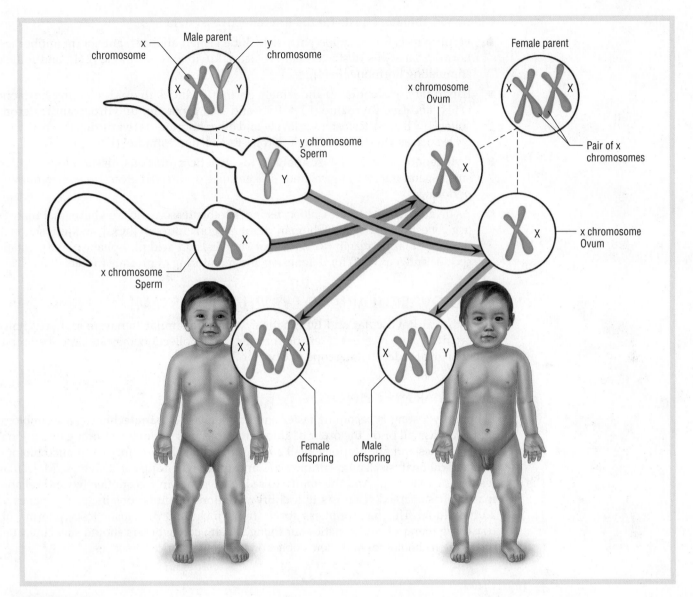

FIGURE 6–30
X and Y Chromosomes

The diagram depicts the offspring when chromosomes from the parents unite.

Disorders of the Reproductive System

- Malignant (cancerous) tumors, cysts
- Sexually transmitted diseases (STDs), such as gonorrhea, genital herpes, syphilis, and **human immunodeficiency virus (HIV)**
- Infertility

Infertility affects more than 6 million people in the United States and is defined as the inability of a couple to conceive a child after one year of regular, unprotected sexual intercourse or the inability to carry a pregnancy to live birth. Assisted reproductive technologies (ART) are procedures that include diagnosis of infertility and processes for *in vitro* fertilization (IVF, fertilization under laboratory conditions) or intrauterine (in the uterus) insemination. The laboratory plays an important role in all processes.[4]

Common Laboratory Tests for the Reproductive System

- Fertility tests for the male partner include semen analysis, antisperm antibodies, hormone analysis (testosterone, prolactin, luteinizing hormone [LH], and follicle stimulating hormone [FSH]).

- Laboratory evaluation of the female partner includes thyroid-releasing hormone (TSH) and free thyroxine (FT_4), FSH and LH, prolactin, dihydroepiandrosterone sulfate (DHEA-S), testosterone levels, and other hormone levels during the menstrual cycle such as FSH, LH, prolactin, progesterone, and estradiol (E2).

- Cytogenetic studies, DNA analysis for genetic mutations, tissue biopsies, Pap smears, and microbiological and viral cultures of infected areas are also commonly performed.

- Aside from fertility studies, blood testing for other reasons includes hormonal analysis (e.g., of estrogen, FSH, LH, human chorionic gonadotropin [hCG], and testosterone), the rapid plasma reagin (RPR) test for syphilis, and acid phosphatase and prostatic specific antigen (PSA) for diagnosing and monitoring of prostate cancer.[4]

CARDIOVASCULAR AND LYMPHATIC SYSTEMS

Since the cardiovascular and lymphatic systems are similar in nature and are vitally important for health care workers performing blood collection, they are described separately in greater depth and scope in Chapter 7.

EMERGING TECHNOLOGY

Laboratory testing is becoming faster and smaller. Use of **nanotechnology** (technology that is ultrasmall or on the order of atomic or molecular scale) is providing exceptional opportunities and applications in all areas of the clinical laboratory from microbiology to chemical analysis. Thus, sample sizes and types will adjust and change. Molecular testing is expanding. And the ability to sequence genes in a cost-effective and reliable manner has enabled scientists to identify variations or mutations in specific genes of an individual. This has countless applications, including diagnostic tests, pharmacology (drug therapy), and genetic counseling. Health care workers should stay abreast of emerging technologies and their impact on their own clinical practices.

Study Questions

For the following questions, select the one best answer.

1 Which layers make up human skin?

  a. striated and visceral
  b. epidermis, dermis, and subcutaneous
  c. muscular and hematopoietic
  d. pharynx, trachea, bronchiole, and alveolus

2 Which of the following body systems provides for CO_2 and O_2 gas exchange?

  a. nervous
  b. muscular
  c. respiratory
  d. reproductive

3 Which of the following are important anatomical structures of the respiratory system?

  a. striated and visceral
  b. epidermis, dermis, and subcutaneous
  c. muscular and hematopoietic
  d. pharynx, trachea, bronchiole, and alveolus

4 The skeletal system provides which of the body's functions?

  a. support, calcium storage, blood cell formation
  b. protection of tissues, temperature regulation
  c. metabolism and peristalsis
  d. ova and sperm cell formation

5 Germ cells are defined as

  a. hair follicles
  b. ova and sperm
  c. mammary glands
  d. neurons

6 Which of the following cell structures is the control center for a cell?

  a. cytoplasm
  b. nucleus
  c. lysosome
  d. mitochondria

7 Which of the following is responsible for skin coloring?

  a. hemostasis
  b. hormones
  c. lymph tissue
  d. melanin

8 What role does DNA play in the human body?

  a. allows for hormonal changes
  b. provides a genetic blueprint
  c. initiates catabolism and anabolism
  d. assists in the digestive process

9 What portion of human body weight is water?

  a. 90 percent
  b. 50 percent
  c. 25 percent
  d. 10 percent

10 Homeostasis refers to which of the following?

  a. chemical imbalance
  b. steady-state condition
  c. balanced chemistry
  d. thousands of genes

Case Study 1

Skin Rash Rosa Costa, age 45, comes to the doctor's office for her routine checkup. She tells the doctor that the previous weekend she had been camping with her family. Rosa then indicates that she has developed an itchy red rash (dermatitis) that is oozing slightly on her right forearm but otherwise she is healthy. When the health care worker goes to take a routine blood specimen from the patient, the irritated portion of Rosa's forearm is near the site where blood is to be taken.

Questions

1 Based on this scenario, what are the next steps for the health care worker?

2 Should the health care worker follow up with a nurse or doctor? Why or why not?

Case Study 2

Special Instructions Ms. Heather Wheatman is a health care worker who recently graduated from her training program at the community college and acquired a position at County General Hospital. One day during her fourth month there, she was informed by a nurse on a floor with patients having orthopedic conditions that any blood collections from patient Bill Davis should be taken while Mr. Davis is in the supine position and that all blood specimens should be taken from the dorsal side of the left hand.

Questions

1 Is the dorsal area the same as the posterior area? Explain similarities or differences.

2 Should Mr. Davis sit up or lie down during the blood collection?

3 An "orthopedic condition" would refer to what type of disorder?

Action in Practice

Muscle Tone Think about the muscular system and what happens when a patient has a cast on his or her arm for a lengthy period of time. The arm becomes smaller and weaker than the arm without the cast. Normally, muscles are well toned, or in a state of partial contraction. Athletes tend to have increased muscle tone—that is, stronger and larger muscle fibers, making their muscles more defined in appearance. When muscles are not used, they tend to lose their tone and become flaccid (soft/flabby). If a patient is required to stay in bed for long periods, his or her muscles may begin to atrophy.

Questions

1 How might a patient feel when getting out of a hospital bed after two days of being bedridden?

2 If you have ever had a cast on an arm or leg, how did you feel when it was removed? Describe the muscle tone in the affected area after cast removal.

3 Why might patients be encouraged to get out of their hospital beds as soon as possible?

Patients Who Need Oxygen A patient in respiratory distress may need supplemental oxygen. Oxygen is delivered to patients in many ways—for example, tracheostomy, intubation (long-term breathing tubes), oxygen mask, nasal cannula (nose tube), and other specialized devices. Health care workers must be aware of what treatments and medications are being administered to patients they serve. If a patient has been intubated, the patient cannot talk because of the tube and because the vocal cords cannot function properly. If a permanent airway is needed, the patient might have a tracheostomy, in which case he or she might not be able to talk or is learning to vocalize. Keen observation of the patient's condition can help avoid any misunderstandings in communication.

Questions

1 The next time you are in a hospital, take note of the numerous ways that oxygen is delivered to patients. How would you feel if your closest relative were intubated?

2 What are the various conditions that reduce oxygen to the lungs?

3 Think about the effects of cigarette smoking on lung disease. How do you react around cigarette smoking?

Fever Infections cause fever. Fever makes your body temperature rise above its normal temperature (98 degrees Fahrenheit or 37 degrees Celsius), a "febrile" condition. It is an attempt by your body to make the environment too hot for the bacteria that have invaded your body. Fever is a response to try to keep your body in a steady state, called homeostasis. It occurs when your brain tricks your body into thinking it is cold, so your body turns up the heat while increasing heart rate and blood pressure. Once the body's internal heater has been turned up, it begins to sweat.

Questions

1 Recall the last time you had fever. What were some of the symptoms you experienced?

2 Describe other ways that your own body keeps you in a steady-state condition. For example, how does your body react if you exercise vigorously, if you are too cold, if you are too hot, if you eat salty foods or drink alcohol, etc.?

COMPETENCY ASSESSMENT

Check Yourself

1 Review Figure 6–14. It is remarkable that our skeletal and muscular systems allow us to move in so many directions. Think about your joint movements while you walk to a chair to sit down. What movements would you go through to prepare to have a blood specimen collected? As you move your arm, then hand/wrist, then ankle/foot, describe the movements of flexion and extension, circumduction, pronation and supination, and dorsiflexion. Say the words as you move your limbs and match the movements with the words. Remember that for some patients, these same easy movements may be painful or impossible because of their medical conditions (e.g., arthritis).

2 Just for practice, go back to the key word list at the beginning of this chapter and read all the terms out loud to yourself. Some of them are easy and some are harder to say. If you have a hard time pronouncing the word, practice it until you can say it easily, without hesitation. Saying them out loud helps you hear your own voice and become more confident in your use of medical terminology.

Competency Checklist: Prefixes

In the space provided, write the definition of these prefixes. Do not refer to the chapter text, and leave the space blank for the words that you do not know. After answering as many as you can, go back to the list to check your work. Note the ones that you missed.

1. a _____	6. ana _____
2. ab _____	7. ante _____
3. ad _____	8. hemi _____
4. ambi _____	9. auto _____
5. an _____	10. poly _____

11. homeo _____
12. brady _____
13. cac _____
14. hydro _____
15. centi _____
16. milli _____
17. contra _____
18. deca _____

19. extra _____
20. hypo _____
21. mal _____
22. dys _____
23. endo _____
24. epi _____
25. uni _____

Competency Checklist: Word Roots

In the space provided, write the definition of these word roots. Do not refer to the chapter text, and leave the space blank for the words that you do not know. After answering as many as you can, go back to the list to check your work. Note the ones that you missed.

1. angio _____
2. angin _____
3. arter _____
4. arterio _____
5. athero _____
6. capillus _____
7. sphygmo _____
8. cardi _____
9. cardio _____
10. vaso _____
11. cyte _____
12. derm _____
13. electro _____

14. embol _____
15. sera _____
16. erythro _____
17. hemo _____
18. infarct _____
19. lipid _____
20. log _____
21. veni _____
22. myo _____
23. phleb _____
24. phlebo _____
25. pulmonar _____

Competency Checklist: Suffixes

In the space provided, write the definition of these suffixes. Do not refer to the chapter text, and leave the space blank for the words that you do not know. After answering as many as you can, go back to the list to check your work. Note the ones that you missed.

1. algia _____
2. blast _____
3. uria _____
4. centesis _____
5. cyte _____
6. rrhage _____
7. dynia _____
8. ectomy _____
9. emesis _____
10. gram _____
11. graph _____
12. tomy _____
13. itis _____

14. philia _____
15. lysis _____
16. megaly _____
17. poiesis _____
18. oid _____
19. scopy _____
20. opsy _____
21. osis _____
22. pathy _____
23. penia _____
24. pexy _____
25. phagia _____
26. phasia _____

Competency Checklist: Identifying Medical Terms

Write the correct medical terms for the following definitions.

1. Inflammation of the joints

   _____

2. Away from the point of reference

   _____

3. Study of diseases of the blood

   _____

4. Excess sugar in the blood

   _____

5. Study of tumors

   _____

6. Instrument used to measure degree of heat

   _____

7. Study of urinary system

   _____

8. Front area of the elbow

   _____

9. Treatment using chemical agents

   _____

10. Hardening of the arteries

    _____

11. Inflammation of the skin

    _____

12. Study of the skin

    _____

13. Inflammation of the liver

    _____

14. Inflammation of the bone and cartilage

    _____

15. Study of blood and blood-forming tissues

    _____

Competency Checklist: Spelling

In the spaces provided, write the correct spelling of these misspelled terms.

1. hemology   _____
2. phlebtomy   _____
3. onclogy   _____
4. proxemal   _____
5. leukomia   _____

6. periphral   _____
7. homatology   _____
8. thorasic   _____
9. anticubile   _____
10. millameter   _____

Competency Checklist: Directional Terms

Define the following directional terms.

1. superior   _____
2. medial   _____
3. proximal   _____
4. posterior   _____
5. anterior   _____

6. dorsal   _____
7. lateral   _____
8. distal   _____
9. medial   _____
10. ventral   _____

Competency Checklist: Body Systems

Name and correctly spell the organ systems described in this chapter, their functions, and at least two methods used in the clinical laboratory to evaluate the system.

1. _____
2. _____
3. _____
4. _____
5. _____

6. _____
7. _____
8. _____
9. _____

REFERENCES

1. Rice, J. *Medical terminology: A word-building approach,* 7th ed. Upper Saddle River, NJ: Prentice Hall, 2011.

2. Ogedegbe, H. O. (2007, May). Review: Renal function tests: A clinical laboratory perspective., *Lab Med, 38*(5): 295–304. www.ascp.org, accessed April 17, 2013.

3. Samuels, M. H. (2001, May). The use of tests for the diagnosis and monitoring of thyroid disease, CE Update. *Laboratory Medicine, 32*(5). www.ascp.org, a, laboratory medicine, May 2001, no5, vol 32, accessed April 17, 2013, www.ascp.org.

4. Rogers, L. C. (2005, January). The laboratory's role in assisted reproduction. *Medi Lab Obser,* January 2005; 12–25.

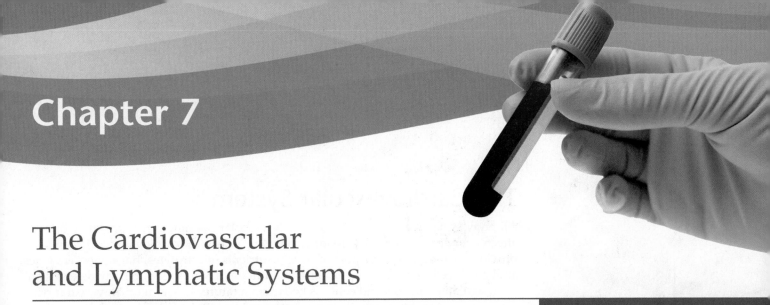

Chapter 7

The Cardiovascular and Lymphatic Systems

Chapter Objectives

Upon completion of Chapter 7, the learner is responsible for doing the following:

1. Define the functions of the cardiovascular and lymphatic systems.

2. Identify and describe the structures and functions of the heart.

3. List pathologic conditions and common laboratory tests associated with the cardiovascular and lymphatic systems.

4. Trace the flow of blood through the cardiovascular system.

5. Describe different types of blood vessels and the properties of arterial blood, venous blood, and capillary blood.

6. Identify and describe the cellular and noncellular components of blood.

7. Describe the differences and similarities between whole blood, serum, and plasma.

8. Locate and name the veins most commonly used for phlebotomy procedures.

9. Define hemostasis and describe the basic process of coagulation and fibrinolysis.

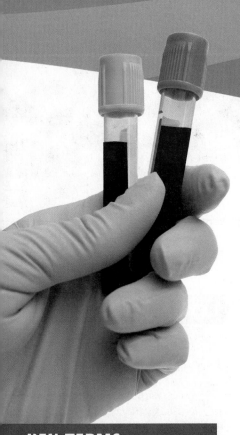

The Cardiovascular System

All body systems are linked by the cardiovascular system, a transport network that affects every part of the body. To maintain homeostasis, the cardiovascular system must provide for the rapid transport of water, nutrients, electrolytes, hormones, enzymes, antibodies, cells, and gases to all cells. In addition, it contributes to body defenses and the coagulation process and controls body temperature. The term **cardiovascular** refers to the cardiac (heart) muscle, the **vascular** system (network of blood vessels that includes veins, arteries, and capillaries), and the circulating blood. Thus, the three primary components of the cardiovascular system (**TABLE 7–1**) are

- Heart
- Circulating blood
- **Blood vessels** (the circulatory system)

TABLE 7–1

The Cardiovascular System: Structures and Functions

Organ/Structure	Primary Functions
Heart	■ Muscular organ about the size of an adult's closed first ■ Contractions push blood throughout the body ■ The average heart beats 60 to 80 times per minute
Arteries	■ Transport blood from the right and left chambers of the heart to the entire body ■ Large arteries branch into arterioles the farther they are from the heart ■ Carry oxygenated blood that is bright red in color ■ Have thicker elastic walls than veins do ■ Have a pulse ■ Are located deep in muscles/tissues
Veins	■ Blood is transported from peripheral tissues back to the heart and lungs ■ Large veins branch into venules in the peripheral tissues ■ Deoxygenated blood is carried back to the lungs to release carbon dioxide ■ Carry blood that is normally dark red in color ■ Have thinner walls than arteries; walls appear bluish ■ Valves prevent the backflow of blood ■ Are located both deep and superficially (close to the surface of the skin)
Capillaries	■ Connect arterioles with venules via microscopic vessels ■ Oxygen and carbon dioxide, nutrients, and fluids in tissue capillaries are exchanged ■ Waste products from tissue cells are passed into capillary blood, then onto removal from the body ■ Carry blood that is a mixture of arterial blood and venous blood
Circulating Blood	■ Oxygen and carbon dioxide, nutrients, and fluids are transported by circulating blood ■ Waste products are removed ■ Nutrients are disbursed ■ Regulates body temperature and electrolytes ■ Regulates the blood-clotting system

The Heart

The human **heart** is a muscular organ about the size of a man's closed fist (**FIGURE 7–1**). The heart contains four chambers and is located slightly left of the midline in the thoracic cavity. The two **atria** are separated by the interatrial septum (wall), and the interventricular septum divides the two **ventricles**. Heart valves are positioned between each atrium and ventricle so that blood can flow in one direction only, thereby preventing backflow.

FIGURE 7–2 traces the flow of blood. The right atrium of the heart receives O$_2$-poor blood from two large veins: the superior vena cava and the inferior vena cava. The **superior vena cava** brings blood from the head, neck, arms, and chest; the **inferior**

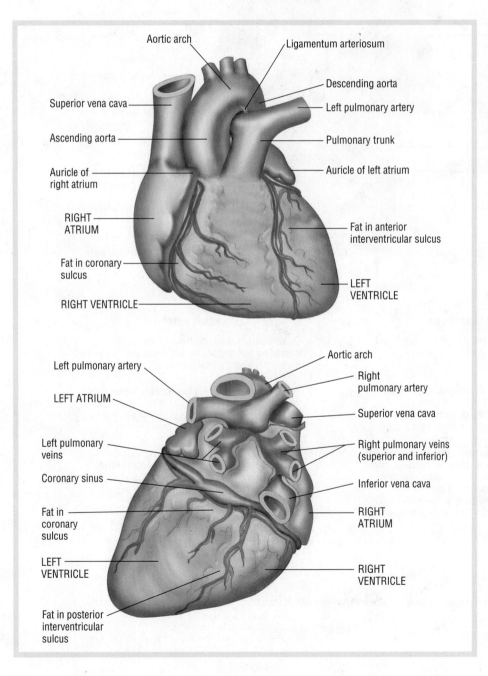

FIGURE 7–1

Superficial Anatomy of the Heart

(*Top*) Anterior (sternocostal) view of the heart showing major anatomic features.
(*Bottom*) Posterior (diaphragmatic) surface of the heart. (Coronary arteries are shown in red, coronary veins in blue.)

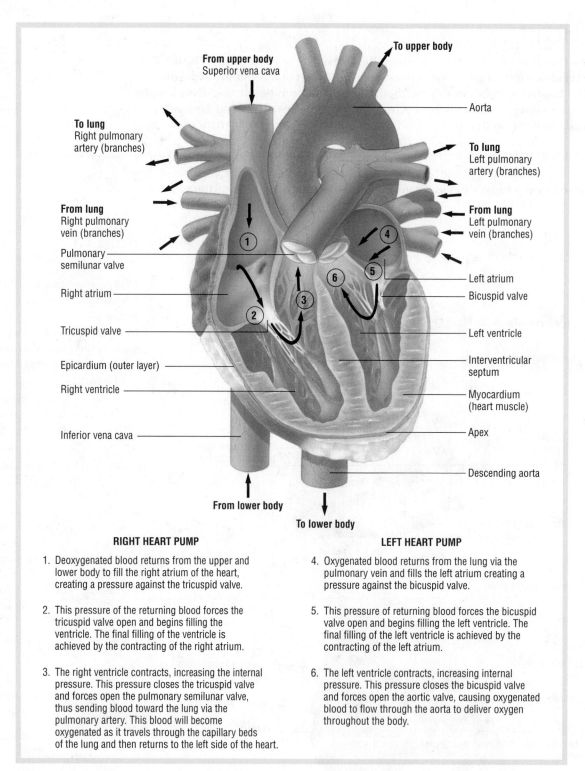

RIGHT HEART PUMP

1. Deoxygenated blood returns from the upper and lower body to fill the right atrium of the heart, creating a pressure against the tricuspid valve.

2. This pressure of the returning blood forces the tricuspid valve open and begins filling the ventricle. The final filling of the ventricle is achieved by the contracting of the right atrium.

3. The right ventricle contracts, increasing the internal pressure. This pressure closes the tricuspid valve and forces open the pulmonary semilunar valve, thus sending blood toward the lung via the pulmonary artery. This blood will become oxygenated as it travels through the capillary beds of the lung and then returns to the left side of the heart.

LEFT HEART PUMP

4. Oxygenated blood returns from the lung via the pulmonary vein and fills the left atrium creating a pressure against the bicuspid valve.

5. This pressure of returning blood forces the bicuspid valve open and begins filling the left ventricle. The final filling of the left ventricle is achieved by the contracting of the left atrium.

6. The left ventricle contracts, increasing internal pressure. This pressure closes the bicuspid valve and forces open the aortic valve, causing oxygenated blood to flow through the aorta to deliver oxygen throughout the body.

FIGURE 7–2

Internal Anatomy of the Heart and Path of Blood Flow

This is a diagrammatic frontal section through the heart showing major structures and the path of blood flow through the atria and ventricles.

vena cava carries blood from the rest of the trunk and the legs. Once the blood enters the right atrium, it passes through the heart valve (right atrioventricular, or tricuspid, valve) into the right ventricle. When blood exits the right ventricle, it begins the **pulmonary circuit**—it enters the right and left pulmonary arteries. Arteries of the pulmonary circuit differ from those of the **systemic circuit** because they carry deoxygenated blood. Like veins, they are usually shown in blue on color-coded charts. (Refer to **FIGURES 7–3** and **7–4**.) These vessels branch into smaller arterioles and capillaries within the lungs, where gaseous exchange occurs (O_2 is picked up and CO_2 is released). From the respiratory capillaries, blood flows into the left and right pulmonary veins and then into the left atrium. The left atrium also has a valve (left atrioventricular, bicuspid, or mitral valve). Blood flows through the mitral valve into the left ventricle. When blood exits the left ventricle, it passes through the aortic semilunar valve and into the systemic

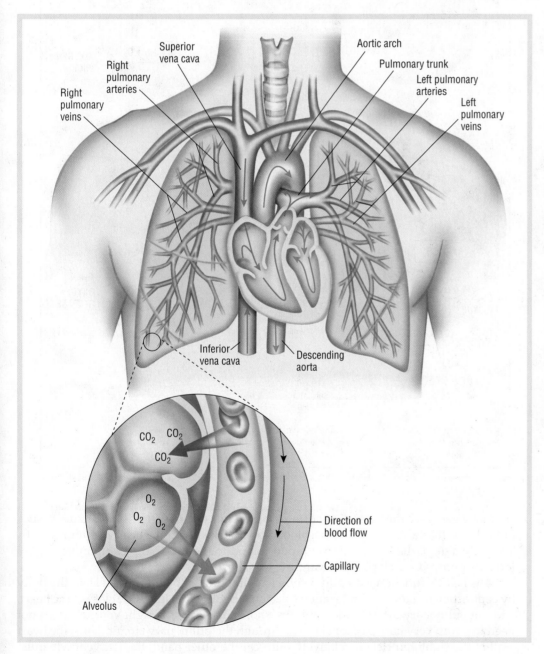

FIGURE 7–3

The Pulmonary Circuit in the Cardiovascular System

The right ventricle of the heart pumps blood into the pulmonary artery (pulmonary trunk), which divides into the right and left pulmonary arteries that go to each lung. In the lungs, the arteries branch extensively into small arteries and arterioles, then to capillaries. The capillaries surround the alveoli so that exchange of oxygen and carbon dioxide can take place. The capillaries flow into veins and finally into the two pulmonary veins that return blood to the heart through the left atrium. This oxygenated blood will then travel to the rest of the body. (Note that the pulmonary veins contain oxygenated blood. They are the only veins that carry blood with a high oxygen content. All other veins of the body carry blood with a low oxygen content.)

FIGURE 7–4

Exchange of Gases in Systemic and Pulmonary Capillaries

Oxygen (O_2) and carbon dioxide (CO_2) molecules are carried in red blood cells by hemoglobin (Hb) molecules. In the systemic or tissue capillaries, O_2 is released and CO_2 is picked up. When the red cell returns to the pulmonary capillaries in the lungs, CO_2 is released and O_2 is picked up.

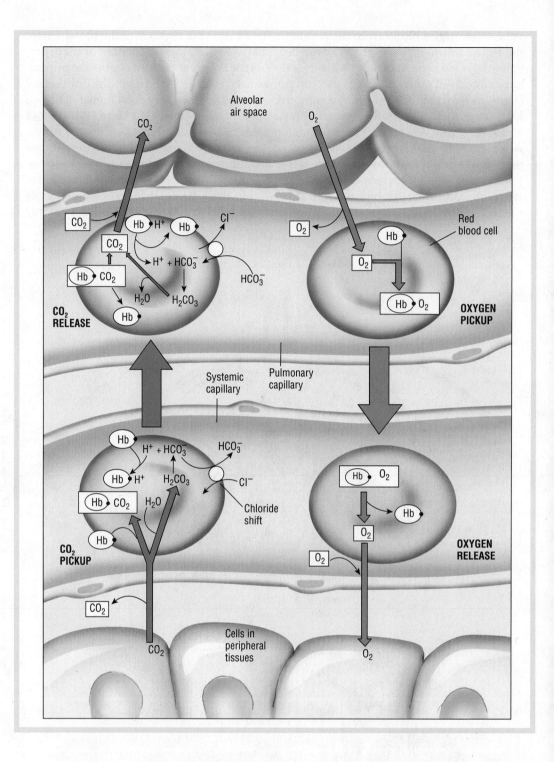

circuit by means of the ascending aorta. The systemic circuit carries blood to the tissues of the body. If a valve malfunctions, blood flows backward and a heart murmur results. The right side of the heart pumps O_2-poor blood to the lungs to pick up more O_2; the left side pumps O_2-rich blood toward the legs, head, and organs.

The heart's function is to pump sufficient amounts of blood to all cells of the body by contraction (systole) and relaxation (diastole). Because the lungs are close to the heart, and the pulmonary arteries and veins are short and wide, the right ventricle does not need to pump very hard to propel blood through the pulmonary circuit. Thus, the heart wall of the right ventricle is relatively thin. On the other hand, the left ventricle must push blood around the systemic circuit, which covers the entire body. As a result, the left ventricle has a thick, muscular wall and a powerful contraction.

BOX 7–1

Word Warning

The terms *palpitation* and *palpation,* as well as the terms *hemostasis* and *homeostasis,* are often confused. These words are important to health care workers who should know the difference and how to use the terms correctly. Practice saying each of the terms and be sure you understand the meanings as they relate to patients and phlebotomy services.

Pal-pi-ta-tion relates to a fast or irregular heartbeat.

Pal-pa-tion relates to touching or feeling (a vein).

Hemo-stasis relates to blood clotting at the site of an injury while maintaining blood flow in other parts of the body. (The opposite of hemostasis is the term **hemorrhage** that means excessive or uncontrolled bleeding.)

Ho-me-o-stasis relates to a steady-state condition as discussed in the previous chapter.

Blood pressure increases during ventricular systole and decreases during ventricular diastole. Blood pressure not only forces blood through vessels, but also pushes it against the walls of the vessels like air in a balloon. Therefore, it can be measured by how forcefully it presses against vascular walls. Refer to Appendix 4 for detailed information about taking blood pressure measurements and other vital signs.

The average heart beats 60 to 80 times per minute. Children have faster heart rates than adults, and athletes have slower rates because more blood can be pumped with each beat. During exercise, the heart beats faster to supply muscles with more blood. During and after meals, it also beats faster to pump blood to the digestive system. During a fever, the heart pumps more blood to the skin surface to release heat. Remember that all responses are designed to maintain homeostasis (**BOX 7–1**). The heart rate (pulse rate) is measured by feeling for a pulse and counting the pulses per minute. Refer to Appendix 4 for more information about measuring pulse rate.

The Vessels and Circulation

Three kinds of blood vessels exist in the human body:

- Arteries
- Veins
- Capillaries

This intricate system travels to every inch of the human body through repeatedly branching vessels that get smaller and smaller as they move away from the heart (arteries) and then get larger again as they return toward the heart (veins). **FIGURES 7–5** and **7–6** provide an overview of the arterial and venous systems, showing the major branches of the vessels. The largest artery (**aorta**) and veins (**venae cavae**) are approximately 1 inch wide. **FIGURE 7–7** shows the capillary connection.

ARTERIES

Arteries are highly oxygenated vessels that carry blood away from the heart (efferent vessels). They branch into smaller vessels, called **arterioles,** and into capillaries. The principal arteries of the body are shown in Figure 7–5. Arteries appear brighter red in color, have thicker elastic walls than veins do, and have a pulse. Refer to **FIGURE 7–8**

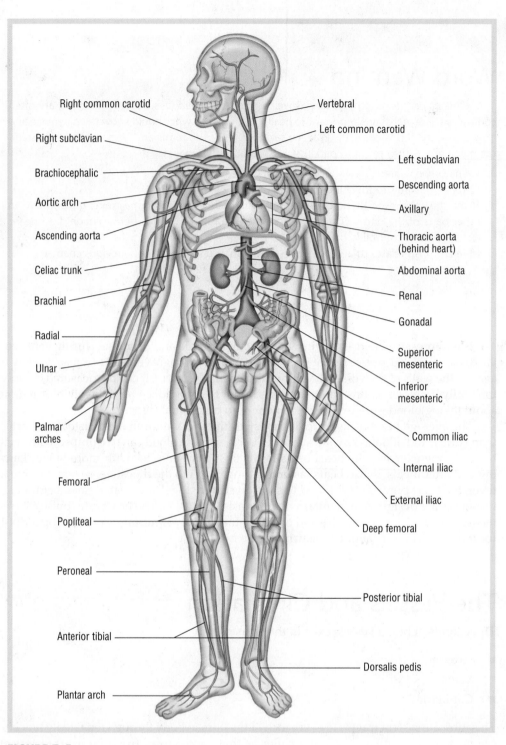

FIGURE 7–5
The Arterial System

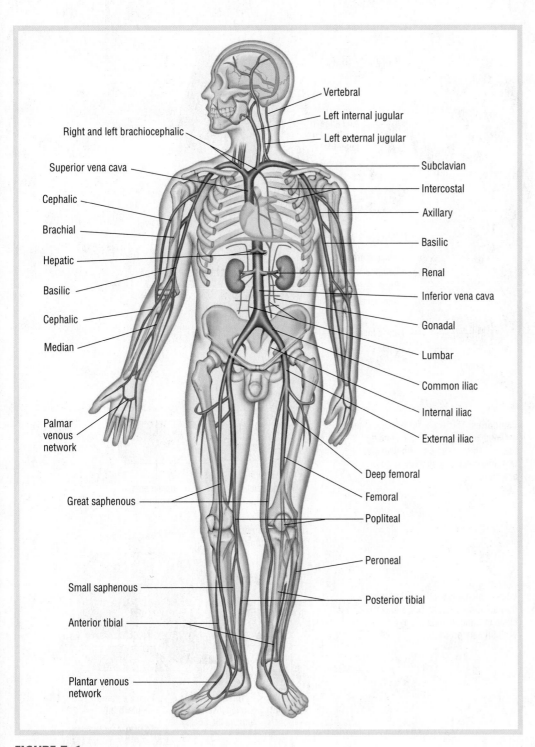

Vertebral
Left internal jugular
Left external jugular
Right and left brachiocephalic
Superior vena cava
Cephalic
Brachial
Hepatic
Basilic
Cephalic
Median
Subclavian
Intercostal
Axillary
Basilic
Renal
Inferior vena cava
Gonadal
Lumbar
Common iliac
Internal iliac
External iliac
Palmar venous network
Deep femoral
Femoral
Great saphenous
Popliteal
Peroneal
Small saphenous
Posterior tibial
Anterior tibial
Plantar venous network

FIGURE 7–6
The Venous System

FIGURE 7–7

The Capillary Connection

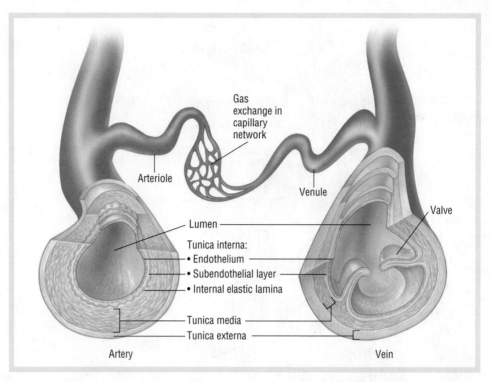

FIGURE 7–8

Anatomic Comparison of Arteries, Veins, and Capillaries

Capillaries: Thin walls permit exchange of blood and fluids from surrounding tissues. They are so small in diameter that only one RBC can pass through at a time.

Veins: Thinner walls than arteries so they are more likely to collapse when blood is withdrawn during a venipuncture procedure.

Arteries: Thicker walls (Tunica externa) than veins; resist the strong pressure of blood being pushed through.

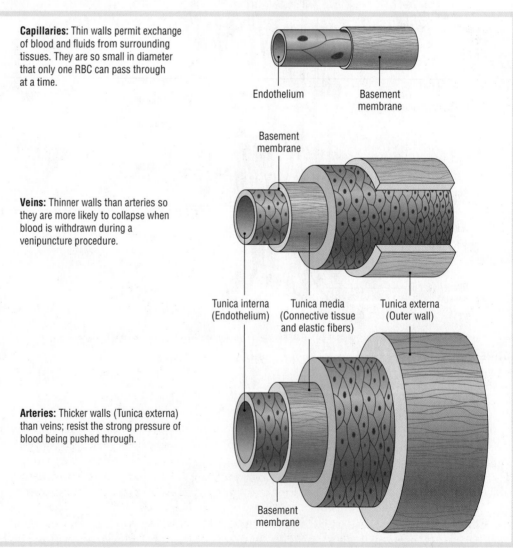

BOX 7–2

What Is "Hardening of the Arteries"?

With age, arterial walls may "harden" (called *hardening of the arteries, arteriosclerosis,* or *athero-sclerosis*). The inner walls of the vessels become rough because of cholesterol or calcium deposits (plaque). As the deposits build, a blood clot (thrombus) may form that clogs the artery further, and the blood supply to tissues is reduced. In serious cases, this lack of blood results in a stroke (if the blood supply in the brain is reduced) or a heart attack (if the blood supply in the coronary [heart] vessels is reduced).[1] (Refer to **FIGURE 7–9**.)

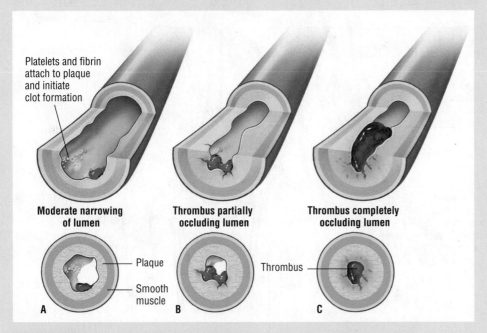

Platelets and fibrin attach to plaque and initiate clot formation

Moderate narrowing of lumen

Thrombus partially occluding lumen

Thrombus completely occluding lumen

Plaque

Smooth muscle

Thrombus

A

B

C

FIGURE 7–9

Thrombus Formation in an Atherosclerotic Vessel

A. The initial clot formation shown in a vessel with yellow plaque buildup. **B.** Partially occluded vessel and thrombus. **C.** Completely occluded vessel.

for a comparison of capillaries, arteries, and veins. Refer to **BOX 7–2** for examples of disorders of the arteries.

VEINS

Blood is carried toward the heart by the **veins** (afferent vessels). It is remarkable that the blood in veins flows against gravity in many areas of the body; these vessels have one-way valves and rely on weak muscular action to move blood cells. The one-way valves prevent backflow of blood. All veins (except the pulmonary veins) contain deoxygenated blood. Veins appear bluish in color under the skin and have thinner walls than arteries, as shown in Figure 7–8.

Health care workers should be familiar with the principal veins of the arms and legs (**FIGURES 7–10** through **7–13**). The antecubital area of the forearm is most commonly

FIGURE 7–10

Venous System of the Upper Torso and Arm

The antecubital area of the arm is where venipunctures are most often performed. The median cubital vein is best for venipuncture because it is generally the largest and best-anchored vein. Others in the antecubital area that are acceptable are the basilic and cephalic veins.

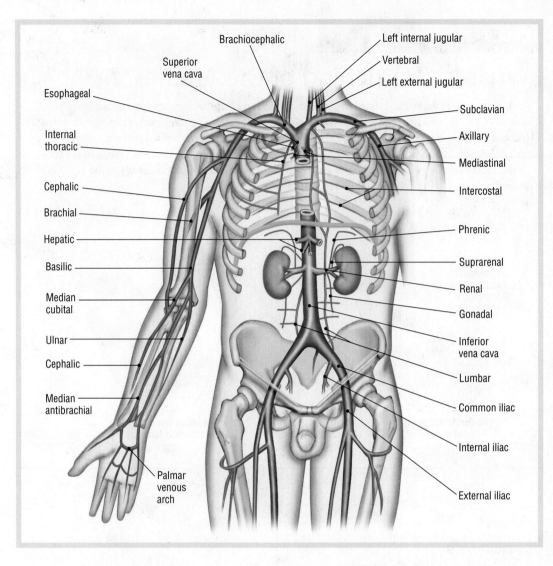

FIGURE 7–11

Major Arm Veins

Note that the *cephalic vein* extends almost the entire length of the arm. The superficial *median cubital vein* serves as a connection between the cephalic and basilic veins. The subclavian, brachial, and axillary veins are deeper veins.

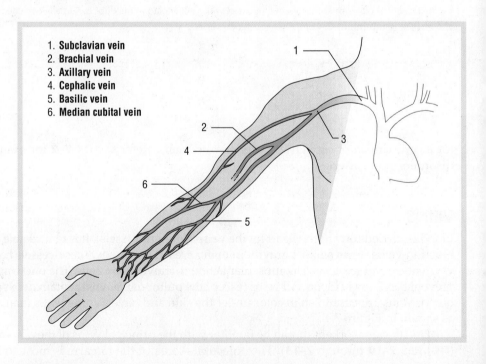

1. **Subclavian vein**
2. **Brachial vein**
3. **Axillary vein**
4. **Cephalic vein**
5. **Basilic vein**
6. **Median cubital vein**

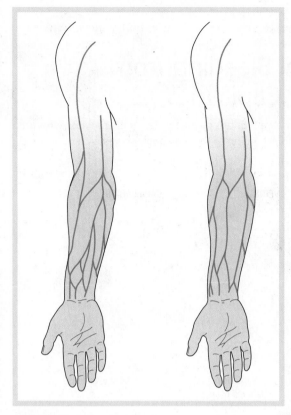

FIGURE 7–12

Variations in Venous Patterns

Since all individuals are unique, the exact location of veins may vary from one to another. This figure depicts variations in venous patterns in the arms of two individuals.

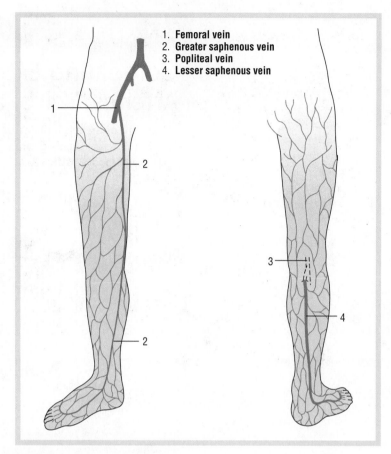

1. Femoral vein
2. Greater saphenous vein
3. Popliteal vein
4. Lesser saphenous vein

FIGURE 7–13

Major Leg Veins

The *femoral vein* is a deep vein. Note that the *greater saphenous vein* is the longest vein in the body. It ascends up the medial side of the leg and the medial thigh and empties into the femoral vein in the groin area. The *lesser saphenous vein* comes up the lateral side of the ankle and enters the deeper *popliteal vein* behind the knee.

used for venipuncture. The **median cubital vein** is best for venipuncture because it is generally the largest and best-anchored vein. Others in the antecubital area that are acceptable are the **basilic vein** and the **cephalic vein.**

CAPILLARIES

Capillaries are tiny microscopic vessels that connect or link arteries (arterioles) and veins (venules) and may be so small in diameter as to allow only one blood cell to pass through at any given time. They are the only vessels that permit the exchange of gases (O_2 and CO_2) and other molecules between blood and surrounding tissues. Capillaries do not work independently but are a part of an interconnected network. Each arteriole ends in dozens of capillaries (capillary bed) that eventually feed back into a **venule** (when gas/nutrient exchange has been completed). Blood in the capillary bed is a mixture of arterial and venous blood (Figure 7–8). Refer to **BOX 7–3** for a comparison of how bleeding is different among vessel injuries.

BOX 7–3

Comparing External Bleeding from Arteries, Veins, and Capillaries

The nature of the job requires that health care workers regularly deal with patients who are bleeding. External bleeding can be described according to the type of blood vessel that is injured and losing blood (**FIGURE 7–14**).[2]

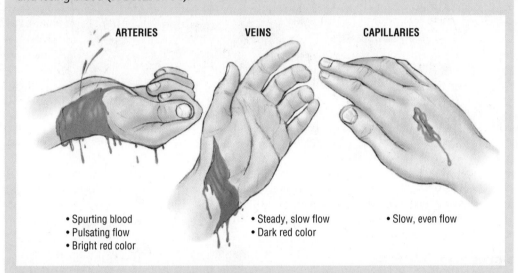

ARTERIES

- Spurting blood
- Pulsating flow
- Bright red color

VEINS

- Steady, slow flow
- Dark red color

CAPILLARIES

- Slow, even flow

FIGURE 7–14

Types of External Bleeding

Arterial blood is bright red in color (due to high O_2 content), and since the pressure is higher in arteries, bleeding is usually quicker, more abundant, and in spurts (with each heartbeat). Arterial bleeding is the hardest to control and usually requires special attention from the nurse and/or doctor. During a venipuncture procedure, if a health care worker accidentally punctures an artery instead of a vein, he or she should follow immediate steps to terminate the procedure and apply pressure to the site. Accidental incidents such as this should be reported to a supervisor immediately.

Venous blood is dark red in color (because it lacks O_2), and bleeding occurs in a steady flow. In normal, healthy adults, venous bleeding is easy to stop by simply applying pressure, because venous pressure is lower than arterial pressure.

Capillary bleeding occurs slowly and evenly because of the smaller size of the vessels and the low pressure within the vessels. Capillary bleeding is usually considered minor and is easily controlled with slight pressure or sometimes bleeding stops without intervention. Capillary blood is a color between the bright red of arterial blood and the dark red of venous blood.

The Blood

Circulating **blood** provides nutrients, oxygen, chemical substances, and waste removal for each of the billions of individual cells in the body and is essential to homeostasis and to sustaining life (**TABLE 7–2**). Any region of the body that is deprived of blood and O_2 soon becomes oxygen deficient, and the tissues may die within minutes. This condition is called **hypoxia.**

Human bodies contain approximately 5 quarts (4.73 liters) of whole blood, which is composed of water, solutes (dissolved substances), and cells. The volume of blood in

TABLE 7–2

Basic Functions of the Blood

Function	Specific Action
Transportation	Carry oxygen (O_2) from the lungs to the tissues
	Carry carbon dioxide (CO_2) from the tissues to the lungs
	Transport waste products to sites such as the kidneys for excretion
	Transport antibodies and white blood cells to defend against pathogenic microbes and viruses
Disbursement of nutrients	Distribute nutrients absorbed in the digestive tract to all organs of the body
	Take nutrients released from fat, muscle, and tissues for use in other parts of the body
Regulation	Regulate the blood pH in all parts of the body
	Regulate electrolyte balance to maintain a "steady state" condition
	Control body temperature by redistribution of heat
Hemostasis	Restrict fluid loss when blood vessels are damaged
	Formation of blood clots to prevent bleeding

an individual varies according to body weight; for instance, adult men usually have 5 to 6 liters of whole blood, whereas adult women usually have 4 to 5 liters (**FIGURE 7–15**). Abnormally low or high blood volumes can seriously affect other parts of the cardiovascular system. Whole blood is normally composed of approximately 3 quarts (2.84 liters), or about 55 to 60 percent, of plasma and 2 quarts (1.89 liters), or about 40 to 45 percent, of cells. Thus, if a blood specimen is withdrawn into a test tube from a vein and centrifuged, about 55 percent will be plasma and 45 percent will be formed elements (cells) (**FIGURES 7–16, 7–17,** and **7–18**). The plasma portion contains approximately 92 percent water and 8 percent solutes. Solutes include proteins, such as albumin (maintains water balance in blood); fibrinogen (for blood clotting); metabolites, such as lipids; glucose; nitrogen wastes; amino acids; and ions, such as sodium (Na), potassium (K), calcium (Ca), magnesium (Mg), and chloride (Cl).

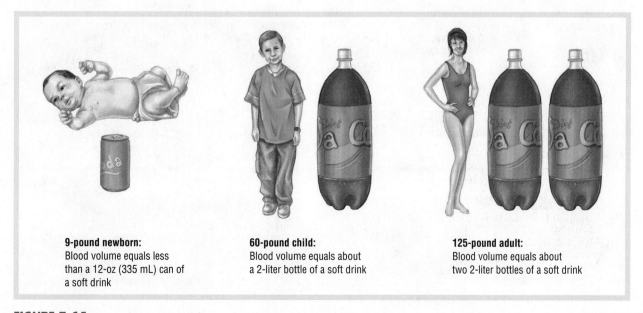

9-pound newborn:
Blood volume equals less than a 12-oz (335 mL) can of a soft drink

60-pound child:
Blood volume equals about a 2-liter bottle of a soft drink

125-pound adult:
Blood volume equals about two 2-liter bottles of a soft drink

FIGURE 7–15
Comparison of Infant, Child, and Adolescent/Adult Blood Volumes

FIGURE 7–16

Health Care Worker Removing a
Blood Specimen after Centrifugation

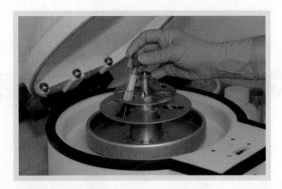

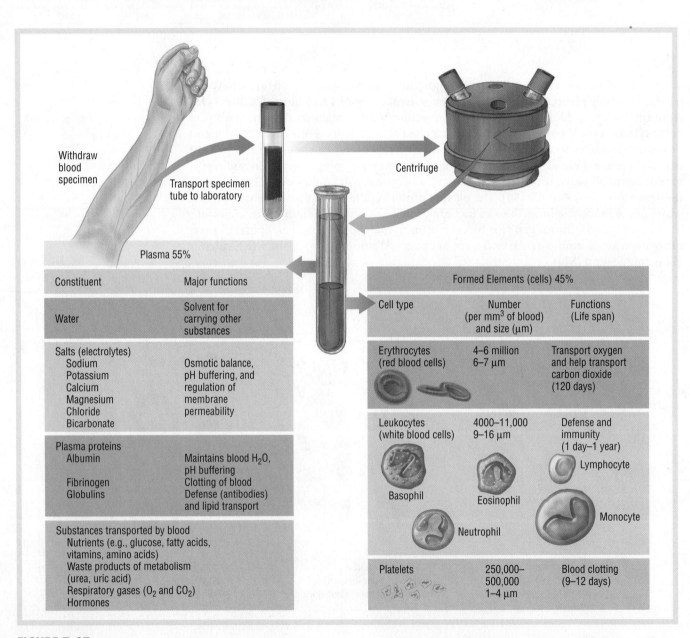

Withdraw blood specimen

Transport specimen tube to laboratory

Centrifuge

Plasma 55%

Constituent	Major functions
Water	Solvent for carrying other substances

Salts (electrolytes)
  Sodium
  Potassium
  Calcium
  Magnesium
  Chloride
  Bicarbonate
	Osmotic balance, pH buffering, and regulation of membrane permeability

Plasma proteins
  Albumin
 	
  Fibrinogen
  Globulins
	Maintains blood H_2O, pH buffering
	Clotting of blood
	Defense (antibodies) and lipid transport

Substances transported by blood
  Nutrients (e.g., glucose, fatty acids, vitamins, amino acids)
  Waste products of metabolism (urea, uric acid)
  Respiratory gases (O_2 and CO_2)
  Hormones	

Formed Elements (cells) 45%

Cell type	Number (per mm^3 of blood) and size (μm)	Functions (Life span)
Erythrocytes (red blood cells)	4–6 million 6–7 μm	Transport oxygen and help transport carbon dioxide (120 days)
Leukocytes (white blood cells)	4000–11,000 9–16 μm	Defense and immunity (1 day–1 year)
Basophil Eosinophil Neutrophil		Lymphocyte Monocyte
Platelets	250,000–500,000 1–4 μm	Blood clotting (9–12 days)

FIGURE 7–17

Basic Composition and Functions of Blood

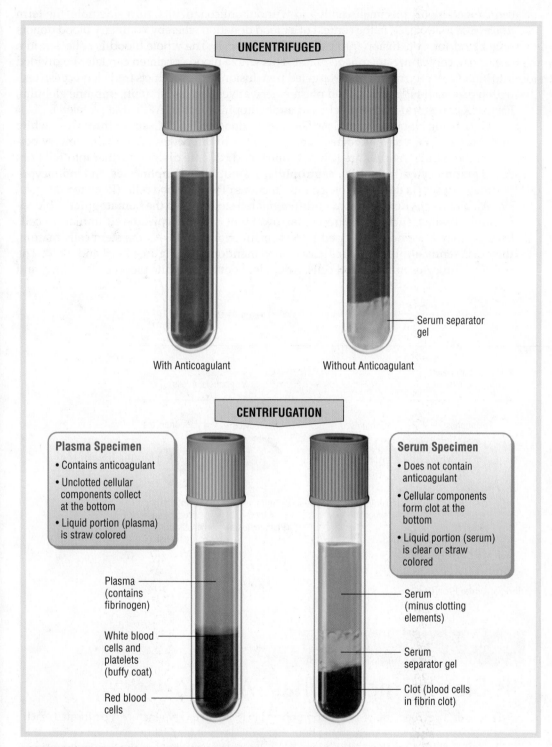

UNCENTRIFUGED

With Anticoagulant

Without Anticoagulant

Serum separator gel

CENTRIFUGATION

Plasma Specimen
- Contains anticoagulant
- Unclotted cellular components collect at the bottom
- Liquid portion (plasma) is straw colored

Serum Specimen
- Does not contain anticoagulant
- Cellular components form clot at the bottom
- Liquid portion (serum) is clear or straw colored

Plasma (contains fibrinogen)

White blood cells and platelets (buffy coat)

Red blood cells

Serum (minus clotting elements)

Serum separator gel

Clot (blood cells in fibrin clot)

FIGURE 7–18

Blood Specimens with and without Anticoagulants before and after Centrifugation

Normally, a blood specimen will begin to coagulate/clot immediately when it is removed from the body (as discussed in the section on hemostasis later in this chapter). Blood specimens can be withdrawn into chemically clean and/or sterile test tubes, or into clean tubes that have premeasured anticoagulants in them that will keep the blood from forming a blood clot. (Refer to Chapter 8 for more information about specimen tubes.) Figure 7–17 depicts the basic composition of blood. Figure 7–18 depicts uncentrifuged and centrifuged blood specimens with and without anticoagulants. As a side note, the term *whole blood* is also used in the context of a blood donation whereby voluntary blood donors give blood for transfusion into patients who need it. The whole blood is collected in a donor bag containing an anticoagulant. This whole blood specimen can later be divided into blood components for more targeted transfusion of the products (red blood cells; fresh frozen plasma [FFP]; plasma; and plasma derivatives such as albumin, immune globulin, Factor IX concentrates, cryoprecipated antihemophilic factor [AFP]; and platelets).

Circulating blood cells are classified as **red blood cells (RBCs or erythrocytes), white blood cells (WBCs or leukocytes),** and platelets (thrombocytes). Approximately 99 percent of the circulating cells are RBCs. White blood cells are divided further into cell lines called **granulocytes (basophils, neutrophils, eosinophils), lymphocytes,** and **monocytes. FIGURE 7–19** shows the morphology and functions of white blood cells. (Refer to **BOX 7–4.**)

All blood cells develop from undifferentiated stem cells in the **hematopoietic** (blood-forming) tissues, such as the bone marrow. Stem cells are considered immature cells because they have not developed into their functional state. As the stem cells mature, they differentiate into the specific cell lines mentioned in Figures 7–19 and **7–20**. The cells (erythrocytes or red blood cells, RBCs, leukocytes or white blood cells, WBCs, and

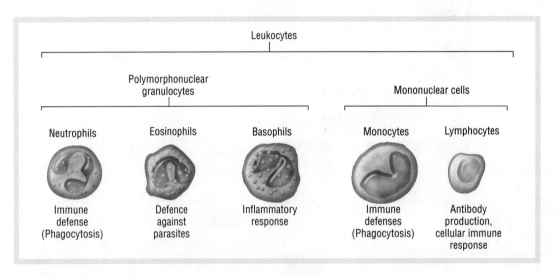

FIGURE 7–19
Morphology and Functions of White Blood Cells

BOX 7–4

Is Blood Thicker Than Water?

The answer is yes, because of all the components in it. When a venipuncture is performed, each test tube can contain anywhere from about 2 to 5 milliliters of blood. In a layperson's terms, this is comparable to about 2 to 5 teaspoons per tube. If you consider just *one drop* of the blood, here is what it contains:

- About 5 million red blood cells
- 200,000 to 400,000 platelets
- 7,500 white blood cells
- Plasma proteins, nutrients, oxygen, carbon dioxide, hormones, electrolytes

This really does make blood thicker than water!

megakaryocytes or platelets) undergo changes in the nucleus and cytoplasm so that when they reach the circulating blood, they will have developed into a specific cell type that is fully mature and functional. The distinguishing features of each blood cell type are clearly visible when staining techniques are used with light microscopy and/or with specialized hematology instruments. Common laboratory tests to assess the blood and cells are covered later in this chapter. Health care workers should be familiar with these blood tests.

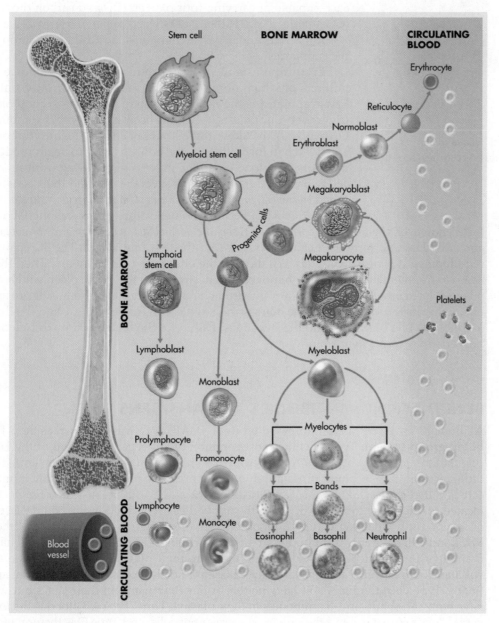

FIGURE 7–20

Hematopoiesis

All cellular elements of the circulating blood found in veins, arteries, and capillaries begin in the bone marrow. Blood cells are considered immature when they are in the bone marrow and mature when they reach the circulating blood (i.e., mature cells can carry out their intended functions of carrying O_2 or CO_2 [RBCs]), providing immunity/defense [WBCs], or helping in blood clotting [platelets]). Note that the pink background area represents the circulating blood. Hematologic analysis in the laboratory can reveal cellular abnormalities if there are too many of any one cell type, or too few, or if they are immature, or if they are abnormally shaped, etc.

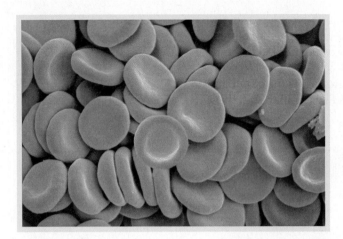

FIGURE 7–21
Erythrocytes

Note the red color of erythrocytes and their unique "donut" or biconcave disk shape. Each cell has a depressed center and no cell nucleus.

Andrew Syred/Science Source

ERYTHROCYTES

Red blood cells measure about 7 μm in diameter with a thickness of 2 μm. Prior to reaching maturity in the bone marrow, normal RBCs lose their nuclei and simultaneously become bi-concaved disks. Their unique and flexible shape enables them to pass through very narrow capillaries and provides for maximum surface area to transfer oxygen and carbon dioxide. Within each mature RBC are millions of hemoglobin molecules, each capable of carrying four oxygen (O_2) and carbon dioxide (CO_2) molecules (**FIGURE 7–21**). Also review Figures 7–3 and 7–4 for details about gas exchange as the RBCs pass through the capillaries.

Erythropoiesis means the production of red blood cells, millions of which normally are formed and destroyed daily. **Erythropoietin** is the hormone (produced in the kidney) that triggers erythropoiesis. When the body is not receiving enough O_2 (hypoxia), the kidneys are stimulated to produce erythropoietin, which in turn activates the bone marrow to begin producing more red blood cells. The process of maturing from a stem cell to a circulating RBC takes several days, and the stages are called *rubriblast, prorubricyte, rubricyte, metarubricyte, reticulocyte,* and *mature RBC.* Because nomenclature differs among laboratories, however, the terms *pronormoblast, basophilic normoblast, polychromatic normoblast,* and *orthochromatic normoblast* can also be used for the first four stages. The life span of red blood cells is approximately 120 days in the circulating bloodstream. Then they begin to fragment and are finally removed and destroyed in the liver, spleen, and bone marrow. As hemoglobin breaks down into iron-containing pigments (hemosiderin) and bile pigments (bilirubin), the bone marrow reuses the iron for new RBCs, and the liver excretes the bile pigments into the intestines. Failure of the bone marrow to function properly may result in anemia.

BLOOD TYPING: ANTIBODIES AND ANTIGENS

All humans have one of the four blood types: A, B, AB, or O; this is known as the **ABO blood group system.** Type O is the most common blood type (45 percent of the U.S. population), followed by types A (41 percent), B (10 percent), and AB (4 percent). The differences in human blood types are due to the presence or absence of protein molecules called *antigens* and *antibodies* (**FIGURE 7–22** and **TABLE 7–3**). The antigens are located on the surface of the RBCs and the antibodies are located in the blood plasma or serum. Individuals with Type A blood will have A antigens on the surface of their RBCs and will have anti-B antibodies in their plasma; individuals with Type B will have B antigens on their RBCs and anti-A antibodies in their plasma; those with Type AB will have both A and B antigens on their RBCs and no antibodies in their plasma; and finally, Type O individuals will have neither A nor B antigens on their RBCs but will have both anti-A and anti-B antibodies in their plasma. Thus, Type AB blood is the universal donor of plasma and the universal recipient of cells; and Type O is the universal donor of RBCs only.[1]

If mismatched blood products are inadvertently given to a patient with a differing blood type than the donor, cross-reactions with opposing antigens may occur. For example, type A blood contains anti-B, which will attack type B red blood cells. Conversely, type B blood contains anti-A, which will cross-react with type A blood cells. Type O blood donors are called universal donors of red cells because their RBCs can be transfused into a recipient with any ABO type (because the donor RBCs do not contain A or B antigens on their surface to react with either the anti-A or the anti-B present in type B or type A blood, respectively).

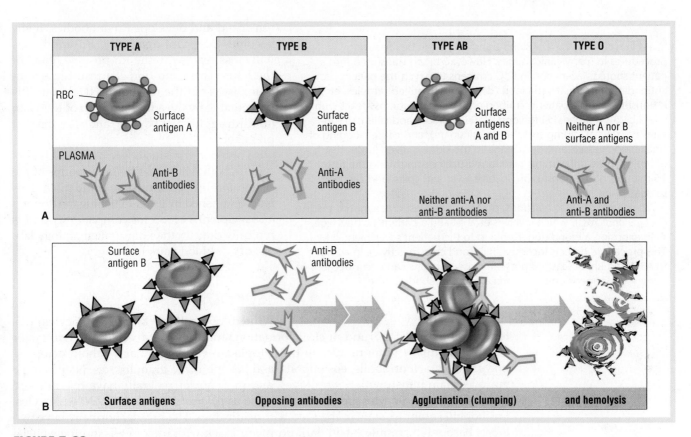

FIGURE 7–22

Blood Typing and Cross Reactions

The blood type depends on the presence of surface antigens (agglutinogens) on RBC surfaces. **A.** The plasma antibodies (agglutinins) that will react with foreign surface antigens. **B.** In a cross-reaction, incompatible antibodies that encounter their target antigens lead to agglutination and hemolysis of the affected RBCs. If this happens in the body, it leads to a transfusion reaction. Transfusion reactions can be life threatening and are most often preventable.

Another blood group system contains the **Rh factor,** in which Rh-positive individuals have the antigen for the Rh factor on their red blood cells, and Rh-negative people do not. About 85 percent of the population have the Rh factor (Rh positive) and 15 percent do not have the factor (Rh negative). In contrast to the ABO system, Rh antibodies are present *only* if the body has been exposed or sensitized to Rh-positive red blood cells, either accidentally by transfusion, during amniocentesis, or during childbirth when an Rh-negative mother is carrying an Rh-positive fetus (the Rh-positive gene came from the father). During delivery when the placenta separates and bleeding occurs, the mother is

TABLE 7–3

Blood Groups and Compatibilities

Type	Antigen	Plasma Antibody	Percentage/ Population	Compatible Donor Blood Groups	Incompatible Donor Blood Groups
A	A	Anti-B	41	A, O	B, AB
B	B	Anti-A	10	B, O	A, AB
AB	Both A and B	No anti-A or anti-B	4	A, B, AB, O	None
O	No A and B	Both anti-A and anti-B	45	O	A, B, AB

Used with permission from J. Rice, *Medical Terminology: A Word-Building Approach,* 7th ed. Upper Saddle River, NJ: Prentice Hall, 2008.

Clinical Alert! Blood transfusions can be life-saving procedures in many clinical cases. However, blood transfused into a patient should never contain RBC antigens to which the patient has antibodies. If mismatched blood (due to misidentified samples, etc.) is transfused into a patient, antibodies of the patient cross-react with specific RBC antigens on the donor's RBCs. Red blood cells can rupture (hemolyze), clump together (agglutinate), and cause clogging of small blood vessels and/or damage to the kidneys, liver, lungs, heart, or brain. These unfavorable reactions usually begin during the first 15 minutes of the transfusion, involve fever and chills, and can lead to death.

To prevent adverse reactions, physicians request **cross-match testing** (or *type and cross*), which involves establishing a patient's blood type, then exposing a blood donor's blood to the patient's (recipient's) blood. This procedure detects incompatibility and cross-reactivity. In addition to ABO and Rh, at least 48 possible cross-reactions can occur because of numerous antigens on the blood cells and antibodies in sera.

sensitized and develops Rh antibodies. If she becomes pregnant again, the Rh antibodies will cross-react with the Rh-positive blood of the fetus. This condition can result in hemolytic disease of the newborn (HDN), but it is preventable by the administration of RhoGam (anti-Rh agglutinins) during and after the first pregnancy.

For blood transfusions to be clinically successful, both ABO and Rh blood groups of the donor and recipient must be compatible. This is accomplished by cross-matching the donor's and recipient's blood for compatibility and is typically done in the immunohematology laboratory or blood bank laboratory.

LEUKOCYTES

White blood cells (WBCs or leukocytes) differ in color, size, shape, and nuclear formation, and they are divided into two major groups: granular (with granules in the cytoplasm) and agranular (without cytoplasmic granules). Neutrophils, eosinophils, and basophils are granulocytes. Neutrophilic granules stain bluish with neutral dyes, and their nuclei generally have two or more lobes. These granulocytes are often referred to as *polymorphonuclear (PMN)* leukocytes. Eosinophilic granules stain orange-red with acidic dyes. Their nuclei normally have two lobes. Basophilic granules stain dark purple or black with basic dyes, and their nuclei are often S-shaped. Agranular leukocytes, lymphocytes, and monocytes have relatively large nuclei (see Figure 7–19). Leukocytes serve as part of the body's defense mechanism. The cells phagocytize (ingest) pathogenic microorganisms. The lymphocytes play a role in immunity and in the production of antibodies.

White blood cells are formed in bone marrow and lymphatic tissues. The exact life span of a cell varies with cell type and is usually from one day to several years. Normally, blood contains 5,000 to 10,000 leukocytes/mm^3, with designated percentages for each cell line (refer to **TABLE 7–4**). The morphological characteristics of WBCs and RBCs are observed by using special laboratory staining techniques, which can be performed manually or by using specialized instrumentation and/or microscopic analysis. This is called a **differential.** Hematology instruments are able to produce automated differentials at a high speed in a cost-effective manner, whereas manual readings require significant expertise and time to interpret microscopic analysis.

White blood cells also have specific cell surface antigens that are expressed at certain times during their development. These antigens can be identified by laboratory methods, including flow cytometry and monoclonal antibodies. Using these laboratory techniques, clinicians can tell more precisely how mature or immature the WBCs in the bone marrow and/or peripheral blood are.

Clinical Alert! Be on the alert for potential complications related to bleeding disorders. Platelet disorders involving low counts (thrombocytopenia) or dysfunctional platelets are often treated by platelet transfusions to restore normal blood-clotting capacity.

In addition, be particularly cautious about patients on anticoagulant therapy such as aspirin, heparin, and coumadin, or the plasma expander dextran, because a simple venipuncture may cause excessive bleeding for these patients. On the other hand, thrombocytosis is a disease characterized by too many platelets. Patients with this condition may exhibit increased or more rapid clot formation.

THROMBOCYTES OR PLATELETS

Platelets (thrombocytes) are much smaller than other blood cells. They are fragments of **megakaryocytes** (*mega* means "big"), which are located in the bone. Normally there are 250,000 to 500,000 platelets/mm^3 in circulating blood. Platelets help in the clotting process by transporting needed chemicals for clotting, forming a temporary patch or plug to slow blood loss, and contracting after the blood clot has formed. Their life span is 9 to 12 days.

TABLE 7–4

Common Hematology, Coagulation, and Immunohematology Blood Tests

Numerous laboratory tests can be done to assess the cardiovascular system. Most of them are performed in a hematology/coagulation laboratory using lavender or blue-top testing tubes, depending on the specific test. The number of RBCs, their morphological traits, and their hemoglobin content can be determined from an anticoagulated blood specimen in the clinical hematology laboratory. Platelets and WBCs can be assessed on the basis of number and morphological features. The results of a WBC differential count enumerate specific cell lines in percentages. Platelet function, as well as each coagulation factor, can be measured from anticoagulated blood specimens in the coagulation section of the clinical hematology laboratory. Tests for blood types and cross-matches for donor blood are done in an immunohematology, transfusion, or blood-banking laboratory.

Serum and plasma constituents, including nutrients, metabolic wastes, respiratory gases, regulatory substances, and protective substances, can all be evaluated from blood specimens in the clinical chemistry laboratory. (This includes cardiac enzymes or cardiac biomarkers that are used to detect signs of a heart attack or coronary artery disease [CAD].) These are listed under the common chemistry tests in TABLE 7–5. These tests, although conducted on plasma or serum, actually assess the substances that are normally carried in the bloodstream yet they relate to the functioning of many other organ systems.

Also, every clinical laboratory should have established reference ranges for the laboratory tests they perform. Reference ranges depend on many factors, including patient age, gender, sample population, and test methods. The few reference ranges listed here are approximate and strictly for educational purposes. They are *not* to be used to interpret patients' clinical data.[3,4]

Refer to Appendix 7 for detailed specimen requirements.

Test	Abbreviation	Reference Range* (Conventional units)	Examples of Clinical Conditions Test Results Increased	Decreased
ABO and Rh type and cross-match	Type and cross	N/A	Checking for compatibility between the blood donor and recipient.	Checking for compatibility between the blood donor and recipient.
Bone marrow examination		Marrow is removed from the iliac crest of the hip. Reference ranges depend on the methods used and many other variables.	Results indicate abnormal numbers and morphological characteristics of bone marrow cells.	
Complete blood count (blood cell indices and cell counts, including RBCs, WBCs, platelets, hemoglobin, and hematocrit)	CBC	CBC refers to all blood cell counts; see individual tests that follow.	Refer to individual tests that follow.	Refer to individual tests that follow.
D-dimer or related tests: fibrin split products or fibrin degradation products	FSP or FDP	Standard reference range is unavailable due to many testing variables.	Positive test indicates recent clotting activity may be due to thromboembolism or disseminated intravascular coagulation (DIC) or other trauma.	
Differential white blood cell count	Diff	Neutrophils 50–70%	*Neutrophilia:* acute bacterial infections, parasitic infections, liver disease	*Neutropenia:* acute viral infections, blood diseases, hormone diseases
		Eosinophils 1–4%	*Eosinophilia:* allergic conditions, parasitic infections, lung and bone cancer	*Eosinopenia:* infectious mononucleosis, congestive heart failure, aplastic and pernicious anemia
		Basophils 0–1%	*Basophilia:* Leukemia, hemolytic anemia, Hodgkin's disease	*Basopenia:* acute allergic reactions, hyperthyroidism, steroid therapy
		Lymphocytes 20–35%	*Lymphocytosis:* acute and chronic infections, carcinoma, hyperthyroidism	*Lymphopenia:* cardiac failure, Cushing's disease, Hodgkin's disease
		Monocytes 3–8%	*Monocytosis:* viral infections, bacterial and parasitic infections, collagen diseases, cirrhosis	*Monocytopenia:* prednisolone treatment, hairy cell leukemia
Erythrocyte sedimentation rate	ESR	Depends on the methods used.	Collagen disease, inflammatory disease, rheumatoid arthritis	Sickle cell anemia, CHF, polycythemia

(continued)

TABLE 7–4

Common Hematology, Coagulation, and Immunohematology Blood Tests (continued)

Test	Abbreviation	Reference Range* (Conventional units)	Examples of Clinical Conditions Test Results Increased	Decreased
Factor assays		Depends on the coagulation factor being tested.		Hemophilia
Ferritin		15–200 ng/mL (men) / 12–150 ng/mL (women)	Excess storage of iron	Microcytic hypochromic anemia; iron deficiency
Hemoglobin	Hgb, Hb	12–18 g/dL	Congestive heart failure (CCHF), chronic obstructive pulmonary disease (COPD), severe burn	Hodgkin's disease, hyperthyroidism, cirrhosis
Hematocrit/ microhematocrit	Hct, HCT	Female: 36–45% / Male: 42–50%	Shock, dehydration, burns	Anemia, leukemia, acute blood loss
Hemogram		Depends on which indices are included.	A hemogram typically refers to all blood cell counts, cellular morphology, and proportions of cells. See individual tests.	
Indices: Mean corpuscular hemoglobin, mean corpuscular volume, mean corpuscular hemoglobin concentration	MCH, MCV, MCHC	MCH = 27–33 pg / MCV = 80–96 fL / MCHC = 33–36%	B_{12} deficiency, folate deficiency, hereditary spherocytosis	Anemia, thalassemia
Serum iron		60–150 μm/dL	Liver necrosis, leukemia, Hodgkin's disease	Iron deficiency anemia
Platelet count		150,000–500,000 $10^3/mm^3$	Cancer, leukemia, splenectomy	Bone-marrow depressant drug, pneumonia infection, possible malignancy, polycythemia, recent splenectomy
Prothrombin time or International normalized ratio	PT or INR		Anticoagulant therapy, liver disease, biliary obstruction	Diuretics, pulmonary embolism, multiple myeloma
Activated partial thromboplastin time	APTT	Depends on the methods used. 60–90 seconds	Bleeding disorders (e.g., hemophilia, disseminated intravascular) coagulation/clotting (DIC) anticoagulant therapy	
Red blood cell count	RBC	Female: 4–5 million/mm³ Male: 5–6 million/mm³	Polycythemia, poisoning, pulmonary fibrosis	Anemia, multiple myeloma, lupus erythemia
Reticulocyte count	Retic count	0.5–1.5% of total RBC count	Acute blood loss	Pernicious anemia
		In pregnancy—slight increase		
		Newborns—increased first week		
Total iron binding capacity	TIBC	Depends on technique used for testing.	Liver necrosis, leukemia, Hodgkin's disease	Hemochromatosis
White blood cell count	WBC	4.4–11 $10^3/mm^3$	Acute infection, leukemia, mononucleosis	Viral infections, bone marrow depression

*Reference ranges are listed in conventional units that are commonly reported in the United States. However, many laboratories also list reference ranges in SI units (Le Systeme International d'Unites, SI), which helps promote global standardization. Typically, this involves a conversion factor (multiplication factor) to convert the conventional unit into an SI unit. For more information on conversions, see the resources at the end of the chapter.

TABLE 7–5

Common Chemistry Tests Performed on Blood

This table lists a few commonly performed laboratory tests. Nutrients, metabolic wastes, respiratory gases, regulatory substances, and protective substances can all be evaluated from blood specimens in the clinical chemistry laboratory. These tests, although conducted on plasma or serum, actually assess the substances that are normally carried in the bloodstream but relate to the functioning of other organ systems besides the cardiovascular system.

Also, every clinical laboratory should have established reference ranges for the laboratory tests they perform. Reference ranges depend on many factors, including patient age, gender, sample population, and test methods, so, in general, they are specific to the laboratory performing the tests. The few reference ranges listed here are approximate and strictly for educational purposes. They are *not* to be used to interpret patients' clinical data.[3,4]

Test	Abbreviation	Reference Range (Conventional units)*	Examples of Clinical Conditions Test Results Increased	Decreased
Blood urea nitrogen	BUN	8–23 mg/dL	Kidney disease, dehydration, GI bleeding	Liver failure, malnutrition
Calcium, total	Ca	9.2–11.0 mg/dL	Hypercalcemia, bone metastases, Hodgkin's disease	Hypocalcemia, renal failure, pancreatitis
Cardiac biomarkers: Troponin I Troponin T Creatine kinase Myoglobin	TnI TnT CK, CK-MB	Individual tests have reference ranges established by the laboratories where they are performed.	Heart damage such as heart attack, myocarditis (heart inflammation), congestive heart failure, severe infections, kidney disease, dermatomyositis	
Chloride	Cl	96–103 mmol/L	Dehydration, eclampsia, anemia	Ulcerative colitis, burns, heat exhaustion
Cholesterol	CHOL	140–200 mg/dL	Atherosclerosis, nephrosis, obstructive jaundice	Malabsorption, liver disease, hyperthyroidism
Creatinine	Creat	0.6–1.2 mg/dL	Chronic nephritis, muscle disease, obstruction of urinary tract	Muscular dystrophy
Glucose fasting blood sugar	FBS	70–110 mg/dL	Diabetes mellitus	Excess insulin
Hepatic (liver) function tests: Alanine aminotransferase Alkaline phosphatase Aspartate aminotransferase Bilirubin Albumin Total protein Albumin/globulin ratio	ALT ALP AST BILI ALB TP A/G Ratio	Individual tests have reference ranges established by the laboratories where they are performed.	Liver disease or damage, including hepatitis, cirrhosis, gallstones, tumors, inflammation, mononucleosis, pancreatitis, obstructive jaundice, or genetic defects that prevent vital liver functions. In newborns, increased bilirubin levels affect developing brain cells and may cause jaundice, mental retardation, physical abnormalities, or blindness.	Malnutrition, hypothyroidism, chronic nephritis, uncontrolled diabetes mellitus, multiple myeloma, autoimmune diseases
Two-hour postprandial glucose (blood sugar)	2-hr PPBS	140 mg/dL	Cushing syndrome, brain damage	Addison's disease, carcinoma (CA) of pancreas
Lactic acid	LDH or lactate	5–20 mg/dL	Acute MI, acute leukemia, hepatic disease	
Potassium	K	3.8–5.0 mEq/L	Renal failure, acidosis, cell damage	Malabsorption, severe burn, diarrhea
Sodium	NA	136–142 mEq/L	Diabetes insipitus, coma, Cushing syndrome	Severe diarrhea, severe nephritis, vomiting
Thyroid tests: Thyroid stimulating hormone Thyroxine (total and free) Triiodothyronine Thyroid antibodies	TSH T4 T3	Individual tests have reference ranges established by the laboratories where they are performed.	Thyroiditis, hyperthyroidism, Graves' disease	Goiter, hypothyroidism
Triglycerides	TRIG	10–190 mg/dL	Liver disease, atherosclerosis, pancreatitis	Malnutrition
Uric acid	Urate	2.7–8.5 mg/dL	Renal failure, gout, leukemia, eclampsia	

GI = gastrointestinal; CA = carcinoma, malignant tumor; MI = myocardial infarction

*Reference ranges are listed in conventional units that are commonly reported in the United States. However, many laboratories also list reference ranges in SI units (Le Systeme International d'Unites, SI) to promote global standardization. Typically, this involves a conversion factor (multiplication factor) to convert the conventional unit into an SI unit. For more information on conversions, see the resources at the end of the chapter.

Abnormalities in the quality or quantity of platelets result in bleeding disorders, which are detected in the laboratory using the bleeding time tests for assessing platelet quality, and the platelet count for assessing the quantity of platelets in the blood. Refer to Table 7–4 for a list of common tests for platelet function and clotting disorders.

PLASMA

The liquid portion of blood and lymph is called **plasma.** Blood cells, dissolved gases, proteins, and other chemical substances are suspended in plasma. Plasma is the medium for transporting constituents in the bloodstream. If a chemical agent called an **anticoagulant** is added to prevent clotting, a blood sample can be separated by centrifugation into the cells and the liquid plasma (review Figure 7–18).

As mentioned previously, plasma is composed of water and solutes, which include nutrients such as glucose, amino acids, fats, metabolic wastes (urea, uric acid, creatinine, and lactic acid), respiratory gases (O_2 and CO_2), regulatory substances (hormones, enzymes), electrolytes (sodium, potassium, calcium, and chloride), clotting substances such as fibrinogen and Factor VIII, and protective substances (antibodies). The cellular portion of the specimen contains WBCs, platelets, and RBCs. If the specimen is centrifuged or allowed to settle, the RBCs (the heaviest) will sink to the bottom of the tube. The WBCs and platelets form a thin white layer above the RBCs, called the **buffy coat.** The thin fluid plasma portion is straw colored and remains on the top. However, if it is mixed or gently inverted, the cells will again become suspended and the entire sample tube will have the appearance of a freshly collected blood specimen.

Some of plasma's substances, such as proteins, cannot pass through the capillary pores because of their large molecular size. The majority of proteins stay in the vascular space, where they exert osmotic pressure. This pressure keeps fluid (blood volume) levels in balance. Proteins in the plasma perform other functions, such as providing energy when the body is not getting enough from regular food intake. In conjunction with electrolytes, proteins help "buffer" the blood. *Buffering* is a term used to describe the body's ability to control the delicate pH of the blood. The pH describes the degree of acidity or alkalinity of a solution on a pH scale of 1 to 14. An "acidic" pH is low (1–7), and a "basic" pH is high (7–14). The normal range of blood pH is narrow and slightly basic, from 7.35 to 7.45. Refer to the pH scale in **FIGURE 7–23**. If the pH in a patient's blood becomes too acidic or too basic, serious complications can result for the patient. In acidosis, carbon dioxide (CO_2) and organic acids build up in the blood, causing it to become acidic. If it is not detected by laboratory testing, blood and tissues can be damaged.

Serum

If a blood specimen is allowed to clot, the resulting liquid portion is **serum** (also straw color) plus blood cells meshed in a **fibrin** clot. Serum contains essentially the same chemical constituents as plasma, except the clotting factors (e.g., fibrinogen) and the blood cells are contained within the fibrin clot (Figure 7–18).

FIGURE 7–23

The pH Scale

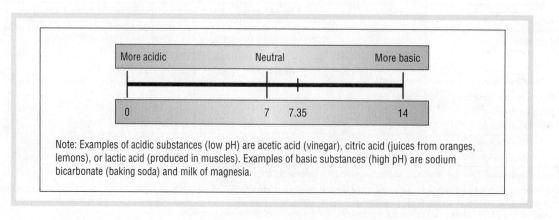

Note: Examples of acidic substances (low pH) are acetic acid (vinegar), citric acid (juices from oranges, lemons), or lactic acid (produced in muscles). Examples of basic substances (high pH) are sodium bicarbonate (baking soda) and milk of magnesia.

Hemostasis and Coagulation

Hemostasis (not to be confused with homeostasis) is a complex series of processes in which platelets, plasma, and coagulation factors interact to control bleeding while at the same time maintaining circulating blood in the liquid state. It enables the human body to retain blood in the vascular system by preventing blood loss. When a small blood vessel is injured, the hemostatic process (clotting response) repairs the break and stops the hemorrhage by forming a plug or blood clot (**FIGURES 7–24** and **7–25**).

This intricate process involves the following phases:

- **Vascular phase**—Once a blood vessel is injured, a rapid constriction of the vessel (**vasoconstriction**) decreases the blood flow to the surrounding vascular bed.
- **Platelet phase**—Platelets degranulate, clump together, and adhere to the injured vessel in order to form a plug and inhibit bleeding.
- **Coagulation phase**—Many specific coagulation factors (including fibrinogen, clotting factors, and calcium) are released and interact to form a fibrin meshwork, or blood clot. This clot seals off the damaged portion of the vessel.
- **Clot retraction**—This occurs when the bleeding has stopped. The entire clot retracts to heal torn edges by bringing them closer together.
- **Fibrinolysis**—When the final repair and regeneration of the injured vessel occurs, the clot slowly begins to break up (lysis) and dissolve as other cells carry out further repair. The entire process is fast, intricate, self-sustaining, and remarkable (**FIGURE 7–26**).

It is important to focus briefly on the **coagulation** process (the third phase), which is a result of numerous coagulation factors. For simplicity, it is divided into two systems: intrinsic and extrinsic. All coagulation factors required for the **intrinsic system** are contained in the blood, whereas the **extrinsic factors** are stimulated when tissue damage occurs. For example, blood vessels are lined with a single layer of flat endothelial cells and are supported by collagen fibers. Normally, endothelial cells do not react with or attract platelets; however, they do produce and store some clotting factors. When the clotting sequence begins due to a vessel injury, endothelial cells react with degranulated platelets in forming the fibrin plug.[1] Bleeding from small arteries and veins can be controlled by the hemostatic process; however, large- or medium-sized veins and arteries require rapid surgical intervention to prevent excessive bleeding.

DISORDERS OF THE CARDIOVASCULAR SYSTEM AND HEMOSTATIC PROCESS

Diseases and disorders in the cardiovascular system are complicated and usually affect more than one area of the body. To summarize the many possible disorders, they are separated into broad categories in **TABLE 7–6**.[1] Also see **TABLES 7–7** and **7–8** for medications and terms related to the cardiovascular system.

Clinical Alert!

- Coagulation tests are performed for a variety of critically important indications (e.g., cardiac, pulmonary, and presurgical work-ups). If small mistakes are made in the collection of specimens, the coagulation testing results are greatly affected. Erroneous coagulation results can cause unnecessary medications to be prescribed for the patient or even delays in surgery. Therefore, health care workers must follow the exact procedures at their institutions for collection of these specimens.

- When a health care worker discovers or anticipates bleeding, it is important to use standard precautions, including gloves, to avoid exposure of the skin and mucous membranes. A mask and protective eyewear or a face shield should also be worn if there is a chance of splattered blood or if the patient is coughing up blood. A gown should be worn if there is a chance that clothing might become contaminated.

ALERT

FIGURE 7–24

Blood Clot

These strands of fibrin trap many erythrocytes to form a blood clot or thrombus.

Source: Susumu Nishinaga/Photo Researchers, Inc.

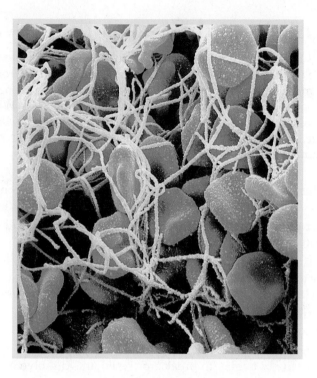

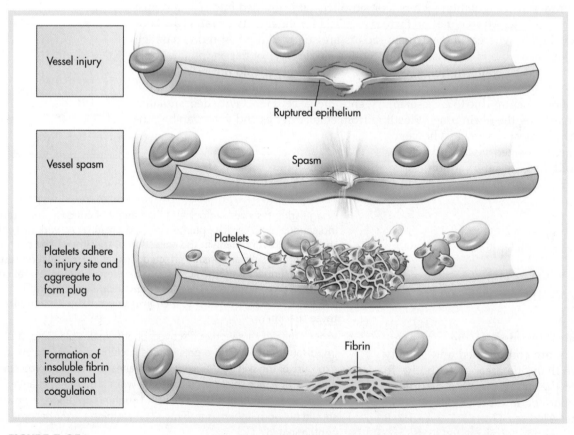

FIGURE 7–25

Hemostasis Overview

The basic steps in hemostasis begin when there is an injury to a vessel wall.

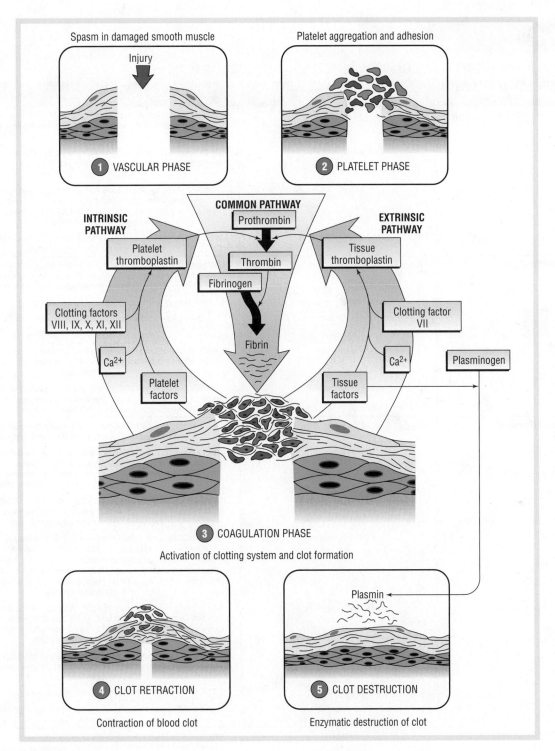

FIGURE 7–26

Details of the Hemostatic or Blood Clotting Process

TABLE 7–6

Disorders of the Cardiovascular System and Hemostatic Process

Category of Disorders/ Disease	General Examples	Descriptions
Disorders of the heart	Cor pulmonale	Serious condition whereby the right side of the heart cannot move blood as effectively as it should and the heart enlarges due to overwork.
	Congestive heart failure	Life-threatening condition in which the heart's pumping action cannot overcome increasing vascular pressure so fluid leaks out of the vessels into the body's tissues.
	Stenotic valves	Valves of the heart are too small so blood flow is restricted. Clots may form in the damaged areas. If the clots detach, they may cause a pulmonary embolus in the lungs or travel to the brain, causing a stroke.
	Valvular insufficiency	Valve passageway is too large or leaking so blood goes backward. Clots may form in the damaged areas.
Vessel problems	Atherosclerosis	Cholesterol deposits (plaque) form on the lining of the vessels resulting in partial or complete blockage of blood flow. Vessels most likely to have plaque buildup are the aorta and coronary arteries.
	Myocardial infarct (MI)	If blood flow is restricted in the coronary arteries a heart attack results.
	Cerebral vascular accident (CVA)	If blood flow to the brain is restricted, it causes a stroke or CVA.
	Ischemia	Reduced blood flow to the tissues.
	Aneurysm	Localized weakened area of the blood vessel wall. In severe conditions, the vessel wall balloons out and may rupture, causing an internal hemorrhage.
	Hemorrhage	Condition in which blood is escaping from a vessel wall. It can be the result of a traumatic cut into the vessel or a leakage of blood into the surrounding tissues. (**FIGURES 7–27** and **7–28**.)
Blood disorders	Polycythemia	Condition in which low levels of O_2 cause the body to produce excessive amounts of RBCs to try to transport more O_2.
	Anemia	Blood condition with lowered RBC count or abnormal or deficient hemoglobin carrying capacity in the RBCs so that the tissues are not receiving enough O_2. Symptoms include pale skin tone (pallor), fatigue, muscle weakness, shortness of breath, chest pains.
		"Iatrogenic" anemia occurs when large quantities of blood are drawn from critically ill patients. This is an adverse outcome for patients and can result in the need for a transfusion.
	Septicemia	Bacterial infection of the bloodstream that can lead to more serious conditions involving sepsis, an inflammatory response to the infection. Blood cultures are most often used to detect the type of bacterial infection present. However, laboratory tests using fluorescent *in situ* hybridization (FISH) provide faster detection and identification than traditional methods.
	Sickle cell anemia	An inherited condition whereby the RBCs and hemoglobin molecules do not form properly. Red blood cells become "sickle shaped"; the body tries to produce more RBCs to compensate and hence clogs up vessels with ineffective cells.
	Leukemia	Usually classified as a bone marrow cancer in which excessive, immature WBCs are produced and do not function properly to fight infections.
	Leukocytosis	High WBC count usually due to infections.
	Leukopenia	Low WBC count usually as a result of taking chemotherapy or corticosteroids.
Disorders in the process of hemostasis	Hemophilia	Inherited conditions that prevent or delay the blood-clotting process. Patients with anemia often require transfusions of blood products, including clotting factors. Excessive bleeding may result in death.
	Thrombocytopenia	Low platelet count that may result in excessive bleeding. It is caused by liver dysfunction, vitamin K deficiency, radiation exposure, or bone marrow cancer.
	Embolus or thrombus	Blood clots caused by damaged vessels or heart valves or by overactive coagulation can result in the clot being transported to another location in the body and causing an obstruction (embolus) or causing an obstruction where it is formed (thrombus).
	Disseminated intravascular coagulation (DIC)	A condition in which small blood clots are widely distributed in the body. It is caused by a hyperactive clotting process. Anticoagulant drugs such as heparin and Coumadin (warfarin), which suppress clotting factors, can be used to prevent clotting problems.

FIGURE 7–27

Medications and Bleeding

Some medications, such as aspirin, can increase bleeding. Always make sure a patient has stopped bleeding after a venipuncture procedure.

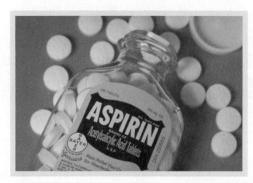

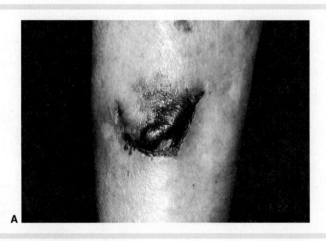

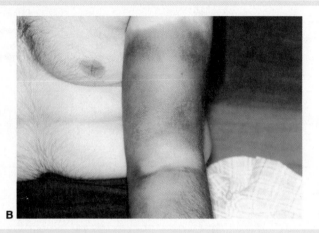

FIGURE 7–28

Hematologic Conditions

A. Traumatic hematoma. **B.** Vein hemorrhage.

Courtesy Jason L. Smith, MD.

TABLE 7–7

Common Drugs for the Cardiovascular System

Drug	Use
Anticoagulants	Used for patients to inhibit blood clot formation. Hemorrhage can occur at almost any site in patients on anticoagulant therapy, so take extra care to monitor bleeding after a venipuncture procedure. Examples: heparin sodium, Coumadin (warfarin sodium), Lovenox (enoxaparin), salicylates or aspirin
Hemostatic agents	Used to control bleeding, can be administered systemically (affecting the entire body) or topically (localized administration on the skin surface). Examples: Proplex (factor IX complement), Amicar (aminocaproic acid), vitamin K, and Surgicel (oxidized cellulose)
Anti-anemic agents (irons)	Used to treat iron deficiency anemia. Oral iron preparations interfere with the absorption of oral tetracycline antibiotics. Examples: Femiron (ferrous fumarate), Fergon, Fertinic (ferrous gluconate), and Feosol (ferrous sulfate)
Epoetin, alfa (EPO)	Used to stimulate the production of red blood cells. It is used in the treatment of patients with chronic renal failure and with HIV-infected patients taking zidovudine (AZT). These drugs are genetically engineered erythropoietin. Example: Procrit
Statins	Used to reduce the production of cholesterol and promote the clearance of low-density lipoprotein (LDL) from the blood by the liver. Example: Lipitor
Other agents	Used to treat folic acid deficiency or vitamin B_{12} deficiency. Examples: Folvite (folic acid), Vitamin B_{12} (cyanocobalamin)

Adapted from J. Rice, *Medical Terminology: A Word-Building Approach,* 7th ed. Upper Saddle River, NJ: Prentice Hall, 2008.

TABLE 7–8

Examples of Medical Terminology Related to the Cardiovascular and Lymphatic Systems

Medical Term	Definition
Agglutination	Clumping process (usually refers to cells).
Anaphylaxis	A strong allergic reaction to substances.
Anemia	Blood condition in which there is a lack of red blood cells, a reduced amount of hemoglobin, or a low volume of packed red cells (**hematocrit**).
Anisocytosis	Unequal size and shape of the RBCs.
Antibody	Means "against the body," or a protein produced in the body that is a response to a foreign substance (antigen).
Anticoagulant	Means "against clots forming" or a substance that prevents blood coagulation.
Antigen	Means "against formation" or a foreign substance that induces the formation of antibodies.
Autotransfusion	Means "self, across, pour, process" or the process of reinfusing a patient's own blood. The patient must donate blood prior to having surgery or other procedures performed. The patient's blood is then stored until needed.
Coagulable	Means "to clot, capable" or capable of forming a blood clot.
Embolus	A blood clot carried in the bloodstream.
Erythrocytosis	Means "red, cell, condition" or an abnormal condition whereby there is an increased number of RBCs.
Erythropoiesis	Means "red cell formation."
Erythropoietin	Means "red, formation, chemical"; refers to a protein secreted by the kidneys that acts on stem cells of the bone marrow to stimulate RBC production (erythropoiesis).
Fibrinogen	Means "fiber formation"; refers to the protein converted to a fibrin clot in hemostasis.
Hematology/hematologist	Means "the study of blood, one who studies blood."
Hematoma	Means "blood, mass" or the accumulation of blood in tissues after blood has leaked out as a result of injury or trauma.
Hemochromatosis	Means "blood, color, condition"; a genetic condition in which iron accumulates in the body tissues.
Hemolysis	Means "blood destruction" or rupturing of the RBCs.
Hyperglycemia	Means "excessive, sugar/sweet, blood condition" or excessive amounts of sugar/glucose in the blood.
Hypoxia	Means low or "deficient oxygen" in the blood and tissues.
Leukapheresis	Means "white, removal"; refers to the procedure whereby the WBCs are removed when a patient donates blood and they can then be reinfused once the other blood components are withdrawn.
Lymph	Clear colorless liquid found in the lymph vessels.
Lymphadenitis	Means "lymph gland inflammation."
Lymphangitis	Means "lymph vessel inflammation."
Lymphedema	Means "swelling" or an abnormal accumulation of lymph in the interstitial spaces.
Lymphoma	Means "lymph mass or fluid collection"; refers to a lymphoid neoplasm (cancer). Lymphomas are classified as Hodgkin's or non-Hodgkin's lymphomas.
Lymphostasis	Means "lymph stand still or stop"; refers to stopping the flow of lymph.
Pancytopenia	Means "all cell lack of" or lack of all cellular elements of the blood.
Petechiae	Minute hemorrhagic spots just under the skin surface that may be an indication of coagulation dysfunction.
Plasmapheresis	Means "plasma removal" or the process by which blood is removed from the body, centrifuged to separate the plasma from the blood and then the cellular elements are reinfused back into the patient.
Polycythemia	Means "many cell blood condition" or too many RBCs.
Sepsis	The body's response to septicemia, a bloodstream infection, which may become serious and include fever, organ failure, shock, or even death.
Septicemia	Also called *bacteremia*, it means "putrefying blood condition" or the abnormal condition in which bacteria are present in the bloodstream (i.e., bacterial infection of the blood).
Splenomegaly	Means "spleen enlargement."
Thrombosis	Means "clot condition" or a blood clot within the vascular system. In venous thrombosis (thrombophlebitis), the thrombus forms on the wall of a vein and can cause inflammation and/or obstruction. Deep vein thrombosis (DVT) occurs when the thrombus forms in deeper veins and can be a complication of hospitalization.
Vasculitis	Means "small vessel inflammation" and can refer to blood or lymph vessels.

Adapted from J. Rice, *Medical Terminology: A Word-Building Approach*, 7th ed. Upper Saddle River, NJ: Prentice Hall, 2008.

Lymphatic System

STRUCTURE AND FUNCTION

The **lymphatic system** has a close and interrelated connection with the cardiovascular system. It consists of lymph, lymphocytes, lymph vessels, lymph nodes, tonsils, the spleen, bone marrow, and the thymus gland. Three main functions of the system are to

1. Maintain fluid balance in the tissues by filtering blood and lymph fluid.
2. Provide a defense and immunity against disease through the lymphocytes.
3. Distribute nutrients and hormones into the bloodstream, remove waste, and absorb fats and other substances from the digestive tract.

About 30 liters of fluid pass from the blood to the tissue spaces each day. Fluid from capillaries enters tissue fluid and flows into lymph vessels and then to the lymph nodes. In the nodes, any pathogens or foreign substances are filtered out and destroyed by WBCs. Fluid then flows from the nodes to collecting ducts and back into the bloodstream. If more than 3 liters were retained in the body's tissue, **edema** (swelling) would result. (The lymph nodes filter lymph fluid, and the spleen filters blood.) Enlarged or swollen lymph nodes are common after infections because they have been working hard to remove waste and unwanted products from the body. Lymphatic organs contain lymphocytes, macrophages, and other cells that provide immunity and protection against infections from microorganisms (**FIGURE 7–29**). For example, there are lymphocytes that play vital roles in immunity. The T-cells (thymus-dependent) provide cellular immunity against bacteria, viruses, fungi, etc. The B-cells (bone marrow-derived) provide humoral immunity, or antibody production in body fluids, including blood. The natural killer (NK) cells attack foreign cells, or normal cells that are infected with viruses, or cancer cells.

DISORDERS

Disorders of the lymphatic system include hematologic malignancies (such as lymphoma and Hodgkin's disease), immune disorders, and infectious processes (**FIGURE 7–30**).

LABORATORY TESTS

Some immune disorders can be analyzed from blood samples, bone marrow, or both. Abnormal lymphocytes may indicate dysfunctions in the lymphatic system. Lymph nodes, however, are often surgically removed or aspirated (called a "fine-needle aspirate") so that cells can be analyzed or cultures performed. Analysis of markers on the surface of the cellular material is also diagnostically valuable. Refer to Table 7–8 for additional medical terms related to the lymphatic and cardiovascular systems.

FIGURE 7–29

Lymphatic System

A. Tonsils, lymph nodes, thymus, spleen, and lymphatic vessels with an expanded view of a lymph node. Lymph nodes range in size from a pinhead to an olive and are located near areas where they are likely to catch pathogens (e.g., near the digestive system, reproductive organs, lungs). Notice that the axillary lymph nodes (armpit) are near the breast. They are frequently removed during a mastectomy (surgical removal of the breast due to cancer). Thus, patients who have undergone a mastectomy lose lymph drainage capabilities on that side. Never collect blood specimens from the mastectomy side. **B.** The lymphatic system is closely entwined into the cardiovascular system.

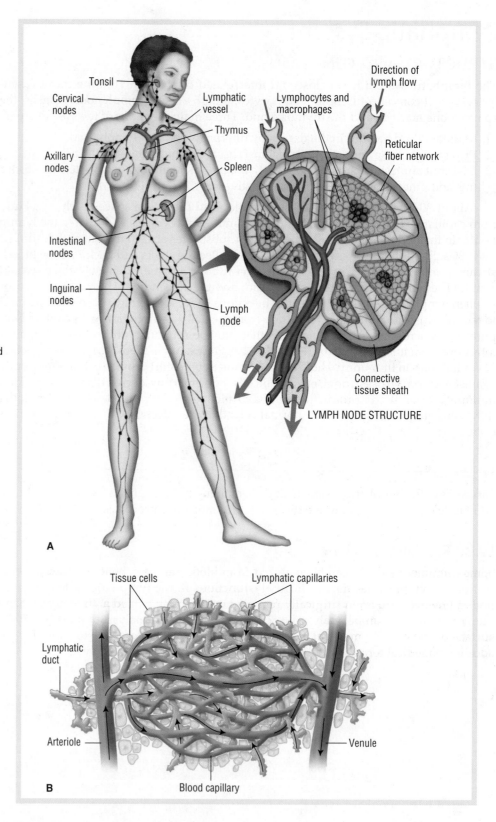

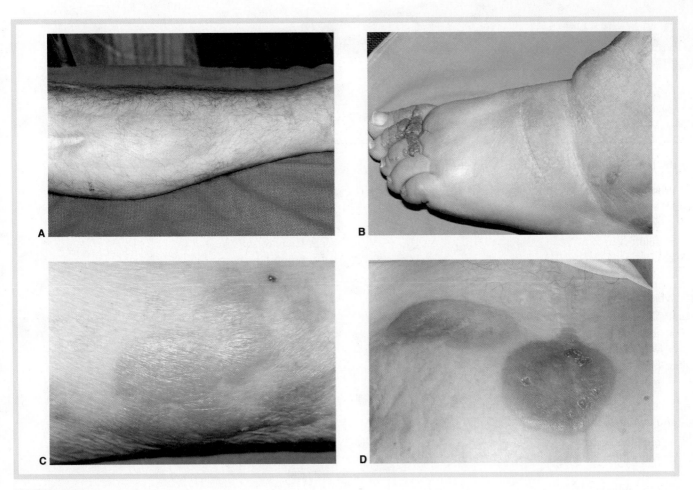

FIGURE 7–30

Disorders of the Lymphatic System

A. Lymphangitis, or inflammation of the lymphatic vessels. **B.** Chronic lymphedema, accumulation of lymph fluid in the interstitial or tissue spaces. **C.** Lymphoma. **D.** Cutaneous T-cell lymphoma.

Courtesy Jason L. Smith, MD.

Study Questions

For the following questions, select the one best answer.

1 Whole blood consists mostly of which of the following?

a. water
b. solutes
c. cells
d. tissue

2 Which type of blood cell is responsible for gas exchange in the circulating blood?

a. red blood cells
b. white blood cells
c. platelets
d. macrophages

3 Which type of blood cell is responsible for defense and immunity?

a. red blood cells
b. white blood cells
c. platelets
d. macrophages

4 The liquid portion of a blood specimen (without an anticoagulant) is called

a. plasma
b. serum
c. cellular components
d. oxygenated blood

5 Which of the following is the preferred vein for venipuncture procedures?

a. popliteal
b. brachial
c. median cubital
d. cephalic

6 Which of the following is the region of the body containing lymph nodes?

a. upper torso
b. lower torso
c. around the heart
d. throughout the body

7 Which type of bleeding is easiest to control?

a. venous
b. capillary
c. arterial
d. systolic

8 Which blood test includes WBC and RBC counts, hemoglobin, and hematocrit?

a. PTT
b. Hgb, Hct
c. blood typing
d. CBC

9 The most common blood type is

a. A
b. B
c. AB
d. O

10 Troponin tests are used to assess

a. RBC size
b. WBC counts
c. heart damage
d. thrombus formation

Case Study 1

Chest Pain Mike Lawrence, age 68, came to the emergency department complaining of chest pains, pains in the left shoulder, and pain radiating down his left arm. The health care worker heard the patient state that he has a pacemaker, he had a stroke a couple of years ago, and he is being treated with anticoagulant therapy. Mike had some bruising on his arms. The health care worker has been asked to collect blood specimens from this patient.

Questions

1 With this limited information, what clues would the health care worker have about Mike's condition?

2 What problems might be anticipated with this patient?

Case Study 2

Axillary Lymph Nodes A 45-year-old woman came to a doctor's office for a routine physical. She had a previous diagnosis of breast cancer and had undergone a mastectomy on her right side 18 months before. The health care worker was asked to collect blood specimens for routine laboratory tests.

Questions

1 Describe the similarities between the blood circulatory system and the lymphatic system.

2 What are the implications of a mastectomy 18 months earlier?

3 From which part of the body should the health care worker collect the blood specimen?

Action in Practice

The Amazing Heart Your heart is amazing because it continues to beat day after day, 24 hours a day, seven days a week, with no vacation. Remember that your heart is about the size of your fist. Pretend that your fist is your heart and mimic the pumping action of your heart by opening your hand fully, then closing your fist tightly. Do this for 60 seconds. (It's not easy after a while!)

Questions

1 Think about how your heart can beat about 100,000 times per day and move about 1,800 gallons of blood each day for years and years.

2 Think of ways that you can keep your heart healthier. Remember that your heart muscle needs a constant flow of blood and nutrients to sustain such a rigorous schedule. The heart uses about 5 percent of all the oxygenated blood from every heartbeat to make sure it has plenty of oxygen and nutrients to function. By eating a low-fat, nutritious diet; getting regular exercise; and controlling stress you will promote a healthier heart.

Becoming a Blood Donor—Know Your Type One way to find out your own blood type is to consider becoming a volunteer blood donor. Seek out your local blood center or hospital blood center and inquire about the different types of donations available. Most often, facilities are available for whole blood donations but some health care facilities have platelet pheresis options available as well. It is a worthwhile endeavor for needy patients, it is gratifying, and you can learn something as well.

Questions

During the donation, pay attention to the following categories. Afterward, write a short story of your experience:

1 The role of the health care worker in screening

2 The actual venipuncture preparation, duration, and procedures

3 The color of the blood and what it looks like going into the donation bag

4 The labels and documentation required for each donation

5 The postdonation procedure

6 How you feel after the donation (emotionally and physically)

COMPETENCY ASSESSMENT

Check Yourself

Describe the properties of arteries, veins, and capillaries and the blood that comes from each blood vessel. Fill in the following table:

Properties	Arteries	Veins	Capillaries
Thickness of vessel wall			
Direction of blood flow			
Color of blood			
Ease of stopping blood flow			

Competency Checklist: Terms Related to the Cardiovascular and Lymphatic Systems

Match the appropriate lettered meaning to the numbered word.

1. Erythrocyte
2. Leukocyte
3. Arteries
4. Venules
5. Capillary
6. Veins
7. Plasma
8. Serum
9. Antecubital
10. Median cubital vein

a. Accumulation of lymph fluid in tissues
b. Small hemorrhagic spots
c. Carbon dioxide
d. Blood-clotting process in the body
e. Leakage of blood into surrounding tissue
f. Deep vessel in the leg
g. Thrombocytes
h. RBC
i. WBC
j. Malignancy of the lymphatic system

11. Basilic vein

12. Saphenous vein

13. Fibrinogen

14. Femoral artery

15. Platelets

16. CO_2

17. Hemostasis

18. Homeostasis

19. Deoxygenated blood

20. Cardiac muscle

21. Hodgkin's disease

22. Hematoma

23. Thrombus

24. Petechiae

25. Lymphedema

k. Thick-walled vessels

l. Blood clot within the vascular system

m. Branching vessels that flow back to the heart

n. Contains a mixture of arterial and venous blood

o. Blood specimen that does not contain anticoagulant

p. Blood specimen that does contain an anticoagulant

q. Best vein to use for venipuncture

r. Alternate vein to use for venipuncture

s. Blood that is carried in the veins

t. The longest vessel in the body

u. Near the bend of the elbow

v. Steady-state condition of the body

w. A blood-clotting factor

x. Heart

y. Thin-walled vessels

Competency Checklist: Structures and Functions of the Cardiovascular and Lymphatic Systems

List and describe the major structures and functions of the cardiovascular and lymphatic systems. Give examples of common laboratory tests and disorders of these systems. Use the following table to organize your answers.

Description Category	Cardiovascular System	Lymphatic System
Major structures and/or organs		
Major functions		
Examples of laboratory tests		
Examples of disorders		

Competency Checklist: Blood Flow and the Hemostatic Process

In general terms, describe the following:

(1) Completed (2) Needs to improve

_____ 1. The flow of blood through the body. Try to begin at the right atrium of the heart and end at the aorta.

_____ 2. The hemostatic process.

REFERENCES

1. Rice, J. (2008). *Medical terminology: A word-building approach,* 6th ed. Upper Saddle River, NJ: Prentice Hall.

2. Colbert, BJ, Ankney, J, and Lee, KT: *Anatomy and Physiology for the Health Professions,* Upper Saddle River, NJ: Prentice Hall, 2007.

3. *Clinical Laboratory Reference 2012–2014.* Table of Reference Intervals, *www.clr-online.com/,* accessed June 4, 2013.

4. *Lab Tests Online, Tests, Conditions & Diseases.* Screening. *www.labtestsonline.org,* accessed June 4, 2013.

RESOURCES

www.clr-online.com Provides critical values for therapeutic drug levels, toxicity levels for drug abuse testing, a table of critical limits, and a table of reference intervals

www.familydoctor.org Provides a dictionary of common medical terms

www.labtestsonline.org Peer-reviewed, noncommercial site provides resources on clinical laboratory testing

www.medilexicon.com Provides a medical dictionary, medical abbreviations, drug database, medical and surgical database, and ICD codes

www.medterms.com Provides easy-to-understand descriptions of medical terms and health news

Chapter 8

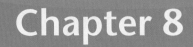

Blood Collection Equipment for Venipuncture and Capillary Specimens

Chapter Objectives

Upon completion of Chapter 8, the learner is responsible for doing the following:

1. Describe the latest phlebotomy safety supplies and equipment and evaluate their effectiveness in blood collection.

2. List the various types of anticoagulants and additives used in blood collection, their mechanisms of action on collected blood, examples of tests performed on the collected blood, and the vacuum-collection–tube color codes for these anticoagulants and additives.

3. Identify the various supplies that should be carried on a specimen collection tray when collecting blood by venipuncture or skin puncture.

4. Identify the types of safety equipment needed to collect blood by venipuncture and skin puncture.

KEY TERMS

acid citrate dextrose (ACD)
additive
antiglycolytic agent
blood-drawing chair
butterfly needle
capillary tubes
citrates
disposable sterile lancet
ethylenediamine tetra-acetic acid (EDTA)
evacuated tube
evacuated tube system
gauge number
glycolysis
glycolytic inhibitor
heparin
holder (adapter)
microcontainers
multiple-sample needles
oxalates
serum separation tube (SST)
sodium fluoride
sodium polyanethol sulfonate (SPS)
specific gravity
sterile gauze pads
vacuum (evacuated) tube
winged infusion set

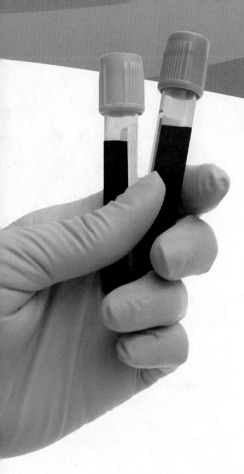

Introduction to Blood Collection Equipment

Health care workers use several types of supplies and safety equipment in the collection of blood and its transportation to the specimen processing center. The collection equipment is used for venipuncture (blood collection from a vein), skin puncture (blood collection from a finger and/or an infant's heel), and arterial puncture. Venipuncture equipment includes vacuum tubes (**evacuated tubes**) and safety-needle collection devices that allow the blood collector to collect a patient's blood, plus a tourniquet to assist in locating a vein, supplies to cleanse the puncture site, labeling supplies, gloves, and special trays for transportation of the blood specimens. **BOX 8–1** lists the equipment used in routine venipuncture procedures.

Venipuncture Equipment

Venipuncture with a **vacuum (evacuated) tube** (VACUTAINER), as shown in **FIGURE 8–1**, is the most direct and efficient method for obtaining a blood specimen.

The **evacuated tube system** requires an evacuated sample tube, the double-pointed needle, and a special safety plastic **holder (adapter)** (**FIGURE 8–2**) with an attached needle cover that is used to cover the needle after blood collection. One end of the double-pointed needle enters the vein, the other end pierces the top of the tube, and the vacuum aspirates the blood. As a result of state and federal laws that require safety-engineered

BOX 8–1

Equipment for Routine Venipuncture

- Antimicrobial hand gel or foam to wash hands
- Safety-needle collection device
- Needles
- Vacuum (evacuated) collection tubes
- Safety syringes
- Safety winged infusion sets (safety butterfly sets)
- Needle disposal container (i.e., sharps container)
- Tourniquet
- 70 percent isopropyl alcohol, chlorhexidine swab sticks
- Disposable gloves
- Gauze pads
- Bandages
- Marking pens and labels
- Specimen collection tray
- Vacuum (evacuated) tube systems

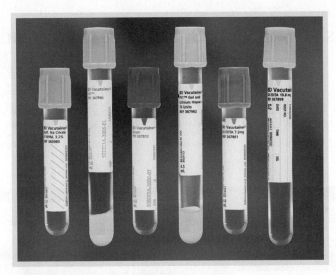

FIGURE 8–1

Vacuum (Evacuated) Tubes

Courtesy and © Becton, Dickinson and Company

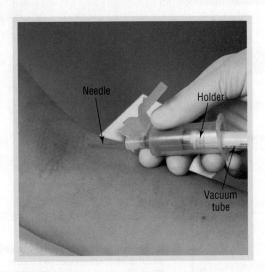

FIGURE 8–2

Vacuum (Evacuated) Tube Holder System and Parts

Courtesy and © Becton, Dickinson and Company

devices, manufacturers have designed different types of safety devices on the needle and/or plastic holder that covers the needle after venipuncture to protect the health care worker from a needlestick injury. Some of the manufacturers have developed both active and passive needle shielding devices. The active device requires the blood collector to "actively" cover the needle with the safety device, whereas the "passive" needle shielding device shields the needle automatically after blood collection. The device shown in Figure 8–2 is an active shielding device. In **FIGURE 8–3**, the BD Vacutainer® Passive Shielding Blood Collection Needle is designed to provide the highest amount of protection against needlesticks during a blood collection. The needle's safety shield releases automatically upon insertion of the first tube, providing protection from the time the first tube is inserted through product disposal.

BD Vacutainer® Passive Shielding Blood Collection Needle

   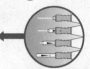

1. Twist and pull needle shield straight off.

2. Perform venipuncture according to your facility's established procedures. Hold device securely.

3. Insert tube. 1st tube releases safety shield to gently rest on patient.

Safety shield is free to move over the needle.

4. Remove needle from patient and safety shield will move forward to fully cover needle. Visually confirm complete shielding.

5. Discard entire assembly into an approved sharps disposal container.

Ordering Information

368636	Passive Shielding Blood Collection Needle	21 G x 1 in. needle	25/Box 200/Case		368637	Passive Shielding Blood Collection Needle	22 G x 1 in. needle	25/Box 200/Case	

Standard Safety Offering

Ordering Information

Ref. #	Description	Packaging
BD Vacutainer® Eclipse™ Blood Collection Needle with Pre-Attached Holder		
368650	With Pre-Attached Holder, 21 G x 1¼ in.	100/Case
368651	With Pre-Attached Holder, 22 G x 1¼ in.	100/Case
BD Vacutainer® Eclipse™ Blood Collection Needle		
368607	21 G x 1¼ in.	48/Box 480/Case
368608	22 G x 1¼ in.	48/Box 480/Case

Ref. #	Needle Gauge	Wing Color	Tubing Length	Configuration	Packaging
BD Vacutainer® Push Button Blood Collection Sets with Pre-Attached Holder					
367352	21		12"	with holder	20/Box 100/Case
368656	23		12"	with holder	20/Box 100/Case
BD Vacutainer® Push Button Blood Collection Sets					
367338	21		7"	with luer	50/Box 200/Case
367344	21		12"	with luer	50/Box 200/Case
367326	21		12"	without luer	50/Box 200/Case
367336	23		7"	with luer	50/Box 200/Case
367342	23		12"	with luer	50/Box 200/Case
367324	23		12"	without luer	50/Box 200/Case
367341	25		12"	with luer	50/Box 200/Case
367323	25		12"	without luer	50/Box 200/Case

Ref. #	Description		Packaging
BD Vacutainer® One Use Holder			
364815	One Use Holder		250/Bag 1,000/Case

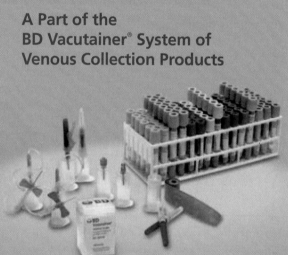

A Part of the BD Vacutainer® System of Venous Collection Products

CAUTION: Handle all biologic samples and blood collection "sharps" (lancets, needles, luer adapters, and blood collection sets) in accordance with the policies and procedures of your facility. Obtain appropriate medical attention in the event of any exposure to biologic samples (e.g., through a puncture injury) since samples may transmit viral hepatitis, HIV (AIDS), or other infectious diseases. Utilize any safety-engineered feature if the blood collection device provides one. Discard all blood collection "sharps" in biohazard containers approved for their disposal.

BD Global Technical Services: 1.800.631.0174
vacutainer_techservices@bd.com
BD Customer Service: 1.888.237.2762
www.bd.com/vacutainer

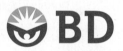 **BD**

BD Diagnostics
Preanalytical Systems
1 Becton Drive
Franklin Lakes, NJ 07417

FIGURE 8–3

Vacutainer Passive Shielding Blood Collection Needle

Courtesy and © Becton, Dickinson and Company

Blood Collection Tubes and Additives

Blood collection tubes are available in different sizes and in safety-engineered plastic to reduce risk of tube breakage and blood spill. The plastic tubes have a silica coat inside or other activating substance in order for clotting to start in the tube and go to completion. Also, the inside of the tubes are sterile. Glass collection tubes are not desirable because the risk of exposure to blood-borne pathogens (disease-causing organisms) is increased due to possible breakage. The external tube diameter and length, plus the maximum amount of specimen to be collected into the vacuum tube, are the two criteria used to describe vacuum tube size (TABLE 8–1). The smaller sizes (e.g., 2 mL) are useful for pediatric and geriatric collections and can be purchased with different types of **additives,** some being anticoagulants. Each vacuum tube is color coded according to the additive contained within the tube (TABLE 8–2). Most manufacturers use these color-coded tubes according to the Clinical Laboratory Standards Institute (CLSI). Since some variations occur among manufacturers, it is important to verify with the manufacturer on its specific color-coded tubes to be used in blood collection.

Many tubes are specifically designed to be used directly with chemistry, hematology, or microbiology instrumentation. In these cases, the tube of blood is identified by its bar code and is pierced by the instrument probe so that the blood specimen is aspirated into the instrument for analyses. Use of these closed systems minimizes laboratory personnel's risk of exposure to blood. In addition, some tubes have plastic tops or screw-on enclosures around the rubber stopper to minimize exposure to blood left on the top of the cap or blood splatters that can occur during cap removal.

The vacuum in these tubes creates a negative pressure that is designed to pull in a precise amount of blood into the tube that is indicated on the tube's label. A normal fill in a blood collection tube should reach the blood volume that is specified by the manufacturer for that tube. A tube should be filled to the indicated volume line. Otherwise, the ratio of blood to additive will be inaccurate and can lead to erroneous results as described in Chapter 9. These tubes can lose their vacuum in several ways, including an overextended expiration date, altitude variations, barometric pressure, pushing the needle into the tube before entry into the vein, storage in inappropriate conditions (i.e., high temperatures), and/or dropping the tube. The expiration dates of tubes should be monitored continuously. Such monitoring is most easily accomplished with an electronic monitoring log for each box of tubes.

In most clinical laboratories, serum, plasma, or whole blood has traditionally been used to perform various assays. Heparinized whole blood has become the specimen of choice for the many clinical laboratory instruments used in STAT (immediate) situations. Using whole blood as a specimen decreases the turnaround time involved in acquiring the test result, because clotting time and centrifugation are not required prior to laboratory testing.

TABLE 8–1

Typical Sizes of Blood Collection Vacuum Tubes for Full or Pediatric Draws

External Diameter × Length (mm)	Draw Volumes (mL)
13 × 75	2.0
13 × 75	2.0 and 3.0
13 × 75	4.0
13 × 100	4.0 and 5.0
13 × 100	6.0
16 × 75	7.0
16 × 100	8.5
16 × 100	10

TABLE 8–2

Specimen Type and Collection Vacuum Tubes

Specimen Type	Collection Tubes (top color/type) from Various Vendors	Additive
Clotted blood/serum	Gray/red or clear	No additive (discard tube)
	Yellow/red	Polymer barrier
	Gold	Clot activator and polymer barrier
	Red	None or clot activator in plastic tube
	Orange	Thrombin (Rapid serum tube)
	Yellow/gray or orange	Thrombin (Rapid serum tube)
	Red/black	Clot activator and polymer barrier
Whole blood/plasma	Green/gray or light green	Polymer barrier and lithium heparin
	Light green	Polymer barrier and lithium heparin
	Light blue	Buffered sodium citrate
	Lavender (purple)	K_3EDTA or K_2EDTA or Na_2EDTA
	Gray	Sodium fluoride and potassium oxalate or sodium fluoride and Na_2EDTA; or sodium fluoride only
	Green	Lithium heparin, sodium heparin, or ammonium heparin
	Royal blue	K_2EDTA-sterile tube for toxicology and nutritional studies
	Pink	Blood Bank K_2EDTA
	Tan	K_2EDTA tube for lead testing
Clotted blood/serum	Royal blue	Clot activator; sterile tube for trace elements, toxicology, and nutritional studies
Whole blood	Lavender (purple)	K_2EDTA or K_3EDTA or Na_2EDTA
	Green	Lithium heparin, sodium heparin, or ammonium heparin
	Black	Sodium citrate for hematology
	Yellow	Sodium polyanethol sulfonate (SPS) or acid citrate dextrose (ACD)

ANTICOAGULANTS AND PRESERVATIVES

Many coagulation factors are involved in blood clotting, and coagulation can be prevented by the addition of different types of anticoagulants.[1] These anticoagulants often contain preservatives that can extend the metabolism and life span of the red blood cells (RBCs) after blood collection. Anticoagulants and preservatives are used extensively in blood donations to ensure the biochemical balance of certain components of RBCs, such as hemoglobin, pH, adenosine triphosphate (ATP), and glucose. Once transferred, anticoagulants, such as **acid citrate dextrose (ACD)** or citrate-phosphate-dextrose (CPD), ensure that the RBCs provide the recipient with the means of delivering oxygen (O_2) to the tissues.

Another major use of anticoagulants and preservatives is in the collection of plasma for laboratory analysis. Specific anticoagulants or preservatives must be used depending on the test procedure ordered. Anticoagulants cannot be substituted for one another or mixed from one vacuum tube to another. Appendix 6 lists the various laboratory assays along with the types of anticoagulants required for each assay.

Coagulation of blood can be prevented by the addition of **oxalates,** citrates, ethylenediamine tetra-acetic acid (EDTA), or heparin. Oxalates, citrates, and EDTA prevent the coagulation of blood by removing calcium and forming insoluble calcium salts. These three anticoagulants cannot be used in calcium determinations; however, **citrates** are frequently used in coagulation blood studies. **Ethylenediamine tetra-acetic acid** prevents platelet aggregation and is therefore used for platelet counts and platelet function tests. Fresh EDTA-anticoagulated blood allows preparation of blood films on microscope slides with minimal distortion of white blood cells (WBCs). **Heparin,** a mucopolysaccharide used in assays, such as ammonia and plasma hemoglobin, prevents blood clotting by inactivating the blood-clotting chemicals—thrombin and Factor X. Refer to Chapter 7 to review the hemostatic process.

In addition, other additives are included in some blood collection tubes to promote clot activation for rapid analysis of the blood. These additives are discussed in further detail later in this chapter.

YELLOW-TOPPED TUBES AND VACUUM CULTURE VIALS

Sterile blood specimens are ordered for blood cultures when the patient is suspected of having septicemia (symptoms of sepsis). A major problem with collecting blood for culture is that the patient's sample can become contaminated with microorganisms from the skin. Thus, the blood must be collected in a sterile container (vacuum tube, vial, or syringe) under aseptic conditions. (See Chapter 15 for blood culture collections.) The additive **sodium polyanethol sulfonate (SPS)** is in the yellow-topped tubes for blood culture specimen collections in microbiology. The SPS is an anticoagulant that reduces the activity of certain antibiotics; it inhibits phagocytosis (defense mechanism to kill microorganisms) in the blood. Thus, the SPS enhances the chances of detecting bacteria in the patient's blood. The collected blood should be gently inverted in the vacuum tube eight times for complete mixing of SPS with the blood. Also, as shown in **FIGURE 8–4**, blood can be collected directly into vacuum vials that contain culture media.

This type of collection minimizes the risk of specimen contamination. The vacuum vials can be purchased with different types of culture media, an unplugged venting unit for aerobic incubation, or a plugged venting unit for anaerobic incubation.

It should be noted that tubes containing ACD (acid citrate dextrose) also use the yellow color code. These tubes are mainly used to preserve blood for donation. Also, ACD is used for specialty blood banking, such as human leukocyte antigen (HLA) typing and DNA testing. The HLA typing is used in paternity (i.e., offspring, children) evaluation and to determine donor compatibility for an organ transplant.

> **Clinical Alert!** There are two important things to remember when using vacuum blood collection tubes:
>
> - These tubes have been designed for a certain amount of blood to be collected into the tube by vacuum as related to the amount of prefilled anticoagulant or other additive in the tube. *Never* add more blood into the tube.
> - If an insufficient amount of blood is collected in the anticoagulated tube, the laboratory test results may be erroneous because of the incorrect blood-to-anticoagulant ratio.

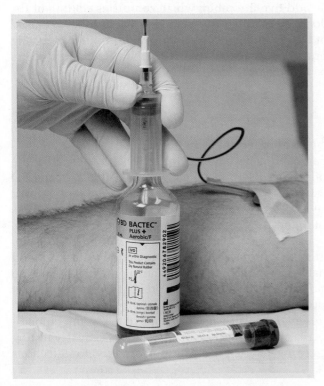

FIGURE 8–4

Collecting Blood for Culture Using the BD BACTEC Culture Vial

Courtesy and © Becton, Dickinson and Company

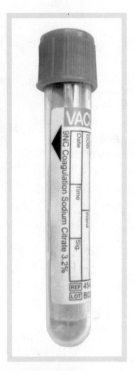

FIGURE 8–5

Light-Blue–Topped Vacuum Tube with Designated Fill Line

Courtesy of Greiner Bio-One, Kremsmunster, Austria.

LIGHT-BLUE–TOPPED TUBES

Many coagulation procedures, such as PT and APTT, are done on blood collected in light-blue–topped vacuum tubes, which contain sodium citrate at various concentrations, dependent on the manufacturer. If a light-blue–topped tube is underfilled, coagulation results will be erroneously prolonged. If the light-blue–topped tube is overfilled, coagulation results will be erroneously shortened. Due to the importance of having the correct amount of blood collected, the blood collection tube manufacturers have light-blue–topped vacuum tubes with designated fill lines. An example is shown in **FIGURE 8–5**. The light-blue–topped tube should be gently inverted three to four times as soon as the blood is collected.

SERUM SEPARATION TUBES (MOTTLED-TOPPED, SPECKLED-TOPPED, AND GOLD-TOPPED TUBES)

Another collection method is to use a **serum separation tube (SST),** such as the BD VACUTAINER Plus Serum Separation Tube or Greiner Bio-One VACUETTE clot-activator serum tube (**FIGURE 8–6**). These tubes contain a polymer barrier that is present in the bottom of the tube. The **specific gravity** (weight compared to water) of this material lies between the blood clot and the serum. After blood is collected in one of these tubes, the tube needs to be gently inverted five to eight times and then allowed to set for 30 minutes prior to centrifugation. During centrifugation, the polymer barrier moves upward to the serum-clot interface, where it forms a stable barrier separating the serum from fibrin and cells. Serum may be aspirated directly from the collection tube, eliminating the need for transfer to another container. These tubes can be used for chemistry, immunohematology, as well as therapeutic drug monitoring (TDM). However, the manufacturer should be contacted to verify that no interferences from specific drugs occur with these types of tubes.

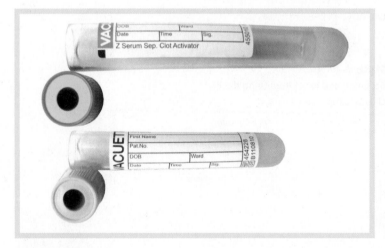

FIGURE 8–6

VACUETTE Serum Tube

Courtesy of Greiner Bio-One, Kremsmunster, Austria.

RAPID SERUM TUBES (RST)

The orange and gray/yellow vacuum-topped tubes have the additive thrombin, which completes clotting of the blood in less than five minutes. These tubes are used for STAT (emergency) laboratory procedures requiring serum specimens. BD VACUTAINER refers to these as the Rapid Serum Tube (RST).

RED-TOPPED SERUM TUBES

The red-topped tubes indicate a tube *without* an anticoagulant or polymer (gel) barrier and is used for the collection of serum. As shown in **FIGURE 8–7**, the BD VACUTAINER red-topped tube has a red stripe down the left side of the label indicating it is a serum tube. Thus, the collected blood *will* clot in this tube. After the blood is collected in the tube, the clotting process begins and takes at least 30 minutes for the fibrin clot to form. Then the tube can be centrifuged so that the serum will be separated from the blood clot in order to test for various analytes in the serum. After centrifugation, if there is no barrier, the serum should be removed to a transfer tube to prevent blood cell contact during transport and storage since the blood cells will falsely alter the patient's true analyte(s) status. If a barrier is present, there is no need to remove the serum immediately. The BD VACUTAINER Plus plastic serum tube can be used for chemistry testing as well as routine blood donor screening and diagnostic testing of serum for infectious diseases.

CLEAR-TOPPED TUBES, WHITE-TOPPED TUBES, AND RED/LIGHT GRAY TUBES

Tubes with tops of clear, white, or red/light gray plastic are used as a discard tube or a secondary specimen tube. They do not contain additives.

GREEN-TOPPED TUBES AND PLASMA SEPARATION TUBES (LIGHT-GREEN, MOTTLED GRAY/GREEN-TOPPED TUBES)

The anticoagulants sodium heparin, ammonium heparin, and lithium heparin are found in green-topped vacuum tubes. These tubes are used in various laboratory assays requiring plasma or whole blood, which are mainly chemistry tests. When a fast turnaround time (TAT) is needed for a STAT test, the green-topped tube is used since the whole blood can be used for testing and the time for clot formation and/or centrifugation is avoided. For potassium measurement, heparinized plasma or whole blood, rather than serum from the red-topped or red-speckled–topped tube, is preferred because sporadic increased potassium levels can occur in serum as a result of potassium released from platelets during blood clotting.[2] The more platelets that a patient has in his or her blood, the greater the difference between the potassium results from the green-topped plasma as compared to the red-topped or red-speckled–topped serum potassium results.

Lithium heparin tubes are used for many assays that include

- Glucose
- Blood urea nitrogen (BUN)
- Ionized calcium
- Creatinine
- Electrolyte studies

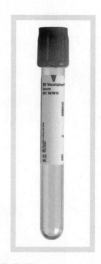

However, lithium heparin is not suitable for tests involving the measurement of lithium or folate levels.[1] Similarly, sodium heparin tubes should not be used for assays that measure sodium concentration. In other cases, a particular procedure will require sodium heparin without lithium, or vice versa.

BD has the PST™ that refers to the Plasma Separator Tube containing lithium heparin and plasma separator gel. These are available from BD in light-green plastic-topped tubes or in tubes that have rubber stoppers the color of mottled gray/green. Greiner Bio-One VACUETTE® tubes have plasma separator tubes in green plastic stoppers.

VACUETTE® Plasma Green-Topped Tubes with Lithium Heparin and Gel has the interior of the tube wall coated with lithium heparin (**FIGURE 8–8**). Heparin activates antithrombins that block the coagulation cascade, producing a whole blood/plasma sample. There is also a barrier gel in the tube indicated by the yellow ring inside the green top. The specific gravity of the gel lies between the blood cells and plasma. During centrifugation, the gel barrier moves upward, where it forms a stable barrier separating the plasma from cells. Plasma may be aspirated directly from the collection tube, which eliminates the need for transfer to another container. These tubes should be gently inverted 5 to 10 times immediately upon blood collection.

The PST tubes are used for plasma determinations in chemistry analysis. With these additives in this type of tube, the time for blood clotting is eliminated. Thus, the PST is used in STAT testing and for patients receiving anticoagulant therapy (i.e., Warfarin, heparin).

Green-topped vacuum tubes should not be used for collections for blood smears on microscope slides that are to be stained with Wright's stain, because the heparin causes the Wright's stain to have a blue background. And, when used for cytogenetic studies, these tubes must be sterile.

Light-green–topped or green/gray-topped tubes have a gel to separate the plasma from the red blood cells and are used for assays that require heparinized plasma.

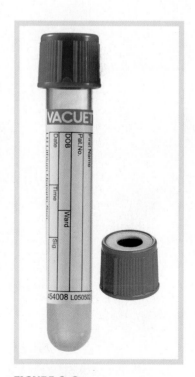

As for other vacuum tubes containing additives and anticoagulants, these tubes should be thoroughly mixed with the blood by eight gentle inversions of the tube immediately after blood collection.

PURPLE (LAVENDER)-TOPPED TUBES

The purple-topped vacuum tubes (containing EDTA) are used for most hematology procedures, such as the complete blood count (CBC), red blood cells (RBCs), white blood cells (WBCs), platelet count, hematocrit, differentials (DIFF), hemoglobin, mean corpuscular hemoglobin (MCH), mean corpuscular hemoglobin concentration (MCHC), and mean cell volume (MCV), among others. Also, this tube is used for molecular diagnostic testing, immunology, and hemoglobin A1c. The EDTA can be ordered as K_2 (spray-dried potassium) attached to EDTA or K_3 (liquid potassium) attached to EDTA. The K_2 is best to use for hematology tests (i.e., CBC, RBC), whereas the K_3 is best for viral markers. The EDTA tube needs to be completely inverted 8 to 10 times after blood collection to avoid the possibility of microclots forming in the tube from lack of proper mixing of the EDTA with the blood (**BOX 8–2**). The purple-topped tubes can also be used for routine immunohematology testing and blood donor screening.

PINK-TOPPED TUBES

Pink-topped tubes contain EDTA with the spray-dried K_2 and are used for blood bank collections and should also be completely inverted 8 to 10 times for complete mixing of the blood with the anticoagulant. This tube has the pink closure and a label that meets the AABB required for blood bank collections. The VACUETTE® pink-topped tube can also be used for viral collections.

GRAY-TOPPED TUBES

Gray-topped vacuum tubes usually contain (1) potassium oxalate and sodium fluoride, (2) Na_2EDTA and sodium fluoride, or (3) only sodium fluoride. This type of collection tube is primarily used for glycolytic inhibition tests. Thus, sometimes **antiglycolytic agent** and **glycolytic inhibitor** are the terms for this tube's additive, meaning that the tube's additive—sodium fluoride—prevents **glycolysis,** the breakdown or metabolism of glucose by blood cells. Thus, gray-topped tubes should not be used for hematology studies since oxalate distorts cellular morphologic features or in enzyme analysis since the enzymes will be destroyed; nor should they be used for Na or K determinations. The gray-topped tubes should be mixed with the blood immediately after collection by inverting completely eight times.

BOX 8–2

Purple-Topped Tubes

If a purple-topped tube is underfilled, the patient will have

- Falsely low blood cell counts
- Falsely low hematocrits
- Staining alterations on blood smears
- Erroneous morphologic changes to RBCs

ROYAL-BLUE–TOPPED AND TAN-TOPPED TUBES

The royal-blue–topped tubes are used to collect samples for nutritional studies and toxicology. This colored tube is the trace element tube. Depending on the laboratory tests that are requested, it is important to check the manufacturer's instructions for the royal-blue–topped tubes since they can be purchased as a serum collection tube or as a plasma collection tube. The tan-topped tube is used for lead testing and contains EDTA.

Clinical Alert! Blood collected in one type of tube with an additive *must NOT* be transferred to another blood collection tube with additive. If adding blood collected from one tube to another tube with the same additive, the blood-to-additive ratio will be erroneous, leading to mistaken laboratory results. Also, if different additives with blood are added together, the mixture will interfere in the laboratory testing.

BLACK-TOPPED TUBES

From certain manufacturers, a black-topped tube with buffered sodium citrate is available for blood collections used to determine the erythrocyte sedimentation rate (ESR).

MOLECULAR DIAGNOSTICS TUBES

Special sterile vacuum tubes for molecular diagnostic studies are available containing different additives (e.g., sodium citrate, sodium heparin, EDTA) as required for the different testing procedures. Manufacturers have different-colored tops for these tubes. For example, Greiner Bio-One has the VACUETTE® K_2EDTA with Gel white-topped tubes (**FIGURE 8–9**). The interior of the tube wall is coated with K_2EDTA. The EDTA binds calcium ions and blocks blood coagulation. These tubes are used for testing plasma in molecular diagnostics and contain a barrier gel that functions as previously described. These tubes should be inverted 8 to 10 times immediately after the blood is collected.

TUBE ORGANIZER

The TIMO™ Tube Management Organizer (**FIGURE 8–10**) is an innovative test tube holder that assists with managing the test tubes during the blood sample collection process. The TIMO™ organizer may be used to collect test tube samples from both patients and blood donors. It holds and organizes test tubes before, during, and after

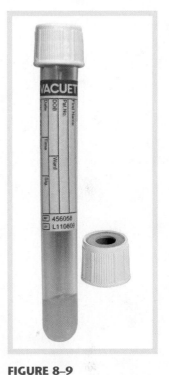

FIGURE 8–9

BD Vacutainer Plus Plastic White-Topped Tube Contains K_2EDTA and Gel (Plasma Separator) for Molecular Diagnostics

Courtesy of Greiner Bio-One, Kremsmunster, Austria.

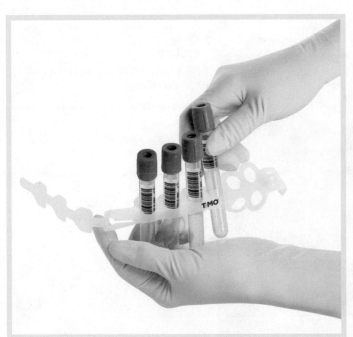

FIGURE 8–10

TiMO™ Tube Management Organizer

Courtesy of ITL Corp.

blood sample collection; provides a simple mechanism to keep one patient or blood donor's set of test tubes together; and ensures test tube management throughout the entire collection process.

Safety Syringes

Some patients' veins are too fragile for blood collection with vacuum tubes, so safety syringes have been generally used for the collection process; however, the safety butterfly needle blood collection sets are becoming the preferred method. Syringes are hazardous and pose an increased risk of accidental needlesticks.[3] Both procedures are covered in Chapter 10.

Syringes are sometimes used for collecting blood from central venous catheter (CVC) lines. This procedure is discussed in detail in Chapter 15. Major parts of the syringe are the needle, safety cover, hub, barrel, and plunger (**FIGURE 8–11**). The barrel and the plunger are made to fit together tightly so that when the plunger is in the barrel and drawn back, a vacuum is created. To fit properly, the needle and syringe must be compatible and are attached by the hub. This vacuum allows blood or other fluids to be aspirated, or sucked, into the barrel as the plunger is pulled back. The barrel of the syringe has graduated measurements in milliliter (mL) or cubic centimeter (cc) increments. Sizes range from approximately 0.2 to 50.0 mL; however, for specimen collection purposes, 5- to 20-mL syringes are most often used. In addition, the health care worker should ensure that the syringe is the correct size for the amount of blood to be collected.

A safety syringe shielded transfer device shown in **FIGURES 8–12** and **8–13** must be used when placing the blood from the syringe into the vacuum tubes for testing

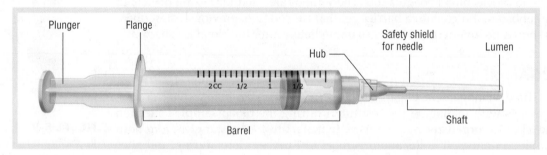

FIGURE 8–11
Example of a Safety Syringe

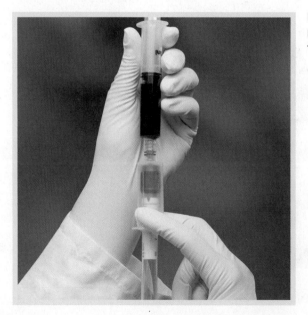

FIGURE 8–12
BD SafetyGlide Needle and BD Blood Transfer Device

Courtesy and © Becton, Dickinson and Company

to avoid possible exposure to the patient's blood.[4] The plunger must *not* be pushed down if the tubes are being filled from the syringe because it is extremely hazardous. Also, pushing the plunger may damage cellular components and cause hemolysis because of the forceful expulsion of blood. The syringe needle should be shielded after blood collection, removed, and discarded in a "sharps" disposal container.[5] The BD Blood Transfer Device is attached to the syringe, and a vacuum tube is inserted into the transfer device. The blood is transferred from the syringe to the tube using the tube's vacuum. Specialized tubes and bottles that may fit the adapter are also available for blood culture collection.

Clinical Alert!

- Safety engineering controls (engineered sharps injury protection) and safe work practices must be used if collecting blood with a syringe.
- Avoid the use of syringes in blood collection if at all possible.
- Needleless safety blood transfer devices must be used to place the blood from the syringe into the vacuum tube.

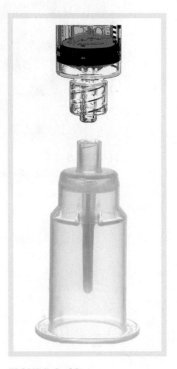

FIGURE 8–13
Greiner Bio-One VACUETTE Syringe Blood Transfer Unit

Courtesy of Greiner Bio-One, Kremsmunster, Austria.

Safety Needles/Holders

The gauge and length of a needle used on a syringe or a vacuum tube is selected according to the specific task. The **gauge number** indicates the diameter of the needle; the smaller the gauge number, the larger the needle diameter and higher the flow rate (**BOX 8–3**).

For example, larger (18-gauge) needles are used for collecting donor units of blood (450 mL or less), whereas smaller (21- and 22-gauge) needles are used for collecting specimens for laboratory assays. When blood is collected from children, a 21- to 23-gauge needle is usually used with a tuberculin, or 3-mL, safety syringe or with a safety butterfly needle blood collection set (safety winged infusion set). The length of the needle depends on the depth of the vein to be punctured. Needles are usually available at either 1- or 1.5-inch. The needle attaches to the safety holder/adapter, or syringe, at its hub.

Needles are sterilized and packaged by vendors in sealed shields that maintain sterility. These sealed shields are packaged in individual containers that are color coded according to the gauge size of the needles and must be twisted apart before the needles are used in blood collection. The needle attaches to the safety holder/adapter, or syringe, at its hub. For example, the BD Eclipse safety-shielding blood needle attaches to a holder (**FIGURE 8–14**).

The BD Eclipse shield is activated immediately after the blood collection tubes are filled and the needle is removed from the vein (**FIGURE 8–15**). When the thumb pushes forward on the shield, as shown in Figure 8–15, an audible click indicates that the safety shield is locked in place. This single-use adapter provides immediate containment of a used needle. Also, shown in Figure 8–3 is the BD Vacutainer® Passive Shielding Blood Collection Needle. The needle's safety shield releases automatically on insertion of the first tube, providing protection from the time the first tube is inserted through product disposal.

BOX 8–3

Needle Sizes Used for Blood Collection

- Larger (16- to 18-gauge) needles are used for collecting donor units of blood (e.g., 450 mL).
- Smaller (21- to 23-gauge) needles are used for collecting specimens for laboratory assays and for children.

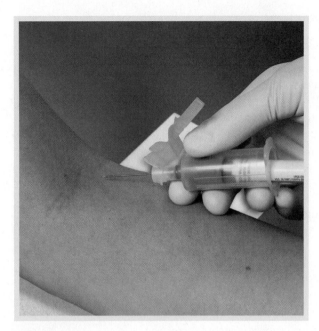

FIGURE 8–14
BD Eclipse Blood Collection Needle Attached to a Holder

Courtesy and © Becton, Dickinson and Company

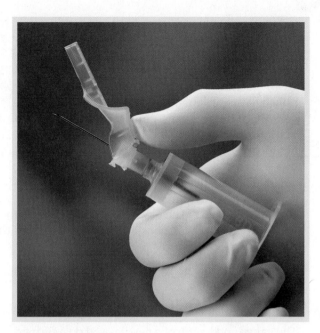

FIGURE 8–15
BD Eclipse Blood Collection Shield Activation for Immediate Containment of the Used Needle

Courtesy and © Becton, Dickinson and Company

Another protective holder that provides effective and immediate containment of a used needle is the Venipuncture Needle-Pro. After removing the needle from the patient's vein, the health care worker activates the needle guard by holding the tube holder and pressing the needle guard against a hard surface so that the guard swings over the needle. Once engaged, both ends of the needle are covered, protecting the blood collector from an accidental needlestick. It reduces the risk of reusing a contaminated holder since it is a one-time-use-only, safety-engineered device.

The Vanishpoint blood collection tube holder features a blood collection tube holder and a small tube adapter. The needle is automatically retracted from the patient when the end cap is closed after the last tube has been removed. It virtually eliminates exposure to the contaminated needle and the possibility of needlestick injury (**FIGURE 8–16**).

FIGURE 8–16
Vanishpoint Blood Collection Tube Holder

Courtesy of Retractable Technologies, Little Elm, TX.

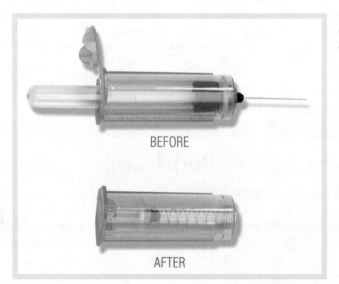

BEFORE

AFTER

The VACUETTE® QuickShield Safety Tube Holder is used to prevent accidental needlestick injuries during venous blood collection (**FIGURE 8–17**). It can be used in conjunction with VACUETTE® blood collection needles. The device is used by pressing the protective cover over the needle with the aid of a stable surface and then disposing the needle and holder into a sharps disposal container.

Sarstedt, Inc., has the S-Monovette® Blood Collection System (**FIGURE 8–18**), which is an enclosed multiple-sampling blood collection system that collects blood using either an aspiration or vacuum principle of collection. Using the aspiration procedure replaces syringe draws for patients with difficult veins and can prevent uncomfortable resticks. All tubes are plastic with screw caps, which minimizes the risk of breakage and aerosol formation when caps are removed. Each needle has an integral holder that does not require assembly before use and cannot be disassembled. Thus, it prevents reuse of the holder.

For any of these blood collection needle and tube holder devices, disposing of the tube holder while it is still attached to the needle ensures that the tube-puncturing needle remains protected during and after disposal.[5] Thus, it significantly reduces the risks of needlestick injuries and blood exposure from the tube-puncturing needle to automatically retract into it after blood collection.

The tip of each needle should be visually checked for damage. A blunt or bent tip can be harmful to the patient's vein and may result in failure to collect blood.

A **multiple-sample needle** is used with vacuum collection tubes and the holder to allow for multiple tube changes without blood leakage within the plastic holder. The multiple-sample needle has a plastic cover over the tube-top puncturing portion of the needle; this cover creates a leakage barrier.

When purchasing phlebotomy supplies from multiple manufacturers, it is important to use needles with holders or syringes that are compatible with the needles to avoid the possibility of leaking blood and blood exposure.

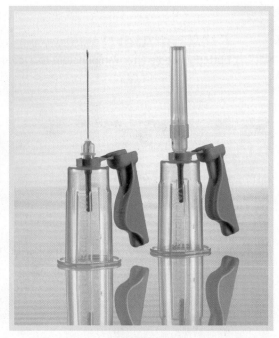

FIGURE 8–17

VACUETTE® QUICKSHIELD Complete PLUS Safety Tube Holder

Courtesy of Greiner Bio-One GmbH, Kremsmuenster, Austria.

THE BUTTERFLY NEEDLE (BLOOD COLLECTION SET)

The safety **butterfly needle,** also referred to as a blood collection set or safety **winged infusion set,** is the most commonly used intravenous device. It is a stainless steel, beveled needle and tube, usually 5 to 12 inches long, with attached plastic wings on one end and a fitting for a multisample Luer adapter or fitting for a syringe attached to the other. The most common butterfly needle sizes are 21- and 23-gauge, and the length of these needles range from ½ to ¾ inches long. The smaller angle of insertion can occur with the shorter needle. The butterfly needle is sometimes used in the collection of blood from patients who are difficult to stick by conventional methods (e.g., geriatric patients, cancer patients, pediatric patients). Refer to Chapter 10 for more details.

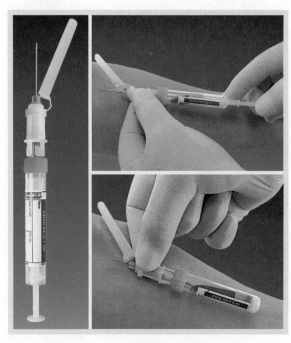

FIGURE 8–18

Sarstedt S-Monovette® Venous Blood Collection System

Courtesy of Sarstedt, Inc., Newton, NC.

Numerous types of safety butterfly needles are available and must be used according to OSHA regulations. Each of these safety needles has a shield that automatically covers the contaminated needle point upon withdrawal from the patient's vein. One example is the MONOJECT ANGEL WING blood collection set. It has a stainless steel safety shield that automatically resheaths the needle during withdrawal from the patient. The system includes multisample needle-shielded tube holders and sets for use in collecting blood specimens directly into blood collection tubes and blood culture bottles, as well as multisample needle-shielded transfer tube holders and

ALERT

Clinical Alert! The safety device *must* be activated on the butterfly needle after venipuncture to avoid needlestick injury.

sets for transferring blood from syringes into collection tubes and blood culture bottles.

BD VACUTAINER Systems *Preanalytical Solutions* has the BD VACUTAINER Push Button Blood Collection Set (**FIGURE 8–19**), which provides immediate protection against needle stick injury when properly activated within the vein and in accordance with the BD directions.

Greiner Bio-One manufactures the VACUETTE® safety blood collection set (**FIGURE 8–20**). It is a winged needle device with a safety shield. Terumo Medical Corp. manufactures the Surshield® Safety Winged Blood Collection Set (**FIGURE 8–21**) that is a safety-engineered butterfly device for blood collection or IV insertion. No matter which type of safety blood collection set is used, it is imperative to use a Luer adapter from the same manufacturer to avoid possible blood leakage and exposure.

The VanishPoint blood collection set (**FIGURE 8–22**) safety device has automated in-vein retraction that effectively reduces the risk of needlestick injuries and blood exposure. The trigger indicator is color coded for needle gauge. Needle retraction clamps the tubing, reducing the risk of exposure to blood. The clear body allows for flashback visualization.

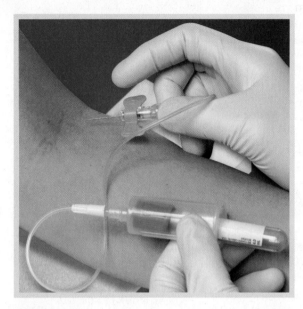

FIGURE 8–19
Blood Collection with BD VACUTAINER Push Button Blood Collection Set

Courtesy and © Becton, Dickinson and Company

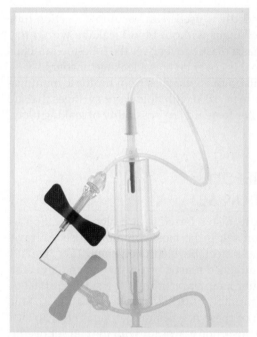

FIGURE 8–20
VACUETTE® Safety Blood Collection Set

Courtesy of Greiner Bio-One, Kremsmunster, Austria.

NEEDLE AND OTHER SHARPS DISPOSAL

Needles, syringes, and lancets (sterile, disposable sharp devices used in skin puncture) must be discarded in rigid, leak-proof, plastic containers, reducing the possibility of needlesticks. Each unit is usually orange or red and is disposable as biohazardous waste (**FIGURE 8–23**). Several sizes of sharps disposal containers are available for use at the bedside, on the cart, in isolation, and on home health care trays. Before beginning a blood collection procedure, note the location of the nearest sharps container.

ALERT

Clinical Alert! *Never* overfill a biohazard sharps container!

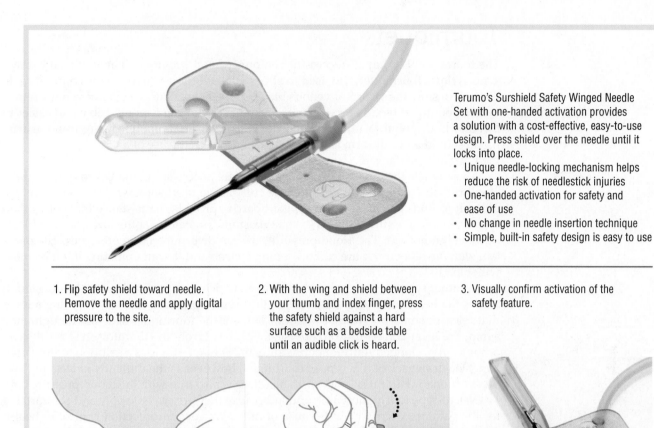

Terumo's Surshield Safety Winged Needle Set with one-handed activation provides a solution with a cost-effective, easy-to-use design. Press shield over the needle until it locks into place.
- Unique needle-locking mechanism helps reduce the risk of needlestick injuries
- One-handed activation for safety and ease of use
- No change in needle insertion technique
- Simple, built-in safety design is easy to use

1. Flip safety shield toward needle. Remove the needle and apply digital pressure to the site.

2. With the wing and shield between your thumb and index finger, press the safety shield against a hard surface such as a bedside table until an audible click is heard.

3. Visually confirm activation of the safety feature.

FIGURE 8–21
Surshield® Safety Winged Blood Collection Set

Courtesy of Terumo Medical Corp., Somerset, NJ.

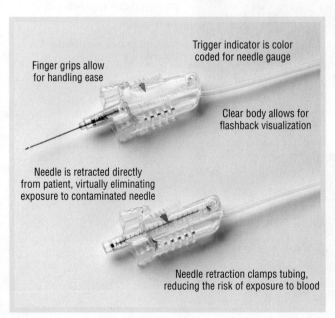

Finger grips allow for handling ease

Trigger indicator is color coded for needle gauge

Clear body allows for flashback visualization

Needle is retracted directly from patient, virtually eliminating exposure to contaminated needle

Needle retraction clamps tubing, reducing the risk of exposure to blood

FIGURE 8–22
VanishPoint® Blood Collection Set

Courtesy of Retractable Technologies, Little Elm, TX.

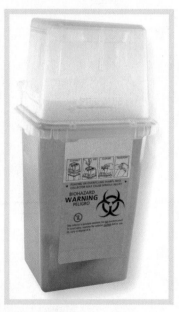

FIGURE 8–23
Sharps Disposal Container with the Required Biohazard Sign

Steve Carroll/Shutterstock.com

Tourniquets

The tourniquet is a key to successful venipuncture: It provides a barrier to slow down venous flow. Tourniquets are used in specimen collection to apply enough pressure to the arm to slow the return of venous blood to the heart. This slowing of venous return causes pooling of blood in the veins, which makes the veins more visible and easier to feel and find. The tourniquet should not restrict arterial blood flowing into the arm. Blood should enter the arm at a normal rate and, with the use of a tourniquet, return to the heart at a slower rate.

Tourniquets that are usually used include the pliable strap, the Velcro type, and the blood pressure cuff. The blood pressure cuff can be used successfully when veins are difficult to find. The most efficient blood barrier provides a resistance that is less than systolic blood pressure but greater than diastolic, or stated another way, so that blood flows in but not out. The blood pressure cuff can determine these pressures. The problem with the blood pressure cuff is keeping it clean and decontaminating it if it is soiled with blood.

Another type of tourniquet is the Seraket, which uses a minature seat-belt design. It allows the health care worker to release the venous pressure partially by using a lever that releases some pressure but not all. Thus, if the tourniquet needs to be tightened again, the lever can be used to adjust it. Because errors in laboratory test results can occur from prolonged tourniquet pressure, the Seraket provides a solution to this problem. One drawback of this type of tourniquet, however, is the difficulty in cleaning and decontaminating it if it is soiled with blood, as is also true with the blood pressure cuff.

Velcro-type tourniquets are popular because they are easy to apply and comfortable for the patient. Alternatively, because of major concern for infection control in health care institutions, many facilities now use a disposable nonlatex tourniquet strap to help prevent cross-contamination (**FIGURE 8–24**). Nonlatex disposable tourniquets are now available as a good option for the blood collector and patient. The Tournistrip is a single-use tourniquet developed in the United Kingdom to fight nosocomial infections. The tourniquet is a plasticized paper band that is fastened using a quick-release seal. If the tourniquets used in the health care facility are not disposable, they must be wiped frequently with 70% isopropyl alcohol and disinfected with a chlorine bleach dilution of 1:10 if contaminated with blood or other body fluids.

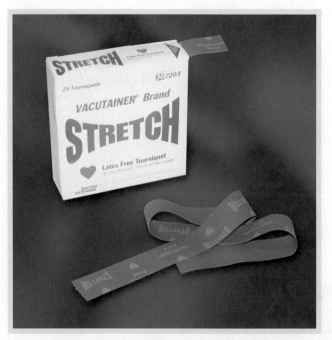

FIGURE 8–24

BD VACUTAINER Latex-Free Tourniquet

Courtesy and © Becton, Dickinson and Company

Venoscope, the Vein Finder

A conventional method to detect a vein for blood collection is the Venoscope II transilluminator. This instrument provides a noninvasive procedure to visualize veins that are difficult to find on all skin types and prevents vein rolling (**FIGURE 8–25**). Additionally, Venoscope has neonatal as well as pediatric and adult transilluminators to noninvasively detect a vein for blood collection (**FIGURE 8–26**). It uses patented LED technology by the high-intensity light illuminating the subcutaneous tissue in the arm that creates a uniform area of orange reflection of the fatty tissue. The light detects the "dark lines" of the veins and makes them easier to find for blood collection.

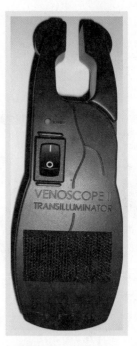

FIGURE 8–25
Venoscope II Transilluminator

Courtesy of Venoscope, L.L.C., Lafayette, LA.

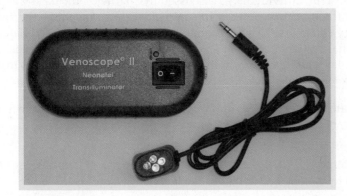

FIGURE 8–26
Venoscope Neonatal Transilluminator

Courtesy of Venoscope, L.L.C., Lafayette, LA.

AccuVein

The AccuVein Vein Viewing System is a noninvasive portable, handheld, lightweight tool that improves patient outcomes for blood collection by a quick location of the veins. The AccuVein AV400 uses two lasers, one infrared and one red, that are rapidly scanned over the skin. Infrared detects hemoglobin, and red projects the vein pattern. The hemoglobin in the blood absorbs infrared light more than the surrounding tissue. The device uses this change in reflection to determine vein location (**FIGURES 8–27** and **8–28**).

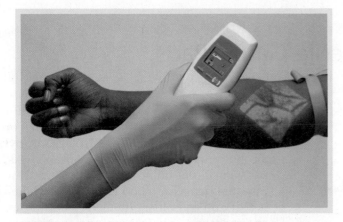

FIGURE 8–27
The AccuVein AV400 Vein Illumination System Helps Practitioners Locate Veins for Venous Access

Courtesy of AccuVein, Cold Spring Harbor, NY.

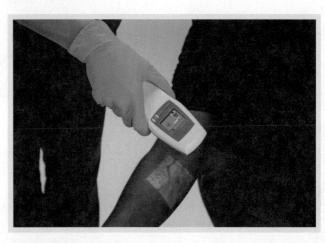

FIGURE 8–28
Courtesy of AccuVein, Cold Spring Harbor, NY.

Gloves for Blood Collection

Safety guidelines have been established for health care workers to help them prevent the possibility of acquiring infections, such as hepatitis or those associated with AIDS. These guidelines include the use of gloves during collection of blood from patients (**FIGURE 8–29**). It is recommended that health care workers not use gloves with talc powder containing calcium, because tubes of patients' blood may become contaminated with this powder, and such contamination can result in falsely elevated calcium values.

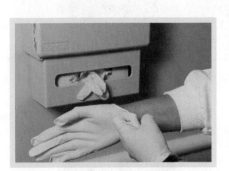

FIGURE 8–29
Use of Gloves

Latex gloves have proved effective in preventing the transmission of infectious diseases to health care workers. However, exposure to latex may result in an allergic reaction in some individuals, as discussed in Chapter 5. Increasing exposure to latex gloves or the lubricant powder in some gloves also increases the risk of developing allergy symptoms. The National Institute for Occupational Safety and Health (NIOSH) has valuable information on its website (www.cdc.gov/niosh/docs/98-113) regarding latex allergy prevention and suggests the following steps to protect oneself from latex exposure:

- Use nonlatex gloves for activities that are not likely to involve contact with infectious materials: housekeeping, maintenance, and so on.
- Use powder-free gloves with reduced protein content.
- "Hypoallergenic" latex gloves do not reduce the risk of latex allergy but may reduce reactions to chemical additives in the latex.
- Use glove liners to avoid contact with the latex gloves.
- When wearing gloves, do not use oil-based hand creams; they can cause glove deterioration.
- Wash hands with mild soap after using latex gloves.
- Frequently clean areas that have been contaminated with latex-containing dust.
- Learn the symptoms of latex allergy.
- Attend latex allergy educational programs.

Because nitrile butadiene rubber is very different from natural (latex), **nitrile gloves** are increasingly being used in health care facilities by health care providers for blood collection and other health care activities. They are a solution to a growing number of people who have developed allergies to the latex proteins that accompany latex gloves. They are available from numerous manufacturers and provide the same needed protection from infectious diseases as latex gloves.

Antiseptics, Sterile Gauze Pads, and Bandages

The health care worker must use antiseptics, **sterile gauze pads,** and bandages for blood collection by either venipuncture or microcollection. Therefore, 70% isopropyl alcohol preparation and iodine swab sticks, pads, or chlorhexidine (for blood cultures) are essential items for blood collection. In home health care and other ambulatory health care environments where soap and water may not be available, a waterless antiseptic agent (**FIGURE 8–30**) should be carried with other blood collection items and used before and after blood collection.

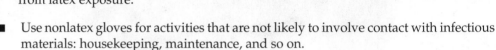

ALERT

Clinical Alert!

- Change gloves between patients' blood collections.
- Do not wash, disinfect, or reuse gloves.
- Over time, latex gloves can become porous if exposed to electrical components or to light. Store them in an appropriate area and discard unused gloves after 3 months.

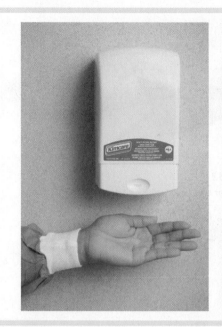
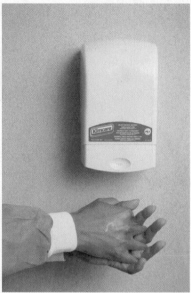
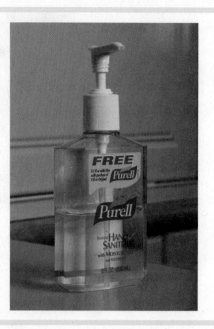

FIGURE 8–30
Waterless Antiseptic Agents: Mounted in Wall Dispensers or Carried with Other Blood Collection Supplies in Travel-Size Containers

Microcollection Equipment

Usually, skin-puncture blood collecting techniques are used on adults and infants when small amounts of blood can be used for diagnostic laboratory testing and also if venipuncture is excessively hazardous for a patient.

A minimal volume of blood should be collected from adults, neonates (newborns), or older infants to avoid the risk of iatrogenic (induced) anemia caused by large amounts of blood loss due to specimen collections.[6,7] Laboratory instruments using skin puncture blood are becoming more prevalent due to the problem of severe blood loss from numerous blood collections in health care settings.

LANCETS AND TUBES

For infants, the Clinical and Laboratory Standards Institute (CLSI) recommends a penetration depth of less than 2.0 mm on heel sticks to avoid penetrating bone.[8] The BD Quikheel lancet (**FIGURE 8–31**) is available for two different incision depths, depending on the needs of the infant. The teal-colored Quikheel Infant lancet has a preset incision depth of 1.0 mm and a width of 2.5 mm, and the purple-colored Quikheel Preemie lancet has a preset incision depth of 0.85 mm and a width of 1.75 mm. This lancet blade retracts permanently after activation to assure safety to the health care worker.

The BD Microtainer Contact-Activated Lancet (**FIGURE 8–32**) is a safety-engineered device that activates only when it is positioned and pressed against the skin, facilitating a consistent puncture depth and providing for the safety of patients and health care workers.

Clinical Alert!

- **Disposable sterile lancets** that are retractable to avoid bloodborne pathogen exposure should be used to puncture the skin for skin puncture collections.

- Surgical blades should not be used for skin puncture due to the hazard to the patient and health care worker.

ALERT

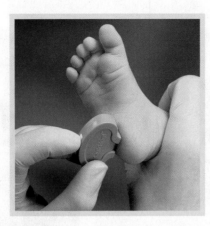

FIGURE 8–31
BD Quikheel Lancet

Courtesy and © Becton, Dickinson and Company

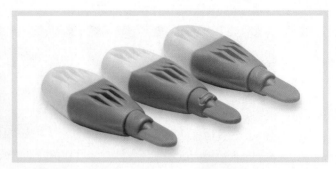

FIGURE 8–32
BD Microtainer Contact-Activated Lancet

Courtesy and © Becton, Dickinson and Company

The Terumo Capiject® Lancet (**FIGURE 8–33**) is a safety-engineered device for skin-puncture blood collection. The Capiject® Lancet is available in an assortment of puncture widths and depths, as well as in a needle lancet for glucose testing.

ITC has produced fully automated, single-use, automatically retracting, disposable devices that provide safety both for the neonate and for the health care worker (**FIGURE 8–34**). Tenderlett Jr. for children, Tenderlett for adults, and Tenderlett Toddler for infants and toddlers are engineered to incise to the least invasive but most effective depth for optimal blood flow. The Tenderlett incises 1.75 mm deep, Tenderlett Jr. incises 1.25 mm deep, and Tenderlett Toddler incises only 0.85 mm deep. The retracting blade of each of these devices eliminates potential injury from an exposed blade contaminated with blood.

Another safety device for microcollection is the MONOJECT Monoletter Safety Lancet for fingerstick collections. The Greiner Bio-One lancet also has a safety microcollection device available for various puncture depths.

The Natus Medical NeatNick lancets (**FIGURE 8–35**) in both preemie and full-term depth controlled sizes has been designed to minimize infant pain through a high-speed nick and precise puncture.

To collect a reliable small-volume blood sample, it is important to use properly designed blood microcollection tubes that are made of plastic or glass tubes coated in a puncture-resistant film for safety. Glass microcollection devices are no longer recommended (i.e., Natelson tubes) due to

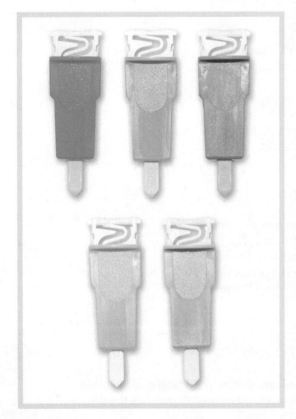

FIGURE 8–33
Terumo Capiject® Lancet

Courtesy of Terumo Medical Corp., Somerset, NJ.

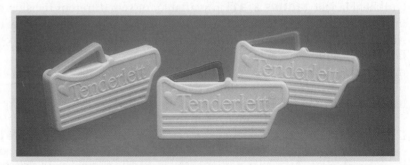

FIGURE 8–34
Tenderlett Automated Skin Incision Device

Courtesy of ITC, Edison, NJ.

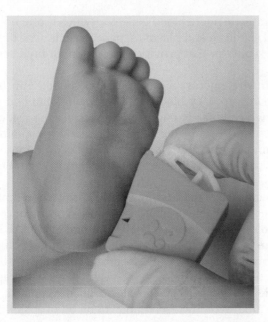

FIGURE 8–35
NeatNick Preemie Lancet

Courtesy of Natus Medical Incorporated

the risk associated with accidental breakage. The **microcontainers** recommended for use for skin puncture collections are listed in **BOX 8–4**.

Microhematocrits are disposable narrow-bore pipettes that are used for packed red cell volume (hematocrit) in microcentrifugation. These plastic or plastic-encased glass tubes also have colored bands; a red band indicates a heparin-coated tube, and a blue band indicates no anticoagulant. After blood collection, these capillary tubes must be sealed at the ends with plastic or clay plugs. The sealant plugs are inserted by using "clay slabs," which create a hazard because they become contaminated with blood and possibly glass fragments. These slabs must frequently be discarded in an appropriate sharps container according to the health care facility's safety policies. Microcollection containers in plastic or glass wrapped, puncture-resistant plastic/film are available for general laboratory collections (e.g., chemistry) and are usually color coded according to the established protocol for blood collection vacuum tube tops. Thus, purple- or lavender-topped tubes contain EDTA, green-topped tubes contain heparin, red- or pink-topped tubes have no additive, and gray-topped tubes have **sodium fluoride** to inhibit blood enzymes that destroy glucose. Some of the manufacturers of microcollection blood tubes produce amber-colored tubes that provide protection for light-sensitive analytes (e.g., bilirubin).

BOX 8–4

Plastic or Plastic-Wrapped Glass Microcollection Devices—Various Types Needed

- Serum or plasma separator devices in different color codes (same colors as for vacuum color-topped tubes described earlier according to additives, e.g., purple—EDTA) gently inverted upon collection with the required number of inversions
- Disposable plastic calibrated microcollection tubes
- Plastic microhematocrit tubes
- Microdilution systems (e.g., BMP LeukoChek)

Covidien manufactures the Samplette micro blood collector, which is offered with a full range of anticoagulants as well as serum and plasma separation gels. One of its collectors is an amber capillary blood separator that provides protection for light-sensitive analytes (e.g., bilirubin).

Electrolytes and general chemistry microspecimens can be collected in the BD Microtainer tube, which has its own capillary blood collector, self-contained serum separator, and Microgard closure, which is safety engineered to reduce the risk of tube leakage and specimen splatter. Each tube is imprinted with two markings, a minimum 250-microliter line and a maximum 500-microliter, to assist in collecting appropriate volumes (**FIGURE 8–36**). These microtainers also have printed lot numbers and expiration dates on each tube.

The BD Microtainer® MAP microtube is the first low-volume collection system to offer both standard, full-size patient identification labels as well as instrument compatibility with most automated hematology instruments. The BD Microtainer® MAP Microtube for Automated Process can run in automated mode with smaller blood volume.

RAM Scientific, Inc., has an unbreakable plastic capillary receptacle system called the SAFE-T-FILL capillary blood collection system. The device consists of a plastic capillary inserted into a microtube receptacle (**FIGURE 8–37**). With the attached receptacle, blood flows directly to the bottom of the tube, avoiding "scooping" of blood droplets. Scooping to collect blood droplets into a microcollection device can cause microclots and other debris from the skin's surface to be collected with the blood into a container. This system makes the blood collection safe and clean. The capillary can then be removed, and the tube is closed with the appropriate color-coded cap.

The Microvette® capillary blood collection system (Sarstedt, Inc.) is another microcollection system that is offered with a full range of anticoagulants and serum separation gel. This system can be used to collect, store, and separate samples in the same unbreakable, disposable container. The Microvette® microcollection plastic containers are available in 200-, 300-, and 500-microliter volumes (**FIGURE 8–38**). The Microvette®

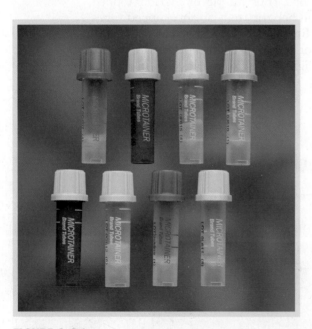

FIGURE 8–36
BD Microtainer Tube

Courtesy and © Becton, Dickinson and Company

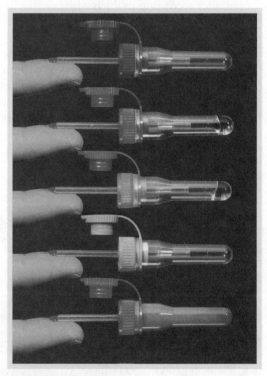

FIGURE 8–37
Safe-T-Fill Capillary Blood Collection Device

Courtesy of Ram Scientific, Inc., Needham, MA.

200 can be used to collect 200 microliters of capillary blood using the end-to-end principle. Blood is collected through a preassembled plastic capillary tube and flows into either a specially designed conical or rounded inner tube, depending on the additive.

Another type of microcollection device is the CAPIJECT® Capillary blood collection tubes (**FIGURE 8–39**). These tubes have color-coded fill lines and caps for volume accuracy and are latex free to avoid latex allergy risk.

Greiner Bio-One MiniCollect Capillary Blood Collection Tubes (**FIGURE 8–40**) have caps with flexible rubber "cross-cuts" that accommodate either a funnel or a coated plastic capillary collection device to collect the specimen without removing the cap. These latex-free tubes have fill-level indicators located on the tube or on the label to indicate blood-to-additive ratio.

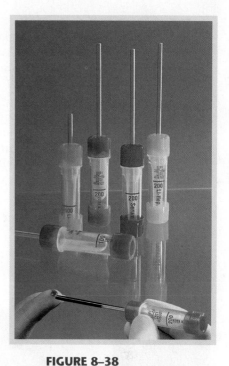

FIGURE 8–38
Microvette® 200 uL Capillary Blood Collection System

Courtesy of Sarstedt, Inc. Newton, NC.

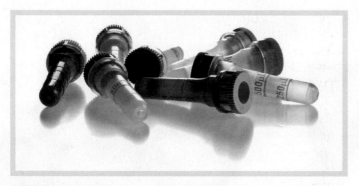

FIGURE 8–39
CAPIJECT® Capillary Blood Collection Tubes

Courtesy of Terumo Medical Corp., Somerset, NJ.

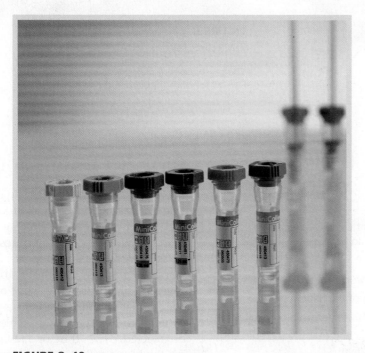

FIGURE 8–40
MiniCollect Capillary Blood Collection Tubes

Courtesy of Greiner Bio-One, Kremsmunster, Austria.

RNA Medical Brand *Safe-Wrap Combo Blood Collection* tubes are Mylar-wrapped glass capillary tubes that contain lithium heparin to prevent the sample from clotting (**FIGURE 8–41**). The Mylar wrapping helps contain both the sample and the glass in the event of accidental breakage. These tubes can be ordered to collect 95-microliter or 65-microliter volumes and are used with the I-STAT System point-of-care system.

The BMP LeukoChek microdilution system, shown in **FIGURE 8–42**, serves as a microcollection and dilution unit for blood samples and, thus, increases the speed and simplicity of leukocyte and platelet counting. These devices are prefilled with buffered ammonium oxalate solution and have been tested to CLIA guidelines. The BMP Leukocyte Test Kit includes:

1. A disposable, self-filling diluting pipette consisting of a straight, thin-walled, uniform-bore, plastic capillary tube fitted into a plastic holder
2. A plastic reservoir containing a premeasured volume of buffered ammonium oxalate solution

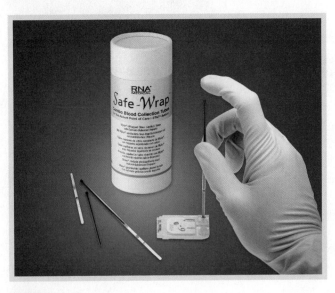

FIGURE 8–41

Safe-Wrap Combo Blood Collection Tube

Courtesy of RNA Medical, Devens, MA.

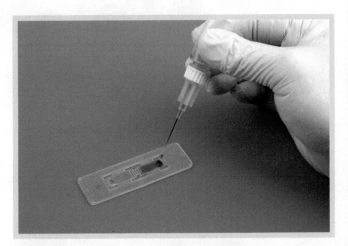

FIGURE 8–42

BMP LeukoChek

Courtesy of Biomedical Polymers, Inc.

ALERT

Clinical Alert ! In an outpatient clinic that requires blood collections, a **blood-drawing chair** should be available for patients. The blood-drawing chair

■ Is needed for maximum safety and comfort of the patient

■ Provides easy accessibility to either arm of the patient

■ Should have an armrest for the patient's use during blood collection

■ Should have an armrest that locks in place so that the patient cannot fall from the chair if he or she becomes faint

■ Should have an armrest that adjusts in an up-and-down position to achieve the best venipuncture position for each patient

Blood-Drawing Chair

There are many chair styles and options available for making phlebotomy procedures easier and safer. Options include recliner-type chairs, or chairs with adjustable armrests, leg extensions, neck pillows or supports, scale mounts, storage cabinets, hydraulic lifts, and foot covers. If blood-drawing chairs are not available, another option is to use the exam table. The patient can lie on the exam table as the blood is collected. Thus, if he or she feels faint during the blood collection, the patient is already in a safe, reclined position. Refer to Chapter 10 for more information about positioning the patient.

Specimen Collection Trays

The health care worker collecting blood specimens needs a specimen tray to take on blood collection rounds (**FIGURE 8–43**). Also, blood collection trays with a cover have been designed for safe transport throughout the various sections of health care facilities. The covered trays help isolate potentially infectious specimens from nonlaboratory personnel (**FIGURE 8-44**). The trays are usually made of a plastic (preferably latex free) that can be sterilized. Each tray should include all necessary equipment. For example, when working in a children's hospital, the tray must contain microcollection equipment, as described earlier. For home health care providers and reference laboratory couriers, the necessary collection supplies, equipment, and collected blood must be carried in an enclosed container with the biohazard symbol shown on the outside. It should be lockable to protect the contents from possible tampering or accidental contamination. It also should have a tight seal to reduce the risk of infection from blood-borne pathogens resulting from spills or accidents. Refer to Chapter 12 for more information about specimen transportation.

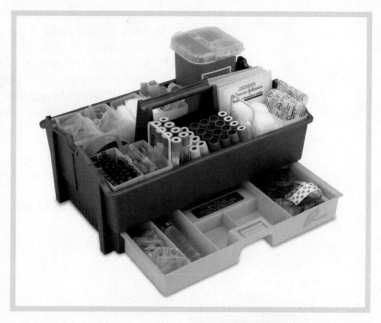

FIGURE 8–43
Specimen Collection Tray

Courtesy of MarketLab,
www.marketlabinc.com

FIGURE 8–44
Covered Specimen Tray for Safe Transport

Courtesy of MarketLab
www.marketlabinc.com

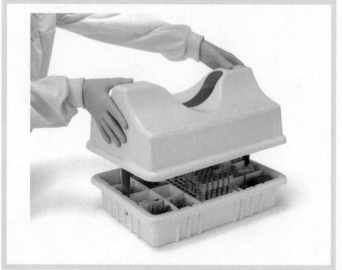

Health care workers who collect blood from adults usually have the following equipment on their trays or in their safety container:

1. Marking pens or pencils
2. Vacuum tubes containing the anticoagulants/additives designated in the clinical laboratory blood collection manual
3. Safety holders for vacuum tubes
4. Safety needles for vacuum tubes and syringes
5. Safety syringes
6. Disposable tourniquet (nonlatex)
7. Safety blood collection sets (butterfly needle assembly)

8. Seventy percent isopropyl alcohol, iodine, and chlorhexidine pads/swabs
9. Sterile gauze pads
10. Bandages
11. Biohazardous waste containers for used needles, holders, and lancets
12. Safety lancets for skin puncture
13. Microdilution devices for fingerstick blood collection
14. Microcollection blood serum and plasma separator tubes
15. Microcollection capillary whole blood collectors with appropriate anticoagulants/additives
16. Disposable nonlatex gloves
17. Appropriate warming device
18. Thermometer
19. Antimicrobial hand gel or foam to clean hands without water and soap

Study Questions

For the following questions, select the one best answer.

1 Which of the following anticoagulants is found in a white-topped blood collection vacuum tube?

a. EDTA
b. ammonium oxalate
c. sodium citrate
d. sodium heparin

2 Which of the following anticoagulants is found in a green-topped blood collection vacuum tube?

a. EDTA
b. ammonium oxalate
c. sodium citrate
d. sodium heparin

3 For capillary collection from newborns, a lancet of which of the following lengths should be used to avoid penetrating bone?

a. 1.75 mm
b. 2.75 mm
c. 3.00 mm
d. 3.25 mm

4 Which of the following blood collection tube tops has sodium fluoride as an additive?

a. light-blue–topped tube
b. gray-topped tube
c. royal-blue–topped tube
d. red-topped tube

5 Which of the following vacuum tubes is used to collect blood for STAT (emergency) laboratory procedures requiring serum specimens?

a. RST
b. EDTA
c. SST
d. ACD

6 The color coding for needles indicates the

a. length
b. gauge
c. manufacturer
d. anticoagulant

7 From the listed needle gauges, which one has the smallest diameter?

a. 19
b. 20
c. 21
d. 23

8 Which of the following is a venipuncture device?

a. Terumo Capiject
b. Tenderlett
c. VACUETTE® QUICKSHIELD
d. BMP LeukoChek

9 Which of the following is an anticoagulant used in blood donations?

a. EDTA
b. ACD
c. Heparin
d. Citrate

10 Specimens for which of the following tests must be collected in gray-topped blood collection tubes?

a. PT
b. trace elements
c. molecular diagnostics
d. glucose

Case Study

Huge quantities of blood are often collected from critically ill patients in the intensive care unit (ICU). Several studies have shown that iatrogenic blood loss due to laboratory testing can result in increased number of hospital deaths due to stress on the cardiovascular and respiratory systems. As an example, Anthony Lopez, an 80-year-old man with a massive heart attack, was admitted to the emergency room (ER) and then the ICU. The first laboratory tests were ordered in the ER for CPK and troponin T and other cardiac assays. Also, a complete blood count was ordered and coagulation tests. Over the next few days, Mr. Lopez developed complications, and as each specialist was consulted, more blood tests were ordered. Blood was collected and more blood was collected. After a week in the ICU, a STAT laboratory requisition for type and cross-match of two units of packed red blood cells was received in the laboratory. Mr. Lopez had developed iatrogenic anemia.

Questions

1 Which vacuum blood collection tube cannot be used to collect for the CPK, troponin T, and other cardiac assays since the additive in the tube would destroy the analytes?

2 Which vacuum blood collection tube should be used for collection of blood for the complete blood count?

3 Which vacuum blood collection tube should be used for collecting the blood to go to the blood bank for type and cross match?

Action in Practice

Ms. Brannon, a phlebotomist in Yoacum's Health Care Clinic, received orders for blood collection from Ms. Sandra Herman for lead testing, CBC, and PT.

Questions

1 What blood collection tubes will Ms. Brannon need to use to collect blood from Ms. Herman for these laboratory tests?

2 What are the anticoagulants/additives in the blood collection tubes that Ms. Brannon needs to use to collect blood from Ms. Herman?

COMPETENCY ASSESSMENT

Check Yourself

1 Which type of tube contains lithium heparin and a plasma separator gel?

2 Larger (17- to 18-gauge) needles are usually used for collecting blood for what purpose?

Competency Checklist: Blood Collection Equipment

This checklist can be completed as a group or individually.

(1) Completed (2) Needs to improve

_____ 1. Describe the use of the BMP LeukoChek in blood collection.

_____ 2. List three safety butterfly needles.

_____ 3. Explain how the BD Blood Transfer Device works.

REFERENCES

1. Clinical and Laboratory Standards Institute (CLSI). (2010). *Tubes and additives for venous and capillary blood specimen collection, approved standard,* 6th ed. (H01-A6). Wayne, PA: Author.

2. Hyman, D., & Kaplan, N. (1985). The difference between serum and plasma potassium (letter). *N Engl J Med,* 642.

3. Rossen J., & Stoker R. (2005). *The compendium of infection control technologies.* Palm City, FL: Biomedical Safety Publishing, LLC.

4. Pugliese, G., & Salahuddin M. (Eds.). (1999). *Sharps injury prevention program: A step-by-step guide.* Chicago: American Hospital Association.

5. Occupational Safety and Health Administration (OSHA), U.S. Department of Labor. (2003, October 15). *OSHA Safety and Health Information Bulletin (SHIB).* Re-use of blood tube holders. Washington, DC: Author.

6. Thavendiranathan, P., Bagai, A., & Choudhry, N. (2005). Do blood tests cause anemia in hospitalized patients: The effect of diagnostic phlebotomy on hemoglobin and hematocrit. *J Gen Intern Med, 20*(6): 520–524.

7. Tilford, J., Simpson, P., Green, J., Lensing, S., & Fiser, D. (2000). Volume-outcome relationships in pediatric intensive care units. *Pediatrics, 106*(2): 289–294.

8. Clinical and Laboratory Standards Institute (CLSI). (2008). *Procedures and devices for the collection of diagnostic capillary blood specimens, approved standard* (Document H04-A6). Wayne, PA: Author.

RESOURCES

www.clsi.org Clinical and Laboratory Standards Institute (CLSI), Wayne, PA.

www.isips.org International Sharps Injury Prevention Society (ISIPS).

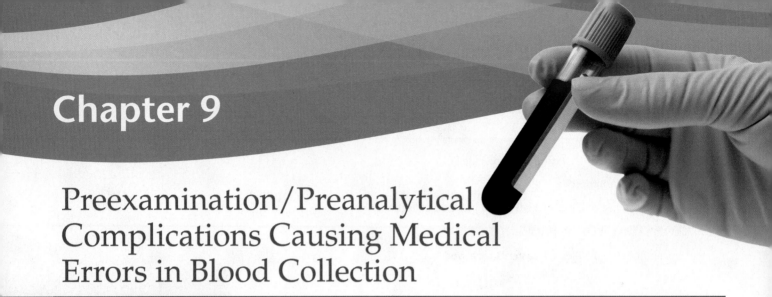

Chapter 9

Preexamination/Preanalytical Complications Causing Medical Errors in Blood Collection

Chapter Objectives

Upon completion of Chapter 9, the learner is responsible
for doing the following:

1. Describe preanalytical (preexamination) complications related to phlebotomy procedures and impacting patient safety.

2. Explain how to prevent and/or handle complications in blood collection.

3. List at least five factors about a patient's physical disposition (i.e., makeup) that can affect blood collection.

4. List examples of substances that can interfere in clinical analysis of blood constituents and describe methods used to prevent these interferences.

5. Describe how allergies, a mastectomy, edema, and thrombosis can affect blood collection.

6. List preanalytical complications that can arise with test requests and identification.

7. Describe complications associated with tourniquet pressure and fist pumping.

8. Identify how the preanalytical factors of syncope, petechiae, neurological complications, hemoconcentration, hemolysis, and intravenous therapy affect blood collection.

9. Describe methods used to prevent these interferences.

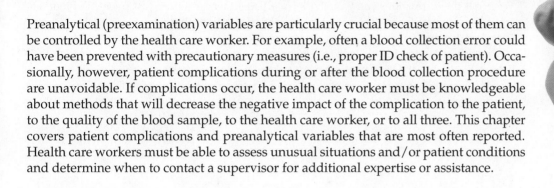

Preanalytical (preexamination) variables are particularly crucial because most of them can be controlled by the health care worker. For example, often a blood collection error could have been prevented with precautionary measures (i.e., proper ID check of patient). Occasionally, however, patient complications during or after the blood collection procedure are unavoidable. If complications occur, the health care worker must be knowledgeable about methods that will decrease the negative impact of the complication to the patient, to the quality of the blood sample, to the health care worker, or to all three. This chapter covers patient complications and preanalytical variables that are most often reported. Health care workers must be able to assess unusual situations and/or patient conditions and determine when to contact a supervisor for additional expertise or assistance.

Categories of Preanalytical Variables

Preanalytical variables that are important to the health care worker when collecting blood are categorized in **BOX 9–1**. Some variables, however, can be controlled by the patient, including physiological variables and those directly related to specimen collection; these, too, can provide a means to avoid preanalytical errors. Uncontrollable variables that include biological influences (e.g., age, sex), environmental influences (e.g., a patient's geographical location, altitude), and underlying medical conditions (e.g., stress, fever) fall into this group of unavoidable preanalytical factors impacting patients' laboratory values. Some major physiological variables that are controllable and can affect the results of laboratory analytes include diet, lifestyle, exercise, posture, circadian rhythm (diurnal variation), travel, and prolonged bed rest.

BASAL STATE

Blood specimens used to determine the concentrations of body constituents such as glucose, cholesterol, triglycerides, electrolytes, proteins, and so on should be collected when the patient is in a **basal state**—that is, in the early morning, approximately 12 hours after the last ingestion of food. The results of laboratory tests on basal state specimens are most reliable. However, several factors—including diet, exercise, emotional stress, obesity, menstrual cycle, pregnancy, diurnal variations, posture, tourniquet application, and chemical constituents (alcohol or drugs)—can cause changes in the basal state. Health care workers need to have a general understanding of these effects and their relationship to laboratory testing.

BOX 9–1

Variables Important in Specimen Collection

- Patient assessment and physical disposition
- Test requests
- Specimen collection
- Specimen transport
- Specimen receipt in the laboratory

> **BOX 9–2**
>
> # Practice Giving Instructions
>
> Write out the instructions you would give to a patient who needs to fast prior to a blood collection procedure. Try to think of the most unusual questions that the patient might ask about eating or drinking.
>
> Practice giving the instructions to a friend or coworker. Practice your communication techniques by double-checking that your listener completely understands; ask specific questions about his or her comprehension of the fasting process and ask for a friendly and constructive critique of your instructions.

DIET

To ensure that the patient is in the basal state, the physician must require the patient to fast overnight. The term **fasting** refers to abstinence from nutritional support such as food and beverages. Some health care workers think that fasting also involves abstinence from water, but it does not. Abstaining from water can result in a patient's dehydration and can impact the "real" basal state laboratory values for patients. The required time period necessary for abstaining usually is 8 to 12 hours. The normal values have been established for laboratories based on the 8- to 12-hour fasting. Before collecting a specimen, the health care worker should ask the patient if he or she has eaten. Blood composition is significantly altered after meals and consequently is unsuitable for many clinical chemistry tests. If the patient has eaten recently but the physician still needs the test, the word *nonfasting* must be included on the requisition and/or directly on the specimen.

When giving dietary instructions, gaining the patient's cooperation is important and is determined by the professional behavior and the competence of the health care worker (**BOX 9–2**). Inadequate patient instructions can cause mistakes in specimen collection. Casual instructions are apt to be taken lightly by the patient or even forgotten. If the health care worker has to explain fasting restrictions to a patient, the instructions should be thorough and clear, with emphasis on the important points of the procedure. Written instructions are also helpful, if available.

If a procedure involves some discomfort or inconvenience, the patient should be informed. For example, if blood is to be collected for a timed blood glucose level determination, the patient needs to fast for 8 to 12 hours, but not beyond 12 hours.[1] The health care worker can inform the patient that several specimens will be collected at timed intervals and that he or she may drink water, but that coffee, chewing gum, and tea should be avoided because they cause a transitory fluctuation in the blood sugar level.

TURBID OR LIPEMIC SERUM

If a patient has recently eaten fatty substances, he or she may have a temporarily elevated lipid (i.e., triglycerides, cholesterol) level, and the serum will appear **lipemic,** or cloudy. **Turbid** serum appears cloudy or "milky" and results from bacterial contamination or high lipid levels in the blood. Turbidity is primarily caused by ingestion of fatty substances, such as meat, butter, cream, and cheese, or can occur when a lipid supplement is included in parenteral nutrition preparations. Because lipemic serum does not represent a basal state and may indicate some chemical abnormalities, documentation about the appearance of the serum may be useful to the physician.

ALERT

Clinical Alert ! Prolonged fasting (i.e., beyond 12 hours) and/or unsupervised fasting to lose weight can cause health hazards, including electrolyte disturbances, heart dysrhythmias, and—occasionally—death.

OBESITY

More than half of adult patients in the United States are overweight. A healthy body weight is based on body mass index (BMI), and for adults the BMI range is 20 to 25 kg/m.[2] **Obese** patients (i.e., patients with an unhealthy accumulation of body fat, or a body mass index of greater than 30 kg/m²) generally have veins that are difficult to visualize and/ or palpate. (Refer to Chapter 10 to view examples of different arm veins.) It is a difficult situation for both the health care workers trying to find a vein and the patient hoping that the blood collector will find one to collect the blood. If the vein is not accessed when first punctured, the health care worker must be careful not to probe excessively with the needle, because doing so ruptures red blood cells (RBCs), increases the concentration of intracellular contents, and releases some tissue-clotting factors. Usually, the patient knows where the "best site" is for venipuncture, so it is helpful to check with the patient prior to selecting the site. Also, there are longer needles available for collections from obese patients.

DAMAGED, SCLEROSED, OR OCCLUDED VEINS

Occluded, or obstructed, **veins** do not allow blood to flow through them; **sclerosed,** or hardened, **veins** are a result of inflammation and disease of the interstitial substances. Veins that have been repeatedly punctured often become scarred and feel hard when palpated. These sites should be avoided because blood is not easily collected from them. However, the Clinical and Laboratory Standards Institute (CLSI) advises against collecting arterial blood specimens as a substitute for venous blood when it is difficult to find a suitable vein for the needed blood specimen. In these situations, skin puncture blood should be used, if possible. Chapter 10 also discusses alternative venipuncture sites.

THROMBOSIS

Thrombi (plural form of *thrombus*) are solid masses derived from blood constituents that reside in the blood vessels. A thrombus may partially or fully occlude a vein (or artery), and such occlusion will make venipuncture more difficult.

ALLERGIES

Some patients are allergic to iodine, alcohol, or other solutions used to disinfect a puncture site. Check for color-coded armbands or posted signs indicating specific patient allergies. If a patient indicates that he or she is allergic to a solution or to latex, all efforts should be made to use an alternative product. Chlorhexidine reportedly has been used as an alternative to decontaminate skin. After application, it can be wiped off with sterile water.[3] In addition, because so many patients and health care workers are allergic to latex, latex-free tourniquets, gloves, and bandages are recommended.

EXERCISE

Effects of exercise on laboratory tests can be categorized as either short-term effects (reported in marathon runners and endurance athletes) or long-term effects (resulting from exercise training programs). Studies suggest that it is difficult to separate the two effects because most endurance athletes go through extensive training programs. In either case, the effects of exercise on laboratory tests depends on the intensity, duration, and frequency of the exercise as well

> **Clinical Alert!** Burned, Scarred, or Tattooed Areas
> Areas that have been burned, scarred, or tattooed should be avoided during phlebotomy. Burned areas are very sensitive and susceptible to infection, and veins under scarred areas are difficult to palpate. Collecting specimens from these sites can be painful and could alter the blood specimens. Tattoos contain dyes that may interfere with laboratory tests. Also, tattooed areas are susceptible to infections and impaired circulation.

ALERT

as the individual's genetic factors, ethnicity, age, gender, hormonal status, and body weight.[4] Many studies about the effects of exercise are inconclusive and/or contradictory, but better data are surfacing as exercise is incorporated more often into daily lives (**FIGURE 9–1**). In general, moderate or excessive exercise has an effect on laboratory test results, but it is up to the physician to interpret the effects. Exercise also has some effects on hemostasis.

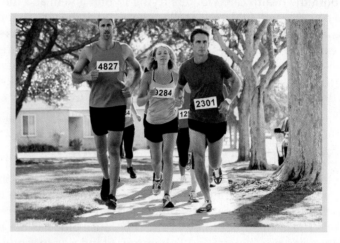

FIGURE 9–1

Blood Analytes Are Affected in Long-Distance Running

© Monkey Business/Fotolia

In a study of marathon runners, laboratory results showed increases in glucose, total protein, albumin, uric acid, calcium, phosphorous, blood urea nitrogen (BUN), creatinine, total and direct bilirubin, alanine transaminase (ALT), aspartate aminotransferase (AST), and alkaline phosphatase 4 hours after the marathon. No change was measured in sodium, potassium, and osmolality after 4 hours, whereas magnesium, chloride, carbon dioxide, and globulin results decreased. Laboratory results for BUN, creatinine, uric acid, ALT, AST, and direct bilirubin remained elevated 24 hours after the race, but glucose, total protein, albumin, globulin, calcium, phosphorous, total bilirubin, and alkaline phosphatase returned to baseline. There was also an increase in white blood cell count, **neutrophilia, monocytosis,** and decreased lymphocytes. Platelets, hemoglobin, mean corpuscular hemoglobin (MCH), mean corpuscular hemoglobin concentration (MCHC), and red blood cell distribution width (RDW) were elevated at 4 and 24 hours, whereas the hematocrit, RBC, and mean corpuscular volume (MCV) decreased. The hematocrit returned to baseline after 24 hours.[5] Patients should be advised to avoid changes in their diet, the consumption of alcohol, and strenuous exercise 24 hours before having their blood collected for laboratory testing.[6]

STRESS

Patients are often frightened, nervous, and overly anxious, especially prior to blood collection. These emotional stresses can cause a transient elevation in the white blood cell (WBC) count, a transient decrease in serum iron levels, and abnormal hormone (e.g., cortisol, aldosterone, renin, thyroid-stimulating hormone [TSH], prolactin) values. Also, mental anxiety can increase blood concentrations of albumin, fibrinogen, glucose, cholesterol, and insulin.[1] In one report, newborns who had been crying violently had WBC counts that are 140% above resting baseline counts. Even mild crying was shown to increase WBC counts by 113%. These elevated counts return to baseline values within 1 hour. Therefore, whenever possible, blood samples for WBC counts should be taken approximately 1 hour after a crying episode.[7] Anxiety that results in hyperventilation also causes acid-base imbalances, increased lactate levels, and increased fatty acid levels.[8]

DIURNAL (CIRCADIAN) RHYTHMS AND POSTURE

Diurnal rhythms, which are body fluid fluctuations during the day, cause some hormone levels to change depending on the time of day (e.g., cortisol, adrenocorticotropic hormone [ACTH], TSH, T4 [thyroxine], plasma renin activity, progesterone, triglycerides, testosterone, catecholamines, bilirubin, aldosterone, insulin, iron). Collecting specimens during the designated time periods is important for proper clinical evaluation; thus, the health care facility's guidelines for timed tests should be followed.

Posture changes are also known to significantly vary laboratory test results of some chemical constituents (e.g., aldosterone and plasma renin activity). This consideration is important when inpatient and outpatient results are being compared. Thus, blood collection should be performed under standardized posture conditions. Changing from a **supine** (or lying) position to a sitting or standing position causes body water to shift from intravascular to interstitial compartments (in tissues). Certain larger molecules cannot filter into the tissue; therefore, they concentrate in the blood. Enzyme, protein, lipid, iron, and calcium levels are significantly increased with changes in position.[9,10] For example, when the patient's sample is collected while he or she is standing, total cholesterol results will be approximately 10% higher, triglycerides 12% higher, and HDL cholesterol 7% higher than in samples collected when the patient is lying down. The standard position for these blood collections is with the patient sitting.[11] These effects can be more pronounced in patients with congestive heart failure and hepatic disorders.

Positional pseudoanemia is a posture-related condition with changes in hematocrit and hemoglobin results. In patients who remain in bed for an extended time with their blood collected for hematocrit and/or hemoglobin during this time, these values are extremely low compared to later in the day when the patients have been sitting or standing up and have their blood recollected for hematocrit and/or hemoglobin. Sitting and standing leads to a net movement of fluid from intravascular to interstitial spaces and increases the hematocrit and hemoglobin values to the normal range. Positional pseudoanemia has to be differentiated from the result of acute bleeding that can lead to "true" anemia.[12] The health care worker can be helpful in providing information on the patient's posture prior to the blood collection for hematocrit and hemoglobin.

If the patient is to receive the correct laboratory values as related to normal values, it is important to collect the blood specimen in the posture in which the normal values were established. As an example, the normal value range for plasma aldosterone is based on the blood specimen collected from the patient in an upright position (standing or seated) for at least two hours before collection. If posture is not controlled in this manner of collection, the correctness of the patient's aldosterone laboratory result is jeopardized, as is subsequent diagnosis and treatment by the patient's physician.

TRAVEL ISSUES AFFECTING LABORATORY RESULTS

Communicating with the patient about recent long-distance travel is a controllable means for the health care worker to possibly avoid erroneous laboratory results. Travel over several time zones affects the diurnal rhythm. As mentioned earlier, several blood analyte values are affected by the circadian rhythm, such as hormonal levels. Five days are required to establish a new stable circadian rhythm after travel across 10 time zones. Also, during a long flight, fluid and sodium retention occurs and takes approximately two days to return to normal.

AGE

Laboratory test results vary considerably during the stages of life: infancy, childhood (pediatric population), adulthood, and older adulthood (geriatric population). For example, blood cholesterol and triglyceride values increase as a person ages. Various hormone levels, such as estrogen and growth hormone (GH) levels, decrease in geriatric women and men.

Clinical Alert ! Venipuncture should never be performed on the same side as a mastectomy (unless approved by the physician), since the patient is more susceptible to infection and some chemical constituents in the blood may be altered. Also, the pressure from the tourniquet could lead to injuries in a patient who has had this type of surgery. If the patient has had a double mastectomy, the back of the hands or fingersticks are alternative methods. However, *the physician should always be involved in determining suitable sites.*

MASTECTOMY

Patients who have undergone a **mastectomy** (the surgical removal of the breast) often have swelling caused by lymph accumulation in the tissues (**lymphedema**) on the side of the surgery because of lymph node removal. The stagnant flow of tissue fluid in the area may make the patient more prone to infections; therefore, the lymphedematous limbs should be protected from cuts, scratches, burns, and blood collection. Refer to Chapter 7 for more detail.

EDEMA

Some patients develop **edema** (an abnormal accumulation of fluid in the intercellular spaces) because of reasons other than a mastectomy (e.g., heart failure, renal failure, inflammation, malnutrition, bacterial toxins, medication, allergic reaction). This swelling can be localized (e.g., fluid leakage from an IV line) or diffused over a larger area of the body. The health care worker should avoid collecting blood from these sites, because veins in these areas are difficult to palpate or locate, and the specimen may become contaminated with fluid. Again, consultation with the physician is needed to determine if and where a blood specimen should be taken.

MENSTRUAL CYCLE

Women normally begin their **menstrual cycle** during puberty (9 to 17 years of age). The menstrual flow lasts between three and seven days and contains normal, hemolyzed, or sometimes agglutinated red blood cells, disintegrated endometrial cells, and glandular secretions. The average blood loss ranges from 44 to 80 mL but may be lessened (if the patient is using oral contraceptives) or increased (if the patient has an intrauterine device, IUD). Menstrual blood loss is the single-most common cause of iron-deficiency anemia in women. This fact reinforces the issue that health care workers need to be careful not to collect more blood than is absolutely necessary so as not to increase the negative effects of additional blood loss during venipuncture.

MEDICATIONS

Blood being collected to determine levels of medications should, in most cases, be collected just prior to the next dose. There are hundreds of medications available, each of which has particular pharmacokinetics (i.e., characteristics related to a drug's metabolism and action, such as time needed for absorption, duration of action, distribution in the body, and method of excretion). Some drugs taken orally reach maximum effective serum concentrations slower than if administered by an IV. Or a drug may be absorbed faster if taken on an empty stomach. Therefore, a health care worker must be knowledgeable of the institutional procedures and/or what the health care team (nursing, laboratory, pharmacy, and physician) requires in terms of when the specimen is to be collected and any additional information needed to help interpret the test results. This may involve notations of the drug name and the time and dates that the drug was administered, in addition to other required information. Refer to Chapter 15 for more information on therapeutic drug monitoring.

INTERFERENCE OF DRUGS AND OTHER SUBSTANCES IN BLOOD

Many prescribed drugs can interfere with clinical laboratory determinations or can physiologically alter the levels of blood constituents measured in the clinical laboratory. The interference of drugs and other substances is so complicated and dependent on the chemical procedures used that only general recommendations are described in this section. Consequently, physicians must work closely with pharmacy and laboratory staff to rule out laboratory test results that are altered because the patient is taking medication.

Drugs administered to alleviate an illness can induce physiologic abnormalities in one or more of the following systems: liver, hematologic, hemostatic, muscular, pancreatic, and renal. The erroneous results may sometimes affect the true clinical diagnosis. Drugs or drug metabolites in blood can also directly cause falsely decreased or falsely elevated values in laboratory analyses (**BOX 9–3**).

Another way that some drugs, including over-the-counter (OTC) drugs such as aspirin, affect specimen collection is in causing the patient to bleed excessively. The most common side effect in patients being treated with anticoagulant drugs such as warfarin or heparin (for management of acute coronary syndromes) is abnormal bleeding. Comprehensive listings of the effects of drugs on laboratory tests have been published.[13] In addition to medications, other substances such as the ingredients in cigarettes may affect several laboratory test results. Through the action of nicotine from the tobacco, the blood concentrations of glucose, growth hormone, cholesterol, and triglyceride increase. Alcohol consumption also can affect laboratory test results, especially hematology results.

The health care worker collecting the blood specimen is the link between the clinical laboratory and the patient. Laboratory tests are often ordered without knowledge of the drugs taken or inhaled (e.g., nicotine) or consumed (e.g., alcohol) by a patient. Yet, as discussed previously, these drugs will lead to falsely elevated or decreased values. Follow-up communication and/or documentation that a patient has taken a medication prior to the blood collection may assist the laboratory personnel and physician in determining the accuracy of the laboratory results.

BOX 9–3

Drug Interference

Interference from medications usually causes falsely elevated values when the true values are in the normal range or the subnormal range. Some drugs, such as acetaminophen (Tylenol) and erythromycin, can increase serum AST and bilirubin levels and, thus, falsely create a clinical interpretation of liver dysfunction without the true presence of an abnormality. Sometimes the acetaminophen can cause liver dysfunction and result in abnormal liver panel results.

Oral medication and intravenous medications or dyes can interfere with laboratory test results. Chemotherapeutic drugs used in cancer treatment can lead to a decrease in blood cellular elements and, therefore, their metabolic and immunologic processes.

Various medications are toxic to the liver, leading to a subsequent increase in the concentration of blood liver enzymes, such as alanine aminotransferase (ALT), alkaline phosphatase (ALP), and lactate dehydrogenase (LD). The production of globulins and clotting factors is decreased in patients with drug-induced toxicity to the liver. Also, these patients may have a possible electrolyte (i.e., sodium, potassium, bicarbonate, chloride) imbalance and elevation of blood urea nitrogen (BUN) levels.

Blood pressure medications such as thiazide diuretics can elevate blood glucose levels and decrease potassium and sodium levels. Pancreatitis can be caused by corticosteroids, estrogens, and diuretics, which cause elevations of serum amylase and lipase values. Aspirin causes **hypobilirubinemia** (a decrease in bilirubin) by expelling bilirubin from the plasma to the surrounding tissue cells.[13]

INFECTIONS

It should always be remembered that many patients have transmittable diseases (e.g., hepatitis) that could be passed from one patient to another. (For precautionary techniques, refer to Chapters 4 and 5.) Also, the health care worker must remember to avoid touching the site for blood collection with his or her finger or any nonsterile materials after the site has been cleaned. To minimize infections from needlesticks, the blood collection equipment (i.e., bandages, needles, tube holders) should not be opened prior to the time of collection from the patient. If the packages are opened ahead of time, they may become contaminated and could lead to an infection in the patient.

VOMITING

Sometimes the thought or sight of blood before or during blood collection causes the patient to experience nausea and possibly vomiting. If this reaction occurs, have the patient take deep breaths and use a cold compress on his or her head. Tissues or a washcloth should be available for the patient to use if he or she needs to clean his or her face and water should be available to rinse the mouth unless the patient is not allowed to have water for some medical procedure. Also, inform the patient's physician or nurse of this complication.

OTHER FACTORS AFFECTING THE PATIENT

Many other factors can affect laboratory test results. Gender and pregnancy, for instance, have an influence on laboratory testing; thus, reference ranges are often noted according to gender. Also, geographic factors, such as altitude, temperature, and humidity, affect baseline values. Collecting blood during home health care visits may entail traveling to regions other than the location of the laboratory. Thus, geographic information may be required in order to be considered in the patient's test results. Follow the health care organization's procedures or consult a supervisor when necessary.

Complications Associated with Test Requests and Identification

IDENTIFICATION DISCREPANCIES

Improper identification is the most dangerous and costly error a health care worker can make. It can lead to errors such as (1) loss of life from an acute hemolytic transfusion reaction, (2) delayed diagnosis and additional blood collection and laboratory testing, and (3) treatment of the wrong patient for the wrong disease. The number-one patient safety goal for the Joint Commission is *improving the accuracy of patient identification* through at least two unique identifiers, one of which can *not* be the patient location.[14] In addition, the specimen containers and tubes must have two unique identifiers, not necessarily the same but linked to the patient identifiers. As discussed in Chapter 10, identification should include a match among the patient's identification band or photo id, his or her verbal confirmation, and the test requisition. Bed labels, water pitchers, or door charts should not be used as a patient identifier. Even armbands are not completely reliable.[15] A study on the use of patient identification armbands in hospitals found that the most frequent errors were missing identification armbands, followed by missing identification armband information, illegible armbands, and conflicting armbands. Refer to Chapter 10 for more details on identification procedures in various circumstances. Sometimes a health care worker is the first to detect a discrepancy between a name on the requisition and the name that the patient verbalizes or the name on the armband. In these cases, the discrepancy should be reported to a supervisor and/or nurse and may result in the prevention of other errors related to that patient.

TIME OF COLLECTION

Timing factors can affect test results. In some cases, such as testing drug levels, the timing of the collection must coincide with the time the dosage was given. Refer to Chapter 15 for further discussion of therapeutic drug monitoring and the glucose tolerance test. Early-morning specimens are most commonly requested in hospital settings because a fasting specimen is preferred (since reference ranges are based on fasting specimens). If a health care worker is running late, the specimen might be collected *after* an inpatient has eaten breakfast and would require a special notation about his or her "nonfasting" condition.

REQUISITIONS

Checking the requisition to match the laboratory tests requested with the appropriate type of collection tube is essential to minimize the amount of blood collected from each patient. Too much blood loss because of excessive specimen removal can result in anemia.

Complications Associated with the Specimen Collection Procedure

TOURNIQUET PRESSURE AND FIST PUMPING

Laboratory test results can be falsely elevated or decreased if the tourniquet pressure is too tight or is maintained too long. The pressure from the tourniquet causes biological analytes to leak from the tissue cells into the blood, or vice versa. For example, plasma cholesterol, iron, lipid, protein, and potassium levels will be falsely elevated if the tourniquet pressure is too tight or prolonged. Significant elevations may be seen with as short as a 3-minute application of the tourniquet (the recommended time for tourniquet application is no longer than 1 minute at a time).[16] In addition, some enzyme levels can be falsely elevated or decreased because of tourniquet pressure that is too tight or prolonged. If it takes longer than 1 minute to find the vein, release the tourniquet for 2 minutes so that the blood in the arm can return to the basal state for more accurate results to be obtained from the blood. Also, pumping of the fist before venipuncture should be avoided because it leads to an increase in the plasma potassium, lactate, and phosphate concentrations.

FAILURE TO DRAW BLOOD

Several factors may cause the health care worker to miss the vein. These factors include not inserting the needle deep enough, inserting the needle all the way through the vein, holding the needle bevel against the vein wall, or losing the vacuum in the tube, as demonstrated in **FIGURE 9–2**. If the needle bevel is against the vein wall or is not inserted deep enough into the vein, the fragile red blood cells will be hemolyzed (rupture of red blood cells) due to the narrowed opening for the red blood cells to enter the needle. To avoid these situations, the needle may need to be moved or withdrawn somewhat and redirected slightly. If the needle is inserted at too high of an angle (greater than 30 degrees maximum), the needle may go through the vein, as shown in Figure 9–2D and Figure 9–2G. In the geriatric patient, the vein may be "tough" during needle entry and may roll; such rolling can cause the needle to slip to the side of the vein instead of properly puncturing it. If this happens, take the vacuum tube off the needle, withdraw the needle slightly while maintaining the bevel under the skin, and anchor the vein as the needle is redirected into the vein. If this second approach is not successful, discontinue the venipuncture from this site and choose another site. Searching by probing for the vein may cause damage to the patient's arm, nerve, and vein, and intense pain. Securely anchoring the vein prior to blood collection is a key factor in blood collection from any patient.

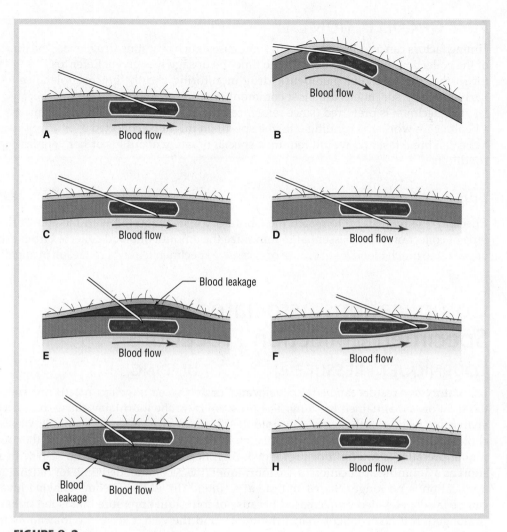

FIGURE 9–2

Needle Positioning and Failure to Collect Blood

A. Correct insertion technique; blood flows freely into needle. **B.** Bevel on vein upper wall does not allow blood to flow. **C.** Bevel on vein lower wall does not allow blood to flow. **D.** Needle inserted too far. **E.** Needle partially inserted, which causes blood leakage into tissue. **F.** Collapsed vein. **G.** Bevel in vein, partially through lower portion of vein, which causes blood leakage into tissue. **H.** Bevel in tissue of obese patient does not penetrate deep enough into vein.

On occasion, a test tube will have no vacuum because of a manufacturer's error, the age of the tube, or tube leakage after a puncture. Consequently, an extra set of tubes should be readily available in case this should happen during venipuncture. Partial-draw tubes are available through some manufacturers and these tubes can be used to collect smaller volumes in difficult-draw patients (i.e., oncology, pediatric). Partial-draw tubes usually fill more slowly because they have lower vacuum by comparison to regular blood collection tubes.[16] Also, needles for evacuated tube systems have been known to unscrew from the barrel during venipuncture. If this happens, the tourniquet should be released immediately and the needle removed.

BACKFLOW OF ANTICOAGULANT

To avoid the risk of backflow of an anticoagulant from a blood vacuum tube into the patient's circulation during a venipuncture procedure, the patient's arm should be placed in a downward position and the tube stopper (top) in the uppermost position. A patient may have an adverse reaction to tube anti-coagulants or other additives. If this should occur, a precautionary measure should be taken, asking (1) the outpatient to lean forward with his or her arm extended in a downward position for the collection and/or (2) the hospital patient to extend his or her arm over the side of the bed as it is supported by the bed to obtain the needed blood specimens. For the hospital patient unable to extend his or her arm over the bed, the alternative is to raise the head of the bed and the patient's arms will be in a downward position for the venipuncture collection.

FAINTING (SYNCOPE)

Syncope is the transient (and frequently sudden) loss of consciousness due to a lack of oxygen to the brain and results in an inability to stay in an upright position. Patients usually recover their orientation quickly, but injuries (e.g., abrasions, lacerations, broken bones) often result from falling to the ground. Syncope may be caused by a variety of factors, including hypoglycemia; hyperventilation; cardiac, neurologic, or psychiatric conditions; and medications. Many patients become dizzy and faint ("get weak in the knees") at the thought or sight of blood. Blood fear (phobia) is a common psychiatric disorder that occurs in 3 to 4% of the general population. Also, patients who have donated blood recently and/or fasting patients frequently become faint. Consequently, the health care worker should be aware of the patient's condition throughout the collection procedure. This can be done by asking ambulatory patients if they tend to faint or if they have ever previously fainted during blood collections. If so, they should be moved from a seated position to a recumbent position. Even for an ambulatory patient without a history of fainting, it is still extremely important to use a blood collection chair with a "locked" armrest to avoid the possibility of a fall if he or she faints.

Throughout the blood collection procedure, communicate and assess that the patient is feeling okay and is not faint. Do not turn your back to the patient—some patients give no signs until they pass out. If a seated patient feels faint, the needle and tourniquet should be removed, the patient's head should be lowered between the legs, and the patient should breathe deeply. If possible, the health care worker should ask for help and move the patient to a lying position. Talking to patients can often reassure them and divert their attention from the collection procedure. Bed-bound patients also experience fainting, or syncope, during blood collection, though rarely. In any case, the health care worker should stay with the patient at least 15 minutes until he or she recovers or until a nurse or physician takes over. A wet towel gently applied to the forehead or a glass of juice or water may help the patient feel better.

HEMATOMAS

When the area around the puncture site starts to swell, usually blood is leaking into the tissues and causing a **hematoma.**

Clinical Alert ! If a patient faints during or after the procedure, the health care worker should try to terminate the venipuncture procedure immediately and make sure that the patient does not fall or become injured. Sometimes, controlling the situation is difficult because of the patient's physical size; however, the health care worker should use common sense about the safest position for a patient. If a patient has fainted and is in a secure position, the health care worker should quickly request assistance from the nursing staff or a physician. A patient who has fainted should recover fully before being allowed to leave and should be instructed not to drive a vehicle for at least 30 minutes. Patients often think they recover very quickly, and after they try to stand up, they collapse again—with a possible injury. An incident report must be filed with the health care facility regarding the fainting incident and any injuries as a result of the fall, the immediate precautions taken, and what instructions were provided to the patient to prevent the possibility of long-term complications (e.g., a car accident after the fainting incident).

ALERT

Clinical Alert ! A hematoma can occur when

- The needle has gone completely through the vein (Figure 9–2D)
- The bevel opening is partially in the vein (Figures 9–2E and 9–2G)
- The patient's vein is fragile, the needle is pulled out of the vein while the tourniquet is still in place
- The health care worker fails to hold firm pressure (or have the patient hold pressure) over the venipuncture site
- A "blind" stick (inability to see or palpate the vein) is performed
- The health care worker probes for the vein.

The swelling of the puncture site results in a large bruise after several days (**FIGURE 9–3**). If a hematoma begins to form, the tourniquet and the needle should be removed immediately, and pressure should be applied to the area for approximately 2 minutes. If the bleeding continues, a nurse should be notified. An ice pack applied to the area can be helpful, but it must conform to the health care institutional policies for proper care of a hematoma.

ALERT

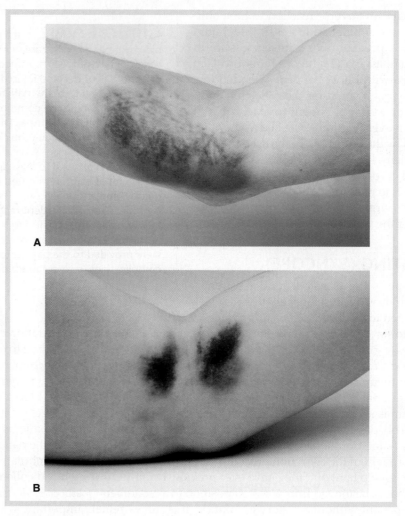

FIGURE 9–3
Patient's Hematoma after Venipunctures

A. © Powered by Light/Alan Spencer/Alamy B. © Julie Thompson/Alamy

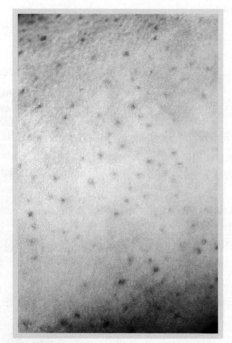

FIGURE 9–4
Petechiae of the Skin in a Patient

CDC Public Image Library

PETECHIAE

Petechiae—small, red, smooth, hemorrhagic spots appearing on a patient's skin—indicate that minute amounts of blood have escaped into skin epithelium (**FIGURE 9–4**). This complication may be a result of a coagulation abnormality such as **thrombocytopenia,** which is a low platelet count, and should be a warning that the patient's puncture site may bleed excessively. Petechiae also occur during febrile illnesses.

EXCESSIVE BLEEDING

A patient usually stops bleeding at the venipuncture site within a few minutes. Patients on anticoagulant therapy and/or those taking high dosages of arthritis medication or other medication, however, may bleed for a longer period. As mentioned earlier, coagulation abnormalities can also cause excessive bleeding. Thus, anytime a venipuncture is performed, pressure must be applied to the venipuncture site until the bleeding stops. If the bleeding continues and a patient leaves an ambulatory clinic, he or she may collapse from fainting or be in shock upon seeing the blood and suffer injury from a fall.

NERVE COMPLICATIONS

If the health care worker accidentally inserts the needle all the way through the vein, selects the wrong vein, or moves the needle excessively or in a sideways position in the vein, he or she may hit the nerve below the vein. If this happens, the patient will most likely have a sharp, electric tingling (and painful) sensation that radiates down the nerve into the hand. The tourniquet should be released immediately, the needle removed, and pressure held over the blood collection site. An ice pack should then be applied to the area to decrease the inflammation if this action conforms to the health care institutional policy. An incident report on the occurrence should be completed and given to the supervisor.

Clinical Alert ! The health care worker must not leave the patient until the bleeding stops or a nurse takes over to assess the patient's situation. In rare instances, the health care worker may accidentally puncture an artery instead of a vein. These cases require that pressure be applied as quickly as possible to stop the bleeding and that a nurse and/or supervisor be notified as soon as possible.

ALERT

SEIZURE DURING BLOOD COLLECTION

A rare but serious complication that may occur during blood collection is a seizure. If a patient begins to have a seizure, the health care worker should immediately release the tourniquet, remove the needle, move the patient to a lying position if he or she has not fallen already, attempt to hold pressure over the blood collection site, and call for help from the nursing station. No attempt should be made to place anything in the patient's mouth unless the health care worker is experienced and authorized to do so.

HEMOCONCENTRATION

Hemoconcentration is a decrease in the plasma volume with an increased concentration of cells and larger molecules (i.e., red blood cells, cholesterol). It is caused by several factors, including prolonged (i.e., longer than 1 minute) tourniquet application; massaging, squeezing, or probing a site; long-term IV therapy; and sclerosed or occluded veins. All of these practices and/or sites for venipuncture should be carefully avoided since the patient's safety is compromised due to the possibility of errors in laboratory test results.

INTRAVENOUS THERAPY

Every time a catheter is used, vein damage occurs. Circulatory blood is rerouted to collateral veins and can result in hemoconcentration. Consequently, patients on intravenous (IV) therapy for extended periods often have veins that are palpable and visible but damaged or occluded (blocked). Whenever a patient has an IV line, the arm with the IV line should *not* be used for venipuncture because the specimen will be diluted with IV fluid. Instead, the other arm or another site should be used if at all possible. If unavoidable, the nurse should shut off the IV for 2 minutes, then the tourniquet should be placed below the IV site, then the lumen through which the blood specimen is to be collected should be flushed with 5 mL of sterile saline and a discard volume withdrawn. Some health care institutions discard the first 5 to 7 ml of blood or more for coagulation studies.

Collecting a blood specimen from above an IV that has been temporarily shut off is not recommended because of the possibility for analyte contamination.[16] It should be documented that the area from which the specimen was collected was below the IV line site. Alternatively, sometimes the nurse or the physician can disconnect the IV line and collect blood from the line that is already inserted. In this situation, the first few milliliters of the specimen should be discarded to remove the IV fluid, and a note should be made on the laboratory requisition that this step was performed. (Refer to Chapter 15 for more detailed information about blood collection from intravenous lines.)

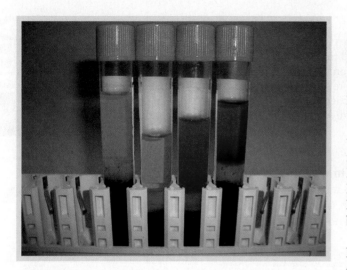

FIGURE 9–5

Normal Serum and Hemolysis

The left tube shows normal serum. Hemolysis is exhibited in the three right tubes.

Courtesy of Greiner Bio-One

HEMOLYSIS

Hemolysis results when RBCs are lysed (the cell breaks apart and is destroyed); hemoglobin is released; and serum, which is normally straw colored, becomes tinged with pink or red (**FIGURE 9–5**). If a specimen is grossly hemolyzed, the serum appears very dark red. Hemolysis may also be the result of physiological abnormalities (e.g., sickle cell diseases, exposure to drugs or toxins, artificial heart valves, some infections).[12,17] Hemolysis causes falsely increased results for many analytes, including potassium, magnesium, iron, lactate dehydrogenase, phosphorus, ammonia, and total protein.[13,18] Hemolysis also shows decreased RBC count, hemoglobin, and hematocrit. Some of the most common causes of hemolysis during blood collection are shown in **BOX 9–4**.

These problems can easily be prevented with appropriate handling. The health care worker should document the fact if he or she notices that a specimen is hemolyzed.

BOX 9–4

Common Causes of Hemolysis during Blood Collection

- The connection of blood collection equipment parts (needle to holder, etc.) is loose.
- The tube choice is not based on the patient's vein (i.e., elderly fragile veins—small tube).
- The syringe plunger is pulled too fast.
- A prolonged tourniquet application (greater than 1 minute) can create hemolysis in the blood sample.
- A too small (25 gauge) or too large (18 gauge) needle is used.
- The needle is readjusted.
- Needle blockage occurs due to the bevel against the vein wall or the improper angle of the needle.
- The tube is shaken or mixed vigorously rather than gently inverted.
- The blood collection is performed before the alcohol has dried at the collection site.
- There is an improper blood collection from peripheral IV catheters or central lines. (The IV cannulas are not designed for withdrawing blood.)
- The syringe collection is made without a quick transfer via the Blood Transfer Device (i.e., BD Blood Transfer Device). Syringe collections can lead to several preanalytical errors compared to using the blood collection vacuum tube systems. Often, the blood being collected in the syringe begins to clot before the blood can be transferred to the vacuum tubes. Hemolysis will result from the pressure of the blood clot in the syringe, as it is being transferred to the vacuum tube via the transfer device even though the plunger is not pushed.
- Sluggish, slow blood collections can result in hemolysis and an underfilled tube.
- There is a lack of proper handling and transport after collection.

COLLAPSED VEINS

Veins collapse when blood is withdrawn too quickly or forcefully during venipuncture, especially when blood is being collected from smaller veins and/or the veins of geriatric patients (Figure 9–2F). Thus, use an evacuated tube with a smaller volume and/or a smaller needle size during the collection process on patients with smaller veins and/or geriatric patients. A collapsed vein should not be probed with the needle.

IMPROPER COLLECTION TUBE

Health care workers should learn which common laboratory tests require which collection tubes. However, there are so many possible laboratory tests and tubes available that workers should also be familiar with how and where to seek information (electronically via laboratory reference manual, etc.) about unfamiliar test and tube requirements. The use of improper blood collection tubes can affect specimen quality, analytical results, and therefore patient safety. Selecting the appropriate tube size for the patient's veins and the intended volume required for the laboratory will assist in obtaining quality specimens. Also, the safety of the patient and blood collector is enhanced with the use of plastic collection tubes. Examples of blood specimens collected in the wrong tube or wrong manner follow:

1. Green-topped tubes containing lithium heparin are not suitable for a patient's lithium studies because laboratory values will be falsely high, suggesting that the patient has a toxic level of lithium when he or she really does not.

2. Sodium heparin is not the anticoagulant of choice for blood to be collected for sodium values.

3. Light-blue–topped tubes with sodium citrate for coagulation testing (e.g., PT, APPT) must *not* be underfilled because coagulation test results will be falsely prolonged, leading to errors in anticoagulant therapy. If the health care worker is collecting blood only for a PT level using the Safety Blood Collection Set/Winged Infusion/Butterfly needle, a "dummy" tube must be collected first with blood before the light-blue–topped tube is used to avoid underfilling of the light-blue–topped tube.

4. Transfusion medicine (blood banking) cannot use the serum separator tubes for antibody screens and cross-matching of blood because a sticky layer is formed between the serum and the red blood cells from the gel of the tubes, leading to false agglutination and false-positive test results.[19]

5. Lavender-topped tubes (ethylenediaminetetraacetic acid [EDTA]) cannot be underfilled because it can lead to

   - Staining alterations on blood smears
   - Falsely low hematocrits, mean corpuscular volumes, and low blood cell counts
   - Erroneous morphologic changes to red blood cells

6. Green-topped tubes cannot be underfilled because inaccuracies may result in some chemistry analysis (e.g., amylase, lipase, potassium, ALT, AST) due to the excessive amount of heparin in the partially filled tube.

7. Red/Gray-topped tubes, gold-topped tubes, and other clot-activator tubes that are underfilled can cause inaccurate results in some immunoassays due to the excessive concentration of clot activator and/or silicone in the partially filled tube.

8. Blood culture bottles cannot be underfilled because the detection of microbiological organisms in bacteremia and septicemia will be delayed as well as the subsequent administration of appropriate antibiotic therapy.

Clinical Alert! A health care worker should *never* combine the blood from two or more underfilled tubes to provide the patient's blood specimen. This behavior leads to twice as much additive and it affects the accuracy of the laboratory results. In addition, the health care worker is exposing himself or herself to the risk of possible blood-borne pathogens.

9. Gray-topped tubes cannot be underfilled because the blood may become hemolyzed from the excessive amount of sodium fluoride in the partially filled tube.

10. Gray-topped blood collection tubes usually contain sodium fluoride and EDTA or potassium oxalate and sodium fluoride. Because sodium fluoride destroys many enzymes, this tube should not be used in blood collection for enzyme determinations (i.e., creatine kinase [CK], alanine aminotransferase [ALT]).

The risk of specimen rejection due to underfilled blood collection tubes can be avoided by following the tube manufacturer's recommendations. These include

- Holding the blood collection tube in place in the tube holder until blood flow has stopped
- Filling the tubes to their stated blood volume and/or filling to the minimum fill indicators on the tubes if indicators are provided

Study Questions

For the following questions, select the one best answer.

1 What is the ideal time for specimens to be collected?

  a. 5 hours after the last ingestion of food

  b. at noon if ingestion of food occurred at 8:00 AM

  c. 10 hours after the last ingestion of food

  d. 16 hours after the last ingestion of food

2 If a patient is taking high doses of Tylenol, which of the following analyte results is most likely to be affected?

  a. serum bilirubin

  b. creatine phosphokinase (CPK)

  c. blood glucose

  d. blood cholesterol

3 If a health care worker collects a venipuncture specimen from an arm site slightly above the patient's IV (in the same arm), what effect does it have on the specimen?

  a. It will increase the red blood cellular counts.

  b. It will increase ammonia levels.

  c. It will dilute the specimen with IV fluids.

  d. It will have no effect.

4 What effect does excessive probing with a needle in the patient's arm have on a venipuncture specimen?

  a. It has no effect at all and the specimen should be acceptable.

  b. Probing is often necessary and alters only the leukocyte count.

  c. It has no effect, but a physician should be notified of the circumstances.

  d. It can rupture erythrocytes and release tissue-clotting factors.

5 Which of the following is a solid mass derived from blood constituents that can occlude a vein (or an artery)?

  a. hemolyzed RBC

  b. hemolyzed WBC

  c. thrombus

  d. triglyceride

6 A physiological abnormality that can cause hemolysis is

  a. performing blood collection before the alcohol has dried at the collection site.

  b. sickle cell disease.

  c. needle readjustment.

  d. shaking blood collection tubes vigorously after blood collection.

7 Which of the following laboratory test results are affected most if the patient is not fasting?

  a. AST and CPK

  b. triglycerides and glucose

  c. cortisol and testosterone

  d. complete blood cell (CBC) count and prothrombin time

8 Which of the following would most likely NOT be an explanation for turbid serum?

  a. bacterial contamination

  b. elevated glucose results

  c. elevated cholesterol results

  d. elevated triglycerides results

9 If the tourniquet is applied for longer than 3 minutes, which of the following analytes will most likely become falsely elevated?

  a. potassium

  b. bilirubin

  c. GGT

  d. parathyroid hormone

10 Emotional stress, such as anxiety or fear, can lead to a decrease of which of the following analytes?

  a. serum iron

  b. WBCs

  c. CPK

  d. RBCs

Case Study

Ms. McKenzie Walters is a health care provider who contracts with local community health clinics to make home health care visits. This morning as she arrived at West Columbia Health Clinic, McKenzie noticed she had four home visits. She quickly threw blood collection equipment in her lockable container and hurried to her first patient, Ms. Margaret Moore, a 92-year-old woman who has type II diabetes and has had a stroke, leaving her as a hemiplegic. Margaret's physician had requested a complete chemistry profile, a CBC and protime, in addition to a physical examination. After checking Margaret's vital signs, McKenzie decided to collect the patient's blood with a winged infusion blood collection set because of the fragility of her veins.

McKenzie prepared the site for blood collection and after opening a 25-gauge safety winged infusion needle set, she inserted the needle into Margaret's vein in her hand and first collected blood in a light-blue topped vacuum plastic tube for the protime, followed by blood collection into a red-speckled–topped vacuum plastic tube. After completing the physical exam and blood collection, McKenzie labeled the tubes, discarded the biohazardous blood collection items in her biohazardous disposal container, and left Margaret's home with the collected blood and health care equipment, including the blood collection items.

Questions

1 Did the health care provider use the proper tubes and order of draw for Margaret's laboratory tests? Explain.

2 Did McKenzie use the correct blood collection equipment? Explain.

Action in Practice 1

An 83-year-old woman, Ms. Suzuki, came to the clinic for her monthly blood collection for a PT test. The health care worker introduced himself and prepared the blood collection equipment. He then checked the right-arm's antecubital area, cleansed the venipuncture site, and inserted a 21-gauge needle with the holder and tube attached. All of a sudden, Ms. Suzuki expressed excruciating pain in her arm and tingling in her hand and fingers. What should the health care worker do?

Action in Practice 2

A 65-year-old woman, Mrs. Garcia, comes for her annual checkup to the oncology clinic. After her visit with her doctor, she is sent to the laboratory to have some routine blood specimens collected. The health care worker correctly identifies her, prepares the site, supplies, and equipment, and inquires about which arm Mrs. Garcia prefers to have the puncture performed on. Mrs. Garcia says, "Well, it doesn't really matter to me but I had my mastectomy done five years ago on this side and they usually stick me over here," as she points to her left arm.

Questions

1 How should the health care worker proceed?

2 Why would a mastectomy make any difference in site selection?

3 Does the length of time after a mastectomy make any difference?

COMPETENCY ASSESSMENT

Check Yourself

1 What laboratory tests will be affected if the green-topped tube is underfilled?

2 Name three laboratory results that will be erroneously affected if the tourniquet is allowed to stay on the arm longer than one minute.

Competency Checklist: Preanalytical Complications

This checklist can be completed as a group or individually.

(1) Completed (2) Needs to improve

_____ 1. Describe how to collect blood from the patient's arm that has an inserted IV line.

_____ 2. Explain why petechiae occurs in some patients.

REFERENCES

1. Guder, W. G., Narayanan, S., Wisser, H., et al. (1996). *Samples: From the patient to the laboratory.* Germany: Git Verlag Pub.

2. Weight Watchers: Welcome brochure. (175 Crossways Park West, Woodbury, NY 11797-2055, 1-800-651- 6000) Available at www .weightwatchers.com, accessed July 17, 2007.

3. Ernst, D. (2003, July). Iodine disinfectant for infants, tips from the clinical experts. *Med Lab Obse, 54.* www.mlo-online.com.

4. Foran, S. E., Lewandrowski, K. B., & Kratz, A. (2003, October). Effects of exercise on laboratory test results. *Lab Med, 34*(10): 736–742.

5. Kratz, A., Lewandrowski, K. B., Siegel, A. J., et al. (2002). Effect of marathon running on hematologic and biochemical laboratory parameters, including cardiac markers. *Am J of Clin Path, 118:* 856–863.

6. Miller, H., & Lifshitz, M. (2007). Pre-analysis. In Henry, J. B. (Ed.), *Clinical diagnosis and management by laboratory methods,* 21st ed. Philadelphia: W. B. Saunders, pp. 20–21.

7. Becton-Dickinson and Company. (1982). *Blood specimen collection by skin puncture in infants.* East Rutherford, NJ: Author.

8. Statland, B. E., & Winkel, P. (1991). Preparing patients and specimens for laboratory testing. In Henry, J. B. (Ed.), *Clinical diagnosis and management by laboratory methods.* Philadelphia: W. B. Saunders.

9. Statland, B. E., Winkle, P., & Bokelund, H. (1974). Factors contributing to intra-individual variation of serum constituents: Effects of posture and tourniquet application on variation of serum constituents in healthy subjects. *Clin Chem, 20:* 1513.

10. Dale, J. (1998). Preanalytical variables in laboratory testing. *Lab Med, 29,* 540–545.

11. McNamara, J. R. (2000). Cardiovascular disease: Laboratory testing adds information to risk profile. *Clin Lab News, 26*(10): 12–16.

12. Giris J., & Satish, R. (2005). Postural pseudoanemia: Posture-dependent change in hematocrit. *Mayo Clin Proc.* 80(95): 611–614.

13. Tryding, N. (2007). *Drug effects in clinical chemistry.* Washington, DC: AACC Press.

14. The Joint Commission 2012 National Patient Safety Goals, 2012 Laboratory Services National Patient Safety Goals. www.jointcommission.org/PatientSafety/NationalPatientSafetyGoals/12_lab_npsgs.htm, accessed December 3, 2012.

15. Renner, S. W., Howanitz, J., & Bachner, P. (1993). Wristband identification errors reporting in 712 hospitals. A College of American Pathologists Q-Probe study of quality issues in transfusion practice. *ArchPathol Lab Med 117:* 573–577.

16. Clinical and Laboratory Standards Institute (CLSI). (2007). *Procedures for the collection of diagnostic blood specimens by venipuncture.* Wayne, PA: Author. Approved Standard, H3–A6.

17. Murphy, M. F, Wainscoat, J., & Colvin, B. T. (2002). Hematological disease. In Kumar, P., & Clark, M. (Eds.), *Clinical medicine,* 5th ed. St. Louis: W. B. Saunders, pp. 424–432.

18. Clinical and Laboratory Standards Institute (CLSI). (2004). *Procedures and devices for the collection of diagnostic capillary blood specimens.* Wayne, PA: Author. Approved Standard, H4–A5.

19. Baer, D: Tips from the clinical experts. Answering your question. *Med Lab Obser,* 2005;37(9)49.

RESOURCES

Frase, C. D. (2001). *Biological variation: From principles to practice.* Washington, DC: AACC Press.

Soldin, S. J., Brugnara, C., & Wong, E. C. (2003). *Pediatric reference ranges,* 4th ed. Washington, DC: AACC Press.

Young, D. (2006). *Effects of preanalytical variables on clinical laboratory tests.* St. Louis: W. B. Saunders.

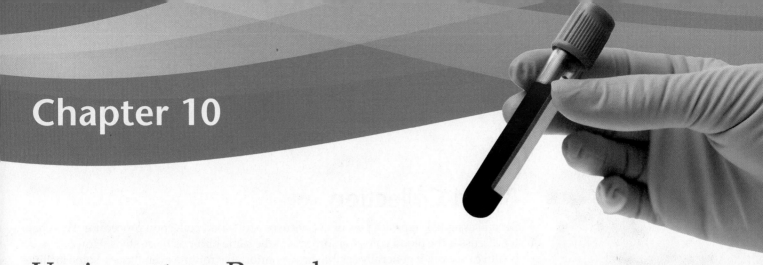

Chapter 10

Venipuncture Procedures

Chapter Objectives

Upon completion of Chapter 10, the learner is responsible for doing the following:

1. Describe the steps a health care worker should take in preparing him- or herself for a venipuncture procedure.

2. List the supplies and equipment used in a typical venipuncture procedure.

3. Describe the detailed steps in the patient identification process and what to do if information is missing.

4. Describe the methods and rationale for hand hygiene.

5. Identify the most appropriate sites for venipuncture and situations when these sites might not be acceptable.

6. Identify alternative sites for the venipuncture procedure.

7. Describe the process and time limits for applying a tourniquet to a patient's arm.

8. Describe the decontamination process and the agents used to decontaminate skin for routine blood tests and blood cultures.

9. Describe the steps of a venipuncture procedure using the evacuated tube method, syringe method, and butterfly method according to the CLSI Approved Standard.

10. Describe the "order of draw" for collection tubes.

11. Describe how to react when the patient has fainted or experiences nausea, vomiting, or convulsions.

12. Define and explain the clinical reason for the terms *fasting*, *STAT*, and *timed specimens*.

KEY TERMS

cleanse/decontaminate

fasting

hand hygiene

physician-patient relationship

therapeutic drug monitoring (TDM)

tourniquet

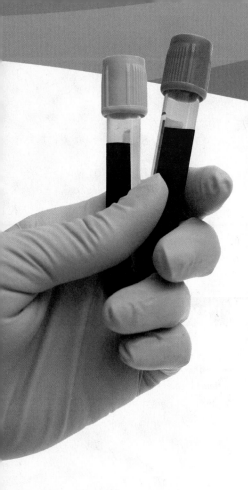

Blood Collection

Several essential steps are part of every successful blood collection procedure. This chapter discusses the blood collection process in the same order as these steps. However, each health care worker generally establishes a comfortable routine even though some facilities vary the sequence of steps based on the characteristics of its patient populations and the type of health care setting. In some cases, steps may occur simultaneously (e.g., while the health care worker is introducing him- or herself, he or she can begin to visually assess the patient's physical disposition). In other cases, a problem may arise that precludes the health care worker from going further in the procedure (e.g., the supplies needed for the venipuncture have expired; the name given verbally by the individual does not match the printed documentation). Each step of the patient encounter must be evaluated carefully by the health care worker in a detailed manner, being careful not to omit any of the essential components (**FIGURE 10–1**). The basic steps involve the following: [1,2]

1. Preparing the health care worker, including **hand hygiene,** cleansing hands through handwashing or use of alcohol-based products, and reviewing laboratory test orders
2. Preparing the work area where the venipuncture will be performed
3. Approaching, identifying, and positioning the patient
4. Assessing the patient's physical disposition, including diet, sensitivity to latex, history of fainting, and/or preference for which arm is to be used
5. Selecting and preparing equipment and supplies, including the correct venipuncture system, gloves, etc.
6. Positioning the patient, applying a tourniquet, and finding a puncture site
7. Choosing a venipuncture method
8. Preparing the puncture site
9. Collecting the specimens in the appropriate tubes and in the correct order
10. Activating needle safety device(s) and discarding contaminated supplies
11. Labeling the specimens prior to transporting them
12. Assessing the patient to ensure bleeding has stopped
13. Maintaining hand hygiene
14. Considering any special circumstances that occurred during the phlebotomy procedure
15. Assessing criteria for specimen recollection or rejection
16. Prioritizing patients and specimen tubes (e.g., STAT requests)
17. Transporting and/or storing specimens appropriately (e.g., at room temperature, chilled/heated, or protected from light)

Health Care Worker Preparation

Before performing any type of specimen collection, the health care worker should have access to protective equipment, phlebotomy supplies, test requisitions, writing pen, and appropriate patient information. If the health care worker is not fully protected, there is a greater risk of health care-acquired infections being transmitted. If the patient information is incomplete on test requisitions, the health care worker may not be able to identify the patient correctly, or the worker may not know in which tubes to collect the blood. If the health care worker does not have the correct phlebotomy supplies, the procedure should not be performed. Workers must learn to seek assistance from authorized resources, including a laboratory supervisor or a nurse before collecting the sample if there are deficiencies in the preparation stage.

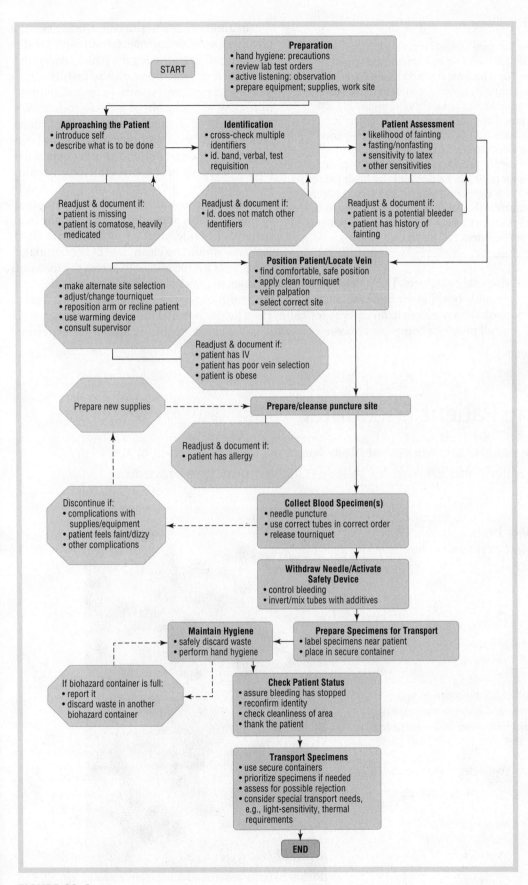

FIGURE 10–1

Flowchart of the Venipuncture Process

Clinical Alert! Health care workers must be familiar with policies regarding precautions for handling blood and body fluids. *All specimens should be treated as if they are hazardous and infectious,* according to the standard precautions described in detail in Chapter 4. Hands should be decontaminated before and immediately after specimen collection procedures. Refer to Appendix 5, "Centers for Disease Control and Prevention (CDC) Guideline for Hand Hygiene in Health Care Settings" and **BOX 10–1**, "Issues in Hand Hygiene." A clean pair of gloves should be put on in the presence of the patient as a safety-conscious gesture for both the patient and the health care worker. Refer to **PROCEDURE 10–2**, "Hand Hygiene and Gloving Technique." A clean, pressed uniform with a laboratory coat also instills a sense of professionalism and cleanliness, which is gratifying to patients and promotes a safer work environment for health care workers.

In addition, the health care worker needs a positive, professional, mental and physical disposition before beginning the patient encounter. A clean and neat appearance instills confidence and professionalism. Refer to Chapter 1 to review an example of a dress code policy. A clear and open mind, free from distractions, aids the health care worker in successful dialogue with the patient and promotes positive patient rapport and more effective listening skills. Refer to **PROCEDURE 10–1**. The health care worker must also prepare the venipuncture workspace, depending on the setting (e.g., patient's bedside, doctor's office, home visit). The area should be clean, free of contaminated items, near a sink, and with access to biohazard disposal containers. The phlebotomy chair, recliner, or patient bed should be in a safe, comfortable position for both the patient and the health care worker. The health care worker should have access to an emergency call system (in the hospital room, clinic setting, or via a cell phone or computer) in case of unanticipated events requiring additional expertise.

PROCEDURE 10–1

Preparing for the Patient Encounter

Rationale   To help the health care worker mentally focus on the importance of the individual patient and prepare for that specific venipuncture procedure.

Equipment/Supplies

- Phlebotomy supplies (**FIGURE 10–2**)
- Personal protective equipment (PPE) (gloves, clean uniform, laboratory coat, etc.)
- Test requisitions/labels
- Writing pen
- Handheld computer bar code reader/scanner (if applicable)

Preparation

1 Prepare and assemble PPE, phlebotomy supplies, test requisitions/labels, writing pen, and appropriate patient information before the patient encounter and prior to the venipuncture process.

2 Keep the work area or counter space clean and free of debris.

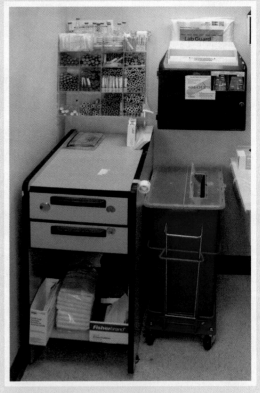

FIGURE 10–2
A Well-Stocked Phlebotomy Workstation

PROCEDURE 10–1

Preparing for the Patient Encounter (continued)

Procedure

3 Present a positive, professional (neat and clean) appearance and temperament (optimistic and open minded) before beginning the patient encounter. Some find it helpful to take a deep, cleansing breath before beginning (**FIGURE 10–3**). As you do this, focus on the individual patient and the requests for that particular person. Use the cleansing breath to center your attention on the upcoming venipuncture task as you temporarily remove yourself from other distracting factors in the workplace (e.g., hallway conversations, TV noise, phones, etc.). Use your keen observations to determine any special circumstances or needs that the patient may have.

4 Arrange and check the phlebotomy supplies, test requisitions, writing pen, and appropriate patient information before beginning the encounter and venipuncture process (**FIGURE 10–4**). Refer to **FIGURE 10–5** to view other types of phlebotomy supply storage options.

5 If the patient information is incomplete on test requisitions, you may not be able to identify the patient correctly, or you may not know in which tubes to collect the blood. In such cases, obtain assistance from a laboratory supervisor or a nurse before collecting the sample.

6 If you or the patient is sensitive to latex products, use nitrile or polyethylene gloves, or other nonlatex gloves. Also, use a nonlatex tourniquet and bandage for the patient during and after the procedure.

7 Help the patient relax and stay calm by professionally explaining the procedure and answering any questions related to the venipuncture.

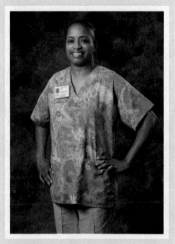

FIGURE 10–3

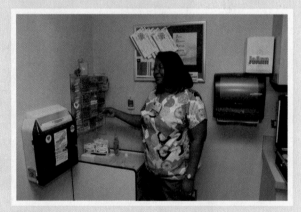

FIGURE 10–4

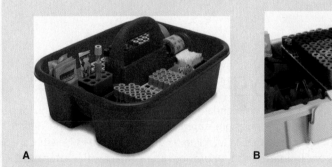
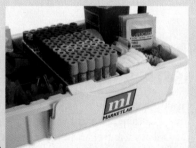
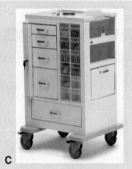

FIGURE 10–5

Phlebotomy Supplies in Commercially Available Carts or Trays

A–E demonstrate the range of storage containers for phlebotomy supplies, ranging from basic trays to mobile phlebotomy carts. Most of them have customizable compartments and removable parts for sanitizing.

Courtesy of MarketLab: www.marketlabinc.com

(continued)

PROCEDURE 10–1

Preparing for the Patient Encounter (continued)

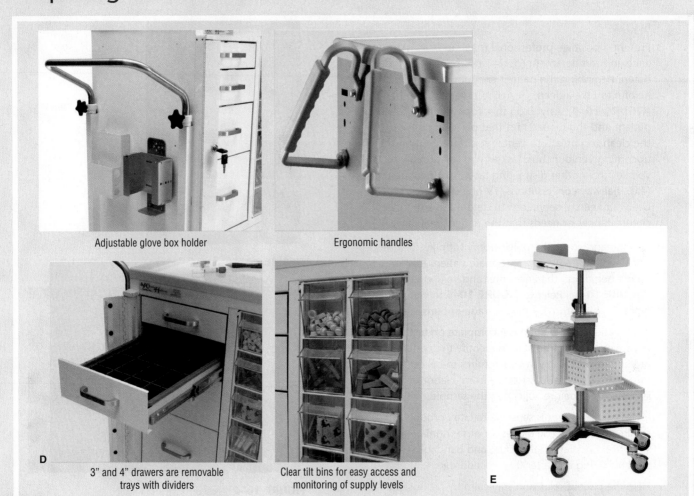

Adjustable glove box holder

Ergonomic handles

D

3" and 4" drawers are removable trays with dividers

Clear tilt bins for easy access and monitoring of supply levels

E

FIGURE 10–5 (*continued*)

BOX 10–1

Issues in Hand Hygiene

Health care workers must know the recommendations and have appropriate training for performing and maintaining hand hygiene. Key issues are summarized here.[3] Refer to Appendix 5, "Centers for Disease Control and Prevention (CDC) Guideline for Hand Hygiene in Health Care Settings." Remember, **cleanse/decontaminate** hands before and after contact with each patient.

Choosing a Hand Hygiene Product

- Consider the efficacy of the antiseptic agents against pathogens.
- Consider how acceptable the products are to personnel who use them (accessibility, ease of use, minimal irritation, etc.). Refer to Chapter 8 for more information about specific products.

BOX 10–1 (*continued*)

- When a soap dispenser is used, soap should not be added to a partially empty container, because the practice of "topping off" can lead to bacterial contamination.

Skin Care

- Hand lotions should be provided to minimize the occurrence of dermatitis associated with frequent hand cleaning.

Other Aspects of Hand Hygiene

- Keep natural fingernail tips less than ¼-inch long. Refer to **FIGURE 10–6**.
- Do not wear artificial fingernails or extenders when caring for patients who are at high risk of acquiring infections. Refer to your health care facility's policy.
- Change gloves between patients; do not wash the same gloves between patients.

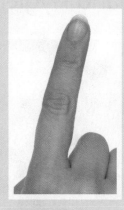

FIGURE 10–6

PROCEDURE 10–2

Hand Hygiene and Gloving Technique

Rationale   To protect the patient and the health care worker from exposure to infectious substances and to prevent the transmission of infectious agents.

Use of gloves does not eliminate the need for hand hygiene, nor does good hand hygiene eliminate the need for gloves. Perform hand hygiene before and after each patient and use new gloves for each patient. See "Reasons for Gloving."

Equipment

Soap and water or alcohol-based hand sanitizer

Preparation

1 Upon entering a patient's hospital room or an outpatient area where a venipuncture procedure is to be performed, locate the hand hygiene method (soap and water or alcohol-based hand sanitizer).

Procedure

2 Decontaminate/sanitize your hands using an alcohol-based hand rub or by washing your hands with antimicrobial soap and water (**FIGURE 10–7**). If your hands are visibly dirty or contaminated with blood or body fluids, always use soap and water.

3 Use the amount of sanitizer or soap that the manufacturer recommends and rub your hands together, thoroughly between fingers and on all sides of your hands (**FIGURE 10–8**).

(*continued*)

PROCEDURE 10–2

Hand Hygiene and Gloving Technique (continued)

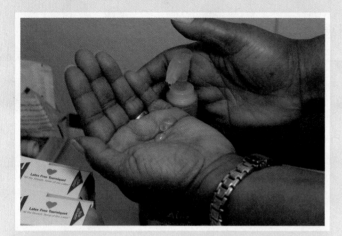

FIGURE 10–7
Cleansing Hands

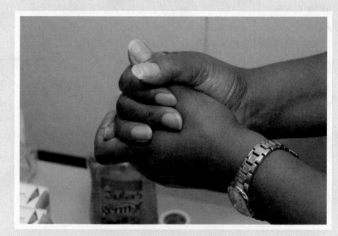

FIGURE 10–8

4 When your hands are dry, slip the fingers of one hand into a clean glove.

5 Pull the glove taut with the other hand so that there is no slack or bagginess of the gloves at the fingertips.

6 Do the same with the other hand (**FIGURE 10–9**).

7 *After the entire venipuncture procedure has been completed,* turn the gloves inside out as you remove them (**FIGURES 10–10** and **10–11**).

8 Discard the gloves with biohazardous materials, unless your health care facility specifies otherwise.

Other Important Factors to Consider

- Remember, if your hands are visibly dirty, contaminated, or soiled, wash them with either an antimicrobial soap and water or a nonantimicrobial soap and water.
- If your hands are not visibly soiled, an alcohol-based hand sanitizer can be used routinely for decontaminating. Apply to the palm on one hand and rub your hands together, covering all surfaces of your hands and fingers, until your hands are dry. Follow the manufacturer's recommendations regarding the volume of product to use (usually a dime-size portion will suffice).[3]

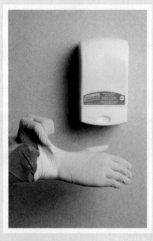

FIGURE 10–9

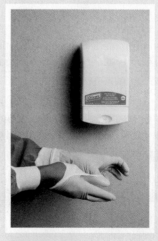

FIGURE 10–10

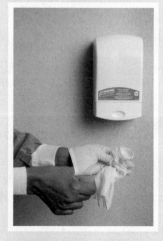

FIGURE 10–11

PROCEDURE 10–2

Hand Hygiene and Gloving Technique (continued)

- If you use an antimicrobial soap and water, first wet your hands with water, apply the amount of product recommended by the manufacturer, and rub your hands together vigorously for at least 15 seconds, covering all surfaces of your hands and fingers. Rinse your hands with water and dry thoroughly with a disposable towel. Use a towel to turn off the faucet.
- Multiple-use cloth towels (hanging or roll type) are *not* recommended for health care facilities.
- Decontaminate/cleanse your hands before and after contact with a patient, blood, or body fluids.
- Cleanse your hands before and after wearing gloves.
- Cleanse your hands before eating and after using a restroom.
- Antimicrobial-impregnated wipes are *not* as effective as alcohol-based hand rubs or antimicrobial soap and water.[3]
- If your workplace does not have the correct gloves (due to skin allergies or size) notify your supervisor so that the appropriate gloves can be ordered.

Reasons for Gloving

- To provide a protective barrier against contamination and exposure when handling potentially infectious materials such as blood and body fluids
- To reduce the likelihood of exposure and transmission of microorganisms from health care worker to patient
- To reduce cross-contamination between patients from the hands of the health care worker

Precautions

As described in Chapter 4, normal human skin is colonized with microorganisms; thus, transmission of pathogens by health care workers from one patient to another can occur easily. Based on studies reported by the CDC, health care workers vary widely in the number of times they actually wash their hands (from 5 times per shift to more than 100 times per shift). There is also great variability in both the duration that workers perform the handwashing process (5 to 24 seconds) and the coverage of surface area on the hands, wrists, and fingers. Adherence to hand hygiene techniques has been shown to significantly reduce outbreaks of infections, including antimicrobial-resistant infections (e.g., methicillin-resistant *Staphylococcus aureus*, MRSA).

Needlestick Prevention Strategies

As noted in previous chapters, the Needlestick Safety and Prevention Act requires specific rules in the workplace to protect health care workers (needlestick prevention strategies, pre- and postexposure follow-up, etc.).[4,5] In addition, many states have enacted legislation related to blood-borne pathogen exposures.[6] Refer to **BOX 10–2**. It is a fact that those who use needles are at increased risk of a needlestick injury. These injuries may lead to serious or fatal infections with blood-borne pathogens such as hepatitis B virus (HBV), hepatitis C virus (HCV), or human immunodeficiency virus (HIV). However, needlestick injuries are preventable with the use of safety devices, precautionary practices, and safe handling/disposal of needles and specimens. In addition, the diseases may be prevented by preexposure vaccination and/or postexposure prophylaxis. Health care workers must report all needlestick injuries as soon as possible so that disease detection and prevention measures can be quickly initiated.[4,5,6]

BOX 10–2

Preventing Needlestick Injuries

Data compiled from various studies by the Centers for Disease Control and Prevention (CDC) indicate that needlestick injuries occur for the following reasons:[4,5,6]

- The type and design of the needle device used
- Recapping a needle
- Transferring body fluids between containers
- Failing to properly dispose of used needles in puncture-resistant sharps containers

What Employers Can Do

- Analyze needlestick and sharps-related injuries in the workplace to identify hazards and injury trends.
- Set priorities for prevention by researching national information about risk factors and interventions.
- Ensure that staff members are trained properly in the safe use and disposal of needles, as well as in universal precautions.
- Modify work practices that pose needlestick injury hazards.
- Promote safety awareness in the work environment.
- Provide high-risk employees with free hepatitis B vaccinations.
- Establish procedures and encourage timely reporting of all needlestick or sharps-related injuries.
- Evaluate the success of the needlestick prevention program and modify the exposure control plan accordingly.

What Employees Can Do

If you are exposed to the blood of a patient, follow these procedures:

- Wash needlesticks and cuts with soap and water. (No scientific evidence shows that using antiseptics or squeezing the wound will reduce the risk of transmission of a blood-borne pathogen; using bleach is not recommended either.)
- Flush splashes to the nose, mouth, or skin with water.
- Irrigate eyes with clean water, saline, or sterile irrigates when appropriate.
- Report the exposure immediately to the responsible department (employee health, infection control, your supervisor).
- Avoid the use of needles when safe alternatives are available.
- Help the employer select, evaluate, and use safety devices.
- Avoid recapping needles.
- Before beginning a procedure, plan for safe handling and needle disposal.
- Assist in coordinating specimen collections to reduce the number of times needles are used on a patient.
- Promptly dispose of used needles in the proper sharps disposal containers.
- Report all needlestick and other sharps-related injuries promptly to ensure follow-up care and to allow for tracking the hazards in the workplace.
- Tell your employer about hazards from needles that are observed in the work environment.
- Participate in blood-borne pathogen training and follow infection prevention practices such as hepatitis B vaccination.
- Follow policies and procedures as established by your employer.

Approaching, Assessing, and Identifying the Patient

INITIAL INTRODUCTION AND PATIENT APPROACH

Several professional and courteous behaviors and phrases can help make the patient–health care worker encounter a smooth interaction. In a hospital setting, health care workers are in and out of many patients' rooms and around the nursing station. Health care workers should speak quietly but professionally and avoid disturbing other members of the health care team who are also busy at work. When entering a patient's hospital room, health care workers should knock on the door (do not pound loudly), greet the patient initially by introducing themself, indicate their department (if required), and state the purpose of the interaction (to collect a blood specimen). Health care workers should be considerate when turning on the lights (use a low level light if the patient is asleep) and with the volume of their voice (avoid a loud voice). Refer to **BOX 10–3**.

Sometimes, the health care worker may need to explain to the patient that the physician ordered the laboratory test(s). The health care worker may also need to explain the procedure as supplies are being set up or as gloves are put on. During setup, the specimen collection tray should not be placed on the patient's bed or eating table. As supplies are being readied and the vein is being palpated, the health care worker may try to alleviate some of the patient's fears. It may be reassuring to purposefully show the patient that the supplies are "new" and "unused." Calming the patient helps to alleviate the fear and anxiety associated with phlebotomy. Chapters 1 and 2 cover verbal and nonverbal cues for detecting apprehension in patients.

If a physician or nurse is consulting with the patient when the health care worker enters the room, the specimen collection procedure should be delayed until the consultation is completed. The **physician–patient relationship,** the private and confidential association based on clinical consultation, has priority over a phlebotomy procedure unless the request is for a timed or STAT specimen, in which case the health care worker may ask permission to proceed.

PHYSICAL DISPOSITION OF THE PATIENT

Factors related to the physical or emotional disposition of the patient often have an impact on the blood collection process or the integrity of the specimen. As mentioned in previous chapters, this relates to the preexamination/preanalytical phase of laboratory testing. If the health care worker is aware of a variable that might affect the laboratory test or the patient encounter, he or she may be able to prepare more adequately for the venipuncture. Sometimes the health care worker can get clues about the patient's disposition upon entering a hospital room. For example, if there is an empty food tray by the patient's bedside, it is likely that the patient has eaten recently, and after confirming the observation with the patient, a notation about the nonfasting condition should be made. At other times, a clue about something unusual may come after talking to the patient or after the identification process has taken place. Health care workers should use keen listening skills and direct observation of the situation and make professional judgments about what modifications or documentation is needed to complete the specimen collection procedure.

The following specific factors may affect the patient's physical and/or emotional disposition:

■ **Diet, alcohol, exercise, and/or smoking**—Many body substances are affected by the ingestion of food and beverages (particularly alcohol) and by smoking. Therefore, it is important to note whether the patient has been fasting; if the patient seems intoxicated; or if the patient is eating candy, chewing gum (containing sugar), or has smoked a cigarette. Diet and alcohol intake have an effect on coagulation activation in people with diabetes and other populations. Smoking elevates plasma fibrinogen, the von Willebrand factor, coagulation factors, thrombin generation, and platelet

BOX 10–3

Typical Health Care Worker–Patient Interaction

The following hospital scenario depicts a health care worker and patient interaction just prior to blood collection. It begins when the health care worker politely knocks on the patient's hospital door and slowly enters the room. Do not use a loud voice because it may startle the patient.

Health care worker: Good morning. I am Ms. Smith from the laboratory. I have come to collect a blood specimen.

Pause to give the patient an opportunity to speak. If the lights are off or dimmed, explain that you need to turn the lights on or seek out a low-level light at first. Doing so gives the patient a moment to adjust to the idea of bright lights if he or she has been asleep. Take note of any hints or signs that the patient may have eaten breakfast.

Health care worker: Could you please state your name and spell it for me. (In general, it is not wise to ask a patient "How are you?" because most patients in the hospital do not feel well.)

Patient: I am John Jones. J-O-H-N J-O-N-E-S.

Health care worker: May I please see your identification (ID) armband?

Check the armband against laboratory requisitions and patient's verbal identification. If all three match, proceed.

Health care worker: This will take only a few minutes. Do you have any questions, Mr. Jones?

Patient: Will it hurt?

Health care worker: It will hurt a little, but it will be over soon. Mr. Jones, when was the last time you ate or drank anything?

Do not use the term fast because some patients may not understand it completely.

Patient: Last night, for dinner.

Health care worker: OK. Have you ever felt faint or fainted during a blood collection procedure?

Patient: No, I haven't fainted, but I don't like this being done.

Health care worker: I can understand your feelings, and a lot of other people feel that way, too. Have you ever had any other problems during a blood collection procedure?

Patient: No.

Health care worker: Mr. Jones, are you allergic to any latex products?

Patient: No, I'm not allergic.

Health care worker: OK, do you have a preference of which arm I use for the procedure?

Patient: No.

Health care worker: OK, now do you have any questions?

Patient: No.

Health care worker: OK, then I'll continue with the procedure.

Proceed with the remainder of the procedure, maintaining a highly professional atmosphere and a respectful attitude as supplies are being readied. At the end of the procedure, ask the patient if he or she feels well. Prior to leaving, say "Thank you."

activation. Moderate ethanol intake inhibits platelet reactivity. Vigorous physical activity leads to coagulation activation, so patients should rest in a comfortable position for 15 to 30 minutes prior to the specimen collection procedure.[7,8]

- **Tendency to faint**—The sight or thought of blood can trigger increased fear and anxiety in some patients. These patients can feel faint or even experience syncope, or "passing out," as the procedure begins, during the procedure, or afterward. The health care worker should ask the patient prior to beginning if the patient has ever had any problems during a blood collection procedure or felt faint or fainted during the procedure. If the answer is yes, then extra care should be taken to have the patient in a safe reclining position (e.g., blood donor chair or bed) when performing the venipuncture. Phlebotomy chairs should have adjustable armrests and a safety bar to prevent patients from falling if they faint. In the event that a patient feels faint, the procedure should be discontinued immediately. Position the patient so that the patient will not fall to the floor. Refer to **FIGURE 10–12**.

- **Latex sensitivity**—Ask patients if they have a latex sensitivity or are allergic to latex products. If the answer is yes, then the health care worker should use nonlatex products (tourniquet, gloves, and bandages).

- **Stress**—Excessively anxious or emotional patients may need extra time to calm down prior to, during, or after the procedure. The health care worker should deal professionally with these emotional needs based on the patient's age, gender, and cultural sensitivities.

- **Age**—Elderly patients have fragile, more "difficult" veins from which to choose the venipuncture site. (Refer to Chapter 13 for more details about the treatment of elderly patients.)

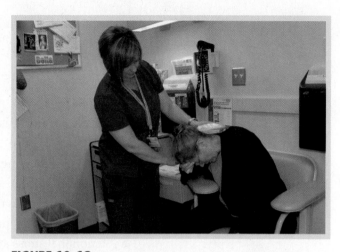

FIGURE 10–12
Health Care Worker Caring for a Patient Who Feels Faint

The health care worker should immediately discontinue the procedure if a patient indicates that she feels faint. If the patient is not already in a reclining position (as in a blood donor-type of chair), use all means to assure that the patient will not incur a self-injury or try to lower the head. In this photo, the arm of the chair was quickly moved in front of the patient and she was asked to lower her head and breathe deeply. A cold compress to the back of the neck or on the forehead is comforting and may prevent the patient from losing consciousness. If the patient has tight clothing around the neck area (a tie or closed collar), ask the patient for permission to loosen the clothing to improve blood flow to the head. Give the patient ample time to recover and dissuade the patient from getting up too quickly. Immediately call for assistance if the patient does not respond. Document the incident and/or report it to your supervisor or nurse.

- **Arm preference**—Some patients prefer that their nondominant arm or hand be used for the venipuncture. Asking the patient "Which arm would you prefer that I use for the blood collection?" can reveal information about personal preference, a previous mastectomy, a scarred or burned area, or a vein site that has been successful in the past. However, health care workers should use their own judgment in selecting the safest puncture site with the highest likelihood of success. It may mean that it is not the patient's preferred site, but a short explanation of the rational for the selection is usually helpful. Blood should never be collected from the same side as a mastectomy, and in the case of a bilateral mastectomy, permission must be obtained from the patient's physician prior to collecting the blood from either side.

- **Weight**—Obese patients may require special equipment such as a large blood pressure cuff for use as a tourniquet or a longer needle to penetrate through fatty tissues to the vein.

As discussed in Chapter 9, many patient variables can influence test results. Health care workers are not expected to evaluate the patient for *all* aspects of these variables prior to each specimen collection procedure. However, they are expected to intervene and act responsibly within their scope of practice as it relates to the specimen collection process. Actions may include documenting a situation, adjusting the patient to be in a more comfortable position, selecting alternative supplies for the procedure, transporting a specimen in a certain manner, and/or seeking guidance from a supervisor about how to proceed. Whatever the case, the factors listed here can introduce preanalytical variability.[7,8]

- Age and gender
- Blood type
- Circadian and seasonal rhythms
- Diet and exercise
- Smoking, chewing gum or tobacco, and alcohol intake
- Medications
- Intravenous lines or vascular access devices
- Menstrual cycle, pregnancy, menopausal status
- Emotional stress and psychiatric disorders

POSITIONING OF THE PATIENT AND THE HEALTH CARE WORKER

Proper positioning is important to both the health care worker and the patient for a successful venipuncture or skin puncture. Efforts to make sure that the patient is comfortable are worthwhile. Patients should not stand or sit on high stools during the procedure because of the possibility of fainting. A reclining (supine) position is preferred; however, another acceptable position for phlebotomy is sitting in a sturdy, comfortable chair with adjustable arm supports and a protective, padded bar to prevent a patient from falling to the floor in case of fainting during or after the procedure. The health care worker can also be positioned in front of the chair to protect the patient from falling forward in the event of fainting. The patient should not have anything (e.g., food, chewing gum, or a thermometer) in their mouth during the venipuncture procedure. **FIGURES 10–13** and **10–14** show phlebotomy-assistive devices and blood collection chairs.

FIGURE 10–13

Devices to Assist in Positioning of the Patient and Supplies

A. A phlebotomy wedge is available to help stabilize the patient's arm. It has an antimicrobial protective vinyl coating that does not absorb liquids and can be wiped clean after each use. B. A hand immobilizer can be useful when hard-to-get hand veins are utilized for phlebotomy. C. These plastic devices come in various sizes, have adjustable straps, and can be disassembled for cleaning. D. Clamps for holding supplies close to the patient during the venipuncture procedure can be attached to bed rails, chair arms, wheelchairs, or countertops.

Courtesy of MarketLab:
www.marketlabinc.com

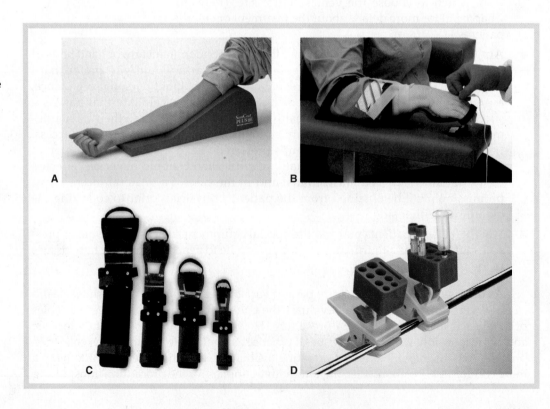

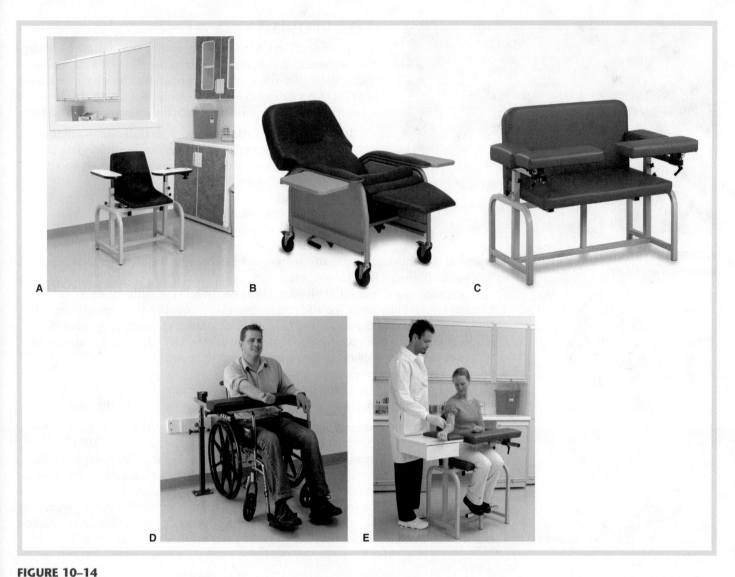

FIGURE 10–14

Blood Collection Chairs

A. A typical phlebotomy chair with adjustable arms. **B.** Recliner-style chair with adjustable arms and/or shelves are available in a variety of styles, often with electronic height adjustments to facilitate comfort and safety for the patient and health care worker. **C.** Extra-wide chairs for large and obese patients. **D.** Some facilities have a mounted wheelchair draw station. It is an adjustable phlebotomy "arm" that enables wheelchair-bound patients to stay comfortable and secure in their wheelchair during the procedure. **E.** Extra-tall chairs are more comfortable for the health care worker because they eliminate back strain. They should be used for patients who have the greatest mobility and are not likely to lose their balance or have trouble getting in and out of the chair. Some chairs have electronic height adjustments so that the health care worker can allow the patient to sit comfortably, then raise the height to a comfortable level during the procedure and then lower it after the procedure.

Courtesy of MarketLab: www.marketlabinc.com

Arm positioning depends on each patient; however, when possible, ask the patient to fully extend the arm in a downward position. Ideally, the position should almost be a straight line from the shoulder to the wrist; however, in reality, most patients have a slight bend in the elbow area. Positioning can also involve a slight rotation of the patient's arm or hand that may help expose a vein and prevent it from rolling as the needle is inserted. A pillow or an arm-resting device may be used for arm support of a weak, bedridden patient or for ambulatory patients to adjust to a more comfortable position. If suitable arm supports are not readily available, the patient's free wrist can be placed under the elbow to straighten the arm a bit more and provide some cushioning during the venipuncture. Collection equipment and supplies should be placed in an accessible spot where they are unlikely to be disturbed by the patient.

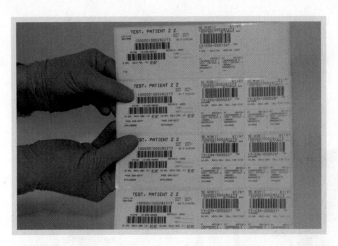

FIGURE 10–15
Requisitions and Labels

TEST REQUISITIONS

As mentioned in Chapter 2, laboratory test requests are usually transmitted electronically or in the form of a paper-based requisition. Electronic requests contain the same required information as paper requisitions. (Refer to **FIGURE 10–15**) In either case, the requisition should contain the following information:[7]

1. Patient's identification information (full name, unique identification or registration number, location, date of birth, or a unique confidential specimen code if an alternative audit trail exists)
2. Patient gender
3. Tests to be performed
4. Date/time of specimen collection or test request, as appropriate
5. Name of the physician or legally authorized person who ordered the tests
6. Test status (timed, STAT, fasting, etc.)
7. Special precautions (potential bleeder, faints easily, latex sensitivity, etc.)
8. Clinical information (note the site of collection if it is not the arm; sometimes additional information is needed to provide more accurate test results, e.g., specimen requests for genetics tests may also include race/ethnicity to allow the laboratory to report detection rates for diseases among specific populations)
9. Source of specimen, when appropriate
10. Billing information (if required by your health care facility)
11. Diagnostic coding and physician signature (if required by your health care facility)

When requisitions are received in a centralized laboratory department, electronically generated labels may also serve as the requisition, as indicated in Figure 10–15.

There are numerous types, colors, and styles of labels (e.g., bar code labels) and requisitions available depending on the practices of each health care facility. Regardless of whether the requisitions are electronic or handwritten on multipart paper forms, health care workers should be familiar with the forms and with their institution's procedures for generating, printing, and using the requisition forms properly. Collection requests should be checked prior to the venipuncture procedure for:

■ Discrepancies

■ Missing information

■ Duplicate test orders

If the health care worker does not understand what test(s) is/are ordered, he or she should consult the laboratory's informational manual and/or a supervisor, laboratory technologist, or nurse prior to the phlebotomy procedure. In some instances, the health care worker may need to consult the ordering physician to clarify orders. Knowing which tests are requested helps the health care worker prepare the patient appropriately and collect the specimen in the appropriate tubes and in the proper order. Failure to do so results in preanalytical or preexamination errors, misleading test results, and repeated venipunctures for the patient. Appendix 6 provides a sample listing of laboratory assays, tube requirements, and reference intervals; however, it should not be used in lieu of the requirements for specific laboratories or health care facilities.

PATIENT IDENTIFICATION PROCESS

Positive patient identification is the most crucial responsibility for which a health care worker is held accountable. **PROCEDURE 10–3** describes the identification process. The 2014 National Patient Safety Goals and Recommendations set by The Joint Commission include improving "accuracy of patient identification." Its recommendations suggest using "at least two patient identifiers" (neither to be the patient's room number) whenever providing care, treatment, or services.[9] Correct patient identification is critical

PROCEDURE 10–3

Basics of Patient Identification

Rationale   To use appropriate patient identifiers for blood specimens, thereby promoting patient safety and accuracy of the laboratory testing results.

Equipment/Supplies

- Completed requisitions/labels
- Bar code scanner/reader, if necessary
- Patient-specific identification armband

Preparation

The actual identification procedure begins after the health care worker has

- Greeted the patient
- Identified him- or herself and stated their department
- Indicated the purpose of the encounter
- Allowed the patient a chance to respond, been given implied consent via a gesture (nod of the head or holding out the arm), and/or noted the patient's refusal for the procedure

The health care worker should not perform a venipuncture against a patient's wishes, or if it is obvious that the patient does not understand the procedure, or if the patient is a child and the guardian does not consent. Follow institutional policies if any of these circumstances occurs and document/report the situations accordingly.

Procedure

Most patients will have their blood collected when they are in a conscious state, so the basic procedure applies to this type of patient, regardless of the setting.

Patient identification involves *at least three steps:*

1 After greeting a conscious patient (**FIGURE 10–16**), ask the patient to state and spell their full name and state their birth date. (You may also request the patient's address and ID number.) *Note:* The room number or bed location must *not* be used as a patient identifier. Refer to the next section, "Special Considerations," for more information.

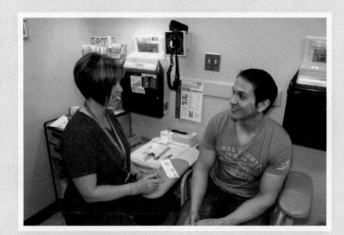

FIGURE 10–16

(continued)

PROCEDURE 10–3

Basics of Patient Identification (continued)

2 Compare the information stated with the information on the laboratory *test requisitions*. If there are discrepancies, report it to the responsible supervisor. Discrepancies in patient identification information must be resolved prior to collecting the specimen (**FIGURE 10–17**).

3 Confirm the information (from steps 1 and 2) with another source of reliable, verifiable identification (e.g., for hospitalized patients it is a printed identification/registration number on the hospital identification armband/bracelet; for outpatients, it may be the same type of identification armband or a driver's license, a nurse in charge of the patient, or the patient's parent/guardian) (Figures 10–17 and **10–18**). If the patient is identified by a nurse or parent, that person's name should be documented as the one who confirmed identity.

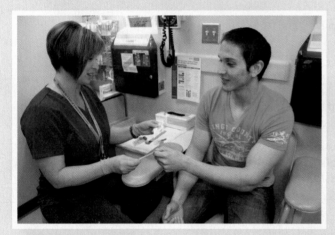

FIGURE 10–17

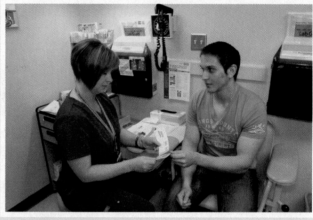

FIGURE 10–18

4 If the tests ordered require a fasting specimen, ask the patient, "When was the last time you ate or drank anything?" Wait for the reply and, if necessary, document the dietary facts accordingly.

5 If any supplies (gloves, tourniquets, bandages, etc.) contain latex, ask the patient about latex sensitivity by saying, "Are you allergic or sensitive to latex products?" Wait for the reply and use alternative supplies/equipment if necessary.

6 It is especially important to ask ambulatory patients about their likelihood of fainting by saying, "Have you ever fainted or felt faint during a blood collection procedure?" Wait for the reply and position the patient in a safe phlebotomy position, recliner, bed, or chair based on the circumstances.

7 Although not always required, it is considerate to ask the patient about arm preference for the procedure. Use good judgment about arm selection and always follow your facility's procedures.

throughout all phases of laboratory testing (preexamination/preanalytical, examination/analytical, postexamination/postanalytical). Correct identification is mandatory for accurate laboratory results on which clinical decisions are made by physicians, nurses, and other members of the health care team. Patient identification errors can occur either at the time of phlebotomy or as the specimen is being prepared for testing—for example, after centrifugation when the specimen is divided into aliquots. The College of American Pathologists requires that each container/aliquot with a patient's specimen be identified. The unique identification for that particular patient can be "text based, bar coded, and so on," depending on the laboratory's discretion so long as "all primary collection containers and their aliquots have a unique label which one can audit back to full particulars of patient identification, collection date, specimen type, etc."[7] The process of identifying patients varies slightly based on the patient's location (inpatient or outpatient or emergency room), the type of patient (pediatric or adult), whether the patient is conscious or unconscious, and the available information at the time (armband or picture identification).

SPECIAL CONSIDERATIONS[1]

Inpatient Identification

Hospitalized patients (except those just entering an emergency room) must wear an identification armband/bracelet indicating their first and last names and a designated hospital number (often called a *unit number* or a *medical record number*). Hospital identification numbers help hospital personnel distinguish between patients with the same first and/or last names. Information on the identification bracelet may also include the patient's room number, bed assignment, and physician's name; however, the key information used for phlebotomy procedures is the name, identification number, birth date, and/or address.

Outpatient/Ambulatory Patient Identification

Ambulatory patients are normally called to a blood collection area from a waiting room. When calling a patient's name in the waiting room, health care workers must be careful to state only the name and not to reveal any confidential clinical information. Alternative methods for dealing with patients in a waiting room may involve the use of a numbering system or paging device. Thus, ambulatory patient identification may be slightly more time consuming because the patients are usually escorted into the specimen collection area first, and they may lack an armband, which would provide an easy visual check. Although not the majority, some ambulatory clinics issue identification bracelets to patients. Many clinics, however, distribute identification cards to patients before any specimens are collected. If this is the case, and the patient has the card available, positive identification can occur in the same manner as with hospitalized patients. These cards can also be used to make an imprinted label for the specimen if an Addressograph/imprint machine is used. If the patient does not have a patient identification armband or card, it is strongly recommended that another form of identification (e.g., driver's license or ID card with photograph) be checked and documented prior to specimen collection. Again, the identification process would involve verbally asking for name, identification number, address, and/or birth date. The verbal information is compared with the requisition and any other form of identity available.

Identification of Patients Who Are Comatose, Semiconscious, or Sleeping

A patient who is sleeping should be awakened before collecting the blood, and the patient identity verified as previously stated. Verbal information should be compared with the information on the requisition and the identification bracelet. If a patient is comatose or semiconscious, a nurse, relative, or friend may identify the patient by providing the patient's name, address, and identification number and/or birth date. Again, this information should be compared with the information on the requisition to confirm identity. Any discrepancy should be reported to a supervisor. Document the individual who verifies identity. Keep in mind that a patient who is semiconscious may move unexpectedly during the procedure.

Identification of Infants and Young Children

It is preferable to use the same identification procedures for both children and adults; however, it is not always practical or feasible. A nurse, guardian, or relative may identify an infant or child by providing the name, address, and identification number, and/

Clinical Alert!

- Do *not* ask, "Are you Ms. Doe?" because an ill patient on medication may mistakenly utter something, nod, or answer yes. Consequently, the best tactic is to ask, "What is your name?" and let the patient reply.

- Do *not* base identity on records or charts placed on the patient's bed or equipment.

- Do not collect a specimen from a patient whose identity is not confirmed or assured or if there is a discrepancy in the identification process. The specimen should not be obtained until identity can be fully verified. Report discrepancies immediately to a supervisor.

or birth date. Again, the name of the verifier should be documented.

Emergency Room Patient Identification

Because all patients must be positively identified, patients who come to the emergency room (ER) unconscious and/or unidentified pose a situation in which the health care worker must be particularly careful. A temporary master identification (e.g., hospital number attached to the patient's body by wristband or other suitable device) may be provided until a positive identification can be made. Using the appropriate test request, ensure that the master identification number is recorded on the requisitions/labels. Complete the necessary labels either by hand or electronically and apply the labels to the specimens. When a permanent identification number is assigned to the patient, the temporary identification number should be cross-referenced to the permanent number to ensure correct identification and correlation of patient and test result information.

Patients with Severe Burns or in Isolation

Occasionally there are special cases, such as patients with severe burns or in isolation, in which the identification is attached to the patient's bed rather than the arm. These are the *only* circumstances in which a health care worker may use a bed-labeled identification tag to confirm identity, and these rare occasions are subject to additional institutional policies. This step should be followed up by a nurse's confirmation and appropriate documentation. Normally, a name card on the bed or door should *never* be used for confirming identity, because sometimes the tags are not changed in a timely manner when patients are discharged and new patients are admitted.

IDENTITY ERRORS ARE PREVENTABLE

Identity errors occur because of inaccurate requisitions, mixed-up paperwork, or failure to follow identification procedures. Collecting blood from the wrong patient can lead to serious consequences, such as incorrect treatment or therapy, and ultimately, may result in death. It is a violation for which health care workers may be counseled, dismissed from their jobs, or even sued. Since patient identification errors can be life threatening for the patient, they pose significant legal liability to both the health care worker who makes the error and to the health care facility that employs him or her. Following the precise procedures each time will prevent mistakes.

As mentioned in Chapter 2, new technology continues to provide enhancements to identification methods. Two-dimensional bar code technologies as well as radio frequency identification systems enable more information (including entire medical records) to be encoded on wristbands and labels. Information can be entered or retrieved from a chip in the wristband for record keeping. In addition, photo identification wristbands have an additional measure of positively identifying a patient, and they have become more reliable, more resistant to tearing or tampering, and more cost effective.[10,11] The more information that is available to identify patients correctly, the less likely identity mistakes become. Each new identification system must be evaluated by the health care facility for accuracy, susceptibility to fraud, usefulness for the end user, cost effectiveness, training involved, compatibility with existing technology, compatibility with electronic medical records, ease of updating records, access and security issues, failure rates, and ability to ensure privacy.

Equipment Selection and Preparation

SUPPLIES FOR VENIPUNCTURE

Supplies for venipuncture differ according to the method used—for example, *evacuated tube system* or *winged infusion/butterfly system*, or syringe method—and the tests that have been ordered. Phlebotomy supplies are usually transported in specially designed carts or trays that should be kept clean and clutter free. Supplies common to most methods of blood collection include the following:

- Gloves—disposable latex and nonlatex alternatives, such as vinyl, polyethylene, or nitrile gloves, gloves without powdered lubricant, or cotton gloves worn underneath latex gloves

- Tourniquet—single use, disposable, and preferably latex-free; blood pressure cuff inflated to 40 mmHg; rubber or fabric-type tourniquets with closure tape, plastic clip, buckle, or other fastener

- Antiseptics, such as alcohol pads, or other skin disinfectants, such as chlorhexidine gluconate swabs

- Nonalcohol antiseptics—for example, chlorhexidine gluconate—if blood alcohol levels are requested

- Chlorhexidine disinfectant prep kits or swab sticks if blood cultures are requested

- Prepackaged gauze pads (do not use cotton balls because of the possibility of the cotton fibers sticking to the blood clot/scab at the puncture site and/or possibly dislodging it)

- Hypoallergenic adhesive bandages and gauze wraps (for more sensitive skin)

- Glass microscope slides, when needed

- Sterile needles with single-use, evacuated tube holders and winged infusion sets

- Plastic capillary tubes with tube sealer

- Sterile syringes and syringe transfer devices

- Blood collection tubes—sterile and evacuated so as to collect a predetermined volume of blood

- Laboratory requisitions or labels

- Ice or refrigerant for specimens that need to be chilled

- Warming devices for dilating blood vessels (not to exceed 42°C)

- Warming device for specimens that need to be kept warm, when needed

- Marking pens

- Puncture-resistant disposal container

- Laboratory test manual (tube requirements for individual tests, specimen handling and precautionary instructions, package inserts for tube use, etc.)

Supplies, which are discussed in more detail in Chapter 8, should be readily available and selected just prior to the procedure.

VENIPUNCTURE SITE SELECTION

It is important to choose the least hazardous site that has the greatest likelihood of successful blood collection by venipuncture. Several techniques can facilitate the selection of a suitable site, including the use of a tourniquet (a tourniquet may not always be necessary if veins are large and easily palpated) and warming the site to increase blood flow to the area. The visibility of veins varies highly with each individual's skin color, weight, physiologic conditions, gender, and physical features. Therefore, the health care worker must rely on the sense of touch (palpation) to locate the vein. The health care worker should palpate and trace the path of veins with an index finger before the venipuncture to establish the safest site for the puncture and to make sure that the vessel is indeed a vein and not an artery. Review Chapter 7 for more details about the differences between veins, arteries, and capillaries. Refer to **FIGURES 10–19, 10–20, 10–21,** and **10–22** to visualize vein placement and variability. Palpating the antecubital area usually helps get an idea of the size, angle, and depth of the vein, and which veins are most prominent in each patient. For some patients, the median cubital vein is more prominent than the cephalic or basilic veins, and in other patients, the reverse is true. Whatever the case, the health care worker must carefully select the most suitable vein. The patient can assist in the process by closing the fist tightly for a short period. (The patient should not open and close the fist rapidly, i.e., pumping the fist, because it can cause localized hemoconcentration.) It is important to remember that patients' veins may also be used for transfusion, infusion, and therapeutic agents. Thus, sometimes physicians request that veins have restricted use ("are reserved") for those purposes only.

If no vein becomes apparent, or "pops up," the patient may be asked to dangle the arm for one to two minutes to allow blood to fill the veins to capacity. Then the tourniquet may be reapplied and the area palpated again. However, the area should not be excessively palpated or tapped because it may compromise test results. The health care worker should never stick a vein unless it can be felt. It is better to defer the patient to someone else who can search for the vein than to take a blind chance.

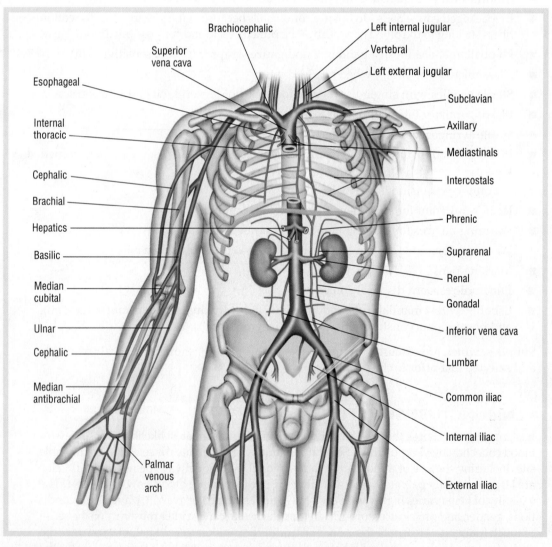

FIGURE 10–19

Venous Circulation of the Arm, Abdomen, and Chest

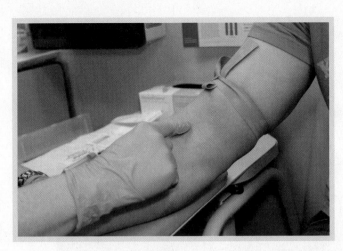

FIGURE 10–20
Palpating the Vein

Arm veins cannot always be seen and even when seen, they vary dramatically among individuals. Learn to find a good vein by feeling or palpating the arm prior to venipuncture.

FIGURE 10–21
Typical Veins of the Arm

A. A human hand and arm labeled with prominent veins. B. Arm of a healthy adult male where the median cubital and basilic veins are visible and also palpable.

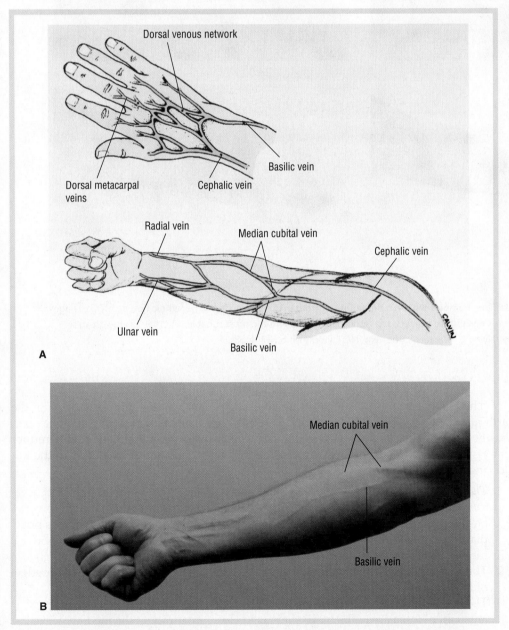

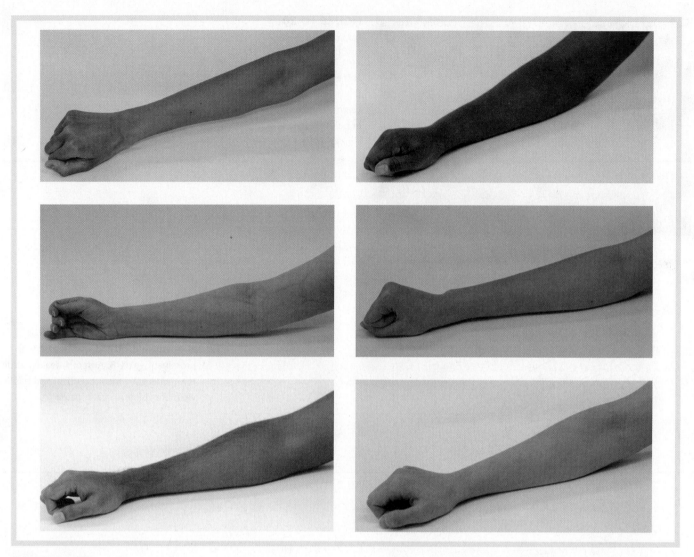

FIGURE 10–22

Vein Variation

Vein patterns are different for every person. The examples shown in this figure are from people of varying races, ethnicities, gender, and ages. Some veins are visible and others are not. For health care workers, the responsibility is to find the most suitable vein that has the greatest likelihood for a successful venipuncture by relying on the feel of the vein, NOT simply on how it looks.

The most common sites for routine venipuncture are in the antecubital area of the arm just below the bend of the elbow. This is where the median cubital, cephalic, and basilic veins lie close to the surface of the skin and are most prominent. In order to reduce the risks of puncturing an artery or injuring a nerve, consider vein selection in the following orders.[12]

1. *The* median cubital, *often referred to as the* median vein, *is the preferred and most commonly used vein for venipuncture* because it is the easiest to obtain blood from, has been reported to be less painful, and is less prone to injury if the needle is not placed precisely in the vein. The health care worker should try to locate suitable median veins on both arms before considering other veins.

2. The second choice of vein should be the cephalic vein, which lies on the outer edge of the arm.

3. The third choice should be the basilic vein, which lies on the inside edge of the antecubital fossa area. The basilic vein is in close proximity to the median nerve

and the brachial artery, so the other choices are usually preferable. Do *not* use the patient's arm veins in the following circumstances:

- Intravenous (IV) lines in both arms
- Burned or scarred areas
- Areas with a hematoma
- Cast(s) on arm(s)
- Thrombosed veins (thrombosed veins lack resilience, feel much like a rope cord, and roll easily)
- Edematous arms (swollen area due to tissue fluid retention)
- Partial or radical mastectomy on one or both sides

4. Veins on the dorsal side of the hands or wrists (i.e., the back side) are acceptable venipuncture sites if the median cubital, cephalic, or basilic veins are inaccessible. Veins in the wrist tend to move, or roll aside, as the needle is inserted; therefore, it may be helpful to have the patient extend the hand into a position that helps hold the vein taut. Do *not* collect blood from the underside of the wrist (palm side of the hand) because tendons and nerves lie very close to the palmar venous network and can easily be injured by the needle (**FIGURE 10–23**). Venipuncture from a hand vein is usually done with a butterfly needle. Refer to Procedure 10–7 later in this chapter for more details about venipuncture from a hand vein.

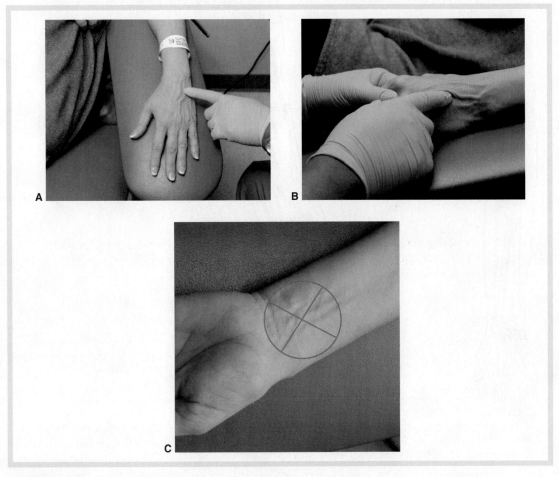

FIGURE 10–23
Dorsal or Backside of the Hand

A. Veins on the dorsal/backside of the hand can be used for venipuncture. **B.** Even though the veins are visible and palpable, they are more prone to rolling sideways during a venipuncture procedure. Note how the vein can be easily pushed to one side. Refer to Procedure 10–7. **C.** Veins on the palm side of the wrist are not acceptable for venipuncture.

Clinical Alert!

- Nerve damage during a venipuncture is rare but has been known to occur due to poor technique, excessive needle probing, sudden movements of the patient, etc. Serious damage can occur if a nerve is accidentally punctured or nicked during the venipuncture procedure. If the patient complains of severe, shooting pain; a tingling sensation; or numbness during the procedure, the tourniquet and needle must be removed *immediately* and the procedure discontinued. Assistance should be sought from a nurse or supervisor. Only a physician can evaluate whether nerve damage has occurred. Nevertheless, the incident should be documented. **FIGURE 10–24** depicts the proximity of nerves in relation to the veins.

- Remember that arteries do not feel like veins. Arteries pulsate, are more elastic, and have a thick wall. Accidental arterial puncture may result in excessive bleeding and hematoma formation. If the health care worker believes an artery has been punctured, the needle should be removed immediately, and direct pressure should be applied to the site for at least 5 minutes or until bleeding has stopped. A supervisor or nurse and the patient's physician should be notified.

- Patients who have had mastectomies often have lymph nodes removed from the same surgical area. Without lymph vessels to remove fluid, swelling occurs on the affected side of the body. Thus, blood should not be collected from the mastectomy side unless approved by the physician.

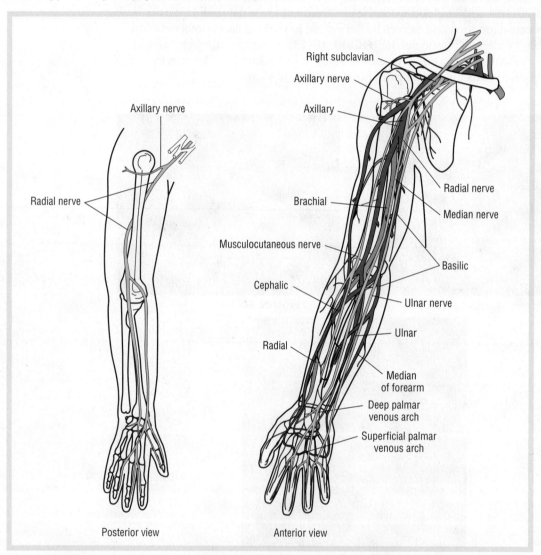

FIGURE 10–24

Arm Veins (blue), Arteries (red), and Nerves (yellow)

Note that several important nerves and arteries pass very close to, or through, the antecubital area where most venipunctures occur. In particular, note the position of the brachial artery and median nerve as they pass through the antecubital area. Both are close to the basilic vein. This is why the basilic vein is not a first choice for a venipuncture site.

5. Ankle and foot veins (on the dorsal, or upper, side) should be used *only* if arm veins have been determined to be unsuitable and with appropriate authorization. Arm veins are preferred sites over foot or ankle veins because coagulation and vascular complications tend to be more troublesome in the lower extremities, especially for diabetic patients. Some hospitals do not allow health care workers to use the lower extremities (foot and ankle) for blood-sampling sites. Other hospitals allow sampling from these sites only after permission is granted from the patient's physician. Venipuncture in small veins is facilitated by the use of a small-gauge safety butterfly needle.

TOOLS TO MAKE DIFFICULT VEINS MORE PROMINENT

The standard method for finding a vein is by palpation in the antecubital area, most often after the application of a tourniquet. Refer to **PROCEDURE 10–4**. However, when veins are hard to find even after using a tourniquet, there are a few tools that assist in making veins more prominent. The tourniquet should not be tight when using these tools. It is important to take the time at the beginning to assure that a suitable vein is located. The following are presented in order from the simplest to more complex and/or time-consuming methods:

- Sometimes the quickest and most effective way to improve the chances of palpating a "good" vein is to ask the patient to position the arm in a downward, relaxed position with fingertips pointing to the floor (for approximately a minute or less). This allows blood to quickly fill the veins to capacity simply by using gravity; it provides a natural, unobtrusive way to increase blood volume in the arm.

- Warming the puncture site helps facilitate phlebotomy by increasing arterial blood flow to the area.

  - If the patient is ambulatory, ask the patient to rinse the arm/hand in warm water for 1 minute.

  - Use commercially available warming packs that are quick and easy to activate and provide localized heat to the potential venipuncture area. The pack should be applied for an adequate amount of time to allow the warmth to penetrate the skin surface. Follow the manufacturer's instructions. Refer to **FIGURE 10–25**.

  - Use a clean towel or a washcloth heated to about 42°C. When the warm towel is wrapped around the site for 3 to 5 minutes, the skin temperature can increase several degrees. The wrap can be encased in a plastic bag to help retain heat and keep the patient's bed dry. The health care worker may leave the warm wrap on the patient while collecting specimens from other patients and then return to the original patient after several minutes.

- Use an assistive device such as the Venoscope Transilluminator or Accuvein Viewing System (refer to Chapter 8 for more details) to show vein pattern and orientation for assistance in vein location (**FIGURE 10–26**).

- Using ultrasound for vein mapping involves high-frequency sound waves to obtain images of veins. Since ultrasound equipment is easily portable, this technique has been used for patients with very difficult veins. It enables vein location when veins cannot be felt or seen from the skin surface. Ultrasound technology has been commonly used for years to evaluate veins that are going to be surgically removed or altered (e.g., for varicose veins, dialysis, etc.). However, applications for venipuncture are usually reserved for special patients whose veins have been damaged by long-term therapy or surgery, or are very difficult to locate. The procedure is not invasive but requires more time and special training to apply the gel and move the ultrasound transducer across

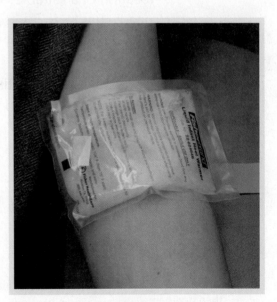

FIGURE 10–25

Disposable Warmer

Use a commercially available warming packet to increase blood flow to the area. In this case, the warmer is a disposable, single-use pack that is also designed for use as an infant heel warmer. Directions for use are printed directly on the pack.

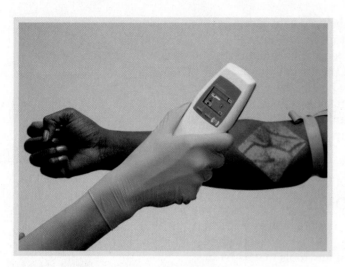

FIGURE 10–26
AccuVein

This is one type of device useful in vein location.

the arm to visualize the veins on a screen. Marks are usually made on the body to identify the location. Marks should not be removed until the doctor has given authorization to do so. Although this is not usually in the scope of duties for many health care workers, it may become more accepted in hospitals for specialized care of specific patients.

TOURNIQUET APPLICATION

A **tourniquet** or blood pressure cuff makes veins more prominent and easier to puncture by slowing down the blood flow toward the heart, thereby causing venous filling. A soft rubber tourniquet about 1 inch (2.5 cm) wide and about 15 to 18 inches (45 cm) long is most comfortable for patients, affordable, and easy to use. Tourniquets come in a variety of colors, as shown in Procedure 10–4.

PROCEDURE 10–4

Use of a Tourniquet and Vein Palpation

Rationale Tourniquet application causes veins to fill with blood, thereby assisting in the location of a suitable venipuncture site and enabling easier blood flow once the needle has been inserted. Palpating the vein helps the health care worker establish size, angle, and depth of the vein. A single-use policy is usually adopted for each tourniquet to minimize the risk of transmitting infections from one patient to the next. However, sometimes one tourniquet can be allotted to one patient for multiple venipunctures. In this case, it should not be shared or used for other patients.

Equipment

- Latex-free, clean, single-use tourniquet
- Gloves
- Alcohol-based hand disinfectants

Preparation

1 Identify the patient properly.

2 Wash or sanitize your hands using appropriate agents, then dry them.

3 Ask the patient to extend the arm fully. Some procedures call for gloving prior to vein selection. However, others allow for vein selection with the health care worker's clean index finger, followed by gloving.

Procedure

4 Use a clean latex-free tourniquet (**FIGURE 10–27**). It is preferable to use a "single-use" tourniquet for each patient.

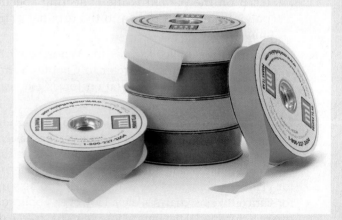

FIGURE 10–27

Courtesy of MarketLab: www.marketlabinc.com

PROCEDURE 10–4

Use of a Tourniquet and Vein Palpation (continued)

5 Stretch the ends of the tourniquet around the patient's arm about 3 to 4 inches (7.5 to 10 cm) above the venipuncture area (antecubital area). Hold both ends of the tourniquet in one hand while the other hand tucks in a section next to the skin and makes a partial loop with the tourniquet (**FIGURE 10–28**).

6 Make sure the tourniquet is tight but not painful to the patient. Do *not* leave it on for more than 1 minute. Do *not* place it over sores or burned skin; however, depending on the policies of each health care facility, it may be placed over a hospital gown sleeve or a piece of gauze. Use alternative types of tourniquets when necessary. (If using a blood pressure cuff as a tourniquet, inflate it to 40 mm Hg and release it at the same time as a tourniquet.)

7 Palpate the antecubital area to locate the safest vein, as mentioned previously (Figure 10–28).

8 Once the vein is selected, begin the decontamination procedure (**PROCEDURE 10–5**). If gloves were not put on earlier, put gloves on and then proceed.

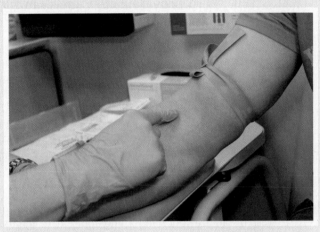

FIGURE 10–28

After the Venipuncture

9 Refer to Procedure 10–6 later in this chapter. When it is time to release the tourniquet, the partial loop should allow for easy release by the health care worker. (For patient comfort and to obtain a good specimen, do not leave the tourniquet on the patient's arm while readying supplies to perform the initial puncture, especially if the process takes longer than 1 minute. If there is a time delay, reapply the tourniquet.) Release it after the needle puncture, when blood has begun to flow into the collection tubes. During the venipuncture, release the tourniquet with one hand, because the other hand will be holding the needle and tubes.

10 Once released, it can remain loosely on the arm or surface of the work area (e.g., bed or blood collection chair) until the procedure is completed (**FIGURE 10–29**). Again, for infection control purpose, tourniquets are designed to be single use or used only on the same patient. Follow the policy for your health care facility.

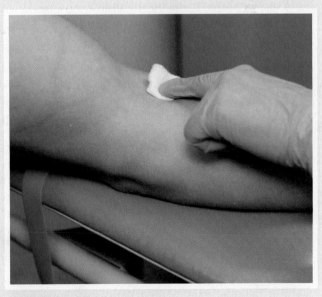

FIGURE 10–29

PROCEDURE 10–5

Decontamination of the Puncture Site

Rationale   To provide a *clean/decontaminated* area of the skin in which to make the needle puncture.

Equipment/Supplies

- Gloves
- Commercially packaged alcohol pads or gauze pads soaked in 70% isopropanol (isopropyl alcohol)
- Blood culture decontamination kits/swabs (e.g., chlorhexidine)

Preparation

1 Identify the patient properly.

2 Wash or sanitize your hands using appropriate agents, dry them, then put on gloves.

Procedure

3 Once the site is selected, cleanse it with a commercially packaged alcohol pad or with a gauze pad soaked in 70% isopropanol (isopropyl alcohol).

4 Rub the site with the alcohol pad, working in concentric circles from the inside out. If the skin is particularly dirty, repeat the process with a new alcohol pad (**FIGURE 10–30**).

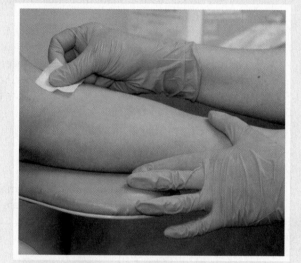

FIGURE 10–30

5 Remember to cleanse the site again if you intend to touch or palpate the site again. Allow the site to air dry (Figure 10–30) or use a sterile dry gauze to wipe once in a downward motion.

6 If blood cultures are requested, additional site preparation is required. Follow your health care facility's standard operating procedures for blood culture collections. Chlorhexidine preparations are primarily used for collecting blood for blood gas analysis and blood cultures. Follow the manufacturer's directions for appropriate decontamination results. However, most prep kit instructions include a two- or three-step scrub procedure, each step taking 30 to 60 seconds, so be prepared to spend more time with this type of cleansing process. Chlorhexidine products are more often used than iodine products because iodine may interfere with some types of analytical instrumentation and some patients are allergic to iodine. If blood cultures have not been ordered, routine venipuncture preparation and cleansing is with alcohol. If a patient is allergic to alcohol, again chlorhexidine cleansers can be used. However, chlorhexidine gluconate is not recommended for infants less than 2 months old.[1] For more detailed information about blood cultures, refer to Chapter 15.

7 After the site has been cleansed, reapply the tourniquet and proceed with the venipuncture procedure.

DECONTAMINATION OF THE PUNCTURE SITE

Once the site is selected, it should be cleansed with a commercially packaged alcohol pad or with a gauze pad soaked in 70% isopropanol (isopropyl alcohol). This prevents microbiological contamination of the patient and the specimen. The health care worker should rub the site, working in concentric circles from the inside out. If the skin is particularly dirty, the process should be repeated with a new alcohol pad. Also, if the health care worker needs to palpate the site again after cleansing it, the worker should cleanse it again. The site should be air dried or may be wiped off using a sterile gauze pad in one downward motion.

Chlorhexidine preparations, povidone–iodine (Betadine) or iodine preparations, and/or multiple isopropyl alcohol preps are primarily used for collecting blood specimens for blood gas analysis and/or blood cultures (see Chapter 15, "Blood Cultures, Arterial, Intravenous (IV), and Special Collection Procedures"). Efforts should be made to remove iodine from the skin with sterile gauze or alcohol after decontamination because excess iodine can interfere with some laboratory tests. Also, since iodine causes skin irritations for some patients and others may be allergic to both iodine and/or alcohol, chlorhexidine has become a commonly used alternative skin decontaminant.[1]

Clinical Alert!

- The cleansed area should never be touched with any nonsterile object.
- The alcohol should be allowed to dry (approximately 30 to 60 seconds), or should be wiped off with sterile gauze after the site is prepared; otherwise, the puncture site will sting, and the alcohol may interfere with test results, such as blood alcohol levels. Therefore, if blood alcohol levels are requested, do not use alcohol for skin cleansing.
- Blowing on the site to hasten the drying process is *not* advised because doing so may recontaminate the site.

Clinical Alert !

The tourniquet should not be left on for more than 1 minute, because it becomes uncomfortable and causes hemoconcentration—that is, blood infiltrates the surrounding tissues, thereby increasing venous blood concentration of large molecules, such as proteins, cells, and coagulation factors. The patient may be allowed to make a fist for a short period but excessive clenching and unclenching also results in hemoconcentration and should be avoided.

Venipuncture Methods

EVACUATED TUBE SYSTEM AND WINGED INFUSION SYSTEM, OR BUTTERFLY METHOD

As mentioned in Chapter 8, blood collection supplies should meet all safety regulations and reduce the risks of occupational exposure. CLSI recommends that venipuncture specimens be collected with a system that enables blood to flow directly into the tubes.[1] Evacuated tube systems and *winged infusion systems* (butterfly) are widely available, equipped with safety devices that comply with this recommendation. **PROCEDURE 10–6** demonstrates a basic venipuncture technique. However, some health care facilities and/or educational training programs may vary their procedures. Health care workers should follow those procedures accordingly.

PROCEDURE 10–6

Performing a Venipuncture Using the Evacuated Tube Method

Rationale   To provide a safe, reliable, effective, and efficient method to obtain blood specimens.

Equipment

- Personal protective equipment (PPE): gloves, clean uniform, laboratory coat, etc.
- Laboratory requisitions and/or labels
- Evacuated specimen tubes and blood culture bottles (**FIGURE 10–31**)
- Sterile, single-use safety needles (for evacuated tube holders and winged-infusion/butterfly sets)
- Tube holders
- Nonlatex tourniquet
- Antiseptics—alcohol pads and/or other skin disinfectants
- Marking pens
- Electronic reader/scanner (if applicable)
- Blood culture decontamination swab kits (chlorhexidine compounds, povidone-iodine, etc.)
- Bandages (hypoallergenic adhesive bandages, gauze pads, and tape)

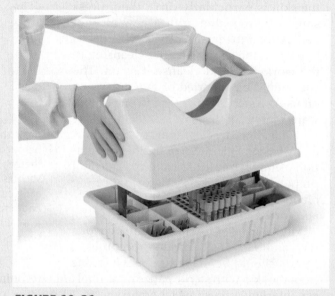

FIGURE 10–31

Courtesy of MarketLab: www.marketlabinc.com

Preparation

Preparation phases prior to venipuncture are described in Procedures 10–1 through 10–5.

1 After greeting, assessing, and identifying the patient (**FIGURE 10–32**), decontaminate your hands, and check the antecubital area for a suitable vein.

2 Assemble supplies and double-check the expiration dates and integrity of the collection tubes. Gently tap the tubes containing additives to remove any additive that may be adhering to the closure/stopper.

3 Offer to answer any questions for the patient while putting on your gloves (if you haven't already done so).

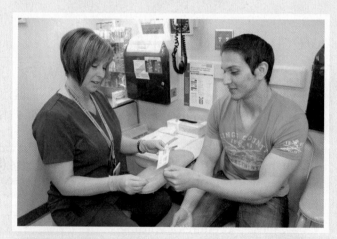

FIGURE 10–32

PROCEDURE 10–6

Performing a Venipuncture Using the Evacuated Tube Method (continued)

4 Position the patient's arm in a straight (or slightly bent) downward manner that is comfortable, apply the tourniquet in the correct location, and cleanse the puncture site (**FIGURE 10–33**).

Procedure

Venipuncture can be accomplished by using either an evacuated tube system or a winged-infusion/butterfly needle system. The steps listed here are typical for either venipuncture system but special considerations for the winged-infusion/butterfly method are described in **PROCEDURE 10–7**. It shows the use of the winged infusion/butterfly needle for smaller veins.

5 After thoroughly going through the preparation and patient identification phases, prepare specific supplies according to the manufacturer's instructions, including attaching a needle onto the appropriate holder when necessary. Be sure that the needle is securely attached so that it does not unthread or detach during use.

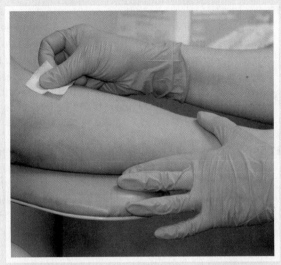

FIGURE 10–33

6 Position the patient's arm so that it is slightly bent from the shoulder to the wrist and is in a downward position (Figure 10–33). Apply the tourniquet and check for potential sites by palpating the vein. Remember, feel for the median cubital vein first (it is usually bigger and anchored better); the cephalic vein (depending on its size) is the second choice (it does not roll and bruise as easily as the basilic); and the basilic vein is third choice. If a suitable vein is not felt, remove the tourniquet and try the other arm or other appropriate sites mentioned in the text. As mentioned earlier, do not leave the tourniquet on for more than 1 minute. Choose a vein that feels the fullest. If needed, use other strategies mentioned previously to improve vein selection (e.g., warming the site and lowering the arm in a downward position).

7 Select the site and cleanse the patient's skin with an alcohol pad in a circular motion from inside to outside. Allow the site to air dry and do not blow on it. Reapply the tourniquet if it was removed and allow the patient to "make a fist" for a brief time if the patient chooses to do so. Some health care workers believe that this makes veins more prominent and easier to puncture. However, vigorous hand exercise or "pumping or clenching" should be avoided because it affects some laboratory values. Prepare the patient by mentioning, "you will feel a stick," or say, "Please remain still while I begin the procedure; you will feel a slight prick." Do not say "This won't hurt." Be mindful that from this step forward, a patient may feel faint and/or lose consciousness. Remember: Do not touch the venipuncture area after cleansing it.

8 Remove the needle cap carefully so as not to touch anything that would contaminate it. Check the needle for defects and replace it if it is defective. If it does touch any surface that is not sterile, replace it with a new needle assembly and discard the old one.

9 Hold the needle assembly in one hand while the thumb of the other hand anchors the vein 1 to 2 inches (2.5 to 5.0 cm) below the puncture site. (Some health care workers use the thumb and forefinger of the free hand to anchor the vein. Others place the last three fingers of the free hand under the elbow to steady the arm even more.)

(continued)

PROCEDURE 10–6

Performing a Venipuncture Using the Evacuated Tube Method (continued)

10 Position the needle so that it is oriented in the same direction as the vein and is at a slight angle (30 degrees or less) with the skin surface. (An angle greater than 30 degrees is too steep and will increase the chances of going completely through the vein and/or of hitting a deeper artery, nerve, or tendons.) With the bevel side up, insert the needle quickly. A slight "pop" should be felt as the needle enters the vein (**FIGURES 10–34**, **10–35**, and **10–36**).

11 While keeping the needle assembly stable in the vein, center the first collection tube in the holder and *gently* push it onto the holder (**FIGURE 10–37**). As the tube is pushed into the holder, the inner needle punctures the diaphragm of the closure. Blood should begin to flow into the tube (**FIGURE 10–38**).

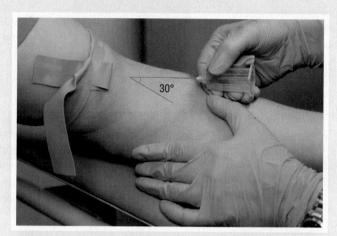

FIGURE 10–34

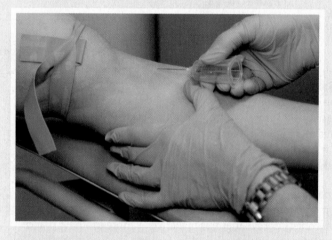

FIGURE 10–35

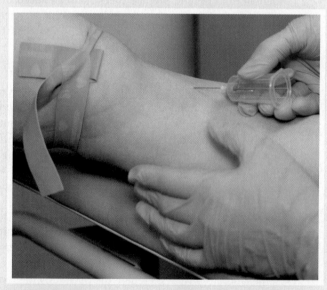

FIGURE 10–36

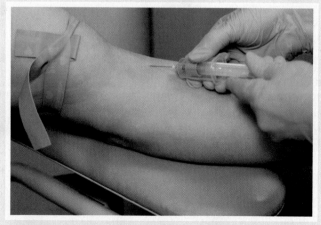

FIGURE 10–37

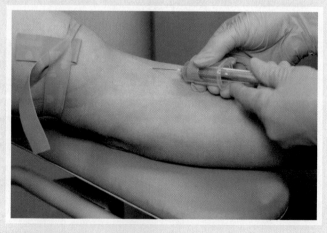

FIGURE 10–38

PROCEDURE 10–6

Performing a Venipuncture Using the Evacuated Tube Method (continued)

12 If blood does not flow, palpate gently above the puncture to feel for the vein and possibly reorient the needle *slightly*. Do not probe!

13 As the blood begins to flow, instruct the patient to open the fist, and release the tourniquet (**FIGURE 10–39**). (The tourniquet can be left on until the tubes have filled if it appears that blood flow is slow and it has *not* been on for over a minute; however, remember that prolonged tourniquet use causes other complications, including an increased risk of a hematoma in patients with fragile veins. Use your best judgment for each tourniquet application, but always remove it *before* withdrawing the needle.) Keep the needle as stable as possible during this step. Carefully push an evacuated tube into the holder so that the tube closure is punctured by the inside needle and blood can enter. Orient the tube in a downward position so as to avoid any possibility of backflow of additives into the patient, which can cause adverse reactions.

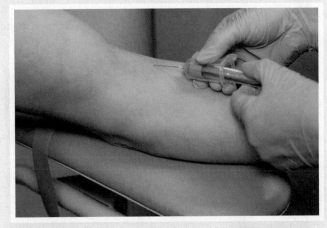

FIGURE 10–39

14 Allow the blood to flow into each collection tube until it stops (when the tube vacuum is exhausted) so that the proper dilution of blood to additive can occur. Watch carefully to see when the blood flow ceases. If multiple sample tubes are to be collected, remove each tube from the holder with a gentle twist-and-pull motion and replace it with the next tube (**FIGURE 10–40**).

During tube transfer, be mindful of these key issues:

- Hold the needle apparatus firmly and motionlessly so that the needle remains comfortable and in the vein during tube changes.

- Keep additive tubes in a downward position.

- Follow the correct "order of draw."

- Always remove the last tube of blood from the tube holder's inner needle before removing the needle from the patient's vein.

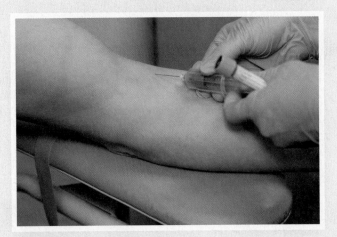

FIGURE 10–40

- Remember that blood stops flowing between tube changes because of the inner needle design, which allows a sleeve to block blood flow if it is not in use.

Tubes with additives should be gently inverted for mixing. A complete inversion means turning the filled tube upside-down then returning it to an upright position. Most additive tubes require 3 to 10 inversions, depending on the manufacturer's instructions. Experienced health care workers can gently mix/invert a full tube in one hand while holding the needle apparatus and waiting for another tube to fill. Some health care workers switch hands to use a dominant hand during tube exchange. Whatever the method, find the approach that is most reliable and comfortable for both patient and health care worker.

(continued)

PROCEDURE 10–6

Performing a Venipuncture Using the Evacuated Tube Method (continued)

15 When all tubes have been filled and removed from the holder, remove the tourniquet if it has not already been done, withdraw the needle, and hold a gauze pad over the site (**FIGURES 10–41** and **10–42**).

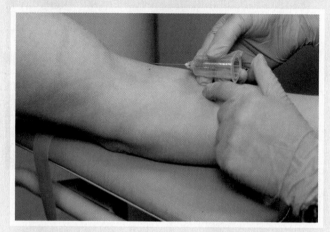

FIGURE 10–41

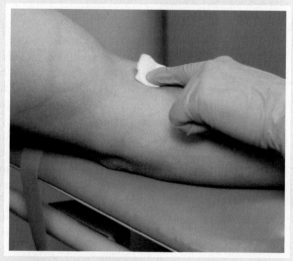

FIGURE 10–42

16 Activate the safety device according to the manufacturer's instructions. This may involve resheathing/covering the needle once it has been withdrawn (**FIGURES 10–43** and **10–44**) or activating a device that covers the needle prior to withdrawal from the vein, as shown in Procedure 10–7. Discard the needle device in an appropriate container (**FIGURE 10–45**).

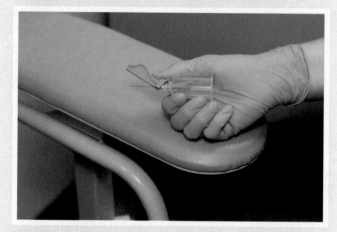

FIGURE 10–43

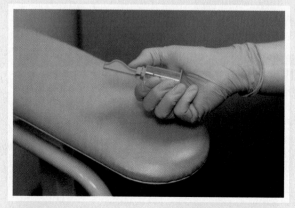

FIGURE 10–44

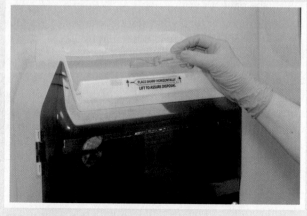

FIGURE 10–45

PROCEDURE 10–6

Performing a Venipuncture Using the Evacuated Tube Method (continued)

17 If the patient is capable (not elderly, or a child, or coma-tose), instruct the patient to apply pressure to the site using the gauze. If necessary, continue gentle inversion of the specimen tubes for complete mixing of additives with the blood. Remember: Do not shake the tubes (**FIGURE 10–46**).

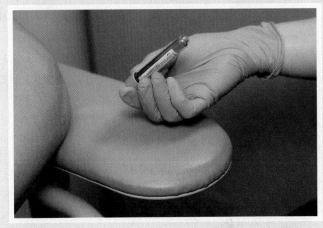

FIGURE 10–46

18 Apply pressure until the bleeding has stopped (or ask the patient to assist), then apply a bandage (**FIGURE 10–47**). In the patient's presence, label specimens appropriately using preprinted labels or handwritten ones (patient's first and last name, identification number, date, time of collection, and health care worker's initials) (**FIGURE 10–48**). Ask the patient to reconfirm identity on the labeled speci-men (**FIGURE 10–49**).

After the Procedure

19 Dispose of contaminated supplies and equipment.

20 Double-check to make sure that the bleeding has stopped.

21 Thank the patient for cooperating and depart with all specimens and remaining supplies.

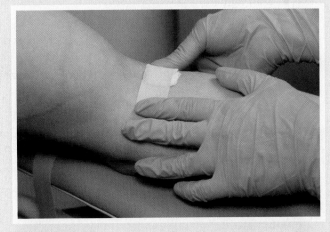

FIGURE 10–47

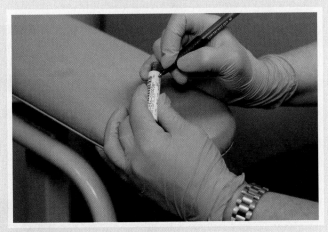

FIGURE 10–48

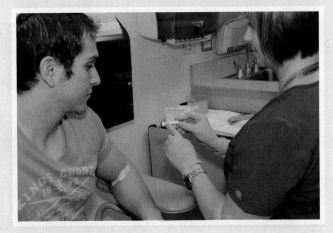

FIGURE 10–49

PROCEDURE 10–7

Hand Vein Venipuncture Using a Winged Infusion/Butterfly Set

Rationale   Winged infusion or butterfly needle devices are useful for venipuncture from smaller veins. Use of this system requires training and practice, and smaller veins require more care as the site is being selected and prepared. Many patients report that these types of devices are less painful, perhaps due to a smaller needle size. However, they are typically more expensive than the traditional venipuncture devices.

Equipment/Supplies

- Personal protective equipment (PPE): gloves, clean uniform, laboratory coat, etc.
- Laboratory requisitions and/or labels
- Evacuated specimen tubes and blood culture bottles
- Sterile, single-use safety needles (for evacuated tube holders and winged-infusion/butterfly sets)
- Tube holders
- Nonlatex tourniquet
- Antiseptics—alcohol pads and/or other skin disinfectants
- Marking pens
- Electronic reader/scanner (if applicable)
- Blood culture decontamination swab kits (chlorhexidine compounds, povidone-iodine, etc.)
- Bandages (hypoallergenic adhesive bandages, gauze pads, and tape)

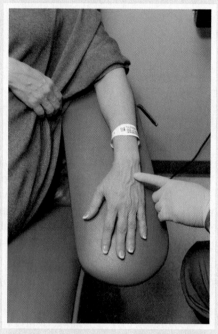

FIGURE 10–50

Preparation

1 Patient greeting and identification, hand hygiene, gloving, and supply preparation are the same as in Procedure 10–6 with the exception of using a butterfly needle device rather than the traditional needle.

2 Check the dorsal side of the hand for a suitable vein (**FIGURE 10–50**).

Procedure

3 Note that hand veins are smaller and may "roll" more easily than veins in the antecubital area of the arm (**FIGURE 10–51**). If the hand is made into a relaxed fist, the veins are slightly more taut and stable (**FIGURE 10–52**).

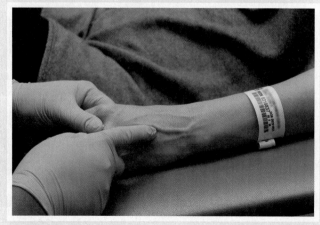

FIGURE 10–51

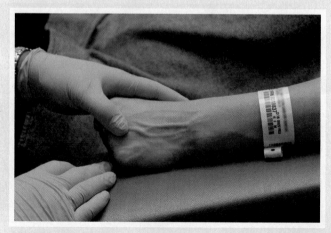

FIGURE 10–52

PROCEDURE 10–7

Hand Vein Venipuncture Using a Winged Infusion/Butterfly Set (continued)

4 When the site is selected, apply the tourniquet. Cleanse the selected site with a 70% isopropanol (isopropyl alcohol) pad as described in previous procedures (**FIGURE 10–53**). Remember: If you intend to touch the site again, repeat the cleansing procedure with a new alcohol pad. You may have to remove then reapply the tourniquet if time exceeds 1 minute. Air-dry the site.

5 Position the needle at a slight angle to the skin. Since hand veins are often closer to the surface of the skin, the angle of insertion is much smaller than for venipunctures in the antecubital area of the arm. Usually, the needle is inserted at a very slight angle, almost parallel to the vein (**FIGURES 10–54** and **10–55**). Note that the health care worker is holding the needle by the "wings," which enables the worker to get a very close and precise needle insertion point.

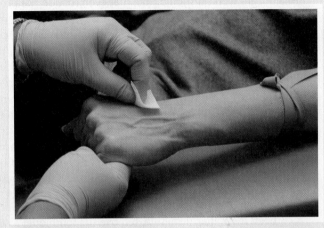

FIGURE 10–53

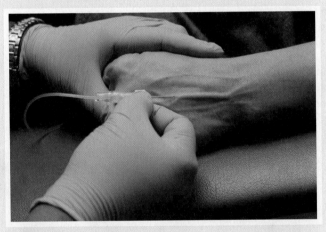

FIGURE 10–54

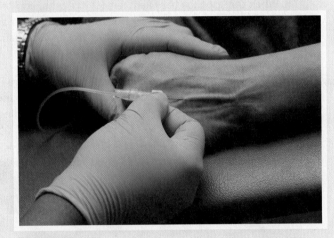

FIGURE 10–55

6 After the needle is in the vein, the blood should begin to fill the tubing and the evacuated specimen tube can be gently pushed into the barrel in the same manner as the previous venipuncture Procedure 10–6 (**FIGURES 10–56** and **10–57**).

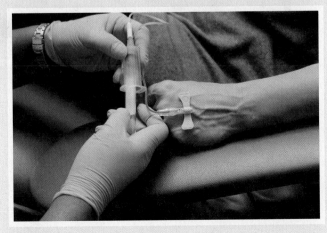

FIGURE 10–56

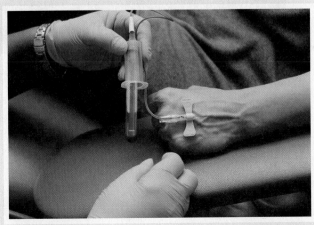

FIGURE 10–57

(continued)

PROCEDURE 10–7

Hand Vein Venipuncture Using a Winged Infusion/ Butterfly Set (continued)

Health care workers should note that even though the procedural steps for the puncture are the same for the evacuated tube system and the winged-infusion system, there may be different steps to follow as the tubes are actually filled. Since the tubing from the winged-infusion system contains air, it will underfill the first evacuated tube by 0.5 mL, thus affecting the additive-to-blood ratio. Therefore, fill a red-topped nonadditive tube prior to any tube with additives. After the first tube, the order of the tube draw should be the same as other methods. When tubes for coagulation are the only ones to be collected, it is suggested that a "dummy" or "discard" tube be collected and discarded. This fills the tubing with blood so that the correct additive-to-blood ratio is obtained for the following coagulation tube. When using the winged-infusion system, hold each tube horizontally or slightly down to avoid transfer of additives from one tube to the next. It is also suggested that small evacuated collection tubes (i.e., 13 × 75 mm or 4 mL) be used with winged-infusion sets to avoid collapsing fragile veins. If using a syringe attached to the Luer adapter, use a small syringe, such as 5 or 10 mL, for the same reason. Use a 21- or 23-gauge needle (not a 25-gauge needle because the small diameter may lead to hemolysis as the specimen is withdrawn).

7 If the procedure is progressing quickly, the tourniquet can be left on while the tubes are filling. However, if it has been more than 1 minute, remove the tourniquet as the tubes fill.

8 When the last tube has filled, remove the tube, and prepare to hold clean sterile gauze to the puncture site. In **FIGURES 10–58** and **10–59**, the health care worker activates the safety device while the needle is still in the vein while removing the needle, and then places clean gauze on the site. Experienced health care workers learn to do this very quickly.

9 The rest of the procedure is identical to venipuncture Procedure 10–6 and includes assuring that the bleeding has stopped, applying a bandage, labeling the specimens correctly, double-checking identity of the specimens, discarding used supplies, and cleaning the surroundings according to institutional policies. Thank the patient for cooperating.

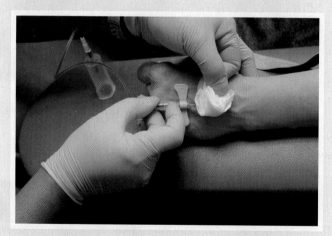

FIGURE 10–58

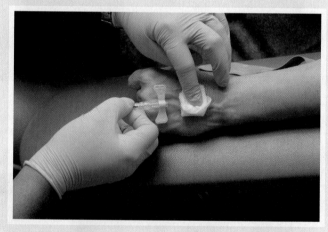

FIGURE 10–59

Each health care worker should make the decision about which procedure to use based on the circumstances of each patient and on the institution's procedures and practices. In most cases, an evacuated tube system is used with a plastic barrel. However, a winged infusion system, also called a *butterfly needle assembly, scalp needle set,* or *baby needle,* can be used for certain patient populations or for particularly difficult venipunctures. This type of method may be useful in the following circumstances:

Clinical Alert! Activating the needle safety device according to the manufacturer's instructions is very important in preventing accidental needlestick injuries. Health care workers should be extra cautious as the butterfly needle apparatus is removed from the patient because it tends to hang loose on the end of the tubing and may sometimes recoil back unexpectedly. If the safety device is not properly activated, it can cause a needlestick injury.

- Patients with small veins (hand or wrist)
- Pediatric patients
- Geriatric patients
- Patients having numerous needlesticks (e.g., cancer patients)
- Patients in restrictive positions (e.g., traction, severe arthritis)
- Patients who are severely burned
- Patients with fragile skin and veins
- Patients who specifically request it because they feel it is less painful
- Short-term infusion therapy

SYRINGE METHOD

As shown in Chapter 8, syringes are typically made of plastic with graduated markings denoting volume in milliliters. Although they are useful for injecting fluids and medications, they are not recommended for routine venipunctures. Syringes pose hazards for accidental needlesticks because their use requires an extra step to transfer the blood specimen into the correct testing tubes and may thus carry over additives from one tube to the next if not handled correctly. In addition, if this transfer step is delayed, clotting may occur in the syringe, rendering the specimen unusable. However, syringes are used in special circumstances because they allow the health care worker greater control of the rate of blood aspiration, which is particularly helpful for fragile veins that collapse easily (**PROCEDURE 10–8**). Follow the organization's policies for when to use the syringe method for venipuncture.

PROCEDURE 10–8

Syringe Method

Rationale Syringes are *not* routinely used for venipuncture because of many safety concerns—issues of accidental cross-contamination of anticoagulants if the blood specimen is injected into multiple evacuated tubes using the same needle and syringe, excessive or forceful withdrawal such that the sample is adversely affected, and potential clotting in the syringe. However, use of a blood transfer device can minimize some of these problems. There are also circumstances when a syringe is helpful, such as for veins that collapse easily. In this case, syringes help because the pressure withdrawing the blood can be more easily and gently controlled.

Equipment

- Personal protective equipment (PPE): gloves, clean uniform, laboratory coat, etc.
- Laboratory requisitions and/or labels
- Evacuated specimen tubes and blood culture bottles
- Safety needles
- Safety syringes and blood transfer devices (**FIGURE 10–60**)
- Tube holders
- Nonlatex tourniquet
- Antiseptics—alcohol pads and/or other skin disinfectants
- Marking pens
- Electronic reader/scanner (if applicable)
- Blood culture decontamination swab kits (chlorhexidine compounds, povidone-iodine, etc.)
- Bandages (hypoallergenic adhesive bandages, gauze pads, and tape)

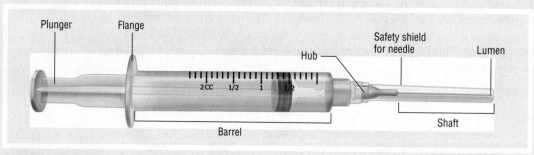

FIGURE 10–60
Example of a Safety Syringe

Preparation

1 After greeting, assessing, and identifying the patient, cleanse hands and don gloves.

2 Assemble supplies and double-check the expiration dates and integrity of the collection tubes. Gently tap the tubes containing additives to remove any additive that may be adhering to the closure/stopper.

3 Offer to answer any questions for the patient while putting on your gloves (if you haven't already done so).

4 Check the antecubital area for a suitable vein. Apply the tourniquet in the correct location, and cleanse the puncture site with an alcohol pad as described previously.

Syringe Method (continued)

Procedure

5 Using a syringe and needle with a safety device, assemble the two. Before the needle is inserted into the puncture site, remove the needle cap and move the syringe plunger back and forth to allow for free movement and to expel *all* air from the barrel of the syringe. Check the needle for defects. (Remember that a syringe can also be attached to a butterfly needle.)

6 Use the same approach for needle insertion as is used for the evacuated tube method (hold the skin taut, check the bevel orientation, and verify the insertion angle). Orient the syringe so that the graduated markings are visible. Say to the patient, "Please remain still. You will feel a slight prick."

7 Do not touch anything that would contaminate the needle. If it does touch any surface that is not sterile, replace it with a new needle assembly and discard the old one. Hold the needle/syringe in one hand while the thumb of the other hand anchors the vein 1 to 2 inches (2.5 to 5.0 cm) below the puncture site. Position the needle/syringe so that it is oriented in the same direction as the vein and is at an angle of 30 degrees or less with the skin surface. Orient the syringe so that you can see the graduated markings that indicate the volume of blood that will be withdrawn. With the bevel side up, insert the needle quickly. A slight "pop" should be felt as the needle enters the vein.

8 Once the needle is in the vein, take care to keep it stable while the syringe plunger is drawn back slowly until the required amount of blood is drawn. Try not to accidentally withdraw the needle while pulling back on the plunger and do not pull hard enough to cause hemolysis (i.e., rupture of the cells) or collapse of the vein.

9 Release the tourniquet as soon as possible after blood begins to flow.

10 After tourniquet release and collection of the appropriate amount of blood, withdraw the entire needle/syringe assembly quickly. Activate the safety device immediately, according to the manufacturer's specifications. Apply a sterile, dry gauze pad to the puncture site and ask the patient to assist in applying gentle pressure.

11 Remove the covered needle (or winged collection set) that is attached to the syringe and discard it appropriately.

12 After applying a syringe transfer device, immediately fill the evacuated collection tubes using the same "order of draw" as for the evacuated tube method of venipuncture (**FIGURE 10–61**).

13 Fill each tube by inserting it into the syringe transfer device. Do *not* push the plunger to expel blood; the tubes will fill because of the vacuum in the collection tube. Carefully watch as the tube fills until it stops. This will assure the correct ratio of blood to additive. Remove the first tube and replace it with the next one. Again, the tubes should be filled in the same order as for the evacuated tube method.

14 Mix additive tubes by gently inverting them according to the manufacturer's instructions.

After the Procedure

15 Discard the syringe attached to the blood transfer device as one unit. Also discard used supplies and label the specimens; check the patient to see that bleeding has stopped.

16 Apply a bandage and instruct the patient to leave it on for at least 15 minutes.

17 If the patient continues to bleed, notify a nurse and/or supervisor.

18 If bleeding has stopped, thank the patient prior to leaving.

(continued)

PROCEDURE 10–8

Syringe Method (continued)

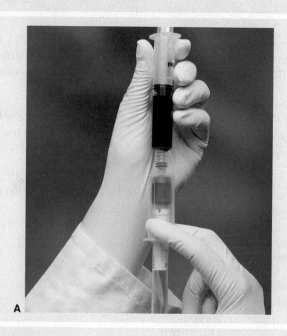

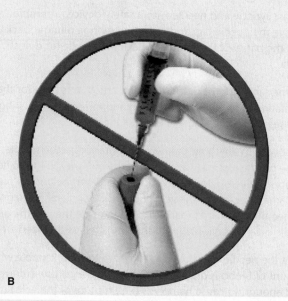

FIGURE 10–61
Blood Transfer Device

A. This image shows the health care worker inserting a tube into the blood transfer device after the needle (with safety device activated) was removed from the syringe and disposed of properly. **B.** This image shows the wrong way to transfer blood from a syringe into a collection tube. Note that the needle might have easily punctured the health care worker's index finger or thumb accidentally while holding the tube.

Courtesy and © Becton, Dickinson and Company

ALERT

Clinical Alert!

- To minimize hazards, a syringe transfer device *must* be used to move the sample from the syringe into the tubes.
- Do *not* remove rubber stoppers/closures on the collection tubes when transferring blood from the syringe.
- Discard the syringe attached to the transfer device as one unit to avoid blood exposure.

FAILURE TO COLLECT BLOOD AFTER A PUNCTURE

The health care worker should not panic if blood does not flow immediately after the puncture is made. The following suggestions may help:[1]

- Change the needle position *slightly, but do* not *probe around at the site.* Try to pull *gently* outward if you think the needle has gone too far, or push *gently* forward if you think the needle has not gone far enough into the vein, or rotate slightly so that the bevel is positioned appropriately in the vein. These should be minute movements so as to minimize the risk of complications.
- Replace the tube with another evacuated tube in case the first one is malfunctioning and/or is lacking a vacuum.

- If you do not have a successful venipuncture attempt after the first try, check for another site. Do *not* make more than two venipuncture attempts on one patient. Seek out another person/supervisor to make another attempt or notify the physician.

Refer to Chapter 9 for more information about preexamination/preanalytical complications during the blood collection procedure.

ORDER OF DRAW FOR BLOOD COLLECTION TUBES

Multiple blood assays are often ordered on patients. There are guidelines for delivery of blood into the proper collection tubes based on the method of venipuncture used, the types of tubes or additives needed for testing, and the specific manufacturer's instructions. A specified "order of draw" is important in reducing the effects of additive carryover or cross-contamination from one tube to the next. Carryover of additives can cause erroneous laboratory results. Each laboratory should document its practices and provide continuing education about the order of draw. The order of draw recommendations from the Clinical and Laboratory Standards Institute (CLSI) are revised periodically due to advances in technology and changes in testing methodology. It is important for health care workers to be aware of the current CLSI standards, the recommendations from manufacturers of the tubes (**FIGURE 10-62**), and the policies and procedures of their own health care facility. The order of draw may vary slightly from one laboratory to another. The Clinical and Laboratory Standards Institute recommends the following specific order when collecting blood in multiple tubes (either glass or plastic) via the evacuated method or the syringe transfer method.[1,13,14]

1. Blood culture tubes (yellow closure) or blood culture vials. Blood cultures are always collected first after special skin decontamination procedures to decrease the possibility of bacterial contamination. (The procedure for collection of blood cultures is discussed in Chapter 15 in greater detail.)
2. Coagulation tube (sodium citrate) (light blue closure).
3. Serum tube, with or without clot activator, with or without gel (red-speckled closure). (Glass, nonadditive serum tubes or plastic serum tubes without a clot activator can be filled before the coagulation tube. However, glass or plastic serum tubes containing a clot activator may interfere with coagulation tests.)
4. Heparin tube (green closure) with or without gel plasma separator.
5. EDTA tube (purple/lavender closure).
6. Glycolytic inhibition tube (gray closure) (potassium oxalate/sodium fluoride; Na_2 EDTA/sodium fluoride, or sodium fluoride only)

Special Considerations for Coagulation Testing[8,14,15,16]

- Remember that plastic or glass serum tubes with a clot activator may cause interference in coagulation testing. However, glass, nonadditive serum tubes or plastic serum tubes without a clot activator can be collected before the coagulation tube (sodium citrate).

- Remember that *if* a coagulation tube is to be collected first and *if* a winged-infusion/butterfly method is being used, then a "discard" tube should be collected *before* the coagulation tube. The discard tube functions to eliminate the air space in the tubing of the winged infusion set so that the correct additive-to-blood ratio can be achieved in the coagulation tube. If a discard tube is not collected first, extra air from the tubing enters the coagulation tube instead of blood, thus making the ratio unacceptable. The discard tube can be a nonadditive tube or a coagulation tube and does not necessarily need to be filled completely; it should be filled just until blood enters the tube so that all air is expelled from the tubing (unless the nonadditive tube will be used for other types of laboratory tests).

- When the syringe method is used to collect a large volume of blood, usually two syringes are used. The blood specimen from the *second* syringe should be used for the coagulation tube since it is less likely to have had time for blood clotting.

- Whenever coagulation tests (prothrombin time [PT]; international normalized ratio [INR]; partial thromboplastin time [PTT]) are the sole tests ordered, accurate results

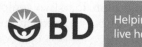

BD Vacutainer® Order of Draw for Multiple Tube Collections

Designed for Your Safety

Reflects change in CLSI recommended
Order of Draw (H3-A5, Vol 23, No 32, 8.10.2)

Closure Color	Collection Tube	Mix by Inverting
BD Vacutainer® Blood Collection Tubes *(glass or plastic)*		
	• Blood Cultures - SPS	8 to 10 times
	• Citrate Tube*	3 to 4 times
or	• BD Vacutainer® SST™ Gel Separator Tube	5 times
	• Serum Tube *(glass or plastic)*	5 times (plastic) none (glass)
	• BD Vacutainer® Rapid Serum Tube (RST)	5 to 6 times
or	• BD Vacutainer® PST™ Gel Separator Tube With Heparin	8 to 10 times
	• Heparin Tube	8 to 10 times
or	• EDTA Tube	8 to 10 times
	• BD Vacutainer® PPT™ Separator Tube K₂EDTA with Gel	8 to 10 times
	• Fluoride (glucose) Tube	8 to 10 times

* When using a winged blood collection set for venipuncture and a coagulation (citrate) tube is the first specimen tube to be drawn, a discard tube should be drawn first. The discard tube must be used to fill the blood collection set tubing's "dead space" with blood but the discard tube does not need to be completely filled. This important step will ensure proper blood-to-additive ratio. The discard tube should be a nonadditive or coagulation tube.

Note: Always follow your facility's protocol for order of draw

Handle all biologic samples and blood collection "sharps" (lancets, needles, luer adapters and blood collection sets) according to the policies and procedures of your facility. Obtain appropriate medical attention in the event of any exposure to biologic samples (for example, through a puncture injury) since they may transmit viral hepatitis, HIV (AIDS), or other infectious diseases. Utilize any built-in used needle protector if the blood collection device provides one. BD does not recommend reshielding used needles, but the policies and procedures of your facility may differ and must always be followed. Discard any blood collection "sharps" in biohazard containers approved for their disposal.

= 1 inversion

BD Technical Services
1.800.631.0174
BD Customer Service
1.888.237.2762
www.bd.com/vacutainer

1 Becton Drive
Franklin Lakes, NJ 07417
www.bd.com/vacutainer

BD, BD Logo and all other trademarks are property of Becton, Dickinson and Company. © 2010 BD
Franklin Lakes, NJ, 07417   1/10   VS5729-6

FIGURE 10–62

Order of Draw and Mixing Requirements for Multiple Tube Collections

Courtesy and © Becton, Dickinson and Company

can be obtained using one tube with an evacuated tube system of collection.[8] (It was thought that if the only tube collected was a coagulation tube, contamination with tissue fluids might initiate the clotting sequence and/or cause erroneous results.) Other types of laboratory coagulation studies may be affected by a single-tube draw, so it is advisable to collect a second tube if other coagulation studies are requested. Each health care worker should use the procedure adopted by the health care facility for these circumstances.

- Since coagulation tests require a specific plasma concentration of sodium citrate (the proportion of blood to liquid sodium citrate dihydrate anticoagulant volume should be 9:1), overfilling the tube causes artificial results indicating short clotting times.

- If a tube is underfilled, the opposite occurs and artificial results indicate prolonged clotting times.

- Be mindful that smaller size evacuated tubes (2 mL or less) may be more sensitive to under- or overfilling than standard 5 mL sodium citrate tubes.

- Additives for molecular coagulation assays vary depending on the testing methodology (DNA extraction techniques), so carefully follow the procedures for tube selection indicated by the facility.

- Immediately after collection, coagulation tubes should be mixed gently to prevent clotting in the tube. However, an excessive number of inversions or vigorous mixing can lead to platelet activation and shortening of clotting times when tested.

Other Issues Related to Filling the Blood Collection Tubes

- During the venipuncture procedure, care should be taken so that the additive or anticoagulant present in one tube does not come into contact with the multisample inner needle as the tubes are changed. To minimize transfer of anticoagulants from tube to tube, the tubes can be gently tapped prior to use to move the additives toward the bottom of the tube; also holding the tube slightly downward during blood collection is recommended. If an anticoagulant is inadvertently carried into the next tube, it may cause erroneous test results. For example, it is recommended that blood for serum iron be collected before other specimens with chelating anticoagulants (e.g., EDTA). This will avoid interference in testing the serum iron level. Also, electrolyte determinations include measurement of potassium (K) and sodium (Na). Since the chelating anticoagulant EDTA is usually bound to potassium or to sodium, it is important to collect specimens that require EDTA *after* a specimen is collected in heparin for electrolytes. The K and Na from the EDTA may falsely elevate the patient's K or Na values.

- *Be attentive to the "fill" rate and volume in each tube.* This is discussed more fully in Chapter 8. Evacuated tubes with anticoagulants must be filled to the designated level for the proper mix of blood with the anticoagulant—that is, the blood-additive ratio.

MANUFACTURERS OF BLOOD COLLECTION TUBES

As mentioned in previous chapters, there are numerous manufacturers of blood collection tubes and related supplies including, but not limited to, Becton Dickinson Vacutainer Systems and Greiner Bio-one. These companies maintain helpful websites (www.bd.com and www.vacuette.com, respectively) that provide educational materials, updates, and recommendations on blood collection devices and how to use them. (Refer to Chapter 8 for other sources.) For example, both companies provide instructions online and a recommended order of draw. Generally speaking, they follow the CLSI guideline but include additional information on specific additive tubes.

SPECIMEN IDENTIFICATION AND LABELING

No foolproof method exists for labeling specimens. However, *specimens should be labeled (adhesive and/or bar code labels) immediately at the patient's bedside or ambulatory setting prior to leaving the patient.* Laboratory procedures should contain explicit instructions on labeling requirements and reconfirmation that the specimen and patient have the same identity. Supervisors should spend ample time not only training new employees in correct identification and labeling practices, but also observing as they perform the steps (**FIGURES 10–63** and **10–64**).

It is acceptable for the health care worker to write directly on the specimen tube/container. Commercial collection tubes may have affixed blank labels for this purpose. Similarly, hospitals and large clinics often use computer-generated

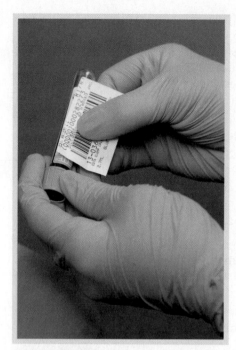

FIGURE 10–63
Labeling the Blood Sample

The phlebotomist should label the blood sample immediately after collecting it so it will not be confused with other samples.

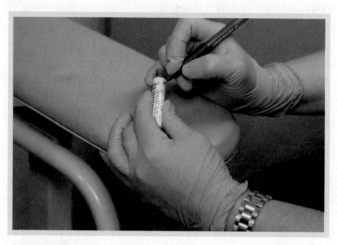

FIGURE 10–64
Initialing the Label

labels for collection tubes; however, capillary tubes, microcollection tubes and vials, or other containers without labels must be identified, either by labeling them directly with a permanent felt-tipped pen, wrapping an adhesive label around them, or placing them into a larger labeled test tube or bag for transport. In some cases, small, electronically generated adhesive labels with printed information are available with and detachable from the requisition form.

Specimen labels should consistently include the following information:[1,2]

1. Patient's name
2. Patient's unique identification number
3. Date of collection
4. Time of collection
5. Identification of the person who collected the specimen
6. Specimen type should be indicated if it is not already on the tube—for example, when an aliquot tube is used and the type of specimen (anticoagulant or serum) is not obvious
7. Assays to be performed (optional)
8. Patient's room number, bed assignment, or outpatient status (optional)

Special Considerations

■ Tubes should not be prelabeled, because if they are not used, they may be erroneously picked up and used for another patient. Also, a different health care worker may complete the venipuncture if the initial health care worker is unsuccessful. In that case, the prelabeled tubes may display the initials of the first health care worker and, therefore, be inaccurate. In addition, if the prelabeled tubes are not used, tearing off the old or unused label may be difficult because of the adhesive; thus, either a new label (from a different patient) would have to be placed on the tube with a partially torn label, or the unused tube would have to be discarded. Either option is unsatisfactory, messy, and wasteful.

- The health care worker should ensure that all the information on the label is complete and correct before leaving the patient's side. The worker should either recheck the identity of the patient and specimens using the armband, or ask the patient to verify that the information on the labeled tube(s) shows the correct identity (**FIGURE 10–65**).

- The date and time are necessary information because physicians need to know exactly when the specimen was collected so that they may correlate results with any medications given or with changes in the patient's condition. Remember that requisitions may indicate only the date and time when a laboratory test was ordered, rather than the date and time it was collected.

- The health care worker's initials are necessary to help clarify questions about the specimen if any arise during any phases of laboratory examination.

- In some cases, the orientation of the label on the actual tube may be specified because of automated processing and analytical requirements.

- If a health care worker cannot obtain a specimen, the worker should document the situation.

> **Clinical Alert!** Bandages are not recommended for infants or very young children because of possible irritation and the potential of swallowing or aspirating the bandage if it comes off.

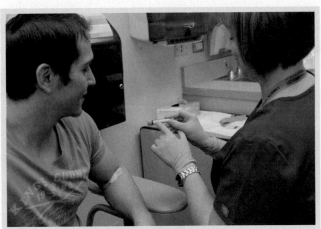

FIGURE 10–65
Confirming Identity of the Blood Sample

CARING FOR THE PUNCTURE SITE

In most circumstances, a dry, sterile gauze should be applied over the puncture site with gentle pressure for several minutes or until bleeding has ceased. (Do not use a cotton ball because the cotton fibers tend to stick to the puncture site and can pull off the blood clot/plug when removed.) If the patient has a free hand, ask the patient to apply the pressure, but the health care worker must monitor the site continuously to check for hematoma development or excessive bleeding. The patient's arm may be kept straight, slightly bent at the elbow, or elevated slightly above the heart. A bandage (hypoallergenic, adhesive) should be applied, and the patient should be instructed to leave it on for at least 15 minutes. However, if the patient continues to bleed, the health care worker should apply pressure him- or herself to the gauze until the bleeding stops. A bandage can then be applied, and the patient should be instructed to leave it on for at least 15 minutes (**FIGURE 10–66**). If the patient continues to bleed, a nurse and/or supervisor should be notified.[1]

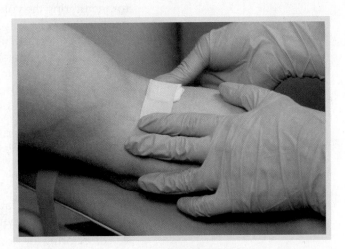

FIGURE 10–66
Applying the Bandage

DISPOSAL OF USED SUPPLIES AND EQUIPMENT

All disposable or contaminated equipment should be discarded into appropriate containers. Paper and plastic wrappers can be thrown into a wastebasket. However, needles and lancets should not be thrown into a wastebasket but into a sturdy, puncture-proof, disposable biohazard container to be autoclaved or incinerated. Any items that have been contaminated with blood should be disposed of in biohazardous disposal containers, as explained in Chapter 4.

Clinical Alert!

Use Once and Discard Immediately

Needles, lancets, syringes, tube holders, and other bloodletting devices (e.g., "sharps") that are capable of transmitting infection from one person to another should be used only *once,* then immediately discarded. Sharps must be discarded in puncture-resistant containers that are easily accessible, located in areas where they are commonly used, and have proper warning labels. "Shearing" or "breaking" of contaminated sharps is illegal and strictly prohibited. Bending, recapping, or removing contaminated needles is not an acceptable practice.

PATIENT ASSESSMENT AT THE END OF THE VENIPUNCTURE PROCEDURE

Before leaving the patient's side, the health care worker must

- Check the puncture site to make sure that the bleeding has stopped and that the patient is recovering from the procedure.
- Apply an adhesive hypoallergenic bandage if the patient is agreeable.
- Ensure that all tubes are appropriately labeled.
- Confirm identity of blood samples with the patient's armband or with the patient's verbal confirmation
- Sanitize hands again.
- Remove or appropriately discard supplies and equipment that were brought in.
- Thank the patient.

The specimen(s) can then be transported in an appropriate container. Considerations for specimen transportation and handling are covered in Chapter 12.

OTHER ISSUES AFFECTING VENIPUNCTURE PRACTICES

Monitoring Blood Volumes Acquired by Venipuncture

In an effort to reduce the incidence of iatrogenic anemia, processes should be in place for monitoring the volume of blood collected from particularly vulnerable patients (e.g., pediatric and critically ill patients).[1] All members of the health care team should strive to reduce the total number of daily phlebotomies and the amount of blood collected daily. One study done in a surgical intensive care unit (SICU) reported daily blood losses of up to 29.5 mL prior to implementing improvement measures. After reorganizing test practices, blood loss volumes decreased by 12.5 mL.[17] Suggestions for reducing and coordinating blood collections include:[19,20]

- Proactive monitoring of test utilization by coordination of laboratory requests among *all* staff physicians working with the patient to reduce duplicate and triplicate laboratory test orders.
- Maintenance of a log of the frequency and volume of blood collected for each patient.
- Organization of laboratory orders by nurses and floor clerks as much as possible to avoid sending frequent requests minutes apart (e.g., batching laboratory test orders).
- Monitoring the number of times that a patient can be punctured. (Generally, a health care worker should not puncture a patient more than twice before calling for a second opinion.)
- Monitoring the number of times that a patient can be punctured in one day. Coordinated efforts should minimize the number of patient venipunctures.
- Reduction of the volume of blood discarded when using blood from IV lines. (Refer to Chapter 15 for more information.)
- Possible modification to laboratory testing panels and better education of physicians to be aware of all the tests on each laboratory panel.
- Notification of the laboratory when multiple timed tests are ordered. For example, if a patient needs a hemoglobin test at 2:00 pm and a glucose test at 3:00 pm, coordinating the times and drawing both specimens during one venipuncture may be possible.

- Reassessment of STAT test orders to make sure they are clinically necessary.
- Coordination of therapeutic drug monitoring among laboratory, nursing, and pharmacy personnel.
- Awareness by the laboratory of patient transfers to coordinate test requests from different floors.

Reducing Hematoma Complications

As mentioned in previous chapters, hematomas are caused by blood leakage into the surrounding tissues (**FIGURE 10–67**). Methods for reducing the likelihood of hematoma formation include the following:

- Strive to insert the needle at the correct angle through the upper vein wall, but not through the lower vein wall. Also, partial vein wall penetration may allow blood to leak into the tissues.
- When collecting blood into multiple tubes, hold the needle very steady when changing tubes so that the needle does not slip out of or completely through the vein wall.
- Remove the tourniquet *prior to* removing the needle from a patient's arm.
- Use the recommended antecubital veins.
- Check for hematoma formation during the procedure and immediately after the needle is withdrawn from the skin and apply pressure to the gauze.

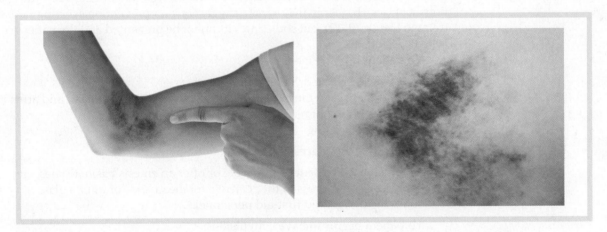

FIGURE 10–67

Hematomas

Courtesy (left) © bertys30/Fotolia / (right) © frenta/Fotolia

Avoiding Specimen Hemolysis

Methods for avoiding specimen hemolysis include the following:

- After decontamination with alcohol, allow the site to air dry.
- Do *not* collect a blood specimen in a site that has a hematoma.
- When using a syringe method, attach the needle securely to the syringe; otherwise, "frothing" may occur, which causes damage to red blood cells. Also, avoid pulling the syringe plunger back too quickly, because it will cause excessive force as the blood enters the syringe, thereby causing cellular damage.
- When mixing blood in tubes containing additives, do not shake the tubes; instead, gently invert them.
- Follow the manufacturer's recommendations to ensure that needles, holders, and transfer devices are compatible.

Providing Clinical Information

Clinical test information provided to the patient by the health care worker is restricted to basic information about the tests that have been ordered and/or the venipuncture procedure. Health care workers should refer specific or detailed queries to the patient's physician who ordered the tests.

Patient Refusal

Every health care facility should have procedures for documenting a patient's refusal to have blood collected. *All patients (or parents/guardians for pediatric patients) have a right to refuse treatment.* The health care worker can explain to the patient that laboratory results are used to help the physician make an accurate diagnosis, establish proper treatment, and monitor the patient's health status, and that the patient's cooperation would be greatly appreciated. If the patient continues to refuse, the health care worker must remain professional and acknowledge the patient's right to refuse. Documentation of the refusal should be made and the patient's physician notified.

Emergency Situations during Phlebotomy Procedures

Occasionally, patients react physically to venipuncture procedures by fainting, feeling nauseous, or having convulsions. In order to provide immediate medical attention, CLSI recommends that at least one member of the staff should have first-aid training (e.g., cardiopulmonary resuscitation [CPR]) to focus on the patient until a physician can reach the patient. All incidents of this nature should be well documented according to institutional policies.[1] Earlier in the chapter, suggestions for preventing syncope were discussed (refer to Figure 10–12), but sometimes it cannot be prevented and the patient completely loses consciousness.

If a patient is nonresponsive:[1]

1. Notify the designated first-aid personnel.
2. If possible, position the patient flat, or if seated, lower the head and arms. (Ammonia inhalants are not recommended.)
3. Loosen tight clothing.

If a patient experiences nausea or vomiting:[1]

1. Try to make the patient comfortable or offer an emesis basin, tissues, etc.
2. Apply a cold compress to the patient's forehead and/or offer a glass of water.
3. Notify the designated first-aid personnel.

If a patient begins to have convulsions:[1]

1. Try to prevent the patient from injury, but do not restrain the movements of extremities completely.
2. Notify the designated first-aid personnel immediately.

Specimen Rejection

Laboratory departments typically have policies in place on the acceptance of specimens for laboratory testing. Since so many variables play a role in the preanalytical process, it is important that the specimen be closely scrutinized prior to any phase of laboratory testing. Part of every quality management program for phlebotomy services should be to evaluate the technical reasons that blood specimens are not suitable and to take action to reduce specimen rejections. Specimens that are unusable for various reasons include the following: [19,20,21]

■ Identity discrepancies between requisition forms and labeled tubes (e.g., names, dates, times)

■ Identity completely lacking or illegible (e.g., unlabeled specimen tubes, label is torn)

- Inadequate volume of blood resulting in unacceptable additive-to-blood ratios
- Hemolyzed specimens (except for tests in which hemolysis does not interfere)
- Specimens in the wrong collection tubes
- Specimens that were improperly transported/stored (chilled, unchilled, frozen)
- Anticoagulated specimens that contain blood clots
- Use of outdated equipment, supplies, or reagents
- Contaminated specimens
- Patient not adequately instructed about diet restrictions
- A timed sample drawn at the wrong time or with the time recorded incorrectly

When a problem arises, the appropriate investigational channels should be followed. The health care worker who drew the specimen and the supervisor should try to solve the problem initially. Errors should be acknowledged and documented with corrective actions and follow-up training. Other personnel may be involved as needed. Communication, honesty, and ethical professional behavior are the keys to an efficient and reliable health care environment. Chapter 9 also discusses complications in blood collection.

Prioritizing Patients

In the course of a day's work at a busy hospital or clinic, a health care worker may have to make decisions about the order in which blood work is obtained from groups of patients. Priorities must be set by the health care facility and adhered to, whether they concern the order in which certain blood tests are drawn on a particular patient or which patients are to be drawn first from among a group. If these distinctions are not made properly, test results can be affected and interpretation of the results may be difficult. Examples of setting blood collection priorities are discussed next.

Timed tests If a test is ordered for a collection at a particular time, the health care worker is responsible for drawing the blood as near to the requested time as possible. Some laboratory values must be based on a specific time because of when a medication was administered (e.g., digoxin), fasting restrictions (e.g., glucose), or circadian rhythm (e.g., cortisol). The most common requests for timed specimens are for glucose level determinations, for which blood should be collected two hours after a meal. The glucose value in the blood is constantly changing, so the blood must not be collected too early, which yields a falsely elevated result, or too late, which yields a falsely normal result.

Timed specimens are also crucial for **therapeutic drug monitoring (TDM).** The laboratory results taken from blood samples for TDM are used in establishing a patient's drug dose. More specifically, TDM is used for the following reasons:[22]

- Monitor or confirm an overdose.
- Determine the dosage of a medication.
- Establish a baseline measurement after a patient has begun or changed to a new drug therapy.
- Check to see that a drug is not interacting with a drug the patient is already taking.
- Check to see if a drug is influenced by the patient's habits; for example, smokers clear theophylline faster than nonsmokers, so their serum drug levels will be lower.
- After a change in the patient's kidney, liver, or gastrointestinal functions.
- Within 6 hours after a seizure recurrence (when using antiepileptic drugs).
- When drug toxicity is suspected. (Some drugs have a narrow therapeutic window such that the amount needed to benefit the patient is often close to the toxic amount.)

■ When the patient is noncompliant with the prescribed medications. (The physician may need the serum level in order to confirm that the patient has not taken the drug or has not taken it as prescribed.)

■ If a patient's condition is not improving after drug therapy. (The serum drug level may be subtherapeutic, so a change in dose may be needed.) Refer to Chapter 15 for more detailed information on drug therapy collections.

Certain natural hormone levels, such as that for cortisol, also increase and decrease with the time of day. For instance, a sample of blood taken at 8:00 AM shows the highest value for cortisol during the day, whereas a sample taken at 8:00 PM usually shows approximately two-thirds the value of the morning sample. Therefore, if a health care worker has difficulty obtaining a blood specimen on a patient at 8:00 AM, someone else should try as soon as possible thereafter, or the test may be canceled until the following day at the discretion of the attending physician.

Aldosterone, another hormone, requires the patient to be in a recumbent position for at least 30 minutes prior to blood collection. Serum or plasma can be used in the analyte determination, but heparin or EDTA should be the anticoagulant if plasma is preferred. Because glass interferes in aldosterone determination, the collecting container should be made of plastic.

Blood collection for a renin-activity test requires an anticoagulated blood specimen from the patient after a three-day special diet and also documentation about whether the patient was in an upright or supine (prone) position when blood was drawn.

Fasting specimens Fasting specimens require that blood be taken from a patient who has abstained from eating and drinking anything (except water) for a particular period of time. Care should be taken that the patient is not unduly inconvenienced by an order for *fasting blood tests.* Fasting levels of glucose, cholesterol, and triglycerides are used for diagnosis and monitoring. If the health care worker finds that a patient has not been fasting, the physician should be consulted to determine whether a nonfasting level will be of benefit. Documentation should then indicate that the patient is nonfasting.

STAT specimens STAT, or emergency, specimens should be acted on immediately because the patient has a medical condition that must be treated or responded to as a medical emergency or health crisis. When blood work is ordered STAT, the specimen must be drawn, delivered to the laboratory, and analyzed without delay.

Study Questions

For the following questions, select the one best answer.

1 A hospitalized patient may *not* be identified by which of the following means?

   a. patient's chart
   b. nurse
   c. patient's armband
   d. verbal confirmation from the patient

2 Identification procedures for a comatose patient may involve which of the following?

   a. positive identification by a volunteer at the hospital
   b. medical record/chart on the bedside table
   c. name tag on the bed
   d. positive identification by a family member

3 The most common sites for venipuncture are in which of the following areas?

   a. the dorsal side of the wrist
   b. the antecubital area of the arm
   c. the middle finger
   d. the middle forearm

4 Palpating the venipuncture site serves which purpose?

   a. provides an indication of the size and depth of the vein
   b. distracts the patient from the discomfort of the procedure
   c. pushes arteries out of the way prior to venipuncture
   d. helps the health care worker determine the age of the patient

5 Using a butterfly needle is beneficial for

   a. heel punctures
   b. routine venipuncture in healthy adults
   c. geriatric patients
   d. patients who have prominent muscles

6 What effect does warming the site have on venipuncture?

   a. prevents veins from rolling
   b. makes blood flow more quickly
   c. causes hemoconcentration
   d. increases localized blood flow

7 How long should the tourniquet be placed around the patient's arm?

   a. approximately 4 minutes
   b. until the needle is removed
   c. until the entire venipuncture is completed
   d. no more than 1 minute

8 What is the best angle for needle insertion during venipuncture?

   a. 5 degrees
   b. 30 degrees or less
   c. 45 degrees or more
   d. 80 degrees

9 Of the following specimens, which should be the first tube collected in the suggested order of draw using the evacuated tube system?

   a. blood culture
   b. lavender-topped tube
   c. light-blue–topped tube
   d. red-topped tube

10 Containers for the disposal of needles and syringes should have which of the following features?

   a. puncture resistance
   b. label with a red and white cross
   c. yellow and black markings
   d. antiseptic solution

Case Study 1

Twice Is Enough A health care worker named Sarah had been an employee for one year at the community hospital. She felt comfortable in her position, and her supervisor told her she was becoming more efficient and productive at her job. She decided that she could improve her productivity even more by moving through the phlebotomy procedures at a faster pace now that she had some experience under her belt. One morning, Sarah encountered a frail, thin patient who mentioned that she had had a mastectomy the previous year. Sarah identified the patient correctly and began to search for a suitable vein. She did not really feel a good one, even after checking both arms. However, she decided to go ahead and stick an arm vein in an area on the nonmastectomy side. She missed the first attempt and the second attempt at a site slightly above the first one. Sarah realized that she should go ahead and get a warming device for the patient. She left the warming device on the patient's arm for about 30 seconds and then wanted to give it one more try. She attempted another venipuncture but missed. She was embarrassed and apologized to the patient, but she felt confident that she could collect the blood so she tried a fourth time on the same arm. After another failed attempt, Sarah left the room in a frustrated manner.

Questions

1 Identify three major problems with this situation.

2 What should Sarah do next?

3 What advice would you give Sarah?

Case Study 2

Getting on Her Nerves George, an experienced health care worker, was closing the clinic just as the last patient showed up to have her blood collected for some routine laboratory work. The patient apologized for being late and mentioned that she was a diabetic and had to stop for an insulin injection prior to arriving. The health care worker proceeded to get the appropriate forms, requisitions, and supplies ready for the venipuncture procedure. The patient preparation and assessment, identification, and site selection process took place without incident, and all was going smoothly until the actual venipuncture occurred into the basilic vein area. Suddenly the patient screamed out in pain and could hardly sit still. George responded, "I know it hurts a little, but if you just wait a few moments, I will be finished with the procedure shortly."

Questions

1 What is the most likely cause of the pain?

2 What should George do?

Action in Practice

Patient Identification Patients frequently have the same or similar names. Sometimes the names may sound alike but are spelled differently. Remember that language differences and/or accents may cause one name to sound like another, resulting in misunderstandings. However, if the identification process is followed carefully and thoroughly, mistakes are preventable.

As a self-assessment exercise, pretend you are tired and at the end of a busy work shift at your clinic. Reflect on the hypothetical names listed here, say the names out loud, and think about how you would react if any of these patients arrived for a venipuncture at the same time:

Lin Dao and Lynn Dow
Mary Gonzales and Maria Gonzalez
Betsy Johnson and Betty Johnston
Jin Liang and Qing Lian

John McLaughlin and James Maclaughlin
Paul Garcia and Raul Garza
Jan Cheung and Jen Chang
John Riley and Jon Reilly

Consider how important each step of the identification process is in these (and all) situations. Next, come up with your own list of similar-sounding names with which you are familiar. Tune-in your eyes and ears to notice different spellings and verbal pronunciations of these names. Remember that if you ever find a discrepancy in the identification process, it should be reported to a supervisor immediately.

COMPETENCY ASSESSMENT

Competency Checklist: Patient Identification

This checklist can be completed as a group or individually.

(1) Completed (2) Needs to improve

_____ 1. List three ways to confirm a patient's identity.

_____ 2. List three methods *that would not be reliable* for confirming a patient's identity.

Competency Checklist: Preparing for the Patient Encounter

This exercise can be done during an actual patient encounter or as a mock encounter. If possible, record a video of the encounter to aid in the assessment critique.

(1) Completed (2) Needs to improve

_____ 1. The health care worker demonstrates a positive, professional appearance.

_____ 2. The health care worker demonstrates positive body language, including a pleasant facial expression and good posture before beginning the patient encounter.

_____ 3. The health care worker has protective equipment, phlebotomy supplies, test requisitions, a writing pen, and appropriate patient information before beginning the venipuncture process.

_____ 4. The health care worker can describe what to do if he or she cannot identify the patient correctly or if information is incomplete.

_____ 5. The health care worker asks questions about latex allergies and likelihood of fainting.

_____ 6. The health care worker looks for signs of patient understanding of the procedure by offering to answer any questions the patient may have.

Competency Checklist: Use of a Tourniquet and Site Selection

Practice on a partner several times before practicing on a patient.

(1) Completed (2) Needs to improve

_____ 1. A clean latex-free tourniquet is used by stretching the ends of the tourniquet around the patient's arm about 3 inches (7.6 cm) above the venipuncture area (antecubital area). The tourniquet is applied tightly but not painfully to the patient. It is not left on more than 1 minute.

_____ 2. The antecubital area is palpated appropriately (not too hard, not too soft, not too much).

_____ 3. Veins are located and identified appropriately. One or more options can easily be identified in the antecubital area.

_____ 4. When it is time to release the tourniquet, the partial loop should allow for easy release by the health care worker using only one hand, because the other hand will be holding the needle and tubes.

_____ 5. Practice applying the tourniquet on the lower arm to identify dorsal hand veins.

_____ 6. Palpate and identify the best option for venipuncture on the dorsal side of the hand.

_____ 7. Release the tourniquet during the appropriate time frame.

Competency Checklist: Cleansing the Puncture Site

Choose a partner to work with. Your partner or supervisor can evaluate the extent to which the site is adequately cleansed.

(1) Completed (2) Needs to improve

_____ 1. After the site is selected, it is decontaminated with a commercially packaged alcohol pad.

_____ 2. The site is rubbed with moderate pressure applied to the alcohol pad, working in concentric circles from the inside out.

_____ 3. Adequate time is allotted for the site to dry.

Competency Checklist: Performing a Venipuncture

The steps listed here are typical for either venipuncture system.

(1) Completed (2) Needs to improve

_____ 1. After greeting and identifying the patient, decontaminating hands, donning gloves, and preparing equipment in the presence of the patient, the health care worker offers to answer any questions for the patient.

_____ 2. The health care worker prepares equipment according to the manufacturer's instructions, including attaching a needle onto the appropriate holder.

_____ 3. The patient's arm is positioned properly.

_____ 4. A clean tourniquet is applied and potential sites are checked by palpating the vein.

_____ 5. If a suitable vein is not felt, the tourniquet is removed and applied to the other arm.

_____ 6. Practice warming the site or lower the arm further in a downward position to pool venous blood.

_____ 7. An appropriate site is selected and cleaned with an alcohol pad in a circular motion from inside to outside. It is allowed to air dry.

_____ 8. The patient is asked to "please close your fist."

_____ 9. The patient is told that he or she will "feel a stick" or "please remain still while I begin the procedure; you will feel a slight prick."

_____ 10. The patient's arm is held below the site, pulling the skin slightly with the thumb.

_____ 11. The needle assembly and arm are held appropriately.

_____ 12. The needle is parallel to the vein and at the appropriate angle.

_____ 13. The patient is instructed to open the fist after blood begins to flow, and the tourniquet is released at the appropriate time.

_____ 14. Evacuated tubes are pushed into the holder in an appropriate manner.

_____ 15. Evacuated tubes are filled in the correct order and until the blood flow stops in each tube.

_____ 16. Each tube is removed from the holder with a gentle twist-and-pull motion and replaced with the next tube.

_____ 17. Tubes are gently mixed/inverted in one hand while holding the needle apparatus and waiting for another tube to fill.

_____ 18. When all tubes have been filled the needle is withdrawn in an appropriate manner.

_____ 19. Bleeding is adequately controlled.

_____ 20. The safety device is activated according to the manufacturer's instructions.

_____ 21. The patient is instructed to apply pressure to the site using the gauze.

Competency Checklist: Order of Draw

The following cases indicate tests requested for laboratory evaluation. Practice numbering the tubes in the correct order of collection for a venipuncture.

(1) Completed (2) Needs to improve

_____ 1. Lavender closure used for hematology tests (CBC), yellow closure used for blood cultures, serum closure used for many chemistry tests

_____ 2. Heparin (green), serum (red speckled), coagulation (light blue)

_____ 3. Blood cultures, coagulation, hematology

_____ 4. Coagulation, serum protein

_____ 5. Heparin, EDTA, serum cholesterol, coagulation

_____ 6. Using a butterfly method: coagulation, hematology

Competency Checklist: Leaving the Patient

This checklist can be completed as a group or individually.

(1) Completed (2) Needs to improve

_____ 1. The health care worker rechecks the puncture site to see whether the bleeding has stopped or if the patient wants a bandage.

_____ 2. The health care worker asks whether the patient is feeling faint.

_____ 3. The health care worker labels all specimens appropriately and reconfirms specimen and patient identity.

_____ 4. Used supplies are discarded appropriately.

_____ 5. Hands are decontaminated after the procedure.

_____ 6. Specimens are readied for transport in a secure fashion.

_____ 7. The health care worker thanks the patient before leaving the room (inpatient setting) and escorts patient to exit point (outpatient setting).

REFERENCES

1. Clinical and Laboratory Standards Institute (CLSI). (2007, October). *Procedures for the collection of diagnostic blood specimens by venipuncture, approved standard,* 6th ed. H3-A6. Wayne, PA: Author.

2. Clinical and Laboratory Standards Institute (CLSI). (2004). *Procedures and devices for the collection of diagnostic capillary blood specimens, approved standard.* H4-A5. Wayne, PA: Author.

3. Centers for Disease Control and Prevention: Morbidity and Mortality Weekly Report. (2002, October 25). *Guideline for hand hygiene in health-care settings, 51*(16). http://www.cdc.gov/handhygiene/guidelines.html, accessed March 14, 2014.

4. Department of Health and Human Services, Centers for Disease Control and Prevention (CDC), National Institute for Occupational Safety and Health (NIOSH). (1999, November). *Preventing needlestick injuries in health care settings.* Publication No. 2000-108. www.cdc.gov/niosh/topics/bbp/sharps.html, accessed March 14, 2014.

5. Department of Health and Human Services, Centers for Disease Control and Prevention (CDC), National Institute for Occupational Safety and Health (NIOSH). (2003, July). *Exposure to blood, what healthcare personnel need to know.* http://www.cdc.gov/ncidod/dhqp/pdf/bbp/Exp_to_Blood.pdf, accessed March 14, 2014.

6. Department of Health and Human Services, Centers for Disease Control and Prevention (CDC), National Institute for Occupational Safety and Health (NIOSH). (2013, January 5). *Overview of state needle safety legislation.* www.cdc.gov/niosh/topics/bbp/ndl-law.html, accessed January 5, 2013.

7. College of American Pathologists, Laboratory Accreditation Program, Laboratory General Checklists. (2007, September 27). www.cap.org, accessed March 14, 2014.

8. Favalaro, E. J., Funk, D. M., & Lippi, G. (2012). Preanalytical variables in coagulation testing associated with diagnostic errors in hemostasis. *Lab Medicine, 43*(2), 54–60.

9. The Joint Commission: 2014 National Patient Safety Goals. www.jointcommission.org, accessed March 14, 2014.

10. Patient Safety & Quality Healthcare: New Products and Services, Trends. (2005, January/February). www.psqh.com/products/prodjf05.html, accessed March 14, 2014.

11. MTB Europe: Technology for healthcare. (2005, December 14). *Information technology: Patient wristband with RFID chip wins award.* www.mtbeurope.info/news/2005/512019.htm, accessed January 5, 2013.

12. Jackson, S. (2003, March 24). Caution: Entering the danger zone, Proper vein selection is key in successful venipunctures. *Advance for Med Lab Prof,* p. 10.

13. Becton Dickinson Vacutainer Systems: BD Vacutainer Order of Draw for Multiple Tube Collections. www.bd.com, accessed March 14, 2014.

14. Greiner Bio-one: VACUETTE Blood Collection System. www.gbo.com, accessed March 14, 2014.

15. Gottfried, E. L., & Adachi, M. M. (1997). Prothrombin time and activated partial thromboplastin time can be performed on the first tube. *Am J Clin Pathol, 107*(6): 681–683.

16. Clinical Laboratory and Standards Institute (CLSI). (2008). *Collection, transport, and processing of blood specimens for testing plasma-based coagulation assays and molecular hemostasis assays, approved guideline,* 5th ed. H21-A5, *28*(5). Wayne, PA: Author.

17. Saxena, S., Belzberg, H., Chogyoji, M., et al. (2003, October). Reducing phlebotomy losses by streamlining laboratory test ordering in a surgical intensive care unit. *Lab Med, 34*(10): 728–732.

18. Madsen Myers, K. (2006). Iatrogenic anemia and the critically ill patient, American Society for Clinical Pathology, Lab Q-P, Phlebotomy No. 4. Continuing education exercise available at 800-267-2727.

19. Rachael, J. L., & Naples, M. F. (1995, March). Creating a workable specimen rejection policy. *Med Lab Observ,* pp. 37–42.

20. Clinical Laboratory and Standards Institute (CLSI). (2010). *Procedures for the handling and processing of blood specimens for common laboratory tests, approved guideline,* 4th ed. H18-A4. Wayne, PA: Author.

21. Garza, D. (2006). Proactive phlebotomy: Error identification and risk reduction, American Society for Clinical Pathology, Lab Q-P, Phlebotomy No. 3. Continuing education exercise available at 800-267-2727.

22. McKenna, R., & Keffer, J. (2000). The handbook of clinical pathology. Chicago: ASCP Press, pp. 255–260.

RESOURCES

www.cdc.gov/niosh The National Institute for Occupational Safety and Health (NIOSH)

www.cdc/handhygiene/guidelines Centers for Disease Control, Hand Hygiene in Healthcare Settings

www.phlebotomy.com Center for Phlebotomy Education

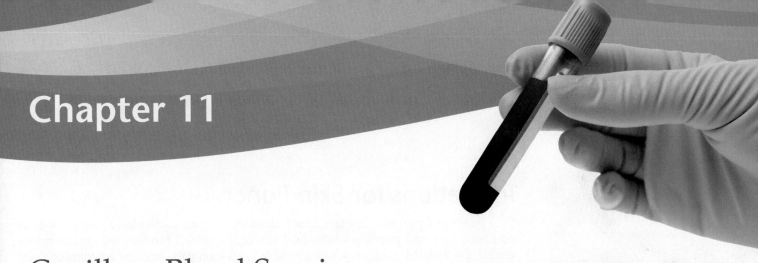

Chapter 11

Capillary Blood Specimens

Chapter Objectives

Upon completion of Chapter 11, the learner is responsible
for doing the following:

1. Describe the reasons for acquiring capillary blood specimens and list laboratory tests
   for which capillary specimens may be collected.

2. Explain why capillary blood from a skin puncture is different from blood taken by
   venipuncture and the impact on laboratory tests.

3. Identify the proper sites for performing a skin puncture procedure and explain why it
   is necessary to control the depth of the incision.

4. Describe the procedure for performing a skin puncture.

5. Describe the procedure for making blood smears and why they are used in the
   laboratory.

KEY TERMS

arterialized capillary blood
capillary action
cyanotic
dehydrated
feathered edge
interstitial (tissue) fluid
peripheral circulation

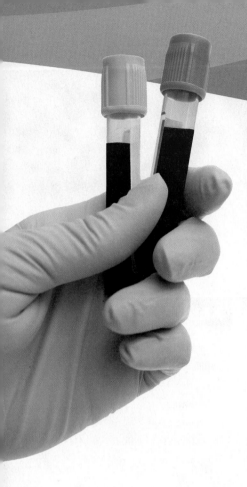

Indications for Skin Puncture

Skin punctures provide capillary blood samples that are particularly useful for both adult and pediatric patients when small amounts of blood can be used for laboratory testing. For pediatric patients it is crucial to withdraw only the smallest amounts of blood needed for laboratory testing to reduce the effects of blood-volume reduction. (Refer to Figure 7–15 in Chapter 7 for a comparison of blood volume for newborns, children, and adults. Remember that a 9-pound newborn has a total blood volume less than a 12-ounce size soda.) Thus, for neonates and infants, use of capillary blood samples is the preferred method of collection. Sample sizes and procedures for obtaining specimen collections from children are in Appendix 7, and pediatric topics are covered in Chapter 13. When the laboratory tests require smaller sample sizes, use of capillary punctures in lieu of a venipuncture can produce several benefits, such as:[1]

- Reducing the likelihood of causing iatrogenic anemia
- Reducing the risk of an accidental sharps injury
- Reducing the risk of injuring adult patients (nerve damage, etc.)
- Reducing the risk of injuries and complications for children and infants (anemia, cardiac arrest, hemorrhage, venous thrombosis, reflex arteriospasm, gangrene of an extremity, damage to surrounding tissues or organs, infections, and injuries from restraining the child during the procedure)
- Being perceived as less painful than a venipuncture (although many patients disagree with this)
- Being less costly in terms of equipment/supplies
- Being faster than the procedure for collecting a venipuncture specimen
- Being easily done for self-monitoring by diabetic patients who can do a skin puncture on themselves

If blood volume requirements are small, skin punctures for adults are often used when the following conditions occur:[1]

- Severe burns on the arms
- Obesity
- Thrombotic tendencies
- Fragile veins (e.g., in geriatric patients)
- "Saving" of veins for therapy (e.g., for oncology patients)
- Self-testing (e.g., diabetic blood glucose screening)
- Point-of-care (POC) testing

Sometimes a skin puncture *cannot* be used because:

- Testing may require larger amounts of blood.
- Swollen sites/fingers may cause **interstitial fluids** (between the tissues) to dilute the blood.

BOX 11-1

Common Laboratory Tests and Capillary Blood Samples

Capillary blood samples are commonly used for the following tests:

- Blood smears for a white blood cell differential (manual method)
- Complete blood count (CBC), hemoglobin and hematocrit (H&H)
- Electrolytes
- Neonatal blood gases
- Neonatal bilirubin
- Neonatal screening (using filter paper or blood spot testing)
- Point-of-care testing (POCT) or home or self-testing (glucose)

Specific laboratory tests for which skin punctures are *not* recommended include:

- Coagulation studies (because of the interstitial fluid)
- Blood cultures (because of volume requirements and sterility concerns about skin contamination)
- Erythrocyte sedimentation rate (ESR) determinations

- The patient may be **dehydrated** and therefore a skin puncture is less likely to produce blood drops.
- The patient may have poor **peripheral circulation** (circulation near the surface of the body).

Laboratory tests commonly performed using capillary blood samples and tests that are not recommended for capillary blood are listed in **BOX 11-1**.

Composition of Capillary Blood

As mentioned in Chapter 7, the composition of capillary blood acquired by skin puncture is significantly different from that of venous blood acquired by venipuncture. It is composed of a mixture of blood from

- Arterioles
- Venules
- Capillaries
- Intracellular and interstitial (tissue) fluids

The exact proportions in a capillary blood specimen from these sources are not known; however, the proportion of arterial blood will be greatest because the arterial pressure in the capillaries is stronger than the venous pressure. Therefore, blood from a capillary blood specimen is actually more like arterial blood than venous blood. Also, because of its mixed composition, capillary blood specimens will have lower values of potassium, total protein, and calcium, and higher values of glucose than venous blood specimens.

Basic Technique for Collecting Diagnostic Capillary Blood Specimens

Many of the steps used for the venipuncture procedure also apply to skin puncture. **FIGURE 11–1** is a flowchart for collecting capillary blood specimens. Basic steps include the following:

1. Greeting, carefully identifying, and assessing the patient
2. Performing hand hygiene and gloving techniques
3. Preparing supplies and the microcollection device
4. Positioning the patient for safety and comfort
5. Verifying diet restrictions, inquiring about latex sensitivity and likelihood of fainting
6. Selecting and assessing the site (if necessary, warming it or lowering arm downward to allow gravity to pool blood in fingertips)
7. Cleaning the site
8. Opening the sterile puncture device within view of the patient
9. Performing the puncture and wiping away the first drop (unless required for POC tests)
10. Obtaining the specimen
11. Applying gentle pressure to the wound using a clean gauze pad
12. Discarding the lancet in a puncture-resistant biohazard container
13. Labeling the specimen, double-checking identity, and preparing it for transportation
14. Assuring that bleeding has stopped, and thanking the patient before leaving

Preparation for Skin Puncture

Skin puncture procedures involve the same preparation steps as discussed for venipuncture procedures in Chapter 10. It is *imperative* that health care workers review the details of these steps because they are essential responsibilities. Such steps include:

- Being emotionally prepared
- Exercising standard precautions
- Using correct hand hygiene techniques and protective equipment
- Using gloves
- Greeting and establishing a rapport with the patient to put him or her at ease
- Ensuring proper patient identification in a variety of situations
- Positioning the patient in a safe, comfortable bed; phlebotomy chair with safety supports; or reclining chair
- Asking about dietary condition (i.e., fasting state)
- Asking about latex sensitivity and likelihood of fainting
- Asking about hand preference or dominance

Supplies for Skin Puncture

Capillary blood specimens are usually collected through the top of a microcollection tube device or by capillary action into a capillary tube. A variety of microcollection tubes and capillary tubes are available commercially with different bore sizes and volume capacities. The tubes and/or their closures can be color coded according to the additives as in larger-size evacuated tubes—for example, lavender for EDTA, green for

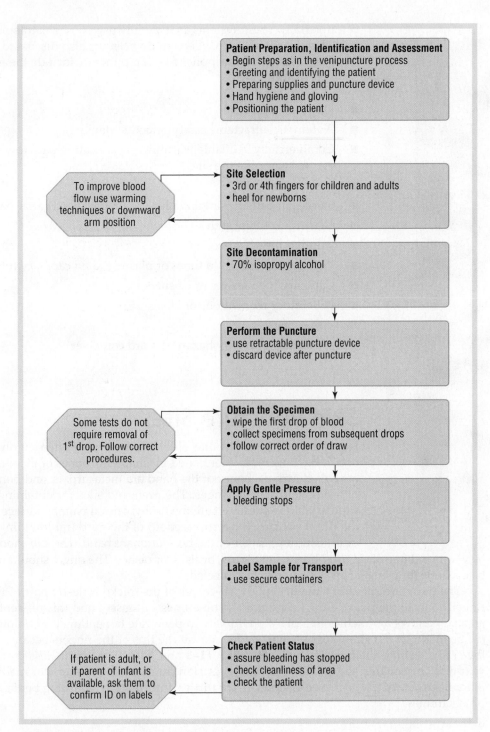

Patient Preparation, Identification and Assessment
• Begin steps as in the venipuncture process
• Greeting and identifying the patient
• Preparing supplies and puncture device
• Hand hygiene and gloving
• Positioning the patient

To improve blood flow use warming techniques or downward arm position

Site Selection
• 3rd or 4th fingers for children and adults
• heel for newborns

Site Decontamination
• 70% isopropyl alcohol

Perform the Puncture
• use retractable puncture device
• discard device after puncture

Some tests do not require removal of 1st drop. Follow correct procedures.

Obtain the Specimen
• wipe the first drop of blood
• collect specimens from subsequent drops
• follow correct order of draw

Apply Gentle Pressure
• bleeding stops

Label Sample for Transport
• use secure containers

If patient is adult, or if parent of infant is available, ask them to confirm ID on labels

Check Patient Status
• assure bleeding has stopped
• check cleanliness of area
• check the patient

FIGURE 11–1

Flowchart: Collecting Capillary Blood Specimens

heparin, pink/red for no additive, and gray for a glycolitic inhibitor. These tubes contain a surface treatment that allows for smooth blood flow into the container. The designs of the capillary blood containers vary from one manufacturer to another. Some allow more exposure to the blood than others, so the health care worker must be particularly cautious when handling open-ended devices. Also available are microdilution systems in which a premeasured amount of reagent is placed in a plastic reservoir that can be punctured by a capillary tube so that the capillary blood specimen is released into the

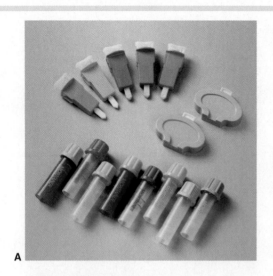

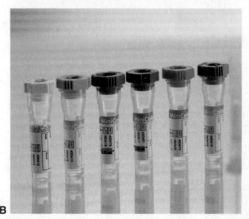

FIGURE 11–2

Capillary Blood Collection Devices and Tubes from Two Manufacturers

A. Courtesy and © Becton Dickinson and Company B. Courtesy of Greiner Bio-One GmbH, Kremsmunster, Austria.

dilution fluid. These systems are typically used for hematological and chemical analyses. Collection devices are also discussed in Chapter 8. In general, supplies for skin puncture include the following (**FIGURE 11–2**):

■ Disposable gloves
■ Automatic retractable safety puncture devices
■ Commercially available warming pack, heating pad, towels, etc., for warming the site
■ Disinfectant pads
■ Sterile hypoallergenic bandages and prepackaged gauze pads
■ Glass microscope slides
■ Diluting fluids as needed
■ Plastic microcollection tubes or plastic-coated capillary tubes
■ Capillary tube sealers or closures
■ Laboratory requisitions or labels
■ A marking pen
■ A puncture-proof biohazard discard container

Skin Puncture Sites

Skin puncture in adults and older children most often involves one of the fingers. As mentioned in Chapter 6, bones of the wrist are called carpals, bones of the hand are metacarpals, and bones of the fingers are phalanges. The preferred sites for obtaining a capillary blood specimen are the fleshy, central palmar surface of the distal phalanx (fingertip section) of the third (middle) finger or fourth (ring) finger of the nondominant hand. The site should be warm and free of calluses, burns, cuts, scars, bruises, or rashes. The finger should not be cyanotic (bluish in color), edematous, or infected.

The puncture should be made slightly off-center of the thickest, fleshy part of the finger because the peak of the fleshy part is sometimes calloused, and this off-center area still allows a puncture in a place least likely to penetrate bone. Punctures should *not* be made on the sides near the nail's edge nor on the tips of the fingers because of the risk of hitting the bone. Refer to **FIGURES 11–3** and **11–4**. For infants less than 1 year old, or neonates, the recommended site for skin puncture is the lateral or medial plantar surface of the heel.[1] See Chapter 13 for further information regarding pediatric phlebotomies.

IMPROVING SITE SELECTION

If the fingers feel cold, it is likely that blood flow (after the skin puncture) may not be abundant enough for an adequate sample. There are a couple of easy ways to improve blood flow so that an adequate capillary blood specimen can be obtained.

Warming the Skin Puncture Site

Warming the skin puncture site, as described in Chapter 10, helps facilitate phlebotomy by significantly increasing arterial blood flow to the area. Capillary specimens from warmed

ALERT

Clinical Alert! Glass capillary tubes can be dangerous because of their potential to break or shatter, putting health care workers at risk for injury. Capillary blood collection devices—such as plastic, glass capillary tubes wrapped in puncture-resistant film, and/or products that avoid the step of pushing tubes into sealant putty—are less likely to break.

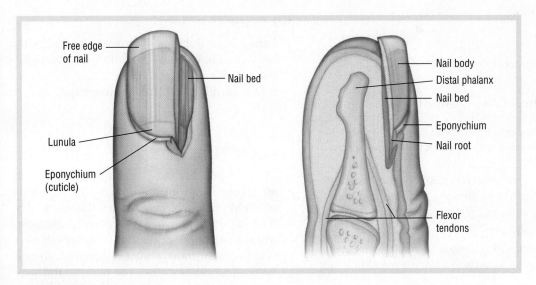

FIGURE 11–3

Structures of the Finger and Nail

Note the positioning of the fingertip bone (distal phalanx) and where it lies in proximity to the edge of the skin. Nails are formed like hair, from a root and grow about 0.1 mm per day.

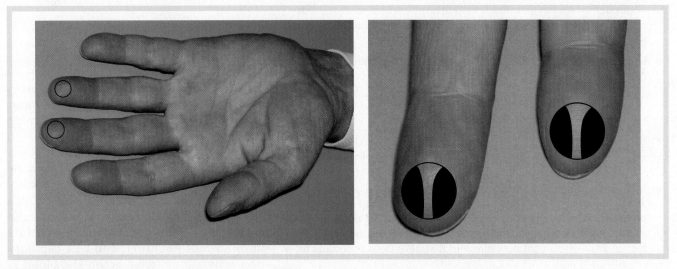

FIGURE 11–4

Sites for Skin Puncture on the Fingers (Fingerstick)

A. The third or fourth finger on the nondominant hand is the preferred choice. **B.** Note that the darkened areas of the circle represent the most suitable puncture sites. However, keep in mind that each patient is different and slight adjustments may be required.

sites can be described as **arterialized capillary blood.** Several easy-to-use methods of warming are commercially available as thermal packs, or a heated surgical towel or a washcloth heated with warm water to 42˚C will not burn the skin and is acceptable. When the towel is wrapped around the site for 3 to 5 minutes, the skin temperature can increase several degrees and arterial blood flow can increase up to sevenfold.[1] Even asking the patient to wash his or her hands in warm water can increase blood flow to the fingertips.

ALERT

Clinical Alert!

The following sites are *not* generally recommended for routine skin punctures:[1]

- Earlobe (even though the earlobe is still used by some, it is not a preferred site due to possible interference with body or ear piercings; also, because of the site's close proximity to the eyes, a puncture device may cause undue anxiety to a patient resulting in a possible jerking of the head)

- Central arch area of an infant's heel and posterior curve of the heel (because of risk of injuring nerves, tendons, cartilage, and bone)

- Fingers of a newborn or infant less than 1 year old (due to the risk of hitting the bone and causing infections)[2]

- The fifth (pinky) finger (because the tissue of this finger is considerably thinner than that of the others and there is a risk of hitting the bone)

- The thumb (because it has a pulse)

- The index (pointer) finger (because it may be more sensitive or it may be calloused)

- Swollen, infected, or previously punctured sites (because accumulated fluid may contaminate the specimen and the site may be bruised, thus causing more pain if it is punctured again)

- Fingers on the side of a mastectomy (because removal of lymph nodes during surgery may result in excessive lymph fluid on the side of the surgery; consult with the ordering physician in the case of a bilateral mastectomy)

- Plantar surface of the big toe (because there is no scientific evidence that supports its use)

ALERT

Clinical Alert!

- Repeatedly puncturing the bone can lead to osteomyelitis, which is an inflammation of the bone due to bacterial infection. Follow your organization's procedures carefully as to the number of times you should puncture a patient and use of the correct puncture device for the situation. Do not puncture sites that have been previously or recently used and/or are sore to the touch.

- Manual, nonretractable lancets are *not* recommended for acquiring capillary specimens because it is harder to control the depth of the puncture; however, they are still used in some facilities. If a sterile lancet is used, it should be carefully removed from its packaging. (If the lancet accidentally touches clothing or brushes against the countertop, it is no longer sterile; and a new device should be opened and used.) Manufacturer's directions should be followed. The finger or heel should be held so as to prevent sudden jerky movements during the puncture. If applicable, remove the protective shield or cap from the lancet. The puncture should be in one continuous movement, perpendicular to the skin. As soon as the lancet has penetrated, it should be quickly removed and immediately discarded into a puncture-proof biohazard sharps container.

Lower the Arm

Sometimes it helps to lower the patient's arm—that is, have the patient simply "dangle" the arm for a few minutes to allow gravity to fill the capillary beds of the fingertips.

CLEANSING THE SKIN PUNCTURE SITE

The skin puncture site should be cleaned with an alcohol pad containing a 70% aqueous solution of isopropanol. Allow the site to dry thoroughly before being punctured, because residual alcohol causes rapid hemolysis and may contaminate glucose determinations. Also, alcohol may sting the patient and prevent formation of rounded drops of blood, which are best for making blood smears on microscopic slides. Iodine tincture preparations are not recommended for disinfecting skin puncture sites because they can falsely elevate potassium, phosphorus, or uric acid determinations.[1]

Skin Puncture Procedure

Microcollection by skin puncture involves many of the same steps used during venipuncture. If the health care worker is performing a heelstick, the infant's heel should be held firmly, with the forefinger at the arch of the foot and the thumb below and away from the puncture site (see Chapter 13 for more details). If a fingerstick is being performed, the patient's finger should be held firmly, with the health care worker's thumb away from the puncture site (**PROCEDURE 11–1**). The best capillary specimens are collected when the blood is freely flowing from the skin puncture. In this case, a capillary tube will fill in approximately 30 seconds, and microcollection tubes will fill within a minute, depending on the exact sizes.

PROCEDURE 11–1

Acquiring a Capillary Blood Specimen (Skin Puncture) Using a Retractable Safety Device

Rationale   To obtain a small amount of blood in a less invasive manner than venipuncture procedures.

Equipment

- Disposable gloves
- Single-use, disposable, sterile puncture device with permanently retractable blade or needle
- Disinfectant pads (70% isopropyl alcohol)
- Warming pads
- Sterile hypoallergenic bandages
- Prepackaged gauze pads (2 × 2 or 3 × 3 inches)
- Glass microscope slides
- Diluting fluids for specified tests
- Plastic microcollection tubes or plastic-coated capillary tubes
- Capillary tube sealers or closures
- Laboratory requisitions or labels
- Marking pen
- Puncture-proof biohazard discard container

Preparation

1 Be emotionally prepared and greet the patient to put him or her at ease.

2 Position the patient in a safe chair, comfortable bed, or reclining chair. Ensure proper patient identification in a variety of situations.

3 Exercise standard precautions and perform hand hygiene and gloving techniques.

4 Prepare supplies and the collection device(s).

5 Verify dietary conditions, that the patient does not have latex allergies, and that the patient is or is not likely to faint.

Procedure

6 Ask about hand preference; check hand dominance. If possible, try to accommodate the patient's preference or use the nondominant hand.

7 Choose a finger that is warm. If possible, select the tip of the third or fourth finger of the nondominant hand (**FIGURE 11–5**). Do not choose fingers that are cold, **cyanotic** (blue in color due to O_2 depletion), or swollen. If the patient's hands are cold, use a commercially available warming device, wrap one hand in a warm towel for 3 to 5 minutes, or ask the patient to wash his or her hands in warm water.

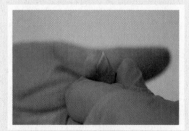

FIGURE 11–5

(continued)

PROCEDURE 11-1

Acquiring a Capillary Blood Specimen (Skin Puncture) Using a Retractable Safety Device (continued)

8 Cleanse the site with an alcohol pad (70% isopropanol) and allow it to air dry. If the finger is visibly dirty, repeat the process with a new alcohol pad until it appears clean (**FIGURE 11–6**).

9 Remove the puncture device and/or lancet from its packaging in view of the patient and follow the manufacturer's instructions. Let the patient know he or she will feel a prick.

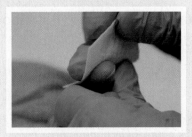

FIGURE 11–6

10 Hold the patient's finger (or heel, in the case of an infant) firmly with one hand, with your thumb away from the puncture site next to the patient's fingernail. With the other hand, position the puncture device on the site (**FIGURE 11–7**). Activate the release mechanism on the retractable safety puncture device and hold it perpendicular to the finger surface. Orient the cut across the fingerprints (perpendicular to the fingerprint grooves) to generate a large, round drop of blood. If the puncture is made along the lines of (i.e., parallel to) the fingerprint, a well-rounded drop will not form and the blood tends to run down the finger.

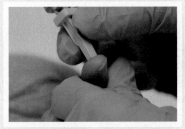

FIGURE 11–7

11 Discard the puncture device in a puncture-proof biohazard container. (If a biohazard container is not within reach, discard the device immediately after completing the collections.)

12 Gently squeeze the finger to expel the first drop (**FIGURE 11–8**). Wipe the first drop of blood away with clean gauze (**FIGURE 11–9**) unless otherwise indicated. (Some point-of-care instruments do not require this step; refer to Chapter 14.) Always follow the manufacturer's instructions.

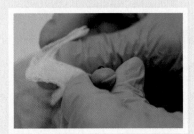

FIGURE 11–8

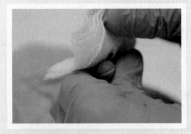

FIGURE 11–9

PROCEDURE 11–1

Acquiring a Capillary Blood Specimen (Skin Puncture) Using a Retractable Safety Device (continued)

13 Collect the second drop of blood by touching it to the tip of the collection device. The blood will flow into the tube by **capillary action,** whereby blood flows freely into the tube on contact, without suction (**FIGURE 11–10**). If the blood becomes jammed in the collection top, gently tap the tube on a hard surface to dislodge it so the blood can flow freely again to the bottom of the tube. Touch the tube to the blood drop as it is formed. Do not "scoop" up the blood.

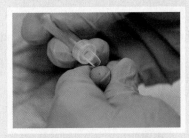

FIGURE 11–10

14 Gently apply pressure to the finger and hold the puncture site in a downward position to encourage the free flow of blood, thereby getting the proper amount of blood. Do not use excessive milking/massaging of the finger or forceful scooping up of blood because that may result in excess tissue fluid and/or hemolysis of the specimen.

15 Each type of microcollection laboratory test has different tube and blood volume requirements. Follow the correct order of draw and appropriate manufacturer's instructions. Gently invert containers with additives to mix the blood with the additives. Carefully and safely seal microcollection tubes with a sealant or with other commercially available devices. When filling capillary tubes, do not allow air bubbles to enter the tubes, because air bubbles can cause erroneous results in many laboratory tests. Blood flow is better and air bubbles are less likely if the puncture site is held downward and gentle pressure is applied

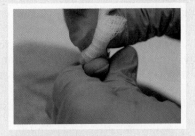

FIGURE 11–11

16 Blood smears can also be made from subsequent drops of blood. Refer to Procedure 11–2, shown later in the chapter.

17 Using a clean gauze pad, apply gentle pressure to the site until bleeding has stopped, usually within a few seconds (**FIGURE 11–11**). Instruct the patient to hold the gauze if the situation allows (**FIGURE 11–12**). The hand may be slightly elevated. (If collecting blood from an infant's heel, apply the gauze pad and elevate the heel until bleeding stops).

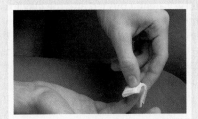

FIGURE 11–12

18 Label the specimens and/or outside containers in front of the patient to verify identity and to prepare them for transport.

19 Discard all other biohazardous supplies prior to removing gloves.

(continued)

PROCEDURE 11–1

Acquiring a Capillary Blood Specimen (Skin Puncture) Using a Retractable Safety Device (continued)

After The Procedure

20 Remove and dispose of gloves in a biohazard container and perform hand hygiene.

21 Ensure that bleeding has stopped, ask the patient to verify that the labels have his or her name, and thank the patient before leaving with specimens and remaining supplies.

Notes

- Retractable puncture devices are currently available on the market and are recommended for many safety reasons instead of a sterile lancet that is not a retractable device.[1] (See Chapter 8 for more information about devices and microcollection tubes.) Some puncture devices are activated "on contact," meaning that the puncture mechanism operates only when it is positioned and pressed against the skin. This minimizes the risk of accidentally activating the device at another time. Others may require the push of a release button. Health care workers should understand and follow the manufacturer's directions for use of each device.

- Puncture devices are made for variable depth and length depending on the patient's age and weight. The average depth of a skin puncture should be 2 to 3 mm for adults, and less than 2 mm for small children and infants, to avoid injuring the bone. Laser devices are also available as skin puncture alternatives. They provide a smaller hole (about 250 µm wide and 1 to 2 mm deep).

- In health care facilities, the puncture devices used are typically small, single-use, disposable devices. However, in home settings, a patient may have a multiuse device in which only the lancet is changed after each use from that single patient. In this case, discard the lancet and clean the multiuse device according to the manufacturer's instructions if it becomes contaminated.

- A free flow of blood is essential to obtain accurate test results. However, do not use excessive squeezing or massaging to obtain blood drops.

- If the blood drop used for the specimen is allowed to remain on the skin too long, some evaporation may occur and the drop may dry out. If this happens, wipe away this drop and use the next one; otherwise, erroneous laboratory values may result.

- If the sample is not adequate and blood has stopped flowing from the puncture site, it may be necessary to repuncture at a *different* site. Warming techniques prior to repuncturing will improve the blood flow to the area. Use a *new* alcohol pad to cleanse the second site, and a *new* sterile retractable lancet for the second puncture. Avoid excessive punctures on one finger or hand.

- Some laboratory tests require the use of capillary tubes that must be sealed with a self-sealing mechanism or by using a clay slab into which the tube is gently pushed and the clay forms a plug to keep the blood from coming out of the tube. Once the tube is pushed into the clay, it should be rotated slightly or twisted as it is being removed so that the clay plug will stay in the tube. These clay slabs may pose a hazard because they become contaminated with blood. They should be discarded at regular intervals in a biohazard container. Some clay sealants are available in punchcard-type trays that have an upper plate to retain the sealant and guide the tube.[1]

ALERT

Clinical Alert! Microcollection tubes must be adequately filled and gently mixed to prevent clotting. Excessive amounts (over-filling) can cause clot formation; inadequate amounts (underfilling) can cause cells to change morphologically because of too much anticoagulant.[1] Do not mix the specimen vigorously because that can cause hemolysis.

Order of Collection

The order of filling microcollection tubes with capillary blood is different than for venipuncture (**FIGURE 11–13**). If multiple laboratory tests have been ordered, the order of collection should be as follows:[1]

- EDTA specimen for hematology tests
- Other tubes with additives
- Nonadditive tubes

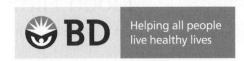

BD Microtainer™ Tubes with Microgard™ Closure
Tube Guide and Order of Draw

Catalog #/Closure Color		Additive	Mix by Inverting	Laboratory Use
365974	Lavender	K_2 EDTA	10x	For whole blood hematology determinations. Tube inversions prevent clotting.
365965	Green	Lithium Heparin	10x	For plasma determinations in chemistry. Tube inversions prevent clotting.
365985	Mint Green	Lithium Heparin and Gel for plasma separation	10x	For plasma determinations in chemistry. Tube inversions prevent clotting.
365987	Mint Green			
365992	Grey	NaFl/Na_2 EDTA	10x	For glucose determinations. Tube inversions ensure proper mixing of additive and blood.
365967	Gold	Clot Activator and Gel for serum separation	5x	For serum determinations in chemistry.
365978	Gold			
365963	Red	No additive	0x	For serum determinations in chemistry, serology and blood banking.

365976
Tube Extender

BD Vacutainer Systems
Preanalytical Solutions
1 Becton Drive
Franklin Lakes, NJ 07417

BD Vacutainer Technical Services: 1.800.631.0174
BD Customer Service: 1.888.237.2762
www.bd.com/vacutainer

BD, BD Logo and all other trademarks are property of Becton, Dickinson and Company. ©2003 BD.
Made in USA   5/03   VS5836-1

FIGURE 11–13
Order of Draw Using BD Microtainer Tubes

Courtesy and © Becton Dickinson and Company

Blood Films for Microscopic Slides

Blood smears are not used in all laboratories because current technologies do not require them. However, some laboratories still use this method for confirmatory purposes or as a backup procedure. **PROCEDURE 11–2** demonstrates the process for making blood films/ smears on microscopic glass slides for performing white blood cell differentials. (Remember from Chapter 7 that blood films are used to determine percentages and morphology of white blood cells.) Red blood cell and platelet morphology can also be assessed. Health care facilities can vary the procedures that they use to make blood smears; appropriate steps should therefore be followed at each facility. It takes a significant amount of practice to learn to make slides that are acceptable for use. Health care workers must be adequately trained to make consistently good slides for microscopic analysis. If the blood films are made at the patient's bedside, they are considered "infectious" until they are stained or fixed chemically in the laboratory. Thus, they should be transported and handled with caution.

PROCEDURE 11–2

Blood Smears/Films for Microscopic Slides

Rationale Blood films on microscopic slides are used to evaluate the morphology (form and structure) of the blood cells. Using this procedure, microscope slides are prepared with a blood drop that is thinned out. The slides are treated with special stains in the laboratory and evaluated under a microscope. Although some facilities no longer use this manual method, it is still used in many cases for detecting cellular abnormalities, for confirmation, and/or for a backup method.

Equipment

- Gloves
- Microscopic glass slides
- Applicator sticks or other commercial devices for placing a drop on the slide
- Drying rack or other clean surface
- Same equipment needed to perform Procedure 11–1

Preparation

1 Prepare and assemble supplies.

2 Identify the patient properly.

3 Wash or sanitize your hands with an alcohol hand rinse; then put on gloves.

4 Perform the skin puncture as directed in Procedure 11–1.

Procedure

5 Blood films/smears can be started by using one of several methods to place the blood drop on the slide.
  - **Directly from the patient's finger:**—Perform the finger puncture in the usual way, wiping the first drop of blood away. Touch the slide to the second drop at approximately 0.5 to 1 inch (1.3 to 2.5 cm) from the end of the slide.

PROCEDURE 11–2

Blood Smears/Films for Microscopic Slides (continued)

■ **From a hematology, anticoagulated (EDTA), lavender-top tube:**—Smears made using blood from an EDTA tube should be done where there is minimal exposure to the blood or blood spills. One method is to use an applicator stick(s) to place the drop on the slide (**FIGURE 11–14**) OR, a commercially available device can be inserted into the EDTA tube and touched to the slide to release a drop (**FIGURES 11–15, 11–16, 11–17,** and **11–18**).

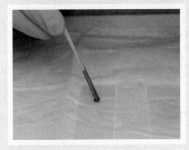

FIGURE 11–14

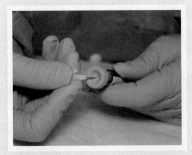

FIGURE 11–15

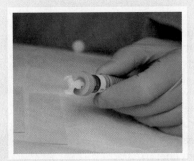

FIGURE 11–16

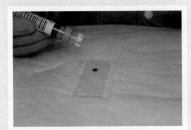

FIGURE 11–17

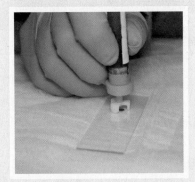

FIGURE 11–18

6 Place the second (spreader) slide in front of the drop of blood and then pull it slowly into the drop, allowing blood to spread along the width of the slide (**FIGURE 11–19**).

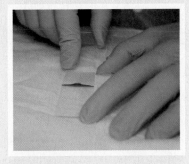

FIGURE 11–19

(continued)

PROCEDURE 11–2

Blood Smears/Films for Microscopic Slides (continued)

7 When the blood spreads almost to the edges, quickly and evenly push the spreader slide forward at an angle of approximately 30 degrees. Do not press downward. The only downward pressure should be the weight of the spreader slide (**FIGURE 11–20**).

8 Allow the slide to air dry; do not blow on it.

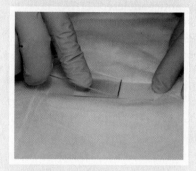

FIGURE 11–20

9 Blood films should have a **feathered edge**, as shown in the last slide labeled in **FIGURE 11–21**. It has a visible curved edge that thins out smoothly and resembles the tip of a bird's feather.

10 No ridges, lines, or holes should be visible in the smear. It should not be too thick either. Errors are often the result of too large a drop, too long a delay in spreading the drop, not moving the spreader slide in a straight line, pressing too hard on the spreader slide, blowing on the slide, or using a chipped slide. In Figure 11–21, the first six blood films are unacceptable for analysis. Again, remember that these slides should be handled carefully.

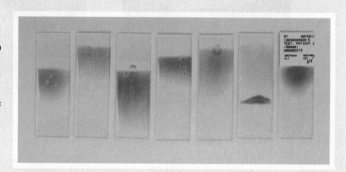

FIGURE 11–21

11 Label the slides and prepare them for safe transport to the laboratory.

After The Procedure

12 Discard any unusable slides and all biohazardous waste in an appropriate container.

13 Wash or sanitize your hands.

14 Recheck identity of the specimens. Thank the patient for cooperating and depart with *all* specimens and *all* remaining supplies.

15 Deliver the slides to the laboratory.

Other Considerations for Capillary Blood Samples

DIFFERENCES IN VENOUS SPECIMEN TEST RESULTS

Due to slight differences between venous and skin puncture blood for many laboratory tests, it is important to note or report on laboratory test results that the specimen was a capillary sample or collected by skin puncture. There *are* differences in the concentrations of glucose, potassium, total protein, and calcium. The concentration of glucose is higher in capillary blood than in venous blood specimens, and the concentration of potassium, total protein, and calcium is lower in capillary blood than in venous blood.[1]

> **ALERT**
>
> **Clinical Alert!** Hemolysis of the capillary blood specimen can cause erroneous laboratory results and is often preventable if good technique is maintained. Hemolysis is caused by[1]
>
> - Not removing residual alcohol at the puncture site
> - Excessive milking of the finger
> - Excessive mixing or agitation of the specimen
> - Increased red blood cell fragility and high packed-cell volume (newborns and infants)

MICROHEMATOCRIT AND OTHER HEMATOLOGY SPECIMENS

The packed cell volume (PCV), or microhematocrit, can be collected directly into a capillary tube containing heparin. The tube should be filled at least two-thirds full and sealed at one end as soon as it is filled. The seal can be sealing clay or commercially available covers.

Hematology specimens can be collected directly into tubes containing the anticoagulants disodium, dipotassium, or tripotassium ethylenediamine tetraacetate (Na_2EDTA, K_2EDTA, K_3EDTA). These specimens are stable for two to four hours for hematologic tests. Since heparin distorts cell morphology and can interfere with staining techniques, specimens for hematology tests should not be collected in heparinized tubes unless the only test needed is the PCV.

BLOOD pH AND BLOOD GAS DETERMINATIONS

The site must be warmed prior to collecting capillary blood for pH and blood gas determinations. This increases arterial blood flow to the area. The heparinized capillary tubes must not contain air bubbles because exposure to air may affect the specimen. The specimen must be quickly sealed after inserting a magnetic mixing bar, or "flea," because the exposure of blood to air (even for short periods of 10 to 30 seconds) can cause significant changes in laboratory values.[3] After inserting the mixing flea, which is a tiny magnetic steel wire, it is drawn back and forth along the length of the tube several times. It is important to remove the flea prior to testing the specimen.[1] This is covered in greater detail in Chapter 13.

Completing the Interaction

DISPOSAL

Used disposable lancets should be placed into a rigid, puncture-resistant biohazard container with a lid.

LABELING

All tubes must be appropriately labeled immediately after capillary blood collection and mixing, and the information on the labels confirmed. This should be done at the patient's bedside before leaving the room. Remember that the health care worker's identity should be available on the specimen label. The specimens can be labeled individually; or, since the specimen tubes are very small, several tubes may be placed together in a larger labeled container. Smaller labels are often available for slides and tubes. Follow the appropriate labeling procedures for each health facility. All supplies and equipment that were brought in should be removed or discarded appropriately.

COMPLETING THE PATIENT INTERACTION

Hand hygiene must be performed after contact with each patient. Before leaving the patient's side, the health care worker must check the puncture site to make sure that the bleeding has stopped, ask the patient if he or she has recovered from the procedure, recheck the identity of the specimens, and then thank the patient. A hypoallergenic adhesive bandage may be applied as needed or requested. Such bandages are not recommended for infants or young children, however, because of possible irritation and the potential of swallowing or aspirating a bandage.

Study Questions

For the following questions, select the one best answer.

1 Which of the following is a preferred site for a capillary puncture?

a. wrist
b. antecubital area
c. third finger
d. thumb

2 Controlling the depth of puncture during a fingerstick prevents which of the following?

a. puncturing a vein
b. bacterial contamination
c. excessive bleeding
d. osteomyelitis

3 A finger puncture should involve which of the following steps?

a. puncturing parallel to fingerprint
b. puncturing along the fingerprint lines
c. puncturing across the fingerprint
d. wiping away the first two drops

4 Skin puncture is *not* useful for patients who have which of the following conditions?

a. obesity
b. burns
c. fragile veins
d. swollen arms and hands

5 Which finger(s) are used most often for skin puncture?

a. thumb
b. second (index) finger
c. third or fourth finger
d. fifth (pinky) finger

6 Blood samples from skin punctures cannot be used for which tests?

a. routine hematology tests
b. glucose testing
c. coagulation studies
d. cholesterol screening tests

7 Capillary blood is more like arterial blood than venous blood for which of the following reasons?

a. the skin has more arterioles
b. arterial pressure is stronger in capillaries
c. there is more arterial blood than venous blood
d. venous pressure is greater in capillaries

8 Plastic microcollection tubes should be filled with blood in which of the following ways?

a. using a syringe to fill the tube
b. allowing the tube to fill by itself using capillary action
c. using suction to pull blood into the tube
d. using the tube to scoop droplets off the skin carefully

9 If alcohol is used to decontaminate the capillary puncture site, which of the following is an essential step?

a. using two alcohol pads for cleansing
b. diluting the strength of the alcohol
c. wiping away the second drop of blood after the puncture
d. allowing the site to air dry prior to the puncture

10 The best angle for using two glass slides to make a blood smear is approximately

a. 10 degrees
b. 15 degrees
c. 30 degrees
d. 90 degrees

Case Study 1

Mastectomy Patient A 55-year-old woman came to have some routine blood tests performed by the skin puncture method. She told the health care worker that she had a mastectomy on her right side about 15 years ago.

Questions

1 Where should the health care worker perform the fingerstick?

2 Why should the health care worker consider the information about the mastectomy important?

Case Study 2

A Young Patient A precocious 5-year-old patient was being seen in a pediatric clinic. The young girl was to have a blood specimen collected for hematology tests. The patient told the health care worker that she hated needles. The health care worker thought about which type of blood collection method she should use for this patient.

Questions

1 What are the options for this patient?

2 Which method seems most appropriate for this patient?

Action in Practice

Action in Practice Think about the last time you had a blood specimen collected. Based on your own experience, make a list of the positive and negative aspects of the venipuncture procedure in comparison to the skin puncture procedure. You may consider interviewing other friends or relatives on their preferences toward each method, the level of pain they experienced with each of the procedures, and their overall impressions of each procedure.

COMPETENCY ASSESSMENT

Competency Checklist: Capillary Blood Collection

Each step must be successfully completed. If one step is not completed successfully, the individual/student should restudy the text and seek guidance from a supervisor or educator. He or she must try again until competency has been achieved.

(1) Completed (2) Needs to improve

_____ 1. Performs patient identification and assessment appropriately

_____ 2. Prepares the appropriate supplies and puncture device

_____ 3. Performs hand hygiene and gloving techniques

_____ 4. Positions the patient appropriately

_____ 5. Selects the correct finger

_____ 6. Cleanses the site appropriately

_____ 7. Uses warming devices or other methods to improve blood flow to the site

_____ 8. Uses a self-retracting puncture device to make an incision across the fingerprint, and then discards the puncture device

_____ 9. Wipes away the first drop of blood

_____ 10. Collects the appropriate specimen in the correct order

_____ 11. Applies appropriate pressure to produce additional drops of blood

_____ 12. Applies gentle pressure to stop the bleeding

_____ 13. Handles the specimens appropriately (e.g., gentle mixing)

_____ 14. Discards all waste in appropriate containers

_____ 15. Labels the specimens appropriately and prepares them for transport

_____ 16. Checks the patient status and reconfirms sample labels/identity are correct

_____ 17. Thanks the patient for cooperating

Competency Checklist: Making Blood Smears for Microscopic Analysis

Many phlebotomists are no longer required to make blood smears or films on microscopic slides. However, it is a skill that is still required in some settings in which phlebotomists are the only ones with this skill. Making suitable microscopic blood films for laboratory analysis requires repeated practice. The skill should be practiced until the phlebotomist becomes proficient.

(1) Completed (2) Needs to improve

_____ 1. Using a practice sample of blood, the phlebotomist is able to make 50 suitable blood smears.

_____ 2. Using blood from a capillary puncture on a patient, the phlebotomist wipes away the first drop of blood.

_____ 3. The glass slide is touched to the finger about 0.5 to 1 inch from the end.

_____ 4. The second slide (the spreader) is placed in front of the drop, which allows the drop of blood to spread along the width of the slide.

_____ 5. The spreader is pushed evenly toward the other end of the slide, causing the blood to flow evenly across the glass.

_____ 6. The blood smear has the shape of a feathered edge.

_____ 7. The slide is allowed to air dry.

_____ 8. The slide is labeled appropriately.

REFERENCES

1. Clinical and Laboratory Standards Institute (CLSI). (2008). *Procedures and devices for the collection of diagnostic capillary blood specimens, approved standard,* 6th ed. H04-A6. Wayne, PA: Author.

2. Phelan, S. E. (1999). Fingersticks on children. *Lab Med, 30*(9): 569–570.

3. Clinical and Laboratory Standards Institute (CLSI). (2004). *Procedures for the collection of arterial blood specimens, approved standard,* 4th ed., H11-A4. Wayne, PA: Author.

RESOURCES

www.ascp.org American Society for Clinical Pathology: ASCP-LabQP, Continuing Educational exercises for phlebotomy

www.phlebotomy.com Phlebotomy Today, e-newsletter

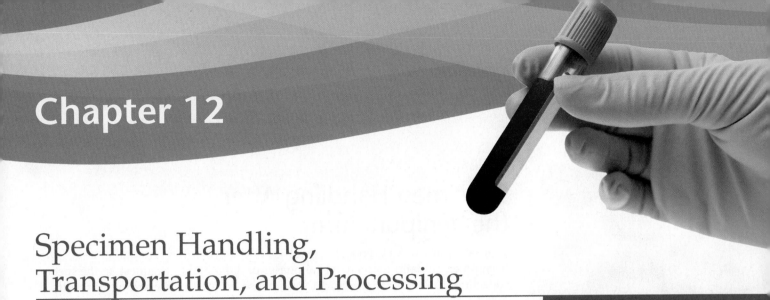

Chapter 12

Specimen Handling, Transportation, and Processing

KEY TERMS

aliquot
critical laboratory value
photosensitive
pneumatic tube systems
thermolabile
turnaround time (TAT)

Chapter Objectives

Upon completion of Chapter 12, the learner is responsible for doing the following:

1. Describe at least three sources of preexamination error that can occur during blood specimen handling.

2. Describe at least three sources of preexamination error that can occur during blood specimen transportation.

3. Describe at least three sources of preexamination error that can occur during specimen processing or storage.

4. Name three methods commonly used to transport specimens.

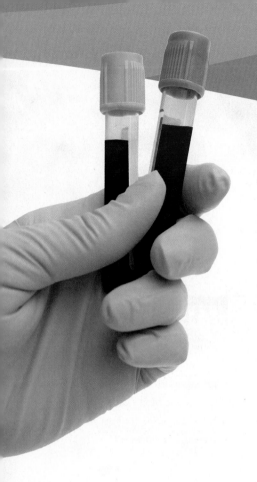

Specimen Handling After the Venipuncture

There are many ways to conceptualize the cycle of performing laboratory tests, flowing from preexamination/preanalytical phases of the initial test request, to the specimen collection, to the examination/analytic phase, to the final reporting of results. The quality and usefulness of laboratory test results depend on the time that specimens are received for processing and how quickly they are analyzed to yield an accurate, reliable test result to help the physician make decisions. The time it takes for a blood specimen to be ordered, collected, transported, processed, analyzed, and a result reported is often referred to as the **turnaround time (TAT).** Blood and other specimens must always be delivered expeditiously. The health care worker has an enormous impact on the TAT and is the vital link in the preexamination phase of laboratory testing.

The preexamination variables that are inherent in phlebotomy duties include the following:

- **Patient variables**—Identification, age, gender, pregnancy, medications, fasting versus nonfasting, diurnal variations, refusal to cooperate, patient unavailable, stress or anxiety, etc.

- **Transportation and handling variables**—Correct filling and mixing of the specimen tubes, specimen leakage, tube breakage, excessive shaking, etc.

- **Specimen processing and storage variables**—Adequacy of centrifugation, sample registration and distribution, delays in processing, contamination of the specimen, exposure to heat or light, etc.

- **Specimen variables**—Hemolysis, inadequate volume in the tube, inadequate mixing of anticoagulant, etc.

A health care worker's duties do not end when the venipuncture procedure is completed. Instead, they continue until the specimen is correctly transported, processed, tested in the clinical laboratory, and ultimately translated into a report. The Clinical and Laboratory Standards Institute (CLSI) defines standards for handling and processing blood specimens after the venipuncture is performed.[1,2] To simplify and break down the process and consider the many variables that might affect laboratory testing, there are basic steps in handling and transporting a specimen prior to processing it once it arrives at a laboratory for analysis:

- **Mixing the specimen** by gentle inversions is important when the tubes contain an additive to ensure even distribution of the additive into the blood. As mentioned in Chapters 10 and 11, this must be done as soon as possible after the blood specimen enters the additive tube. It should be done gently to avoid damage to blood cells, which can result in hemolysis. If the specimen is not mixed adequately, tiny clots may form within the specimen tube and lead to erroneous test results, particularly for hematology tests. If gel separation tubes are not mixed thoroughly, clotting may be incomplete. Keep in mind that specimen tubes without additives do not require mixing.

- **Labeling the specimen correctly** involves three steps. First, the label should be placed on the tube immediately after collection, without delay. It should be oriented correctly on the tube. (Remember: The label should include the patient's first and last names, the identification number, the date and time of collection, the name/initials of the person collecting the specimen, and any optional information—test ordered, volume requirements, physician's name, etc.). Many labels are compatible with laboratory instruments such that the bar code is scanned by the analyzer and test results are electronically linked. Thus, there are often requirements about orientation and placement of the label on individual specimen tubes. **FIGURE 12–1** depicts one example of a manufacturer's recommendations for orientation of the label. Note that the specimen tubes with misaligned, wrinkled, or overlapped labels have the potential of being misread.

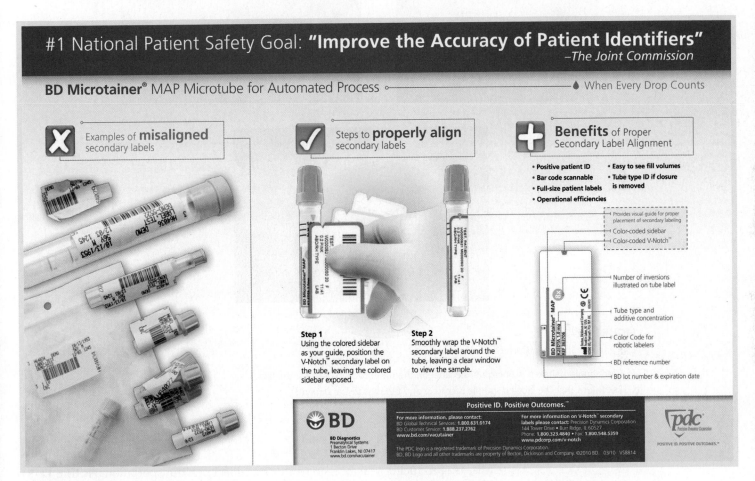

FIGURE 12–1

Example of Manufacturer's Guide for Label Alignment on Tubes

Courtesy and © Becton, Dickinson and Company

Second, the health care worker must sign or initial each labeled specimen, according to the instructions at the health care facility. And third, whenever possible, the labeled tube should be compared to the patient's identification bracelet or the patient can verbally verify that the label information is correct (**FIGURE 12–2**).

■ **Placing the blood specimen in a biohazard bag** or rack or other safety-conscious carrier. Most laboratories require the use of a leakproof plastic bag for enclosing and transporting the primary specimen tube (i.e., the blood samples taken directly from the patient). This bag protects the health care worker from pathogenic

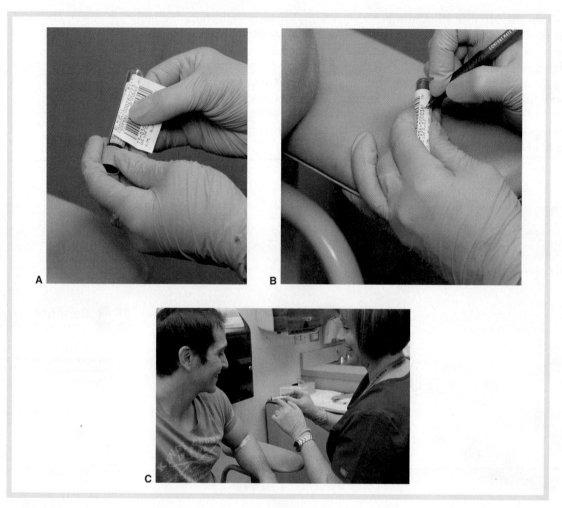

FIGURE 12–2

Labeling the Specimen Correctly

A. Care should be taken in lining up the label on the tube. B. Sign or initial the label.
C. Reconfirm that the labeled sample is correct and belongs to the patient.

(disease-producing) microorganisms during specimen transportation (**FIGURE 12–3**). The transport bag may have a pouch on the outside for the laboratory requisition or other forms, thus eliminating the potential for contamination. If possible, the blood specimens in evacuated tubes and microcollection tubes should be maintained in a vertical (upright) position with the tube cap or closure on top to promote complete clot formation and to reduce the possibility of agitating the sample, which may cause hemolysis. Handling blood specimens in a gentle manner also reduces the chances of hemolyzing the specimens.

■ **Transportation to the appropriate laboratory** should occur *as soon as possible* from the time of collection so that the specimen can be processed appropriately (i.e., so that serum or plasma can be separated from the blood cells). If there are significant delays in transportation, interfering factors can affect the test results. Glycolytic action (the breakdown of glucose) from the blood cells, which interferes with the analysis of various analytes (such as glucose, calcitonin, aldosterone, phosphorus, and enzymes), can occur. Also, rough handling and agitation of the specimen may be more likely if there are delays, and can have an effect on coagulation tests (for example, platelet activation and shortened clotting times).

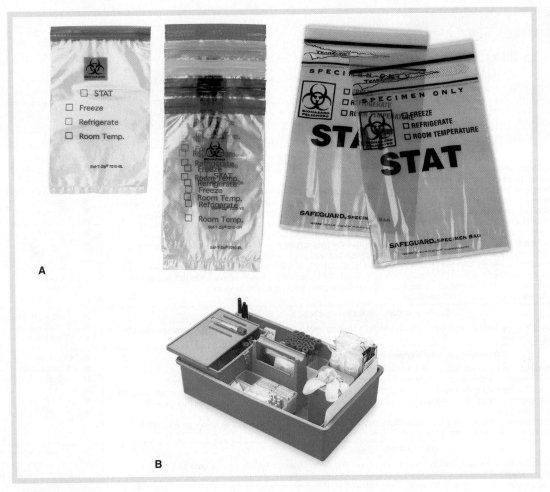

FIGURE 12–3

Specimen Transportation

A. Specimen bags. B. Specimen rack included in the phlebotomy tray.

Courtesy of MarketLab Inc. www.marketlabinc.com

■ **Special handling procedures** are needed for specific laboratory tests. Some require cooling to slow metabolic processes, some require transport at body temperature (37°C) to prevent precipitation or agglutination, and others require protection from light to prevent the analyte from breaking down. Specific examples are mentioned in **TABLE 12–1.**

■ **Microbiological specimens** are also frequently transported along with blood specimens. Specimens include blood cultures, throat cultures, and urine specimens for microbiological culture. They also need to be transported to the laboratory as quickly as possible so that the specimens can be transferred to culture media or incubated appropriately, and the urine analyzed. This enhances the likelihood of detecting pathogenic bacteria. Blood culture specimens are usually collected directly into culture media, which minimizes possible contamination and speeds the contact with the culture media. (See Chapter 15 for more information on blood cultures.) Since culture media provides nutritional ingredients for bacterial growth, the sooner they are incubated, the sooner bacteria will grow, and the sooner positive results can be detected.

■ **Specimen transportation to/from remote sites** occurs from remote reference laboratories as well as ambulatory sites, including home health collections. The health care worker must still follow the handling guidelines according to standard precautions.

TABLE 12–1

Special Handling Requirements

This table reflects the CLSI recommendations for special handling during transport of blood specimens when specific tests are requested.[1,2,3,4] Laboratory procedures are constantly changing and being updated or modified; consequently, health care workers should be familiar with these tests as well as the policies and procedures used by their own facility in handling, transporting, and processing specimens. These are general requirements but are subject to change in different settings.

Special Handling Requirement	Laboratory Tests
Specimens that are thermolabile and require chilling ■ **Thermolabile** means that the substance is sensitive to higher temperatures, and specimens being tested for these substances need to be chilled immediately. ■ Chilling a specimen inhibits blood cell metabolism and stabilizes most constituents. ■ Chilling can be accomplished using commercially available products or by the use of an ice water slurry (mixture of ice and water; do not use large chunks of ice because of the likelihood of freezing the specimen) **(FIGURE 12–4)**. ■ *Special note for blood gas specimens*: Delivery speed is essential to prevent the loss of blood gases from the specimen. If the sample will be analyzed within 30 minutes, use of a plastic syringe is recommended and the transport can occur at room temperature. However, if analysis is delayed, then glass syringes can be used and cooled as soon as possible after collection. The cooling action decreases the loss of gases from the specimen. ■ Some analytes are negatively affected by chilling, such as potassium (K). If a potassium test is ordered and collected in the same tube with other analytes that require chilling, it should be tested within two hours or collected in a separate tube. Chilling for more than two hours causes K to leak out of the cells, causing a false elevation. ■ Specimens for electrolytes should not be chilled.	■ Ammonia ■ Blood gases (see Special note below) ■ Catecholamines ■ Gastrin ■ Lactic acid ■ Parathyroid hormone ■ Pyruvate
Specimens that require transport at 37°C ■ These specimens require either a commercially available controlled heat source or a heating block for transportation and handling purposes.	■ Cold agglutinins ■ Cryofibrinogen ■ Cryoglobulins
Specimens that are photosensitive and should be protected from light ■ **Photosensitive** means that the substance is sensitive to light and will decompose after exposure to bright light. ■ Chemical constituents in blood that are light sensitive, such as bilirubin, will decompose if exposed to light. ■ Blood collected for light-sensitive chemical analysis should be protected from bright light with a commercially available amber/brown biohazard bag, an aluminum foil wrapping around the tube, or a transport container that does not allow light to enter (see Figure 12–4). ■ Recent studies have suggested that exposure to light may not affect folate and B vitamins, so follow your facility's procedures for protecting specimens as needed.	■ Bilirubin ■ Beta-carotene ■ Folate ■ Porphyrins ■ Vitamin A ■ Vitamin B$_6$
Plasma-based coagulation assays[4] ■ Temperature fluctuations for coagulation tests should be avoided during transport. Use of ice or cold packs is not recommended because of possible cold activation of clotting factors and platelet disruption. ■ Ideally, transportation should occur within one hour of collection. However, acceptable time delays vary depending on the test ordered; for example, PT assays may be acceptable even after a delay of up to 24 hours. However, if monitoring unfractionated heparin therapy, the delay should not exceed one hour if collected in sodium citrate. Therefore, follow your facility's procedures for transport and handling coagulation specimens. ■ Specimens should be stored capped. ■ PT specimens can remain uncentrifuged or centrifuged with the plasma on top of the cells at room temperature (up to 24 hours). Specimens for APTT from patients who are not on heparin therapy can remain uncentrifuged or centrifuged with plasma on the cells at room temperature for up to four hours from the time of collection. If specimens contain unfractionated heparin, they should be kept at room temperature and centrifuged within one hour of collection. Again, follow your facility's procedures. ■ For molecular hemostasis assays, the ideal DNA extraction would occur from fresh specimens. However, anticoagulated, whole blood (EDTA or citrate) can be stored at room temperature for up to 8 days or at 2 to 8°C before the DNA is extracted. Laboratories should also follow manufacturers' directions and provide up-to-date information to all personnel who are involved in transporting these specimens. ■ Coagulation specimens may be rejected if they are clotted in the wrong additive, if the tube is overfilled or underfilled, if there are time delays, or if transported at the wrong temperature. Follow all procedures accordingly.	■ Acceptable time delays can vary depending on the specific coagulation test performed.

The health care worker should use the same safety equipment used in a hospital environment (e.g., closed venipuncture system, gloves, disposable laboratory coat, plastic blood collection tubes, and a biohazardous disposal container). In addition, all blood collection equipment and specimens should be transported in an enclosed or lockable container to avoid spills in the unlikely event that the health care worker is in a car collision. The container should have a biohazard warning label on it and notification procedures in case of an accident. Cold packs should be used in the container for transport during hot weather, or, the reverse, the vehicle should be heated in freezing weather. The container should be placed in a protected part of the car (such as the floorboard or secured in the seat) to prevent accidental tumbling and to prevent direct exposure to heating or cooling vents. For home collection, the health

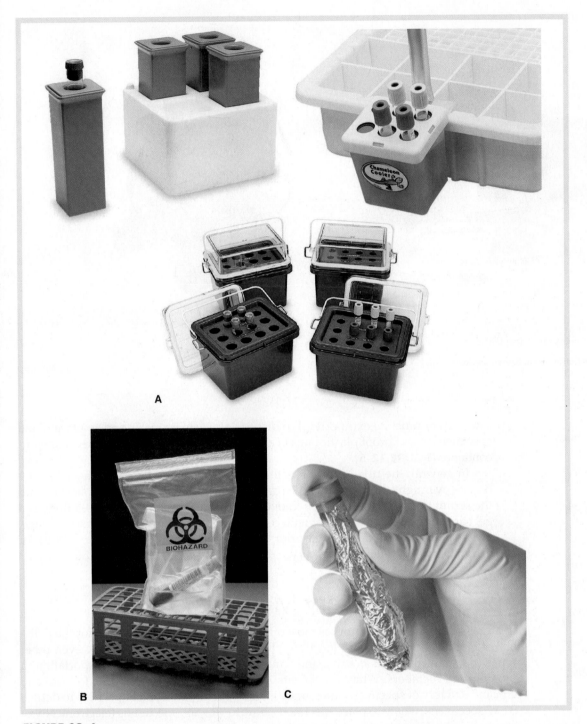

FIGURE 12–4

Chilling Specimens

A. Transportation racks designed specifically for transporting specimens that need to be cooled. *(Courtesy of MarketLab Inc. www.marketlabinc.com)* B. Specimen in an ice slurry. C. Specimen wrapped in foil for protection from light.

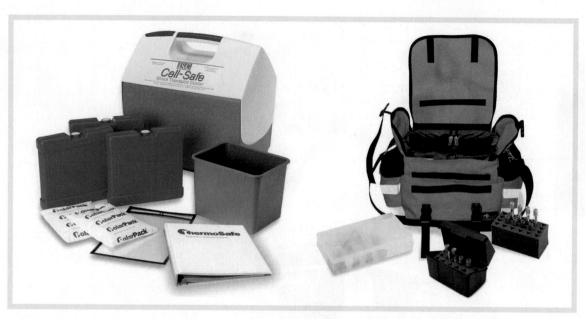

FIGURE 12–5

Transport Containers for Longer Distance.

Courtesy of MarketLab Inc. www.marketlabinc.com

care worker must be extra careful to dispose of waste properly and to place blood specimens in leakproof plastic bags in an upright position inside a labeled transport container (**FIGURE 12–5**).

In general, the rule of thumb is that blood specimens for chemistry tests that require overnight shipping should be centrifuged within two hours of collection and the serum or plasma should be removed from contact with cells (unless there is a gel barrier that prevents contact with cells). Sometimes, it is necessary to centrifuge, separate, and freeze the plasma prior to shipping. Follow specific procedures for each facility or reference laboratory.

Specimen Delivery Methods

In larger facilities, the laboratory is most often the department responsible for the delivery of blood specimens to the location where they will be analyzed. However, other types of specimens, such as urine and sputum, may be delivered by transportation or nursing staff members. Whatever the site, guidelines should be available for safe and efficient delivery of specimens; these may include a schedule of pickups, how to deliver STAT specimens, where to place specimens, how to "log in" specimens (electronically or manually), etc. Appropriate documentation procedures and open communication among all departments are the keys to successful and efficient specimen delivery.

Commercial courier services are also used to transport specimens to or from off-site areas, such as reference laboratories, blood-drawing stations, or remote clinics. Again, considerations before and during transportation should include adequate packaging and handling. This is especially true in hot or cold temperatures.

HAND DELIVERY

Many specimens are hand-carried and require guidelines for timeliness of delivery to the laboratory. A log sheet or data entry for specimens that are hand delivered to the laboratory is commonly used. For health care workers in a hospital setting, the blood collection trays or carts are typically arranged to hold specimens awaiting delivery to the laboratory using test tube racks, a holder for microscopic slides, plastic holders, cups, and/or a leakproof container for ice water. Many commercially available carriers and racks provide a safe, effective method to transport specimens. Figures 12–3 and 12–4 showed numerous carrying trays specifically designed for phlebotomy collections.

PNEUMATIC TUBE SYSTEMS

Pneumatic tube systems are commonly used to transport patient records, messages, letters, bills, medications, x-rays, and laboratory test results. Considerations in the use of these systems for transporting specimens are mechanical reliability, distance of transport, speed of carrier, control mechanisms, landing mechanism, radius of loops and bends, shock absorbency, sizes of carriers, cleaning methodology, and laboratory assessment of chemical and cellular components in transported specimens versus hand-carried specimens. If specific documentation does not already exist, the pneumatic tube system should be carefully evaluated for these effects on laboratory results. However, the CLSI reports that many studies have documented the validity of laboratory results after this type of transport and suggests that tests most affected (lactate dehydrogenase, potassium, plasma hemoglobin, and acid phosphatase) are due to the disruption of the red cells. Also, specimens for coagulation testing should be protected from vibrations and shock to avoid platelet activation during transport.[4] However, the majority of analytes are not usually affected, and this is an efficient means of specimen transport. It is recommended that blood specimen tubes be placed in the pneumatic tube with shock-absorbent inserts padding the sides and with the tubes separated from one another to prevent spillage or breakage. Plastic clear liners are also commercially available so that if leaks do occur, they are visible and are contained to prevent contamination of the tube system, the carrier, and the personnel handling the specimens (**FIGURE 12–6**).

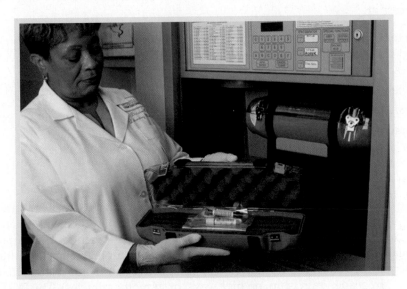

FIGURE 12–6

Pneumatic Tube System to Transport Blood Specimens

Notice the shock-absorbent padding to protect the specimens from vibrations and the biohazard bag to contain accidental breaks, spills, or leaks.

TRANSPORTATION BY AUTOMATED CARRIER

Some manufacturers provide transport systems that are motorized and/or computerized. Delivery of specimens can occur by means of a small container car attached to a network of track that is routed to appropriate sites in the laboratory, nursing stations, or other specimen collection areas. Again, a thorough evaluation of such automated delivery systems needs to include the same factors mentioned for pneumatic tube systems. When plans are made to renovate a laboratory area so that it includes this type of transport system, extra space above the ceiling tiles should be considered because the transport vehicles require a sizable right-of-way.

Processing the Specimen on Arrival at the Clinical Laboratory

When the blood samples arrive at a clinical laboratory, they are processed to be prepared for the examination/analytical procedures. Many blood specimens with additives (EDTA/lavender/purple stopper tubes for hematology tests) are simply mixed gently prior to being analyzed. They are placed on a tray that feeds directly into an analyzer. However, other specimens require more processing and are divided into smaller portions, or **aliquots,** for testing on multiple analyzers. Processing steps can be thought of in three phases: precentrifugation (after the specimen is collected but before centrifugation), centrifugation (while the specimen is in the centrifuge), and postcentrifugation (after centrifugation of the specimen but before removal of an aliquot of serum or plasma for testing).[1] There are currently hundreds of laboratory assays, chemical reagents, and manufacturers' instructions for testing specimens. With all the data, it is not surprising that some evidence on specimen variables may be conflicting. However, **BOX 12–1** summarizes basic CLSI recommendations for handling and processing blood specimens. Aliquot preparation is hazardous and can be error prone because it is not always standardized. Larger facilities often use automated instrumentation for aliquot preparation; however, it is common to find laboratory staff (including phlebotomists) who are responsible for accomplishing this task. Suggestions for improving the aliquoting process are:[5]

- Try to design the process in discrete observable steps in which a deviation is considered serious; for example, pour off serum one tube at a time into the cuvette that is placed directly onto the analyzer.
- Review the steps by direct observation, including peer review.
- Randomly retest aliquots against original tubes.
- Reinforce training through repetition.

SHIPPING BIOHAZARDOUS SPECIMENS

With the expanded worldwide transport of specimens and the increased attention to security, many air carriers, couriers, customs agents, and federal and state agencies have become more cautious in monitoring transport of hazardous agents. The primary source for regulations governing the specimen and biological shipments in the United States is the Department of Transportation (DOT). It regulates shipments transported in commerce (i.e., by plane, train, ship, on highways, or in motor vehicles). The DOT's guidelines do not include shipments on private property, whether by motor vehicle or other means.

BOX 12–1

Recommendations for Handling and Processing Blood Specimens

This overview summary of essential recommendations is adapted from the CLSI approved guideline titled *Procedures for Handling and Processing of Blood Specimens.*[1,2] The guidelines are much more detailed and provide numerous references and resources for further information. Since every laboratory is under pressure to balance transportation, time, test accuracy, and specimen rejection issues, each laboratory should undergo its own assessment of processing/handling specimens by reviewing published clinical studies in the literature, following the manufacturer's recommendations, and/or evaluating its own practices. Conclusive evidence from these sources may warrant adjustments for specimen handling when testing for specific analytes; so health care workers should follow the policies and procedures from their own health care facility.

Specimens in Which No Centrifugation Is Required

Not all specimens require centrifugation or additional processing prior to analysis except for gentle mixing (specimens for hematology or coagulation testing). Typically, the hematology specimens are placed on an automatic mixing tray and/or placed directly into an analyzer. *Tubes with additives should be gently inverted 5 to 10 times (according to the manufacturer's instructions) to mix the specimen with the additive.* This should be done first at the patient's side prior to transportation, and then the specimens can be gently mixed again prior to analysis.

- It is preferable to perform CBC, differentials, reticulocyte counts, and nucleated RBC (NRBC) counts on blood specimens as soon as possible. However, data suggest that some hematology parameters may be reliable even after three or four days using specific instrumentation. Specifically, white blood cell, red blood cell, hemoglobin, and platelet counts for specimens up to three days old and reticulocyte count and percentage from specimens up to four days old are reliable with a suggestion to add a comment about the age of the specimen. Nucleated red blood cells and differentials are *not* reliable if the specimen is older than one day.[6] It is preferable to make blood smears from EDTA specimens within one hour of collection to minimize the likelihood of changes in cellular morphology.

Precentrifugation

Precentrifugation refers to specimen handling/processing after collection and prior to centrifugation. For specimens that do require centrifugation, the general rule of thumb is that *serum or plasma should be removed from cells as soon as possible and not exceed two hours from the time of collection.* This means that processing should proceed without delay.

- Anticoagulated specimens (plasma specimens) can be centrifuged immediately after collection.
- Specimens without anticoagulant additives (serum specimens) should be clotted prior to centrifugation, which usually takes 30 to 60 minutes at room temperature (22 to 25°C).
- Clotting time is affected (often delayed) by anticoagulant therapy that the patient may be taking (Coumadin, warfarin, heparin, etc.).
- Chilling the specimen will delay clotting.
- Clotting may be accelerated by activators such as glass or silica particles, thrombin, and snake venom/thrombin. They may reduce clotting times to 15 to 30 minutes.
- Because some analytes are photosensitive, they should be kept wrapped with aluminum foil or placed in an amber specimen container to shield the specimen from light for as much of the processing as possible.
- Some laboratories still use the practice of removing the tube closure to "rim the tube" with a wooden applicator stick. This releases a blood clot attached to the tube closure or to the sides of the tube. However, this practice *is not recommended* because of the aerosol dangers and it may cause hemolysis. It is not necessary since there have been many manufacturer improvements in the tube/closure systems in recent years.

Centrifugation

Centrifugation refers to specimen handling/processing during centrifugation. It causes the specimen to rotate at high speeds, thereby creating a centrifugal force that causes heavier elements to sink to the bottom of a test tube and lighter substances to stay on top of the specimen tube. Thus, solid elements (cells) flow to the bottom, and the liquid portion of the specimen (serum or plasma) stays at the top. The centrifugation time and speed are critical parameters that each manufacturer and laboratory establishes. Each laboratory should have procedures in place for the equipment that it uses for centrifugation (BOX 12–2). Although the procedures take a significant part of the turnaround time of the laboratory processing phase, it is important to comply with them because reduced

(continued)

BOX 12–1 (*continued*)

centrifugation time can result in an incomplete barrier gel formation and residual blood cell elements in the plasma or serum, thereby causing analytical interference.[7,8] Manufacturers' specifications generally indicate the speeds and times of centrifugation. Refer to **FIGURE 12–7** for an example of specimens in a centrifuge.

- Serum specimens should be allowed to clot before centrifugation. Complete clotting takes 30 to 60 minutes; however, be mindful that patients on anticoagulant therapy (heparin, Coumadin) and chilled specimens will take longer to clot. Incomplete clotting before centrifugation can leave fibrin residue in the serum, which would interfere with analyses.

- Tubes should be centrifuged with stoppers/caps in place. Removing the stopper can expose the health care worker to contaminated aerosols and cause evaporation of the specimen, loss of gases in the specimen, possible contamination with glove powder (some powders contain calcium that may interfere with calcium levels), etc.

- Specimen tubes should be balanced in the centrifuge, whereby tubes of the same size and volume are placed opposite one another in the centrifuge holders. Tubes that are not balanced are more likely to break, which is very hazardous to health care workers, and causes another specimen to be collected from the patient.

- The centrifuge should have a top that secures appropriately, and it should not be opened until the centrifuge has stopped completely (**FIGURE 12–8**).

- Since centrifuges generate internal heat, they should be temperature-controlled so that heat-sensitive analytes are protected.

- Specimens should not be centrifuged more than once; and specimens that contain separation devices should never be recentrifuged.

- Many types of gel and nongel devices are available to enable a barrier to form between the serum/plasma and the blood clot/cells during centrifugation. They all have a particular viscosity and specific gravity that is between the clot/cells and the serum/plasma.

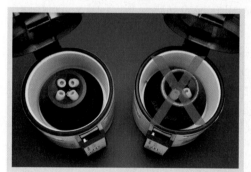

FIGURE 12–7

Centrifuge with Blood Specimens

Blood specimens should be loaded into a centrifuge in a "balanced" orientation, whereby there is a tube directly across from another tube. These centrifuges are fixed-angle centrifuges. The first shows four blood specimen tubes appropriately balanced. The second centrifuge is not balanced because the tubes are oriented adjacent to each other rather than across from each other. This has the potential to cause inadequate centrifugation. Always follow the manufacturer's instructions for placement of tubes, time, speed, and calibration of the instrument.

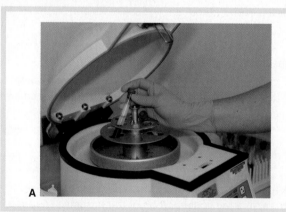
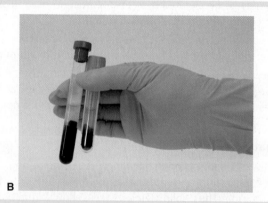

FIGURE 12–8

Specimens in a Centrifuge

A. Removing the specimen after centrifugation. B. Note the centrifuged samples: On the left side (red top) the sample has a clot on the bottom with serum above and on the right side the sodium citrate (light blue top) sample shows plasma with cells on the bottom.

BOX 12–1 (*continued*)

These gels and nongels may be incorporated into the tube as an additive, or they may be added just prior to centrifugation. Whatever the case, the manufacturer's directions should be followed precisely.

Postcentrifugation

Postcentrifugation refers to specimen handling/processing after centrifugation and prior to removal of serum or plasma. *Serum or plasma should be physically separated from cells as soon as possible and no longer than two hours from the time of collection (unless there is conclusive evidence that longer times do not affect specific test results.)*

The serum or plasma that is separated from the cells must be handled according to specified testing procedures, but in general, sera (plural form of *serum*) can remain at room temperature (22°C) for testing, be refrigerated (2 to 8°C), be stored in a dark place, or be frozen (at or below –20°C), depending on the prescribed laboratory method. All specimen refrigerators and freezers should be marked appropriately with biohazard labels. Many studies have been done to test stability of specimens at varying temperatures for varying time durations. Evidence suggests that separated serum/plasma should remain at 22°C for no longer than eight hours. If testing cannot be completed within eight hours, the specimen should be refrigerated.

- Unless manufacturers' directions instruct otherwise, if testing is not completed within 48 hours, the separated serum/plasma should be frozen at or below –20°C. Frost-free freezers are not suitable for storage because they automatically go through freeze/thaw cycles that can potentially activate coagulation factors.[4]

- Aliquot preparation occurs when the specimen must be subdivided into multiple tubes for testing on different instruments. The same identification information or code should be placed on each aliquot specimen (**FIGURE 12–9**).

(*continued*)

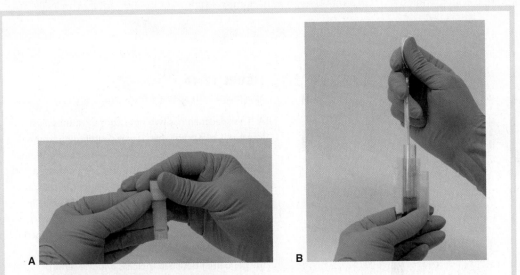
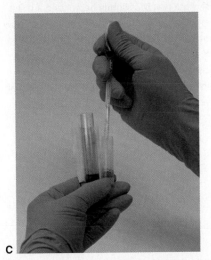
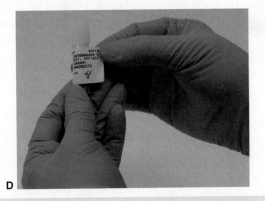

FIGURE 12–9
Aliquot Preparation

A. Aliquot tube. B. Holding the empty tube adjacent to the sample tube allows for minimal distance during serum transfer. C. A single-use, disposable pipette is commonly used for transferring the serum without cells. D. Labels should be appropriate for the size of the aliquot tube.

BOX 12–1 (*continued*)

- Since storage temperatures can affect analytes, consider all tests ordered to ensure that there is proper storage for each of the analytes being tested.
- Serum/plasma should not be repeatedly frozen and thawed because of destruction or deterioration of some analytes.
- Serum/plasma may be left in contact with a gel, barrier, or separator device as recommended by the manufacturer.
- The tube should be inspected after centrifugation to check for a complete barrier between the serum/plasma and the cells.
- The tube should be stored in an upright position with a secure closure.
- Serum/plasma and whole blood should be kept covered at all times to avoid contamination, evaporation, changes in concentration, accidental spills, and/or creation of aerosols.
- Excessive agitation causes hemolysis of the specimen when the RBCs rupture as a result of the rough handling. Hemolysis causes chemical interference with the laboratory assays listed: elevated for LD, AST, potassium, plasma hemoglobin, iron, ALT, phosphorus, total protein, albumin, magnesium, acid phosphatase; decreased for T_4. Refer to **FIGURE 12–10**.
- Some specimens appear lipemic. In these cases, follow the procedures for one's own health care facility. In some cases, the lipemic specimen can be airfuged in an ultracentrifuge to remove the triglyceride r-rich lipoproteins.[8]
- Plunger-type filters are sometimes used to separate serum/plasma from the clot/cells after centrifugation. The device (a plastic tube with a filter on the end) is inserted into the centrifuged blood tube and slowly moved into the specimen. The serum/plasma flows into the tube while the filter acts as a barrier to keep the clot/cells out. It is recommended that filters be used only if they can fully prevent backflow (particulate matter passing into the filtered serum/plasma). Refer to **FIGURE 12–11**.
- For potassium, ACTH, cortisol, catecholamines, and lactic acid, a shorter time is recommended for removal of the sera from the cells.
- Many studies have been conducted on the effects of time on analytes' stability. Some show that analytes such as albumin, alkaline phosphatase, ALT, bilirubin, calcium, cholesterol, CK, creatinine, magnesium, phosphorus, sodium, total protein,

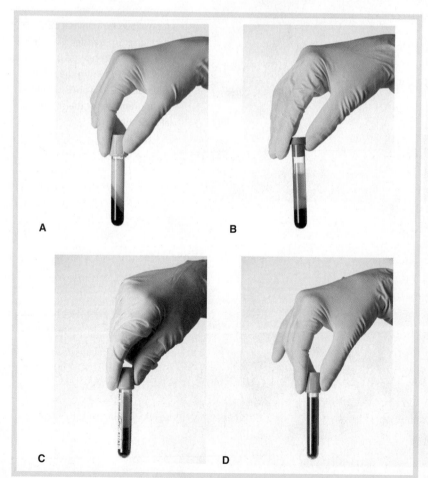

A
B
C
D

FIGURE 12–10

Specimens with Special Conditions.

A. This specimen has two noteworthy features. First, it was not balanced when it was centrifuged, so the barrier between cells and plasma is slanted and thinner than it would be if it had been properly positioned. This mistake can often lead to leakage of the cells into the plasma. Second, the specimen is lipemic; it is cloudy and milky, which indicates a high level of lipids in the blood. B. This specimen was centrifuged properly, as evidenced by the correct shape of the gel barrier between the cells and the serum. However, note that it is slightly hemolyzed. C. This specimen does not contain a barrier but notice how it separates into cells and plasma. D. This specimen is grossly hemolyzed. The plasma portion is hardly distinguishable from the cellular portion because of the deep red hemolysis. This was likely the result of excessive mixing and agitation.

BOX 12–1 (*continued*)

triglycerides, T3, T4, urea nitrogen, and uric acid may *not* be affected even if the serum is not removed for 48 hours; others demonstrate stability for longer periods.

■ Some analytes *are affected* significantly after two hours if the serum/plasma is not removed; glucose level decreases, potassium increases, and LD increases.

■ Analyte stability is also affected by temperature.

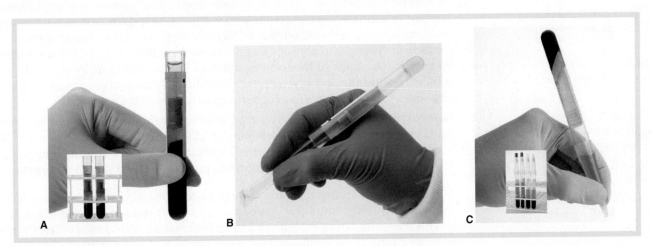

FIGURE 12–11
Commercially Available Plunger-Type Devices for Separating Fibrin and Cellular Materials from Plasma or Serum

Courtesy of MarketLab Inc. www.marketlabinc.com

BOX 12–2

Using the Right Centrifuge

The laboratory bench-top centrifuge is a key piece of equipment for every clinical laboratory. When used correctly, the centrifuge not only separates serum and plasma but can enhance productivity by reducing turnaround time. Some laboratories use large-capacity centrifuges in which many tubes are spun in batches. However, sometimes it is more efficient to use high-speed, low-capacity centrifuges (smaller in size) in a location closer to the processing and testing area instead of larger centrifuges in a centralized location that might require more transportation time. Consider the following aspects when deciding on the most appropriate centrifuge:[7]

■ **Type of tubes** Some models allow only a few tube sizes; others have adaptors/inserts for varying tube sizes.

■ **Rotor** The most common types of rotors are horizontal and fixed angle. This makes a difference when spinning gel tubes in that a horizontal rotor will have a flat gel barrier, which is preferable for chemistry and immunoassay testing. If spun with a fixed angle rotor, the gel barrier will have a slanted angle that may create problems with some chemistry analyzers.

■ **Spin time** Depending on the model, the revolutions per minute (RPMs) vary, as do the acceleration and deceleration times.

■ **Capacity** Smaller bench-top models usually range from 4 to 12 tubes. However, if adaptors are used for larger or smaller tubes, fewer may be accommodated.

■ **Noise level and proximity to other instruments** Sometimes in a busy laboratory, the noise level from numerous analyzers and centrifuges can be too loud. In this case, a separate area or sound barrier should be designated for the centrifuge.

■ **Training for centrifuge operators** Because centrifuges vary widely in their design, adaptor/inserts for different tubes, and rotors (e.g., fixed angle for coagulation versus swing buckets for chemistry), each operator should be adequately trained for proper use according to the manufacturer's instructions.

The DOT has collaborated with the World Health Organization (WHO) and the United Nations (UN) Committee of Experts as well as the Centers for Disease Control and Prevention (CDC) to establish guidelines designed for safety and security. The Department of Transporation has defined a two-tiered classification for infectious substances:[9]

- **Infectious substances** Infectious material is known or reasonably expected to contain a pathogen. A *pathogen* is a microorganism (including bacteria, viruses, rickettsiae, parasites, fungi) or other agent, such as a proteinaceous infectious particle (prion), that can cause disease in humans or animals

- **Category A** This is a classification of an infectious substance in a form capable of causing permanent disability or life-threatening or fatal disease in otherwise healthy humans or animals when exposure to it occurs. An exposure occurs when an infectious substance is released outside of its protective packaging, resulting in physical contact with humans or animals. Classification must be based on the known medical history or symptoms of the source patient or animal, endemic local conditions, or professional judgment concerning the individual circumstances of the source human or animal. Category A poses a higher degree of risk than Category B.

- **Category B** This is a classification of an infectious substance not in a form generally capable of causing permanent disability or life-threatening or fatal disease in otherwise healthy humans or animals when exposure to it occurs. This includes Category B infectious substances transported for diagnostic or investigational purposes.

For clinical laboratories that ship specimens to other laboratories or locations, it is the responsibility of the individual preparing the specimen to assure that it is done correctly. This means ensuring that the specimen is classified and labeled correctly, placed in the proper type of packaging with related labels, and is accompanied with correct documentation. If any of these items are not done according to regulations, the shipment can be rejected, delayed, and/or the shipper can be fined.

It is the organization's and/or employee's responsibility to comply with the following requirements:[9,10]

- Provide information and training to all employees who are involved in the preparation of specimens for transport. The training should be specific to all the substances that will be shipped from the laboratory.

- Use package materials that meet strength and absorbency requirements. (Packing materials must pass stringent testing to ensure it will not leak contents under stress such as cold, heat, rain, pressure, and drops from various heights.)

- Properly identify, classify, pack, mark, label, and document accordingly.

- Make advance arrangements with all carriers of the specimens.

- Receive confirmation of prompt delivery.

- Notify all carriers of all shipping details.

- Follow up immediately if a problem is reported.

General packing requirements for infectious substances being shipped by passenger or cargo aircraft involve the following (also refer to **FIGURE 12–12**).

- Packaging *must* include a primary, leak-proof receptacle or package; a secondary leak-proof container such a sealed plastic bag; a rigid outer package; appropriate package markings; and the name and telephone number of the person responsible for the shipping in durable, legible ink.

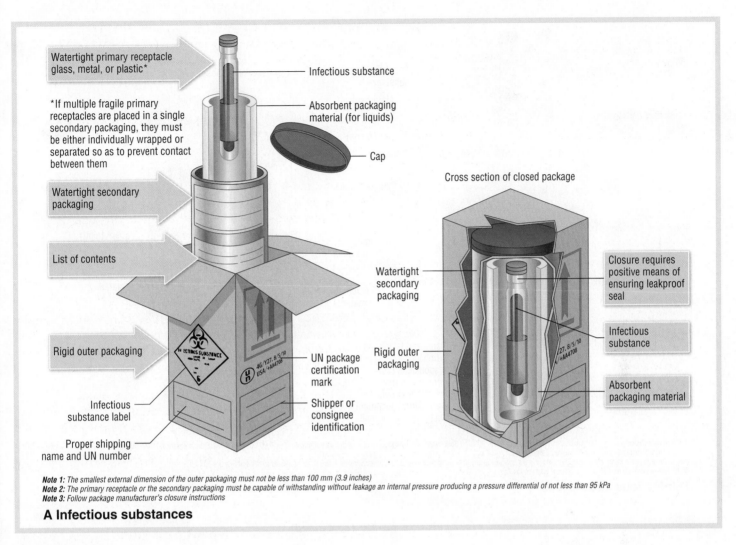

Watertight primary receptacle glass, metal, or plastic*

Infectious substance

*If multiple fragile primary receptacles are placed in a single secondary packaging, they must be either individually wrapped or separated so as to prevent contact between them

Absorbent packaging material (for liquids)

Cap

Watertight secondary packaging

List of contents

Rigid outer packaging

Infectious substance label

Proper shipping name and UN number

UN package certification mark

Shipper or consignee identification

Cross section of closed package

Watertight secondary packaging

Closure requires positive means of ensuring leakproof seal

Rigid outer packaging

Infectious substance

Absorbent packaging material

Note 1: *The smallest external dimension of the outer packaging must not be less than 100 mm (3.9 inches)*
Note 2: *The primary receptacle or the secondary packaging must be capable of withstanding without leakage an internal pressure producing a pressure differential of not less than 95 kPa*
Note 3: *Follow package manufacturer's closure instructions*

A Infectious substances

FIGURE 12–12

Safe Transporting of Infectious Substances

A. Example of packaging for Category A specimen shipment.

(*continued*)

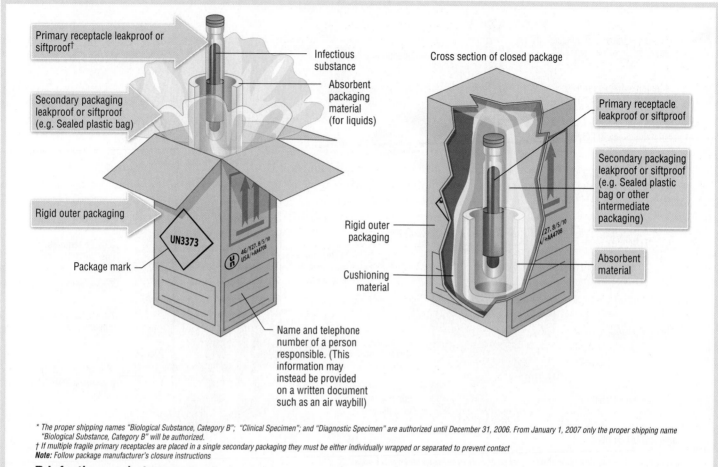

Primary receptacle leakproof or siftproof†

Secondary packaging leakproof or siftproof (e.g. Sealed plastic bag)

Rigid outer packaging

Package mark

UN3373

4G/Y27. 8/5/10 USA/+AA4708

Infectious substance

Absorbent packaging material (for liquids)

Name and telephone number of a person responsible. (This information may instead be provided on a written document such as an air waybill)

Cross section of closed package

Primary receptacle leakproof or siftproof

Secondary packaging leakproof or siftproof (e.g. Sealed plastic bag or other intermediate packaging)

Rigid outer packaging

Cushioning material

Absorbent material

27. 8/5/10 /+AA4708

* The proper shipping names "Biological Substance, Category B"; "Clinical Specimen"; and "Diagnostic Specimen" are authorized until December 31, 2006. From January 1, 2007 only the proper shipping name "Biological Substance, Category B" will be authorized.
† If multiple fragile primary receptacles are placed in a single secondary packaging they must be either individually wrapped or separated to prevent contact
Note: Follow package manufacturer's closure instructions

B Infectious substances

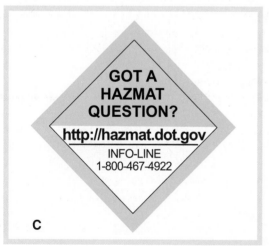

GOT A HAZMAT QUESTION?
http://hazmat.dot.gov
INFO-LINE
1-800-467-4922

C

FIGURE 12–12 (*continued*)

B. Example of packaging for Category B specimen. C. Where to learn more

For more information refer to "Transporting Infectious Substances Safely", Federal Register, U.S. Department of Transportation, Pipeline and Hazardous Materials Safety Administration, www.dot.gov, accessed March 26, 2014

- The inner primary receptacle must be a leak-proof, watertight secondary packaging container, with an absorbent material between the primary and secondary containers that is capable of absorbing all contents of the primary receptacle, and some cushioning material.

- Multiple primary specimen tubes must be individually wrapped, separated, and supported to avoid contact among them.

- The rigid outer package must be marked with "Infectious Substances" labels, and appropriate information must appear, including the name and telephone number of the responsible person.

- When specimens are refrigerated or frozen, careful attention to the manufacturer's instructions is needed so that complete compliance is observed.
- A specimen received from an outside source should be immediately identified, logged in, and checked for sample integrity.

When packages are received at the health care facility, they should be thoroughly inspected to make sure storage criteria have been maintained. This includes taking the temperature, making sure ice has not melted and thawing has not occurred for frozen specimens, and checking the packaging for damage. (For blood components, the FDA requires that they be checked for viability before being transfused into a patient, and that procedures are in place for ensuring that the temperature has been maintained during transport.)

There are serious fines and legal ramifications for failure to comply with these requirements. The DOT has two branches that may inspect laboratories for compliance: the Pipeline and Hazardous Materials Safety Administration (PHMSA) and the Federal Aviation Administration (FAA). The FAA focuses on laboratories that ship specimens by air, and the PHMSA inspects any facility that ships hazardous materials by any means of transport. Accurate and current training records, records retention, and proper packaging materials are keys to compliance. Fines and sanctions usually relate to improper training, poor record keeping, the shipper's failure to follow the manufacturer's instructions for packaging, or altering the packaging in a way that it does not meet the DOT requirements. It is imperative that laboratory personnel check for the most recent DOT regulations for shipping specimens to assure that safety and compliance are upheld.[9,10]

Reporting Laboratory Results

WRITTEN REPORTS

Both The Joint Commission and the College of American Pathologists (CAP) state that laboratory results should be confirmed, dated, and accompanied by permanent reports that are available in the laboratory, as well as on the patient's medical record via an electronic transmission or a hard copy. The CAP also states that each report should contain adequate patient identification, the date and hour when the procedures were completed, and be authorized electronically or manually by the laboratory personnel performing the procedure. When electronic reports are used, laboratory documentation on instrument-generated worksheets by personnel performing the procedures is sufficient. The CAP has suggested that health care personnel consider the following data for laboratory test results:

1. Identification of patient, patient location, and physician
2. Date and time of specimen collection
3. Description, source of specimen, and labeled precautions
4. For paper copies, compactness and ease of shipment/mailing
5. Consistency in format
6. Clear understandability of instructions or orders
7. Logical location in patient's medical record for reference laboratory reports
8. Sequential order of multiple results on single specimens
9. Listing of reference ranges or normal and abnormal/critical values
10. Assurance of accuracy of request transcription
11. Administrative and record-keeping value

Any unique institutional requirements for an acceptable laboratory result/report should be stated in the laboratory procedure manual (hard copies or electronic versions) and may include criteria such as quality control (QC) limits and/or delta checks—that is, QC that allows for detection of clinically significant changes in laboratory results. (Remember that QC records for supplies or reagents are additional, in that they include expiration dates and storage or stability information.) Results can be documented in one or more ways: manual recording of test results, laboratory-instrument–printed reports, and electronically generated reports.

VERBAL REPORTS

The use of verbal and telephone reports has declined because of easier, more reliable computer access and the concern for privacy. Verbal reports, although useful for reporting STAT results and critical values, are more prone to error because of miscommunication or insufficient information. The health care worker giving out the verbal report should request a verbal read-back from the individual receiving the report. This can reduce the risk of giving incorrect information. Verbal reports should also be accompanied by documentation with the following information: patient name and identification number, name of person receiving the report, date and time, information given, and name of person issuing the report, as shown in **FIGURE 12–13**.

```
PATIENT NAME:                              PATIENT ID #:
PHYSICIAN:
PERSON REQUESTING INFORMATION:
DATE OF TEST RESULTS:

INFORMATION GIVEN:


DATE & TIME OF INQUIRY:

REPORTED BY:
```

FIGURE 12–13

Sample Form Used for Reporting Verbal Laboratory Results

Reporting laboratory results is a serious responsibility, and each health care facility has policies for who is authorized to do so and under which conditions. Compliance with HIPAA regulations ensures that patients' privacy and confidentiality wishes are maintained. Only employees who are authorized to do so should complete the required documentation when appropriate.

COMPUTERIZED REPORTS

Various computer-transmission devices can provide a rapid online report system and are more reliable than verbal reports. Hospitals may have computers located in each patient unit. After the tests have been completed and verified in the laboratory, the results can be immediately displayed in each patient unit. A printer can be attached to each terminal to generate a temporary hard-copy report as needed. However, steps must be taken to ensure the privacy and confidentiality of patient results as they are reviewed and after they are printed.

A health care facility's computer system can easily provide daily laboratory reports and cumulative reports for the patient's medical record. All reports should be available at times convenient for making clinical decisions by the medical staff.

The business office of the health care facility also receives data online regarding laboratory procedures. This office must be notified of all laboratory charges, according to data requested and procedural codes for patient billing. It is financially advantageous to send reports promptly.

ALERT

Clinical Alert! A **critical laboratory value** is a test result that "represents a pathophysiologic state at such variance with normal as to be life-threatening" unless action is taken by the patient's physician. According to the Clinical Laboratory Improvement Act (CLIA), health care workers are required to report critical values to physicians in a timely manner.[11] In many laboratories, critical laboratory values are repeated and/or verified by an authorized supervisor prior to releasing the information. Reporting these results means paging or telephoning a physician at home and/or during off-hours. Although this can be an unwelcome task, it is important for the patient's welfare and to avoid liability risks. All laboratories should have policies about what should be done when results are in a critical range.[11]

Study Questions

For the following questions, select the one best answer.

1 Which one of the following would be considered a preexamination/preanalytical error?

a. reporting a critical lab value on the wrong patient
b. testing the wrong aliquot for a glucose test
c. underfilling the aliquot container
d. changing a result without documenting it

2 Which blood specimen should be chilled during a 45-minute transport?

a. porphyrins
b. cold agglutinins
c. cholesterol
d. blood gases

3 Which blood specimen should be kept warm during transport to the laboratory?

a. cholesterol
b. blood gases
c. porphyrins
d. cold agglutinins

4 Which of the following analytes should be protected from light?

a. porphyrins
b. blood gases
c. cholesterol
d. glucose

5 Which analyte is photosensitive?

a. glucose
b. bilirubin
c. cholesterol
d. albumin

6 Which of the following practices will likely cause hemolysis?

a. taking the top off the test tube
b. shaking the tube to mix the contents
c. gently mixing the tube
d. covering the tube with aluminum

7 After blood collection, when should plasma be centrifuged?

a. as soon as possible
b. 10 minutes
c. 30 minutes
d. 60 minutes

8 Serum should be removed from blood cells after which time period?

a. 10 minutes
b. 30 minutes
c. 60 minutes
d. 120 minutes

9 A specimen should be protected from light for which of the following determinations?

a. bilirubin concentration
b. hemoglobin level
c. glucose level
d. blood cultures

10 A specimen should be chilled for which of the following analyses if there is a significant delivery delay?

a. complete blood count (CBC)
b. bilirubin level
c. blood gas
d. glucose level

Case Study 1

Potassium Results and Preanalytical Error A patient was seen in one of the clinics adjacent to the hospital. She had her venipuncture procedure and had tubes collected for routine hematology tests and chemistry tests. Her laboratory results were normal except for the potassium result, which had abnormally increased. The laboratory supervisor suspected that it was a result of preanalytical error.

Questions

1 What could have occurred during the transportation and handling phases of the specimen to make the potassium elevated?

2 How can this be prevented?

Case Study 2

Hemolysis and Recollect Ellen, a new intern, was collecting a blood specimen for a new patient. She performed the venipuncture procedure correctly and after completion of the procedure, she shook the tubes to mix the additives. She labeled them properly and delivered them to the laboratory. A few hours later, as Ellen was looking for test results on the blood specimen that she had collected, she saw the comment that the specimen had been hemolyzed. She followed up to see if the patient had been punctured again for a second specimen. The health care worker assigned to the floor had performed the recollect and delivered the specimen to the laboratory.

Questions

1 What mistake did Ellen make after collecting the blood specimen?

2 How could this be prevented in the future?

3 What should the patient be told about the recollect?

Action in Practice

Recall the last time you or someone you were with had a blood specimen collected by venipuncture. Jot down notes about the procedure that you remember.

Questions

1 Did the health care worker correctly fill all the tubes?

2 Did the health care worker mix the specimens as they were being collected or after the venipuncture?

3 Did the health care worker label the specimens prior to leaving?

4 Did the health care worker place the specimen tubes in an upright rack?

Competency Checklist: After Venipuncture, Before Delivery to the Laboratory

This checklist can be completed as a group or individually.

(1) Completed (2) Needs to improve

_____ 1. Name the steps after a venipuncture but before delivering the specimen to the laboratory.

_____ 2. Name analytes that are photosensitive.

_____ 3. Name analytes that are thermolabile.

_____ 4. Name analytes that must be warmed.

Competency Checklist: Centrifugation Issues

This checklist can be completed as a group or individually.

(1) Completed (2) Needs to improve

_____ 1. Name specimens that do not require centrifugation.

_____ 2. Describe the importance of centrifugation time and speed.

_____ 3. Describe why tubes should be balanced in a centrifuge.

_____ 4. Describe the differences in centrifugation practices between serum specimens and plasma specimens.

Competency Checklist: Postcentrifugation

This checklist can be completed as a group or individually.

(1) Completed (2) Needs to improve

_____ 1. List three factors that affect analyte stability.

_____ 2. List the causes of hemolysis in a blood specimen.

_____ 3. Describe the lag time between the centrifugation and the removal or separation of serum/plasma from cells.

_____ 4. Describe three methods of storage for blood specimens and the temperatures for each.

_____ 5. Define the term aliquot and the reasons for preparing a sample aliquot.

REFERENCES

1. Clinical and Laboratory Standards Institute (CLSI). (2010, April). *Procedures for the handling and processing of blood specimens for common laboratory tests, approved guideline,* 3rd ed. GP-rr-A4, formerly H18-A4. Wayne, PA: Author.

2. Clinical and Laboratory Standards Institute (CLSI). (2007). *Procedures for collection of diagnostic blood specimens by venipuncture, approved standard, approved guideline,* 6th ed. GP41-A6, formerly H3-A6. Wayne, PA: Author.

3. Clinical and Laboratory Standards Institute (CLSI). (2004). *Collection of arterial blood specimens, approved standard,* 4th ed. GP43-A4, formerly H11-A4. Wayne, PA: Author.

4. Clinical and Laboratory Standards Institute (CLSI). (2008). *Collection, transport, and processing of blood specimens for testing plasma-based coagulation assays and molecular hemostasis assays, approved guideline,* 5th ed. H21-A5. Wayne, PA: Author.

5. Warner, S. (2007, June 1). *Specimen Process Control, Advance Newsmagazines for Administrators of the Laboratory. http://laboratory-manager. advanceweb.com,* accessed March 26, 2014.

6. De Baca, M. E., Gulati, G., Kocher, W., & Schwarting, R. (2006). Effects of storage of blood at room temperature on hematologic parameters measured on Sysmex XE02100. *Lab Med, 37*(1): 28–34.

7. Yu, M. (2013, March 11). Beyond serum and plasma, today's centrifuges play an important role in reducing waste and improving productivity. *Advance for Medical Laboratory Professionals. http://laboratory-manager .advanceweb.com/,* accessed July 1, 2013.

8. Lippi, G., Salvagno, G. L., Montagnan, M., & Guidi, G. C. (2007). Preparation of a quality sample: Effect of centrifugation time on stat clinical chemistry testing. *Lab Med, 38*(3): 172–176.

9. U.S. Department of Transportation, Pipeline and Hazardous Materials Safety Administration. (2006, October 1). *Transporting infectious substances safely, www.dot.gov,* accessed January 31, 2014.

10. Creighton, D. (2012, December 12). Specimen transport compliance, *ADVANCE. http://laboratorian.advanceweb.com,* accessed March 26, 2014.

11. Dalton-Beninato, K. (2000). Critical value notifications are never welcome news. *Lab Med, 31*(6): 319–323.

RESOURCES

www.cdc.gov/od/ohs/biosfty/biosfty.htm Centers for Disease Control and Prevention: Biosafety

www.cdc.gov/od/ohs/pdffiles/DOTHazMat8-14-02.pdf Standards for Transporting Infectious Substances

http://www.iata.org/whatwedo/cargo/dgr/Pages/index.aspx International Air Transport Association: Safe Handling of Dangerous Goods

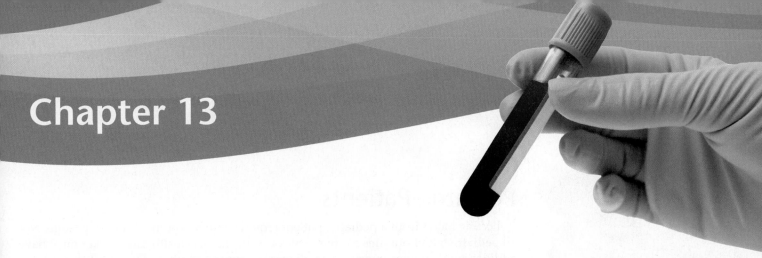

Chapter 13

Pediatric and Geriatric Procedures

Chapter Objectives

Upon completion of Chapter 13, the learner is responsible for doing the following:

1. Describe fears or concerns that children in different developmental stages might have toward the blood collection process.

2. List suggestions that might be appropriate for parental and health care worker behavior during a venipuncture or skin puncture.

3. Identify puncture sites for a heel stick on an infant and describe the procedure.

4. Describe the venipuncture sites for infants and young children.

5. Discuss the types of equipment and supplies that must be used during microcollection and venipuncture of infants and children.

6. Explain the special precautions and types of equipment needed to collect capillary blood gases.

7. Describe the procedure for specimen collection for neonatal screening.

8. Define five physical and/or emotional changes that are associated with the aging process.

9. Describe how a health care worker should react to physical and emotional changes associated with the elderly.

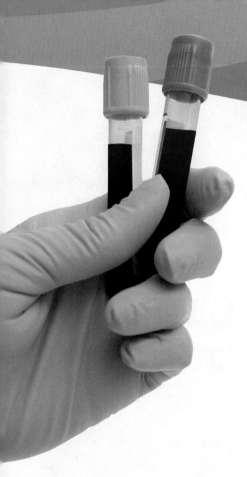

Pediatric Patients

Collecting blood from a pediatric patient requires much expertise and knowledge. Not all **pediatric phlebotomies** are fingersticks, so the novice health care worker must have additional knowledge specific to pediatric anatomy and physiology. Children are not just little adults and should not be treated as such. There are differences that relate to the anatomy and physiology of children (**FIGURE 13–1**). The health care worker needs to be familiar with special types of equipment available, observe the various techniques as they are performed by a health care worker experienced in pediatric phlebotomy, and practice the techniques to develop the necessary skills. The health care worker must also develop competence in relating psychologically with children of various ages and developmental stages.

Performing venipuncture on young patients is technically and emotionally challenging for the health care worker because of the patients' small size and because children are less emotionally and psychologically prepared to cope with pain and anxiety. Therefore, a successful outcome requires the use of good interpersonal skills in preparing the child and the concerned, apprehensive parents.

With proper training in technique and an understanding of pediatric developmental characteristics, the delicate task of collecting blood from a frightened child need not cause fear or dread in the health care worker. Phlebotomy skills should be perfected on older children first; then when confidence is attained, venipuncture can be attempted on younger children. When learning the techniques, the health care worker should remember to ask for help if needed and allow adequate time to develop the necessary skills. Many pediatric hospitals employ child life specialists who are trained in helping children cope with hospitalization and painful procedures. If a child life specialist is available, he or she can play an important role in assisting the child and parent through the procedure.

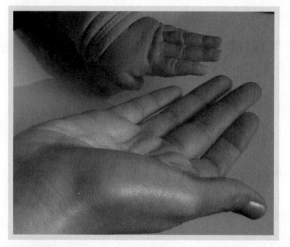

FIGURE 13–1
A New Generation

Note the differences between the mother's and baby's hands related to sizes, proportions of the fingers, and skin features.

Age-Specific Care Considerations

Age-specific care considerations are shown in **TABLE 13–1**. It describes not only the fears and concerns of the pediatric patient at various ages, but also suggests **parental involvement** and comfort measures and provides competencies and tips for the health care worker.

Preparing Child and Parent

The timing of the preparation depends on the child's age; generally, the younger the child, the closer the explanation should be to the time of the procedure.[1] Preparing the child and the parent for the blood collection procedure involves the following steps:

1. A calm, confident approach is the first step in obtaining the cooperation of the child and parent. Introduce yourself. Be warm and friendly, establish eye contact with both the child and the parent, and show that you are concerned about the child's health and comfort. When you interact with a pediatric patient and his or her parent, provide a sense of trust and confidence.

TABLE 13–1

Age-Specific Care Considerations and Competencies

Age	Fears and Concerns	Communication	Comfort	Safety	Parent Behavior
0–6 months	Totally dependent on and trusts parents and other adults.	Introduce yourself to caregiver. Explain procedures.	Keep patient warm. Warm site of puncture if needed. Parent may hold child. Use a very gentle approach. Use of a distraction, such as light pen, key ring, or bell, may minimize fear.	Keep side rails up during procedure. Do not leave any supplies or discarded items on bed. Encourage parent to hold or cuddle infant after procedure. Use appropriate microcollection supplies and equipment and methods to alleviate pain from phlebotomy.	Parent may hold child as an aid to the health care worker and to provide comfort.
6–12 months	Fear of strangers. Fear of separation from parent. Limited language use.	Introduce yourself to caregiver. Talk slowly to infant. Try to make eye contact with infant.	Keep patient warm. Warm site of puncture if needed. Allow familiar health care worker to perform procedure. Allow parent to be in close proximity. Allow child to use pacifier and/or hold teddy, blanket, or other comforting items.	Do not separate from caregiver unless absolutely necessary. Keep side rails up. Do not leave any supplies or discarded items on bed. Encourage parent to hold or cuddle infant after procedure. Use appropriate microcollection supplies and equipment and methods to alleviate pain during phlebotomy.	Parent may assist by holding, explaining to, and comforting the child. Parent may help identify comforting toy.
1–3 years	Self-centered. Fear of injury. Fear of long separation from parent.	Introduce yourself to both child and caregiver. Child will understand simple commands and may choose to cooperate. Take it slowly; do not rush patient, he or she needs time to think about your requests. Allow child to touch supplies but dispose if they become contaminated. Ask parent to explain procedure in familiar terms.	Keep patient warm. Warm site of puncture if needed. Allow familiar health care worker to perform procedure. Allow parent to be in close proximity. Allow child to use pacifier and/or hold teddy, blanket, or other comforting items.	Try not to separate from parent unless absolutely necessary; if needed, reinforce that it is only for a short period of time. Keep side rails up. Do not leave supplies or discarded items on bed. Use appropriate microcollection supplies and equipment.	Parent may assist by holding, explaining to, and comforting the child. Parent may help identify comforting toy. Encourage parent to praise child after procedure.
3–5 years	Self-centered. Fear of injury. Enjoys pretending and role playing (**FIGURE 13–2**).	Introduce yourself. Talk to child in simple terms. Allow child to touch equipment. Try using familiar cartoon characters (Disney, Sesame Street) in the explanation. Perhaps use toys to demonstrate procedure. Child may pretend he or she is the doctor and will "help" with the procedure. Provide tokens for bravery and let child choose own bandage.	Allow child to have familiar things or people nearby. Give child time to verbalize his or her fears.	May tolerate separation from parent. Able to recognize danger and obey simple commands. Needs close supervision. Keep side rails up. Do not leave supplies or discarded items on bed. Use appropriate microcollection supplies and equipment.	Parent may be present to provide emotional support and to assist in obtaining the child's cooperation. Encourage praise for bravery.

TABLE 13–1

Age-Specific Care Considerations and Competencies (continued)

Age	Fears and Concerns	Communication	Comfort	Safety	Parent Behavior
6–12 years	Less dependent on parents. Fear of losing self-control. More willing to participate. Tries to be independent. Curious.	Introduce yourself. Child may be interested in health concepts— "why" and "how." Explain "why" the blood is needed. Involve child in the procedure and show the child the equipment and supplies that will be used for the blood collection.	Try not to embarrass the child but offer her/ him a comforting toy or familiar object. Take it slowly, allow time for repeat questions. Allow child some input on decisions (e.g., color of bandage).	Side rails should be left up after procedure. Do not leave supplies or discarded items on bed. Use appropriate microcollection supplies and equipment.	Child may ask parent to leave room.
13–17 years	Actively involved in anything concerning the body. More independent. Embarrassed to show fear. Needs privacy. May act hostile to mask fear.	Introduce yourself. Use adult vocabulary; do not "talk down." Explain procedure thoroughly. Ask if he or she would like to help with the procedure. Ask what might make the teen more comfortable. Allow time for questions or to handle supplies.	Maintain privacy. Take extra time for explanations and or preparation. Offer the teen the opportunity to have parent close by. Allow the teen time to recover after the procedure if he or she has cried.	Use same strategies as adult. Use appropriate collection supplies and equipment depending on the size of the individual and the physical and emotional tolerance to procedure.	Child may not want parent to be present.
Children with special problems or mental challenges.	Fears are similar to the behaviors of the developmental level. Need relaxed, gentle approach.	Use strategies that are appropriate for the developmental stage.	Use strategies that are appropriate for the developmental stage.	Use strategies that are appropriate for the developmental stage.	Use strategies that are appropriate for the developmental stage

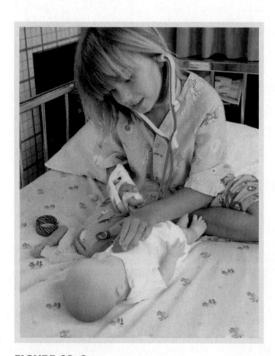

FIGURE 13–2

Age-Appropriate Play to Adjust to Health Care Needs

2. Correctly identify the patient by using at least two patient identifiers.[2] The patient should have an identification bracelet with his or her name and hospital number or birth date. Verify these identifiers. A hospitalized infant usually has the identification bracelet on his or her ankle. Newborns who are not yet named are usually identified by their last names (e.g., Baby Boy Smith, Baby Girl Jones) and identification number. If the mother is still in the hospital after delivery, the baby may wear an identification band that is cross-referenced to the mother. Keeping identifications straight is always crucial, but especially so when specimens from twin babies must be collected and labeled.

3. Find out about the child's past experience with blood collections. Ask whether the child has ever had blood collected. The child and the parent can then tell you about any experiences with past procedures and provide you with valuable information about the approaches that worked effectively for the child and those that were not as successful.

4. Develop a plan. Ask the parent how cooperative his or her child will be. Parents are excellent predictors of their child's behavior and possibility for distress. Usually, the younger child with poor venous access will experience more distress. A successful plan involves not only the parent's suggestions about what will be most helpful but also the health care worker's knowledge of pediatric phlebotomy techniques. If possible, allow the child to have some control by offering a choice of which arm or finger he or she prefers for blood collection.

5. Place yourself at the child's eye level to explain and demonstrate the procedure (**FIGURE 13–3**). When explaining what you will be doing, use words appropriate for the child's age. Use of a doll, puppet, or stuffed animal in the demonstration can help you relate to the child in a nonthreatening manner. If the child has a favorite doll, blanket, or toy, he or she should be encouraged to hug it for comfort and support.

6. Establish guidelines. Tell the child and the parent that the procedure will most likely be successful on the first attempt. If not, it will be attempted only once more by another health care worker.

7. Be honest when a child asks if the puncture will hurt. Tell the child that if the procedure hurts too much, it can be momentarily stopped, but that the quicker the procedure is performed, the less painful it will be. Instruct the child to say when he or she feels the pain or "hurt." Tell the child that saying "Ouch" or making faces is acceptable, but that he or she must make an effort to keep the arm absolutely still. Reassure the child that the blood will be collected as quickly as possible so that the pain will be brief.[1]

8. Encourage parent involvement.[1] Explain how the parent can assist by holding, distracting, and soothing his or her child before and during the procedure (**FIGURE 13–4**). Some parents, however, may be reluctant to participate because they do not want to be a part of a procedure that will cause their children pain. If the parent does not wish to assist but is willing to be in the room, ask him or her to maintain eye contact with the child to reduce stress. If, after discussing his or her role, the parent is still reluctant to be in the room, respect his or her wishes. If the parent does not wish to participate, you may ask another health care worker to assist.

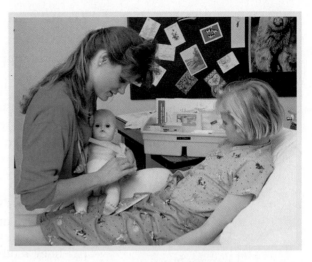

FIGURE 13–3
Talking to a Child at Eye Level

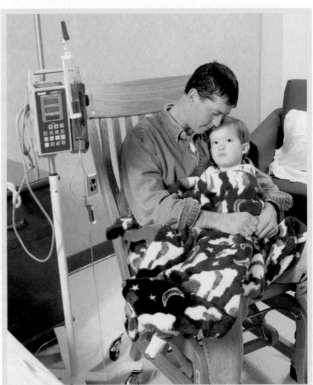

FIGURE 13–4
Parent's Role in Pain Management

PSYCHOLOGICAL RESPONSE TO NEEDLES AND PAIN

Children especially fear needles, and an emotionally upset child has difficulty separating fear from actual pain. Children 1 or 2 years old may have extreme reactions to painless procedures, such as taking a temperature. Children 3 to 5 perceive pain as a punishment for bad behavior. They may react aggressively. Children ages 6 to 12 are more likely to relate pain to past experiences. Many children perceive that a "shot," or needle, hurts more than anything else that has ever happened to them. The 13- to-17-year-old children are more independent and embarrassed to show fear. They usually need privacy and may act hostile to mask fear. With proper preparation, the child and the parent can develop coping skills to help lessen the fear and thereby diminish the "hurt."

The following parental behaviors and examples will have a positive effect on relieving the child's distress.[3,4]

Clinical Alert! It is not unusual for a sick or injured child to act younger than he or she really is. If a child who is 6 years old behaves like a 3-year-old, use strategies appropriate for a 3-year-old.[3]

ALERT

Parental Behaviors	Examples
Distraction	"Look at Mommy"; "Tell the nurse about your doll."
Emotional support	Hugging, stroking hair, patting, and talking in a soothing voice.
Explanation	"We need to take a tiny bit of blood from your finger"; "You will feel a little prick"; "Mommy will help you hold your arm still so that we can finish quickly."
Positive reinforcement	"You did a great job at holding your arm still!"

DISTRACTION TECHNIQUES

Children age 3 and older respond well to distraction techniques to help them cope and lessen distress. Distraction helps the child refocus on a more pleasant experience. A parent or another health care worker can provide the distraction. Some examples of distraction are blowing bubbles, pinwheels, counting, reading a book or looking at a video, listening to music, singing, or talking in a gentle voice about something enjoyable. School-age children may respond to strategies such as picturing themselves in a pleasant setting or participating in the procedure.[3,4]

ROOM LOCATION

For psychological reasons, the best room location for a painful procedure is a treatment room away from the child's bed or playroom. For a hospitalized child, the bed should be a safe, secure place to rest and sleep, not a place associated with pain. If the child shares a room with another child, performing the procedure at the bedside can be upsetting to the roommate as well. If the child cannot be moved to a treatment room, privacy should be maintained by drawing a curtain between the beds and speaking in a calm, quiet manner.

EQUIPMENT PREPARATION FOR A FRIENDLIER ENVIRONMENT

Just the sight of needles, syringes, and a person in a white laboratory coat can be frightening to a child. Nurses and other health care providers working with children frequently wear bright, colorfully printed uniforms or smocks to create a child-friendly environment. Equipment, too, can be modified to appear less threatening. As an example, prepare the phlebotomy equipment and supplies prior to entering the child's room so that the child does not become even more anxious by watching the preparation. Use shorter needles if possible, and keep threatening-looking supplies (such as needles) covered and out of sight. If the hospital policy requires goggles or face shields for blood-exposure precautions, put this equipment on after greeting the child. Praise the child throughout the procedure. At the completion, reward the child with a colorful bandage, a sticker, an age appropriate toy, or with parental permission, a lollipop. If no parent is present to assist in relieving the anxiety, you or the nurse may cuddle, rock, and offer a pacifier to an infant or gently stroke or talk softly to sooth a small child.

Positions for Restraining a Child

Holding the child may be required to ensure that the child does not move the limb during blood collection. Restraining techniques should be compassionate and safe and be performed quickly. A supportive parent who has been properly instructed can assist with restraining while providing comfort to the child.

Two preferred methods of restraining a child to immobilize the arm are the vertical position (**FIGURE 13–5**) and the horizontal, or supine, position (**FIGURE 13–6**).[3,4] In both cases, the parent's face is in close proximity to the child's, thereby providing a comforting and secure feeling. The vertical technique, which works well for toddlers, requires the child to be held on the parent's lap. As the parent hugs and holds the child's body and the arm not being used, the health care worker can firmly hold the other arm to perform the procedure.

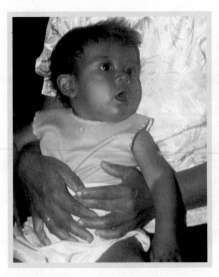

FIGURE 13–5
Vertical Position for Restraining a
Child to Perform Blood Collection

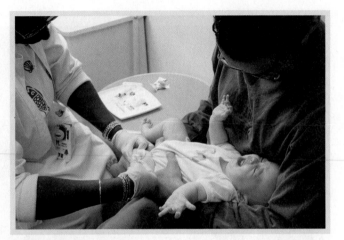

FIGURE 13–6
Supine (Lying) Position for Restraining a Child to Perform Blood
Collection

In the horizontal position, an older child lies supine, with the health care worker on one side of the bed and the parent on the opposite side. The parent gently but firmly leans over the child, restraining the closest arm and the body while holding the opposite, extended arm securely for the health care worker.

Neonates and infants age 3 months and younger usually do not require restraint and can be managed by the health care worker alone. Swaddling helps comfort an upset newborn from the pain of the procedure (**FIGURE 13–7**).

Combative Patients

At times, a child will become uncooperative even after the proper steps have been followed to gain cooperation. Children may become combative—kicking and thrashing—if force is used. Because sharps are involved in blood collection, the health care worker must be certain that the procedure can be performed safely. Using force to the point of potential physical injury is unethical and unprofessional. If a parent or guardian is available and willing to assist, the procedure may be performed quickly and without injury. Otherwise, other health care workers can assist with the uncooperative child by immobilizing him or her to protect the health care worker and patient from injury during the blood collection. However, if at all possible, avoid forceful restraining unless it is needed to protect the patient and oneself. If the risk of injury to the child or the health care worker is high, the blood collection attempt should be discontinued, and the nurse or the physician notified. In such instances, alternative coping measures or pharmacological intervention may be necessary prior to the next attempt.

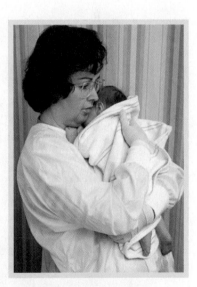

FIGURE 13–7
Swaddling a Newborn

Decreasing the Needlestick Pain

A topical anesthetic (pain reliever), an **eutectic mixture of local anesthetics (EMLA)**, can be rubbed on the skin when a needlestick is going to be used for venipuncture to a child. This local anesthetic is ideal for use prior to venipuncture or starting intravenous (IV) therapy because it does not require a needle. It is applied to the skin as a patch or a cream that is then covered with a transparent adhesive dressing (**FIGURE 13–8**).

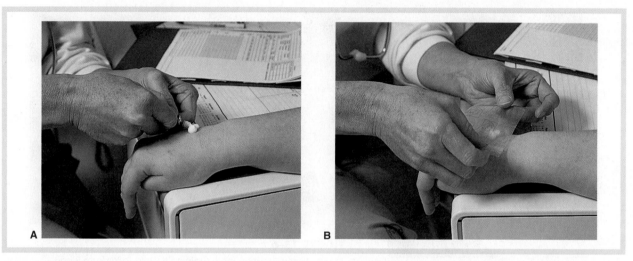

FIGURE 13–8

Using a Topical Anesthetic

When a needlestick is planned, EMLA can be used to anesthetize the skin where the needlestick will occur. A. Apply a thick layer of the EMLA cream over intact skin (half of a 5 g tube). B. Cover the cream with a transparent adhesive dressing for 45 to 60 minutes.

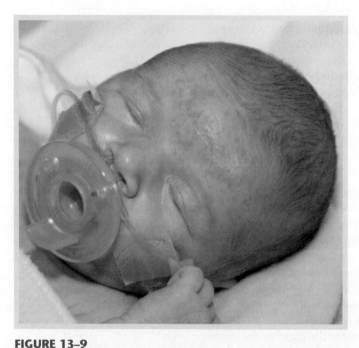

FIGURE 13–9

Use of Pacifier

Suckling on a pacifier has a calming effect on newborns.

Optimal anesthesia occurs after 45 to 60 minutes and may last as long as two to three hours. Drawbacks to the use of EMLA are cost, the need to apply it 60 minutes prior to the procedure, and the need to know in advance of the location of the vein to be used. Two separate locations may be anesthetized if the child has difficult veins from which to obtain blood. Do not use EMLA if the child is allergic to local anesthetics.[2,6,7]

ORAL SUCROSE

Sucrose (a sugar) is effective in reducing pain and crying time during a procedure for an infant up to 6 months of age. A 25% solution of sucrose can be prepared by mixing four teaspoons of water with one teaspoon of sugar. The sucrose can be carefully administered by oral syringe, dropper, nipple, or on a pacifier. A **sucrose nipple** is given 2 minutes before heel sticks, and its action lasts about 5 minutes. Infants given pacifiers (**FIGURE 13–9**) or sucrose have also been shown to be more alert following the procedure, to be less fussy, and to cry for a shorter duration.[5,7]

Precautions to Protect the Child

Premature infants, newborns, and children who are chronically ill or have extensive burns are more susceptible to infections. To protect these children from potentially harmful microorganisms, some hospitals may require protective precautions. In these cases, PPE—gowns, gloves, and masks—will be worn as indicated before entering the room. Remove the PPE according to policy and dispose of it in the appropriately marked container. Wash your hands or sanitize them according to policy. Alcohol-based waterless rubs, foams, or rinses are as effective as handwashing if the hands are not soiled.[8] Put on a clean gown and gloves before attending to the next infant or child.

> **Clinical Alert!** Puncturing deep veins in children may cause cardiac arrest, hemorrhage, venous thrombosis, damage to surrounding tissues, and infection.

Latex Allergy Alert

Some children may be allergic to latex. Usually, a sign posted on the hospital door will note the child's allergy, or the child may wear a bracelet indicating a **latex allergy** or a latex alert. Several brands of nonlatex gloves should be available for use with children who have this allergy. Children with spina bifida and those with congenital urinary tract abnormalities or neurogenic bladders are particularly sensitive to latex. If a tourniquet is used, it should also be latex free.[9]

Pediatric Phlebotomy Procedures

Two methods are used to obtain blood from infants and children: microcapillary skin puncture and venipuncture. The previously described steps for preparing the child and the parent should be taken before the procedure is performed.

MICROCAPILLARY SKIN PUNCTURE

Skin punctures are useful for pediatric phlebotomy when only small amounts of blood are needed and can be adequately tested. It is particularly important to collect only the smallest amounts of blood necessary from neonates, infants, and children and consolidating the blood collection tests so that the effects of **blood volume** reduction are minimal.[10] Overcollecting blood during phlebotomy causes anemia and may require packed cell transfusion in an infant. Studies have shown that patients lose 4 mg of iron for every 10 mL of blood collected.[11]

A 10 mL sample taken from a premature or newborn infant is equivalent to 5 to 10% of the infant's total blood volume. Calculation of blood volume is based on weight and can be made for any size person if the weight (in kilograms) of the individual is known. The total blood volume of a person is calculated by multiplying weight (kg) by the following blood volumes:

115 mL/kg	Premature infants
80–110 mL/kg	Newborns
75–100 mL/kg	Infants and children
70 mL/kg	Adults

> **Clinical Alert!** Small infants can become anemic if too much blood is taken.

> **Clinical Alert!** A 3 kg infant (approximately 6.6 pounds) will have a total blood volume of between 240 to 330 mL. It is important to monitor how much of this is withdrawn each day.[2] The table in Appendix 7 provides the amount of blood that can be collected from patients at any one time based on weight and the maximum cumulative amount of blood that can be collected during a given hospital stay of one month or less.

Clinical Alert! Do not obtain blood by skin puncture from the toes or the central area of an infant's heel, as this may result in injury to nerves, tendons, and cartilage; do not use fingers of infants under 1 year of age or a previously punctured site. If an infant has compromised circulation to the extremity, as in shock, or has edema, bruises, rashes, or infection at the heel, use another site (i.e., venipuncture procedure).

When performing skin punctures, collect the hematology specimens first to minimize platelet clumping, then collect for chemistry and blood bank specimens. Each laboratory has approved procedures for phlebotomy, including the volume of blood that is required for each test; these procedures should always be followed. Always record the amount of blood collected.

Skin Puncture Sites

The heel is the most desirable site for skin puncture of the infant or neonate (**PROCEDURE 13–1**). The most medial (inside) or most lateral (outside) section of the plantar, or bottom, surface of the heel should be used (**FIGURE 13–10**).

Do not use (1) the central area of the infant's heel for blood collection, (2) the fingers of an infant or newborn, (3) the earlobes, or (4) the posterior curvature of the heel. For children age 1 and older, the palmar surface of the distal phalanx (fingertip section) of the third (middle) or fourth (ring) finger, ideally of the nondominant hand is most frequently used, as the thumb has a pulse and the index finger may be more sensitive. The fifth finger is not used because the skin is too thin. The plantar surface of the great toe is *not* recommended for skin puncture. Using the proper pediatric size skin-puncture device, make an incision that is less than 2.0 mm deep (**FIGURE 13–11**). Major blood vessels lie 0.3 to 1.6 mm beneath the skin at the dermal-subcutaneous junction in newborns.[12,13] If an incision goes deeper, the **calcaneus** or heel bone may be hit and may lead to osteomyelitis and/or **osteochondritis**.[14,15]

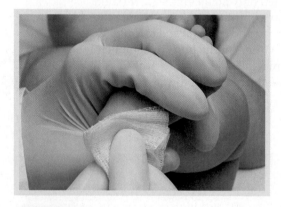

FIGURE 13–10

Courtesy of BD VACUTAINER Systems, Preanalytical Solutions, Franklin Lakes, NJ.

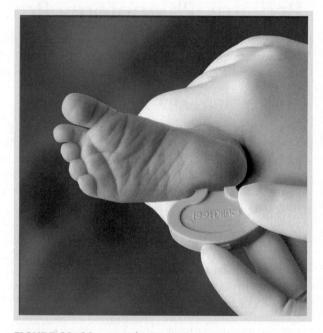

FIGURE 13–11
Performing a Heel Stick on an Infant

Courtesy and © Becton, Dickinson and Company

PROCEDURE 13–1

Heel Stick Procedure

Rationale   To perform a blood collection from the infant's heel.

Equipment

The following equipment is necessary for pediatric skin puncture:

■ Sterile, automatic, disposable pediatric skin-puncture safety devices in different manufacturers' incision depths (0.65 to 0.85 mm for premature neonates, 1.0 mm for larger infants) (Please see Chapter 8, "Blood Collection Equipment for Venipuncture and Capillary Specimens" for photo examples.)
■ 70% isopropyl alcohol swabs
■ Sterile 2" × 2" gauze sponges
■ Plastic capillary collection tubes and sealer or caps
■ Microcollection containers
■ Glass slides for smears
■ Puncture-resistant sharps container
■ Disposable gloves (nonlatex if child is allergic)
■ Compress (towel or washcloth) to warm heel if necessary
■ Marking pen
■ Laboratory request slips or labels

Preparation

1 Prepare and assemble supplies. Do *not* place the specimen collection tray on the infant's bed or in the bassinet.

2 Introduce yourself to the parents, explain the procedure, and use appropriate comfort techniques.

3 Identify the infant properly. Identify the infant by name, address, and identification number and/or birth date and compare with the laboratory test request form. If the infant is not wearing an identification bracelet, the name of the person who performs this identification procedure must be documented in the medical records and charts.

Procedure

4 Wash or sanitize your hands with an alcohol hand rub, then put on gloves. If required, don a gown and a mask.

5 Inspect the selected area and assess it for proper warmth. If it is cool or a blood gas specimen is to be collected, prewarm the foot with a warm, wet towel or a chemical heel-warming pack, according to policy. Wipe the heel dry after removing the warm towel.

6 Position the baby in a supine (lying) position with the knee at the open end of the bassinet. This position allows the foot to hang lower than the torso, improving blood flow. When the baby is in an acceptable position for this procedure, clean the intended incision site on the heel with an antiseptic swab. Allow the heel to air dry. Do not touch the incision site or allow the heel to come into contact with any nonsterile item or surface (**FIGURE 13–12**).

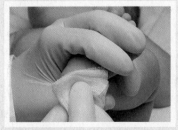

FIGURE 13–12
Courtesy of ITC, Edison, NJ.

(*continued*)

PROCEDURE 13–1

Heel Stick Procedure (continued)

A CLOSER LOOK

Heel Warming

Rationale

The amount of blood that can be obtained from a single **heelstick** is limited; therefore, to obtain an adequate sample, prewarming the heel may be indicated. Prewarming the heel increases blood flow and arterializes the specimen. This step is essential for collecting specimens for **capillary blood gas analysis.**

Procedure

A Prepare and assemble supplies: a warm, wet towel and a plastic bag or chemical heel-warming pack.

B Warm the site with a commercially available warming pack or wrap a warm, wet towel at a temperature no more than 42°C around the infant's foot. If the temperature of the towel exceeds 42°C, it may burn the infant.

C Encase the towel in a plastic bag to help retain heat and to keep the patient's bed dry. Use caution if the towel is heated in a microwave oven, because heating is uneven and the towel may have hot spots.

D Prewarm the site for 3 to 5 minutes.

E Depending on the institution's policy, call in advance to prewarm the infant's heel.

7 Remove the appropriate Tenderfoot puncture device from its blister pack, taking care not to rest the blade slot end on any nonsterile surface (**FIGURE 13–13**).

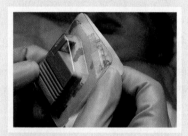

FIGURE 13–13
Courtesy of ITC, Edison, NJ.

8 Remove the safety clip. *Note:* The safety clip may be replaced if the test is momentarily delayed; however, prolonged exposure of any Tenderfoot device to uncontrolled environmental conditions before use may affect its sterility. Once the safety clip is removed, do *not* push the trigger or touch the blade slot (**FIGURE 13–14**).

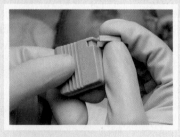

FIGURE 13–14
Courtesy of ITC, Edison, NJ.

PROCEDURE 13–1

Heel Stick Procedure (continued)

9 Hold the infant's foot firmly but gently to prevent sudden movement. Holding the foot too tightly may cause bruising and restrict blood flow. Also, it can lead to erroneous laboratory test results.

10 Raise the foot above the baby's heart level and carefully select a safe incision site (avoid any edematous area or site within 2.0 mm of a prior wound). Place the blade-slot surface of the device flush against the heel so that its center point is vertically aligned with the desired incision site (**FIGURE 13–15**).

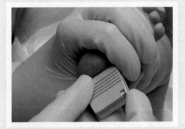

FIGURE 13–15
Courtesy of ITC, Edison, NJ.

> **Clinical Alert!** Avoid excessive milking or squeezing, which causes **hemolysis** and dilutes the blood with interstitial and intracellular fluid.

ALERT

11 Ensure that both ends of the device have made light contact with the skin, and depress the trigger. After triggering, immediately remove the device from the infant's heel and dispose of it in the biohazard sharps container (**FIGURE 13–16**).

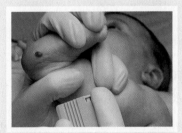

FIGURE 13–16
Courtesy of ITC, Edison, NJ.

12 Using only a dry sterile gauze pad, gently wipe away the first droplet of blood that appears at the incision site (**FIGURE 13–17**).

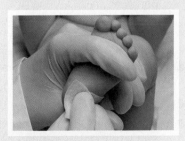

FIGURE 13–17
Courtesy of ITC, Edison, NJ.

(continued)

PROCEDURE 13–1

Heel Stick Procedure (continued)

13 Taking care not to make direct wound contact with the collection container or capillary tube, fill to the desired specimen volume (**FIGURE 13–18**). Take care *not* to scoop blood into the microtube, as this technique can lead to hemolysis.

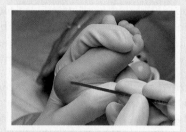

FIGURE 13–18
Courtesy of ITC, Edison, NJ.

14 After blood collection, gently press a dry sterile gauze pad to the incision site until bleeding has ceased. This step will help prevent a hematoma from forming (**FIGURE 13–19**).

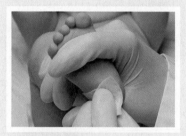

FIGURE 13–19
Courtesy of ITC, Edison, NJ.

ALERT

Clinical Alert!

Complications from HeelStick

Some complications associated with neonatal heelsticks include cellulitis, osteomyelitis of the calcaneus, abscess formation, tissue loss, scarring of the heel, and calcified nodules. Calcified nodules occur most commonly in infants who, as preemies (premature babies) or neonates, received multiple heel sticks. In neonates, these nodules appear as small depressions, which progress to firm nodular lesions that appear 4 to 12 months later, migrate to the skin surface, and disappear by 18 to 20 months.

15 Label the specimen container and verify identification. Record the time of collection.

After the Procedure: Care of The Heel

16 Elevate the heel slightly above the body and ensure that bleeding has stopped.

17 Check the infant's heel puncture site for late bleeding or inflammation.

PROCEDURE 13–1

Heel Stick Procedure (continued)

> **Clinical Alert!** Use of an adhesive bandage over skin-puncture sites is not recommended for children under 2 years old. Infants have delicate skin that may be irritated by the adhesive strip, and an older infant might remove it and put it in his or her mouth. Bandages can also be swallowed by older children.

ALERT

Clean Up

18 Dispose of the used skin-puncture device in a sharps container with a biohazard label.

19 Check the infant's bed for any equipment or trash left behind.

20 Discard blood-soaked gauze sponges, grossly contaminated items, and gowns or gloves used in isolation rooms in biohazardous waste containers.

21 Dispose of gowns and gloves that are not from isolation rooms in the regular trash.

22 Wash or sanitize your hands after removing the gloves.

CAPILLARY BLOOD GASES

Arterial blood is the specimen of choice for blood gas analysis (i.e., pH, pCO_2, pO_2, oxygen [O_2] content, total carbon dioxide [TCO_2] content of the blood, and O_2 saturation [O2SAT]). However, capillary (skin puncture) blood is most often collected from infants and small children for blood gas analysis since it is a safer procedure than arterial blood collections (**PROCEDURE 13–2**). Skin puncture blood is less desirable as a specimen because it contains blood from capillaries, venules, and arterioles, and fluids from the surrounding tissue. In addition, common collection methods for capillary blood gas specimens employ an open collection system in which the specimen is temporarily exposed to room air, allowing for a brief exchange of gases (both O_2 and CO_2) before sealing the specimen from the air. The air exposure must be minimized to avoid falsely elevated blood oxygen levels.

PROCEDURE 13–2

Collection for Capillary Blood Gas Testing

Rationale   To perform a blood collection for capillary blood gas analysis.

Blood for **capillary blood gas analysis** is often collected from small children and babies for whom arterial punctures can be too dangerous. They are collected from the same areas of the body as other capillary samples, such as the lateral posterior area of the heel or the ball of the finger.

Equipment

- Sterile, automatic, disposable, pediatric skin-puncture safety devices in different manufacturers' incision depths (0.65 to 0.85 mm for premature neonates, 1.0 mm for larger infants)
- Heparinized safety plastic capillary tube
- 70% isopropyl alcohol swabs
- Sterile 2" × 2" gauze sponges
- Plastic capillary collection tubes and sealer
- Microcollection containers
- Glass slides for smears
- Puncture-resistant sharps container
- Disposable gloves (nonlatex)
- Warming packs or compresses (towel or washcloth) to warm heel if necessary
- Marking pen
- Laboratory requisitions or labels
- Minute metal filing
- A magnet

Preparation

1 Prepare and assemble supplies.

2 Introduce yourself to the parents (if they are present), explain the procedure, and use appropriate comfort techniques.

3 Identify the infant properly. If the infant is not wearing an identification bracelet, identify the infant by name, address, and identification number and/or birth date and compare this information to the laboratory test request form.

4 Warm the site according to the institution's procedures.

Procedure

5 Wash or sanitize your hands with an alcohol hand rinse; then put on gloves. If required, don a gown and a mask.

6 Use a heparinized safety plastic capillary tube for the collection (**FIGURE 13–20**).

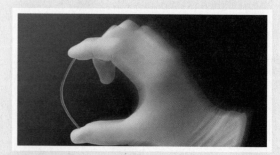

FIGURE 13–20

SAFE-T-FILL Blood Gas Capillary Tube—100% Plastic for Safety

Courtesy of Ram Scientific, Inc., Needham, MA.

PROCEDURE 13–2

Collection for Capillary Blood Gas Testing (continued)

7 Insert a minute metal filing (also referred to as *mixing wires*) into each capillary tube before collecting blood to help mix the specimen while it is entering the tube (**FIGURE 13–21**).

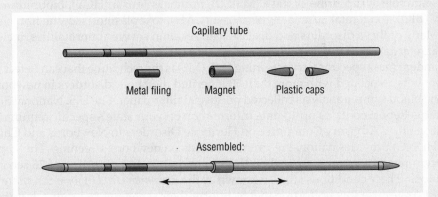

FIGURE 13–21
Capillary Blood Gas Tube, Metal Filing (wire), and Plastic Caps

Clinical Alert! The specimen must be collected with no air bubbles, which can distort the values obtained from the specimen.

ALERT

8 Perform the capillary (skin) puncture as previously mentioned and wipe away the first drop of blood.

9 When the tube is full, seal the ends with plastic caps, and use a magnet to draw the metal filing (wire) back and forth across the length of the tube to mix the specimen completely.

10 Label the tube and prepare it for immediate transfer to the laboratory. Notify laboratory personnel of the urgent blood gas test to be performed.

11 Press the skin puncture site with a clean gauze sponge until the bleeding stops.

After the Procedure: Care of The Heel

12 Elevate the heel slightly above the body and ensure that bleeding has stopped.

13 Check the infant's heel puncture site for late bleeding or inflammation.

Clean Up

14 Dispose of the used skin-puncture devices in a sharps container with a biohazard label.

15 Check the infant's bed for any equipment or trash left behind.

16 Discard blood-soaked gauze sponges, grossly contaminated items, and gowns or gloves used in isolation rooms into biohazardous waste containers.

17 Dispose of gowns and gloves that are not from isolation rooms in the regular trash.

18 Wash or sanitize your hands after removing the gloves.

19 Deliver the sample immediately to the laboratory. Delays of more than 15 minutes at room temperature (or more than 60 minutes at 4°C), will affect the results.

NEONATAL SCREENING

In the United States, newborns are routinely screened for a variety of metabolic and genetic defects by analysis of blood collected on a special filter paper. Screening newborns is important for the early detection, diagnosis, and treatment of certain genetic, metabolic, and infectious diseases. It is now possible to screen for more than 50 inherited disorders.[16] Some of the disorders that are tested through **neonatal screening** include **phenylketonuria (PKU),** congenital **hypothyroidism,** galactosemia (GAL), sickle cell disease, maple syrup urine disease (MSUD), homocystinuria (HCY), biotinidase deficiency (BIO), congenital adrenal hyperplasia (CAH), toxoplasmosis, cystic fibrosis, and HIV. Many of these disorders and diseases can result in severe abnormalities, including mental retardation, if not discovered and treated early.[17]

Tandem mass spectrometry screening (MS/MS) is the technique that can detect blood components associated with more than 50 inherited metabolic disorders in newborns in just one blood sample analysis collected on special filter paper. The U.S. National Screening Status Report contains up-to-date information on your state's specific requirements. The Secretary's Advisory Committee on Heritable Disorders in Newborns and Children (SACHDNC) provides national recommendations on newborn screening. This committee recommends a screening panel of 31 core conditions and reporting of 26 secondary conditions. These conditions are also known as the *Recommended Uniform Screening Panel (RUSP).* States use this uniform panel to inform their screening programs, but it is not enforced by law. In some states, a neonate may be screened for only a few disorders, whereas another state may require screening for more than 30. The National Newborn Screening Task Force recommends more education and standardization among states for newborn screening procedures and policies. The following websites should be reviewed for more specific information: the Health Resources and Services Administration (HRSA) through the links at https://genes-r-us.uthscsa.edu/resources/consumer/StatePages/Texas.htm and the American Academy of Pediatrics (AAP) at www.aap.org.[17]

Blood-spot testing for screening is performed before the newborn is 72 hours old (PROCEDURE 13–3). The AAP states that the optimal time for collection from a healthy newborn is as close to hospital discharge as possible. If the blood specimen is collected before the newborn is 24 hours of age, because of early discharge from the hospital, a second specimen for screening must be collected before age 2 weeks. In classic galactosemia, symptoms occur within the first two weeks of life.[18] Filter specimens must be obtained from newborns prior to any blood transfusions for valid test results. Blood cells from a transfusion provide normal enzymes that may invalidate screening results.

PROCEDURE 13-3

Collection of Capillary Blood for Neonatal Screening

Rationale | To perform a capillary blood collection for newborn screening specimens. The heel of the neonate is the most frequently used site for collection of blood for screening.

Equipment

The following equipment is necessary for newborn screening blood collection:

- Sterile, automatic, disposable, pediatric skin-puncture safety devices in different manufacturers' incision depths (0.65 to 0.85 mm for premature neonates, 1.0 mm for larger infants) (Please see Chapter 8 for photo examples.)
- 70% isopropyl alcohol swabs
- Sterile 2" × 2" gauze sponges
- Newborn screening cards (usually kept in the hospital laboratory or the nursery) (Do not use cards that are beyond the expiration date on the filter paper!)
- Puncture-resistant sharps container
- Disposable gloves (nonlatex)
- Warming packs or compresses (towel or washcloth) to warm heel if necessary
- Marking pen
- Laboratory requisitions or labels

Preparation

1 Prepare and assemble supplies (**FIGURE 13-22**).

2 Introduce yourself to the parents (if they are present), explain the procedure, and use appropriate comfort techniques.

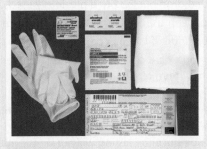

FIGURE 13-22
Courtesy of Wadsworth Center, New York State Department of Health

3 Identify the infant properly. If the infant is not wearing an identification bracelet, identify the infant by name, address, and identification number and/or birth date and compare this information with the laboratory test request form. Fill out the information on the newborn screening card, as shown in **FIGURE 13-23**.

4 Warm the site according to the institution's procedures.

Procedure

5 Wash or sanitize your hands with an alcohol hand rinse; then put on gloves. If required, don a gown and a mask.

6 To prevent contamination, do not touch with hands or gloves any part of the filter paper circles before, during, or after collection. Do not allow the filter paper to come in contact with substances such as alcohol, formula, water, powder, antiseptic solutions, or lotion.

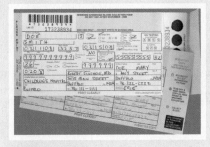

FIGURE 13-23
Courtesy of Wadsworth Center, New York State Department of Health

(continued)

Collection of Capillary Blood for Neonatal Screening (continued)

Circles are printed on the filter paper portion of the card, as shown in **FIGURE 13–24**.

7 Perform the capillary (skin) puncture as previously mentioned and wipe away the first drop of blood with a sterile gauze sponge.

8 Allow another large blood drop to form.

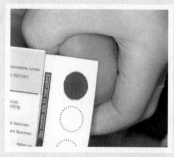

FIGURE 13–24
Courtesy of Wadsworth Center, New York State Department of Health

9 As shown in Figure 13–24, lightly touch the printed side of the filter paper with the blood drop and fill each printed circle (**FIGURE 13–25**). Allow the blood to soak through and completely fill the circle with a single application of the large blood drop.

- If the circle does not fill entirely, wipe the heel and express another, larger drop to a different circle. Do not add a second drop of blood to a previously used circle.
- The filter paper must not touch the skin puncture site.
- Only use one side of the filter paper.
- Dry blood spots on a clean, dry, flat, nonabsorbent surface for a minimum of 4 hours.
- Direct application of blood from the heel to the card is the technique of choice. Most newborn screening laboratories will not accept blood spots collected by a capillary tube since the testing will not be accurate.

10 Press the skin puncture site with a clean gauze sponge until the bleeding stops.

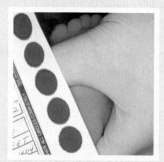

FIGURE 13–25
Courtesy of Wadsworth Center, New York State Department of Health

After the Procedure: Care of The Heel

11 Elevate the heel slightly above the body and ensure that bleeding has stopped.

12 Check the infant's heel puncture site for late bleeding or inflammation.

Clean Up

13 Dispose of the used skin-puncture devices in a sharps container with a biohazard label.

14 Check the infant's bed for any equipment or trash left behind.

15 Discard blood-soaked gauze sponges, grossly contaminated items, and gowns or gloves used in isolation rooms into biohazardous waste containers.

16 Dispose of gowns and gloves that are not from isolation rooms in the regular trash.

Collection of Capillary Blood for Neonatal Screening (continued)

17 Wash or sanitize your hands after removing the gloves.

18 Correctly complete all the information on the screening card so that follow up can be done if the results are abnormal.

19 The blood spots must not be touched or smeared. The screening card (blood specimen) needs to air dry on a nonabsorbent horizontally level open surface for at least three hours at a regulated temperature between 18 degrees C to 25 degrees C. Each patient's blood specimen must not touch another blood specimen for this screening procedure. Also, these blood spots must not be exposed to direct sunlight or stacked.

20 After sufficient drying, the screening card should be placed in an appropriate envelope and sent to the laboratory within 24 hours.

Interferences in Newborn Screening Collections

It is important to be cautious and careful in the blood collection and transfer to the filter paper for the newborn screening.[18] Many interferences can result from poor blood collection techniques. The most common include the following:

- Blood specimen not properly dried before mailing
- Filter paper circles not completely filled, not saturated with blood, or not *all* circles filled
- Contamination of filter paper circles before or after blood collection by substances such as hand lotion, powder, alcohol, antiseptic hand solution, or touching of areas with gloved or ungloved hands
- Blood applied to both sides of filter paper
- Excess blood applied (usually occurs with a capillary tube)
- Heel stick squeezed or milked, resulting in "tissue-diluted" specimens
- Alcohol not wiped off heel stick site before puncture is made

FINGERSTICK ON CHILDREN

Use a pediatric safety skin-puncture device designed for the age and size of the child. An automatic skin-puncture device controls

ALERT

Clinical Alert!

A fingerstick to obtain blood for routine laboratory analysis is usually preferred for children older than age 1 (**FIGURE 13-26**). Also, a fingerstick may be necessary if a child has damaged veins from repeated venipuncture or if the veins are covered with bandages or casts. Do not perform a fingerstick if the extremity has compromised circulation, is edematous, or is infected.

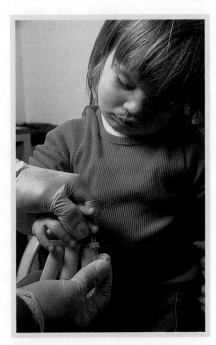

FIGURE 13-26
Collecting Blood via Fingerstick from a Toddler

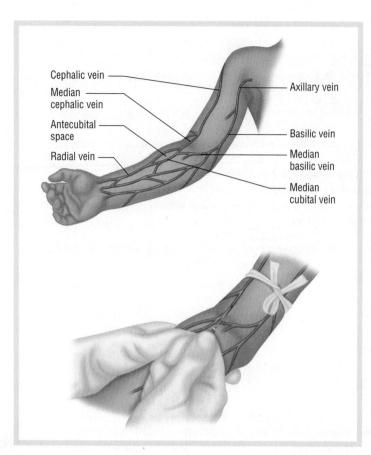

FIGURE 13–27
Veins in the Arm

the puncture depth, which should not exceed 2.0 mm in small children. The distance from the skin surface to bone or cartilage in the middle, or third, finger is between 1.5 and 2.4 mm. Automatic puncture devices are available in sizes that incise to depths of 0.85 mm for preemies, 1.25 mm for infants, and 1.75 mm for toddlers. For a detailed description of the blood collection procedure and supplies, refer to Chapter 11, "Capillary Blood Specimens," and Chapter 8, "Blood Collection Equipment for Venipuncture and Capillary Specimens."

VENIPUNCTURE ON CHILDREN

Venipuncture on children is used when larger quantities of blood are needed for sampling. The veins of the antecubital fossa, or the forearm (**FIGURE 13–27**), are the most accessible and are chosen for most toddlers and children. If a venipuncture is done on a child younger than age 2, the site should be limited to a superficial vein. Some studies have indicated that venipuncture, when performed by a skilled health care worker, appears to be the method of choice for blood sampling for neonates, since it is less painful and can provide adequate blood for testing.[19,20] Other sites used for venipuncture are the medial wrist, the dorsum of the foot, the scalp, and the medial ankle. Always check the policy at your facility before performing venipuncture on foot or ankle veins. If the neonate or child is receiving fluid or medication intravenously, the distal veins should be avoided for phlebotomy and preserved for IV therapy. Venipuncture is indicated for blood sampling for routine laboratory tests, erythrocyte sedimentation rate (ESR), blood cultures, cross-matching, coagulation studies, and drug and ammonia levels. Do not use veins in an extremity, an area with edema or infection, or if an IV line is present. Avoid deep veins in a child with hemophilia or other bleeding disorders.

Precautions

Remove the tourniquet before withdrawing the needle. Apply pressure with the gauze sponge for 3 minutes to prevent a hematoma. Do not use alcohol pads to apply pressure, as they will cause stinging and prevent hemostasis. Equipment of choice for venipuncture on a small child is a winged safety butterfly needle.

Equipment for Venipuncture

The equipment necessary for a pediatric venipuncture includes the following:

1. Winged safety infusion (butterfly) needle (21 gauge × 1 inch or 23 gauge × 3/4 inch)
2. Syringes slightly larger than the volume of blood needed
3. Paper tape
4. 70% isopropyl alcohol swab in a sterile package
5. 2" × 2" gauze sponges
6. Appropriate specimen containers
7. Pediatric-size tourniquet (nonlatex)
8. Sterile disposable gloves (nonlatex)
9. For blood culture:

   ● Bottles, both aerobic and anaerobic. For smaller children, use a special pediatric bottle. The required volumes are for children ages 2 to 12, 2 to 4 mL; for infants under age 2, 1 mL.

   ● Alcohol swabs.

   ● Chlorhexidine gluconate swabs (use for infants older than 2 months).

10. Bandage strip (for use only with older children)
11. Marking pens
12. Biohazardous waste container

Procedure

The procedure for performing venipuncture on children is similar to that for adults (see Chapter 10). The differences include the necessary preparation of the child and the parent, assistance in restraining the child, and the use of special pediatric-size needles or safety winged infusion sets. After the child is securely positioned, place the tourniquet proximal to the selected vein to distend it. If necessary, the limb may be lowered, rubbed gently, or warmed to promote dilation of the vein. Disinfect the site thoroughly. Allow the alcohol to dry completely. Then hold the two wings of the infusion set together in the dominant hand as the other hand pulls taut the skin below the puncture site. After inserting the needle, and when blood appears in the tubing, release the wings of the infusion set. The skin will hold the needle in place, or paper tape can be used to secure it. Gently aspirate the syringe until the required amount of blood is collected. Release the tourniquet and apply pressure over the puncture site with a gauze pad as the infusion set is quickly removed. Ask the parent or the nurse to hold pressure on the site until the bleeding stops. A colorful bandage strip may be used on an older child. Remove the syringe from the safety butterfly set after the needle safety guard has been engaged. Then attach the syringe to a safety syringe shielded transfer device (see Figure 8–12, page 258) for safe transfer of blood to the collecting tubes.

Scalp Vein Venipuncture

Scalp veins may be used on infants when access to other veins is difficult or undesirable. The health care worker must have appropriate blood collection training for this procedure. **FIGURE 13–28** shows the scalp veins used for peripheral vascular access. Additional equipment required for this procedure includes a disposable razor and a large, flat rubber band. A 23-gauge safety winged infusion set (butterfly needle) is preferred for the venipuncture.

The appropriate procedures should be followed: handwashing and gloving, preparing the infant, and positioning with an assistant to provide restraint. If the scalp veins are not readily visible through the hair, a disposable razor may be used to shave the hair

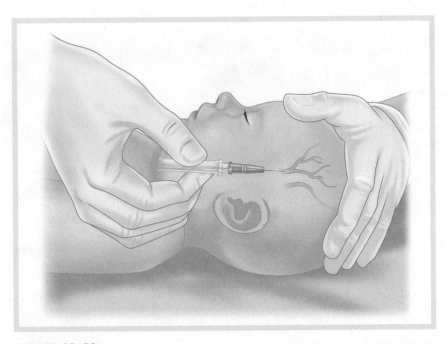

FIGURE 13–28
Infant Scalp Veins

carefully in the frontal or parietal scalp area. A prominent vein may be found proximally with a finger pressed on the scalp to occlude the vein. Feel for a pulse with the forefinger and not the thumb to prevent hitting an artery. If a vein cannot be located with the finger, a large, flat rubber band may be placed around the upper head as a tourniquet. (Placing a gauze pad under an area of the band helps in removing it after the procedure.) Disinfect the scalp with an iodine preparation, chlorhexidine, or alcohol; allow the scalp to dry; and then wipe it with sterile gauze. After the scalp is inspected for the desired vein, release the tourniquet to permit refilling of the veins. Reapply finger pressure or the rubber band. Hold the skin taut with the nondominant hand distal to the site to be punctured.

Next, hold the infusion (butterfly) set with the two wings folded together and the bevel of the needle up. Position the needle at a 15-degree angle over the vein in the direction of the blood flow. Puncture the skin, and slowly advance the needle until blood begins to flow into the tubing of the needle set. Attach the syringe. Gently and slowly aspirate the blood to prevent hemolysis or occlusion by the vein wall. When sufficient blood is collected, release the finger tourniquet or rubber band. Place the sterile gauze pad over the puncture site, and apply pressure before quickly removing the needle. Apply additional pressure for several minutes to ensure that the bleeding has stopped. The remaining iodine or chlorhexidine is removed with a sterile saline solution or water to prevent absorption. Fill the collecting tubes in the usual fashion with the safety syringe shielded transfer device. Comfort the infant by stroking softly or by offering a pacifier with sucrose, if permitted. Be sure all used supplies are removed from the bed area.

COLLECTING BLOOD FROM IV LINES

The number of children receiving central venous catheters (CVCs) for the administration of medications and quick and painless withdrawal of blood has increased dramatically.[21] Hospitalized children or infants who are undergoing IV therapy (**FIGURE 13–29**), whether for total parenteral nutrition (TPN), administration of an antibiotic, or chemotherapy, often have poor veins. They may have a heparin or saline lock or a CVC when long-term access is required (**PROCEDURES 13–4** and **13–5**). Some blood tests can be performed with blood collected from these lines, but some hospitals limit the number of times a line can be accessed. Usually, managers of health care facilities require nursing or laboratory personnel to take specialized training courses prior to allowing them to collect blood from a central venous line. Please see Chapter 15 for additional information on the collection of blood from IV lines.

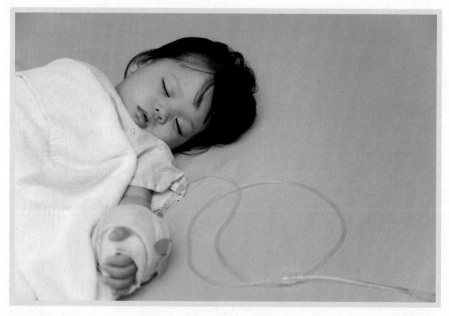

FIGURE 13–29

Intravenous Line in Infant

jomphong/Shutterstock

PROCEDURE 13–4

Procedure for Heparin or Saline Lock Blood Collection

Rationale To collect blood for laboratory tests through a heparin or saline lock.

Equipment

- Personal protective equipment, gloves (recommended nonlatex, sterile gloves for aseptic technique), mask, clean uniform, laboratory coat, etc.
- Laboratory requisition forms and pen
- Evacuated tubes and labels for the specimen
- Transfer device for syringe to evacuated tube blood transfer
- Syringe filled with 3 to 4 mL of normal saline
- Syringe filled with 2 to 3 mL of heparinized flush solution; 100 μ/mL (1 mL for heparin lock)
- 5-mL syringe for discard
- 10-mL syringe for blood specimen
- Small blood collection tubes
- Needleless cannula for gaining access to heparin lock
- Isopropyl alcohol, iodine or chlorhexidine swabs (check hospital's policy)
- Sterile double stopcock for central line
- Sterile intermittent injection port or Luer-Lok catheter cap
- Sterile 4" × 4" gauze sponge
- Biohazard container for wastes
- Alcohol wipes

Preparation

1 Check the patient's chart for the physician's order to collect blood through a heparin or saline lock.

2 Obtain laboratory requisitions and labels that reflect the patient location and tests for which blood is needed.

3 Check the labels against requisitions and the patient's identification bracelet, as described in Chapter 10.

4 Explain the test to the parent and the child (if old enough to understand).

5 Wash or sanitize your hands with an alcohol hand rinse, don gloves (nonlatex if the patient has latex allergy), and prepare and assemble equipment and supplies next to the patient. The procedures may involve the following steps but are subject to differences among hospitals and must be performed by authorized personnel only and under institutional guidelines.

Procedure

6 Identify the patient.

7 Disinfect the catheter injection port with an alcohol, iodine, or a chlorhexidine swab and let dry.

8 Check the patency of the line by attaching the syringe with normal saline and flushing with a small amount.

9 Attach a needleless cannula to the discard syringe, and insert it into the cap of the lock.

10 Gently withdraw approximately 2 to 3 mL of fluid and blood; remove the syringe and discard in a sharps biohazard container.

11 Insert another needleless device and syringe to collect the blood sample. When a sufficient amount of blood has been obtained, withdraw the syringe and fill the collection tubes using a safety syringe shielded transfer device.

12 Clean the cap or injection port of the heparin lock with an alcohol swab, then insert the syringe with the heparinized flush solution, injecting slowly.

PROCEDURE 13–5

Procedure for Central Venous Catheter Blood Collection

Rationale To collect blood for laboratory tests through a CVC.

Equipment

- Personal protective equipment, gloves (nonlatex, sterile gloves for aseptic technique), mask, clean uniform, and laboratory coat
- Laboratory requisition forms and pen
- Small evacuated tubes and labels for the specimens
- Transfer device for syringe to evacuated tube blood transfer
- Syringe filled with 3 to 4 mL of normal saline
- Syringe filled with 2 to 3 mL of heparinized flush solution
- 5-mL syringe for discard
- 10-mL syringe for blood specimen
- Needleless cannula for gaining access to heparin lock
- Isopropyl alcohol, iodine or chlorhexidine swabs (check hospital's policy)
- Sterile double stopcock for central line
- Sterile intermittent injection port or Luer-Lok catheter cap
- Sterile 4" × 4" gauze sponge
- Biohazard container for wastes
- Alcohol wipes

Preparation

1 Check the patient's chart for the physician's order to collect blood through a CVC.

2 Obtain laboratory requisitions and labels that reflect the patient location and tests for which blood is needed.

3 Check the labels against requisitions and the patient's identification bracelet, as described in Chapter 10.

4 Explain the test to the parent and the child (if old enough to understand).

5 Wash or sanitize your hands with an alcohol hand rinse, put on mask and gloves (nonlatex), and prepare and assemble equipment and supplies next to the patient. The procedures may involve the following steps but are subject to differences among hospitals and must be performed by authorized personnel only and under institutional guidelines.

Procedure

6 Stop all CVC intravenous fluids. Clamp all CVC access ports.

7 Open a sterile 4" × 4" gauze sponge, and place it under the catheter port to serve as a sterile field.

8 Option 1—Through injection port:
   a. Clean port with iodine swab or chlorhexidine swab. Allow to dry then wipe with alcohol swab.
   b. Aseptically insert syringe with saline using needleless system. Unclamp catheter. Flush central line port with normal saline. Remove and discard syringe and needleless system access.

PROCEDURE 13–5

Procedure for Central Venous Catheter Blood Collection (continued)

   c. Aseptically insert the next syringe using needleless system. Withdraw enough blood to clear the volume of the catheter. This amount will vary with different catheters. The manufacturers of the catheters specify a flush volume to determine the discard volume. Remove and discard syringe and needleless device in biohazardous waste container.

   d. Aseptically insert the next syringe using the needleless system. Withdraw appropriate volume of blood for blood sample. Remove syringe and needleless system and insert blood sample into appropriate evacuated tubes using the safety syringe shielded transfer device.

9 Option 2—Catheter hub to syringe hub:

   a. If CVC is a triple lumen device, use the access port closest to the child. Clamp the catheter; then remove the intermittent injection cap after vigorously scrubbing the connection with iodine, chlorhexidine, or 70% alcohol for 30 seconds (Check hospital's policy.). Allow to dry.

   b. Disconnect the IV tubing from the catheter and cover with a sterile capped needle.

   c. Aseptically connect the discard syringe and collection syringe to the sterile stopcock ensuring a tight seal; attach to the port.

   d. Unclamp the catheter, open the stopcock to the discard syringe, and withdraw 3 to 5 mL of fluid based on catheter volume. Close that port; then open the stopcock port to the collection syringe and aspirate the required amount of blood. Close that port, and remove the syringe.

   e. Attach the syringe with the heparinized solution to the port. Gently aspirate to clear the stopcock of air, holding the syringe vertically to allow bubbles to rise. Tap the syringe to free any bubbles sticking to its side.

   f. Flush the catheter with 5 mL of saline, close that port, and then open the port to the heparinized solution and flush with 5 mL.

   g. Reclamp the catheter and remove the stopcocks.

   h. Clean the connection site of the catheter with a new alcohol pad; then attach a new Luer-Lok cap.

   i. Attach the safety syringe shielded transfer device to the syringe and fill the collection tubes.

10 Discard used items in the appropriate containers.

After the Procedure

11 Determine that IV fluids are infusing properly at the rate set by the unit nurse. *Note:* If a pump is being used, make certain the pump is on and the alarm is on. If the rate of IV flow appears altered, notify the unit nurse immediately.

12 Make sure the pediatric patient is in a safe and comfortable position, with the bed down, siderails up, and bedside table and call light accessible to him or her. As mentioned earlier, discard all used equipment and supplies in appropriate containers.

13 Always immediately label the blood specimens and indicate that these specimens were collected by a line draw. Dispatch to the laboratory in the usual manner.

14 Remove gloves and mask, and wash or sanitize your hands.

15 Thank the parents and the pediatric patient for cooperating and depart with all remaining supplies. Do not leave anything at the patient's bedside.

16 Document completion of the procedure and any problems.

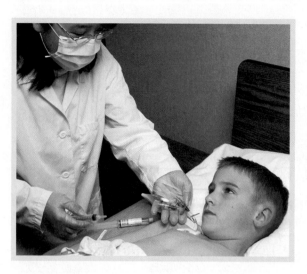

FIGURE 13–30

Collecting Blood from a Central Line

The health care worker uses sterile techniques and carefully examines the central line to plan access from the correct port for blood collection.

Confirm the amount of blood that can be collected based on the child's weight. Check with the nurse in charge or the doctor to verify the policy.

In an effort to reduce sharps injuries as mandated by OSHA, latex or silicone membrane ports on CVCs are recommended. These ports allow penetration with a needleless access device and can be easily disinfected before each entry, thereby reducing the risk of bacterial entry. When accessing a latex/silicone membrane port or a connector, the following steps are considered essential: (1) perform hand hygiene; (2) establish a sterile workspace using sterile gauze; and (3) prepare the access port with 70% alcohol, using sufficient friction and allowing the surface to dry[22,23] (**FIGURE 13–30**).

Geriatric Patients

The elderly, or **geriatric,** population comprises approximately 5% of the U.S. population and uses 31% of the nation's health care services (**FIGURE 13–31**). In 25 years, the geriatric population will have reached over 20% of the total U.S. population.[24,25] Physical conditions, such as arthritis, **Parkinson's disease** (a disease causing tremors), **Alzheimer's disease (AD)** (a disease that causes loss of intellectual abilities and mood disorders such as depression and combativeness), and other debilitating diseases in elderly persons will continue to increase point-of-care testing by skin puncture because of the difficulty of obtaining blood by venipuncture. In addition, this patient population will increasingly need point-of-care testing and other health care services in their homes, nursing homes, rehabilitation centers, and other long-term–care facilities (i.e., where the length of stay is more than 30 days) (**FIGURE 13–32**).

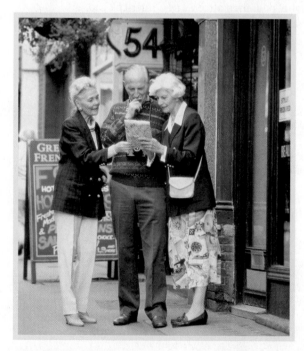

FIGURE 13–31

Increasing Geriatric Population in the United States

The number of elderly citizens is rapidly increasing because of the advancing age of the Baby Boomer generation.

Source: Ron Chapple/Getty Images

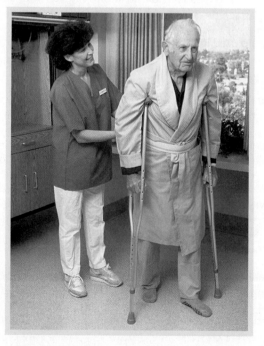

FIGURE 13–32

The Need for Health Care Workers

Increasing numbers of health care workers will be necessary to provide care in the expanding numbers of health care facilities.

The process of aging presents physical and emotional problems that can be challenging for health care workers. Some of these physical problems are depicted in **FIGURES 13–33** and **13–34**. Whatever the case; treat elderly individuals with the utmost respect and dignity. It is important to establish eye contact. Be sensitive to the patient's needs and don't forget to smile. Physical problems that are common in older individuals include the following:

- Hearing loss may cause embarrassment and frustration. Repeating instructions or facing the patient to speak in the "good" ear may be necessary for the patient to truly understand a procedure. If possible, reduce outside noise as much as possible. Do not shout. Speak slowly and clearly. Also, if the patient does not understand you the first time, rephrase the statement.

- Failing eyesight is common. Take care to guide the elderly individual to the appropriate seat for blood collection or to the bathroom for urine collection. Also, in the hospital, assist the elderly patient with his or her glasses if he or she wants them during the blood collection.

- Loss of taste, smell, and feeling can accompany the aging process. Elderly people may lack an appetite, which may lead to malnourishment and dehydration. They may tend to drop things or not be able to make a fist because of muscle weakness. Make a note of these clues, particularly if the patient is homebound without a caregiver.

- Memory loss can affect the patient's ability to take medications or to remember the last time he or she ate. These factors may interfere with the interpretation of laboratory results. Including family and friends in the discussion of the last meal eaten by the patient can assist in determining if the blood specimen is a fasting specimen.

- Skin tissue becomes thinner, thereby making venipuncture more difficult. Hold the skin extra taut so that the vein does not "roll." Also, do not "slap" the arm when trying to locate the vein. This causes bruising. Use of heated compresses can be helpful. A tourniquet may not be necessary for venipuncture. If it is used, it should be applied loosely to avoid bruising and harm to the fragile veins. If the tourniquet is used, release it as soon as blood appears in the collection tube to prevent excessive pressure in the vein.

- Muscles become smaller, so the angle of penetration of a venipuncture needle may need to be more shallow.

- The elderly have increased susceptibility to accidental hypothermia (a subnormal drop in body temperature) that can make them feel cold. Thus, specimen collection may require warming of the site.

- They may also experience increased sensitivities and allergies. Ask patients whether they have any allergies.

- Emotional problems that are associated with aging include the possible loss of career, spouse, close friends, or relatives and can be reflected by depression or anger at life in general. Remember to address elderly persons with dignity and respect by using Mr., Mrs., Miss, etc. Also respect the patient's privacy.

CONSIDERATIONS IN HOME CARE BLOOD COLLECTIONS

If specimens are to be collected in homes, all procedures are similar except take extra care to do the following:

- Take extra supplies and equipment, including biohazard containers for disposables and a temperature-regulated specimen transport container, into the home. Identify the closest bathroom in case it is needed.

- Positively identify the patient if possible. If not possible, develop and follow the procedures of the health care organization.

- Place the patient in a comfortable, preferably reclining, position in case of fainting.

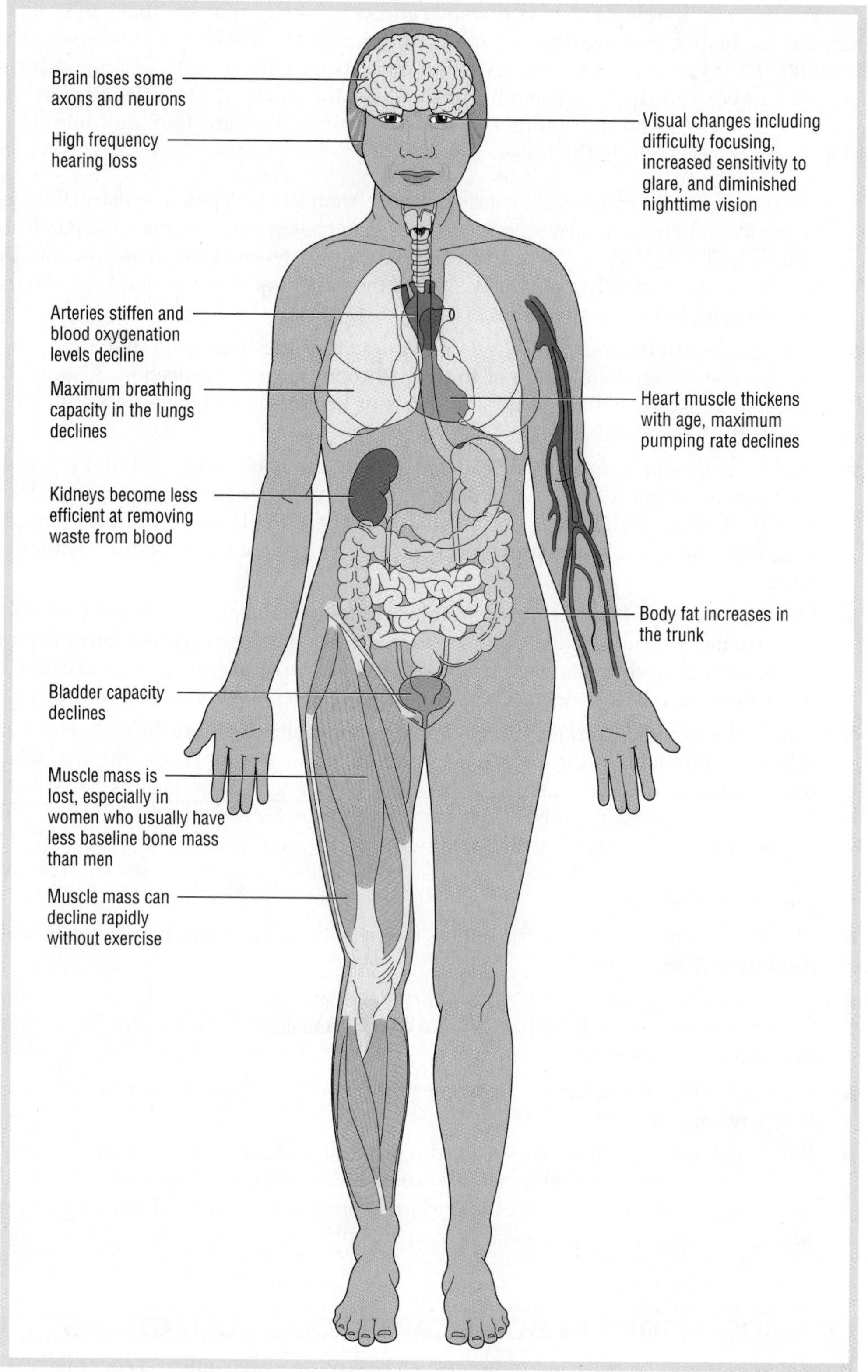

FIGURE 13–33
Normal Changes of Aging

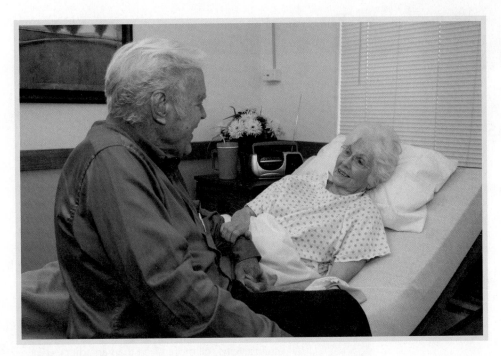

FIGURE 13–34

Elderly Patients Use About a Third of All Health Services in the United States.

Note how this couple has characteristics that a health care worker can observe and be sensitive to. Signs of hearing and sight impairments include the hearing aid and glasses, skin appears to be fragile, and hands appear as if the patient may have arthritis or other joint disorders.

- Carry a hand disinfectant with other supplies and equipment and use the disinfectant on your hands before collecting blood.
- Wait for the puncture site to stop bleeding, because many elderly patients take medications that prolong bleeding (i.e., Coumadin and heparin).
- Carefully inspect the area after the procedure to ensure that all trash and used supplies have been properly discarded.
- Carefully label the specimens and place them in leakproof containers with the biohazard sign on the container. Check the appropriate temperatures for transport.
- When working in high-crime areas, take security precautions, travel with a mobile phone, and carry maps or GPS to avoid getting lost on the way to or from the patient's home.
- Carefully document delays in returning specimens to the laboratory.

Chapter 10, "Venipuncture Procedures," and Chapter 11, "Capillary Blood Specimens," also provide procedures that apply to the elderly patient. In blood collections, factors to consider for older patients include the types of blood collection equipment to use. For example, using a safety butterfly needle and small evacuated tubes is usually more appropriate for the elderly patient's fragile veins. Consider the physiological situation of each geriatric patient in the decision to obtain a quality blood specimen for laboratory tests.

Study Questions

For the following questions, select the one best answer.

1 Which is the preferred site for a heel stick?

a. anteromedial aspect
b. medial or lateral aspect
c. posterior curve
d. previous puncture site

2 Which of the following describes the behavior of a 6- to 12-month old infant undergoing a painful procedure?

a. fears separation from parent
b. is embarrassed to show fear
c. fears injury to body
d. wants privacy

3 Which of the following is a debilitating disease causing loss of intellectual abilities and mood disorders, particularly in elderly individuals?

a. Alzheimer's disease
b. Parkinson's disease
c. arthritis
d. depression

4 Which of the following is an acceptable intervention to alleviate pain in pediatric blood collection?

a. xylocaine injection
b. EMLA application
c. ice pack
d. lidocaine application

5 The preferred technique for restraining a child is

a. vertical with child sitting in parent's lap
b. total sedation
c. mechanical restraint
d. vertical with parent leaning child against the wall

6 Which is the *best* location for performing a phlebotomy on a hospitalized child?

a. bedside in a chair
b. playroom
c. treatment room
d. in his or her bed

7 Performing blood collection on a child is challenging because

a. a child is less emotionally mature than an adult
b. a child's veins roll more often than an adult's veins
c. smaller equipment must be used
d. a child's blood clots more quickly

8 Warming the heel does which of the following?

a. arterializes blood
b. dramatically decreases blood flow
c. prevents hemolysis
d. hastens hemostasis

9 Methods of distracting a child to alleviate anxiety include:

a. showing the child where the venipuncture will occur
b. providing the samples of blood collection equipment to be used
c. music
d. pinching an alternate site

10 Which of the following is an important step in preparing the child and the parent for a phlebotomy?

a. assess their past experience with blood drawing
b. perform the phlebotomy slowly to avoid pain
c. ask the parent to leave the room
d. use lidocaine to decrease the pain of the blood collection

Case Study

Mr. Frank McGuire is a 90-year-old former industrial worker who has lost 30 pounds over the past 4 years, resulting in a frail body. He has been diagnosed as having Parkinson's disease as well as congestive heart failure. Mr. McGuire is having his blood collected in the nursing home where he now resides; his physician has ordered a potassium level, a hemoglobin level, and a PT/INR test because he is on Coumadin.

Questions

1 What is the proper "order of draw" for the collection of blood for these assays?

2 What is the most appropriate blood collection equipment to use?

3 How should the patient be approached for the blood collection?

Action in Practice

Two health care workers oversee blood collection in the newborn nursery on the weekends. On Sunday morning, the clinical laboratory scientist (CLS) overseeing the clinical chemistry section noticed that the bilirubin value for Baby Sullivan was as follows:

Day	Time	Bilirubin Value (mg/dL)
Friday	8:30a	13
Saturday	8:05a	12
Sunday	7:30a	3

Knowing that the ultraviolet light on newborn Baby Sullivan could not make the bilirubin value decrease that dramatically from Saturday to Sunday, the CLS called in the health care worker who had collected the Sunday morning blood sample to ask him questions regarding the collection.

Questions

1 Which type of microcollection container should have been used to collect the bilirubin specimen?

2 Does taking the blood immediately to the clinical laboratory for testing make any difference?

COMPETENCY ASSESSMENT

Check Yourself

1 List the equipment that is needed on a blood collection tray in order to perform a fingerstick on a 2-year-old child.

2 After you have introduced yourself in a confident manner and then properly identified the patient (a 3-year-old child), describe the age-specific steps to prepare the child and parent for the blood collection procedure.

Competency Checklist: Pediatrics and Geriatrics

This checklist can be completed as a group or individually.

(1) Completed (2) Needs to improve

_____ 1. List blood collection equipment necessary for a capillary blood gas collection from a newborn infant.
_____ 2. Identify four physical problems that are common in the elderly that can challenge blood collection efforts.
_____ 3. List three important considerations in blood collection from within an elderly patient's home.

REFERENCES

1. London, M. L., Ladewig, P. A., Ball, J., & Bindler, R. (2011). *Maternal and child nursing,* 3rd ed. Upper Saddle River, NJ: Prentice Hall.

2. Clinical and Laboratory Standards Institute (CLSI). (2008). *Procedures and devices for the collection of diagnostic capillary blood specimens, approved standard.* Document H04-A6. Wayne, PA: Author.

3. Markenson, D. (2002). *Pediatric prehospital care.* Upper Saddle River, NJ: Prentice Hall.

4. Cavender, K., Goff, M. D., Hollon, E. C., & Guzzetta, C. E. (2004). Parents' positioning and distracting children during venipuncture: Effects on children's pain, fear, and distress. *J Holist Nurs. 22:* 32–56.

5. Stevens B., Yamada, J., Lee, G. Y., & Ohlsson, A. (2013) *The Cochrane collaboration.* The Cochrane Library, Issue 1: Sucrose for analgesia in newborn infants undergoing painful procedures (Review). New York: Wiley and Sons.

6. Gradin, M., Eiserafy, F., Alsaedi. S., et al. (2009, May–June). Oral sucrose and a pacifier for pain relief during simple procedures in preterm infants: a randomized controlled trial. *Annals of Saudi Medicine, 29*(3): 184–188.

7. Lindh, V., Wiklund, U., Blomquiat, H. K., & Hakansson, S. (2003). EMLA cream and oral glucose for immunization pain in 3-month-old infants. *Pain, 104*(1–2): 381–388.

8. Centers for Disease Control and Prevention. (2002, October 25). CDC guideline for hand hygiene in health-care settings. *MMWR Rec and Rep, 51* (RR-16).

9. Shriners Hospitals for Children, Patient Education. (n.d.). *Latex allergy in children.* www.shrinershq.org/_pvw253fa4/hospitals/chicago/patient_info/default.aspx, accessed November 7, 2007.

10. Valentine, S. L., & Bateman. S. T. (2012, January). Identifying factors to minimize phlebotomy-induced blood loss in the pediatric intensive care unit. *Pediatr Crit Care Med, 13*(1): 22–27.

11. Hicks, J. M. (2001). Q & A: Blood volumes needed for common tests. *Lab Med,* (2): 187.

12. Reiner, C. B., Meites, S., & Hayes, J. R. (1990, March). Optimal depths for skin puncture of infants and children as assessed from anatomical measurements. *Clin. Chem., 36*(3): 547–549.

13. Jain, A., & Rutter, N. (1999, May). Ultrasound study of heel to calcaneum depth in neonates. *Arch Dis Child Fetal Neonatal Ed, 80*(3): F243–F245.

14. Vertanen, H., Fellman, V., Brommels, M., & Viinikka, L. (2001, January). An automatic incision device for obtaining blood samples from the heels of preterm infants causes less damage than a conventional manual lancet. *Arch Dis Child Fetal Neonatal Ed, 84:* F53–F55.

15. Meites, S., Hamlin, C, R., & Hayes, J. R. (1992). A study of experimental lancets for blood collection to avoid bone infection of infants. *Clin. Chem, 38:* 908–910.

16. McDowell, G. (2005). *Newborn screening beyond PKU.* Burlington, NC: Lab Corp, Inc. CME, p. 1.

17. National Newborn Screening and Genetics Resource Center, U.S. National Screening Status Report. http://genes-r-us.uthscsa.edu/resources/newborn/screenstatus.htm, updated 2012–2013, accessed April 9, 2013.

18. Clinical and Laboratory Standards Institute (CLSI). (2007). *Blood collection on filter paper for newborn screening programs, approved standard,* 5th ed. Wayne, PA: CLSI Document LA4-A5.

19. Ogawa, S., Ogihara, T., Fujiwara, E., Ito, K., Nakano, M., et al. (2005). Venipuncture is preferable to heel lance for blood sampling in term neonates. *Arch Dis Child Fetal Neonatal Ed., 90*(5): F432–F436.

20. Shah, V., & Ohlsson, A. (2011). Venipuncture versus heel lance for blood sampling in term neonates. *Cochrane Database Syst Rev.,* accessed as up-to-date, July 8, 2011.

21. Carson, S. M. (2004). Chorhexidine versus povidone-iodine for central venous catheter site care in children. *J Ped Nursing, 19*(1): 74–80.

22. Kilbride, H., Powers, R., Wirtschafter, D., et al. (2003, April). Evaluation and development of potentially better practices to prevent neonatal nosocomial bacteremia. *Pediatrics, 111*(4).

23. HICPAC/CDC Guidelines for the Prevention of Intravascular Catheter-Related Infections. www.cdc.gov/hicpac/pdf/guidelines/bsi-guidelines-2011.pdf, accessed March 27, 2013.

24. Nixon, R. G. (2003). *BRADY geriatric prehospital care.* Upper Saddle River, NJ: Prentice Hall.

25. Federal Interagency Forum on Aging Related Statistics. (2012). Older Americans 2012: Key indicators of well-being. www.agingstats.gov, accessed April 10, 2013.

RESOURCES

American Federation for Aging Research. (2004). *Biology of aging, theory of aging information center. www.infoaging.org*, accessed November 20, 2007.

Coffin, C. M., Hamilton, M. S., Pysher, T. H., et al. (2000). Pediatric laboratory medicine: Current challenges and future opportunities. *Am J Clin Pathol, 117:* 683–690.

Lindh, V., Wiklund, U., Blomquiat, H. K., & Hakansson, S. (2003, July). EMLA cream and oral glucose for immunization pain in 3-month-old infants. *Pain, 104*(1–2): 381–388.

Lindh, V., Wiklund, U., & Hakanssom, S. (2000). Assessment of the effect of EMLA during venipuncture in newborn by analysis of heart rate variability. *Pain, 86:* 247–254.

MacLaren, J. E., & Lindsey, L. (2005). A comparison of distraction strategies for venipuncture distress in children. *J Ped Psychology, 30*(5): 387–396.

Panlener, J. (2003, May). Successfully meeting the challenge of Pediatric Sample Size in laboratory medicine. *Childx,* Summary of symposium. *www.childx.org/sample_size.htm*, accessed November 7, 2007.

Saint, S. (2001). Prevention of intravascular catheter-associated infections. In K. G. Shojania, B. W. Duncan, K. M. McDonald, & R. M. Wachter (Eds.), *Evidence report/Technology assessment No. 43, Making health care safe: A critical analysis of patient safety practices.* Rockville, MD: Agency for Health Care Research and Quality, pp. 163–183.

Chapter 14

Point-of-Care Collections

Chapter Objectives

Upon completion of Chapter 14, the learner is responsible for doing the following:

1. List two other terms that are synonymous with point-of-care testing.

2. Identify four analytes whose levels can be determined through point-of-care testing.

3. Describe the most widely used application of point-of-care testing.

4. Define quality assurance and its requirements in point-of-care testing.

With new and emerging technology, laboratory testing services and results delivery have expanded beyond the laboratory to the hospital bedside, the home, the nursing home, exercise or health clubs, and any other direct-contact patient setting. The terms used for these direct laboratory services include:

- Point-of-care testing (POCT)
- Decentralized laboratory testing
- Onsite testing
- Alternate-site testing
- Near-patient testing
- Patient-focused testing
- Bedside testing

Point-of-care testing has become a popular means of meeting the demands for faster laboratory testing. The demand for POCT is increasing because rapid turnaround of laboratory test results is necessary for prompt medical decision making.

The International Organization for Standardization (ISO) seeks to harmonize the health care industry practices of several countries for better interoperability and to provide a vocabulary that can be commonly shared between health care industries. It has defined (ISO 22870) point-of-care testing. The requirements of ISO 22870:2006 apply when POCT is carried out in a hospital, clinic, and by a health care organization providing ambulatory care.

Point-of-care testing instruments, meters, and other devices use small amounts of uncentrifuged blood specimens, allowing the use of fingersticks over the risk of venipuncture. Also, some POCT specimens are urine and saliva. A wide list of analytes are available through POCT, and some of those are shown in **BOX 14–1**.

The rapid increase in the use of POCT in health care institutions and home health care has led to concern about the quality and risks associated with point-of-care testing. For example, blood gas analyzers carried between patient hospital rooms in one health

BOX 14–1

Frequently Used Point-of-Care Tests

- Brain natiuretic peptide (BNP)
- Electrolytes and blood gas analytes
- Glucose
- Hemoglobin A1c
- Hemoglobin
- Infectious diseases (i.e., HIV)
- Influenza A and B
- Lipids (cholesterol, HDL cholesterol, LDL cholesterol)
- Pregnancy
- Triglycerides
- White blood cell (WBC) count

care facility were contaminated with infectious organisms and antibiotic-resistant organisms.[1] Also, blood glucose testing analyzers have been linked to the transmission of hepatitis B in long-term health care facilities in three states.[2] Health care workers using POCT analyzers need to be aware of the potential risks to patient safety to ensure appropriate test results. Point-of-care testing involves instrument calibration and quality control to ensure accuracy and reliability of the tests' results. Thus, the operators of the POCT instruments need to learn the steps in the instrument calibration, quality assurance, and use of the instruments before actually performing patient testing using the devices.

Glucose Monitoring

One of the most widely used applications of point-of-care testing is blood glucose monitoring, in which commercially available instruments, such as those shown in Procedure 14–1, are used to determine blood glucose levels. Such determinations allow the physician to choose appropriate treatment regimens for patients with **diabetes mellitus,** a chronic disease in which the pancreas cannot produce enough **insulin** or cannot use the insulin that it does produce. Insulin is a chemical that is released into the bloodstream by the pancreas when glucose levels in the blood increase after meals. Insulin causes the glucose to be absorbed from the blood into the body tissues, where it is used for energy. Because of the lack of insulin in patients with diabetes mellitus, glucose is not properly absorbed by the tissues, and the glucose levels within the blood increase.

During the past decade, small glucose-monitoring instruments, such as the ones described in **TABLE 14–1** and shown in **FIGURE 14–1**, have become commonplace in the

TABLE 14–1

Blood Glucose Monitors

Instrument (Manufacturer)	Features	Test Time	Volume
Accu-Chek Aviva (Roche Diagnostics Corp.)	2000 tests' battery life	5 seconds	0.6 µL
Ascensia DEX2 Diabetes Care System (Bayer Diagnostics)	Electrochemical assay; 100 tests	10 seconds	3–4 µL
One Touch Ultra 2 (Life Scan)	7-, 14-, and 30-day averages	5 seconds	1 µL
FreeStyle (Abbott Diabetes Care)	Electrochemical assay; 250 tests	5 seconds	0.3 µL

FIGURE 14–1

Blood Glucose Monitor

Many types of glucose meters are available today.

Courtesy of Vicente Barcelo Varona/Shutterstock

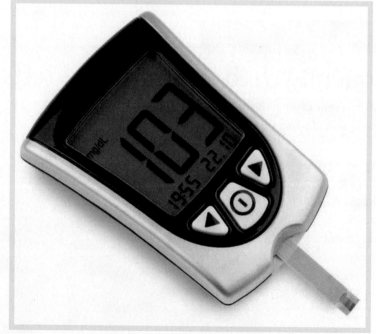

home, in the nursing home, and at the hospital bedside. These "rapid" methods require whole blood samples collected by skin puncture from the finger, heel (for infants), or a flushed heparin line. As with any blood collection procedure, appropriate infection control and safety protocols must be followed (e.g., wearing gloves), and disposal of potentially contaminated waste must be part of the quality control and safety guidelines (see Chapters 4 and 5). These bedside procedures are handy for quick screening in a hospital or outpatient setting.

To perform the blood glucose determinations, health care providers need to gather the appropriate supplies (**PROCEDURE 14–1**) and must be aware of all the quality control procedures that are required to obtain accurate and precise results.[3,4] The timing of the reaction is critical, and most of these instruments call the time to the attention of the operator by buzzing, sounding an alarm, or digitally displaying the glucose result. Also, the health care provider needs to know which type of blood—blood from a fingerstick and/or blood from venipuncture—can be used to perform glucose determinations with the point-of-care instrument and the patient age group for whom the blood instrument can be used.

As an example, the HemoCue β-Glucose Analyzer (**FIGURE 14–2**) can obtain test results from capillary, venous, or arterial whole blood. It uses a microcuvette rather than a test strip and does not require blotting. Also, it can be used to monitor blood glucose in neonates as well as adults and children.

Another example of a glucose analyzer is the advanced blood glucose monitoring system from Nova Biomedical, the Nova StatStrip® point-of-care glucose monitor (**FIGURE 14–3**) that provides accurate glucose results in 6-second analysis time. Its small 1.2 microliter sample size results in easy sample acquisition and minimal pain for the patient. Sample types include capillary, venous, arterial or neonatal whole blood.

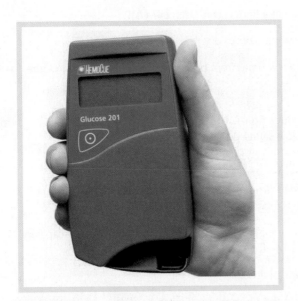

FIGURE 14–2
HemoCue® Glucose 201 Analyzer

Courtesy of HemoCue America, Brea, CA.

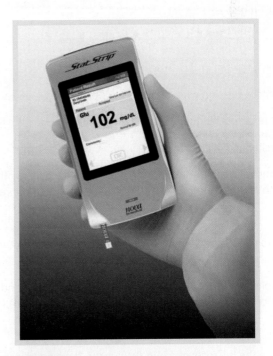

FIGURE 14–3
StatStrip® Glucose Analyzer

Courtesy of Nova Biomedical, Waltham, MA.

PROCEDURE 14–1

Obtaining Blood Specimen for Glucose Testing (Skin Puncture)

Rationale To select the optimum treatment procedure for patients with diabetes mellitus.

One of the most widely used applications of point-of-care testing is blood glucose monitoring, in which commercially available instruments, such as the one shown in this procedure, are used to determine blood glucose levels. Such determinations allow the physician to choose appropriate treatment regimens for patients with diabetes mellitus.

Equipment

- Gloves
- Safety automatic lancet
- Antiseptic for hand cleansing
- 3 alcohol/acetone or alcohol preps
- Sterile gauze pads
- Hemocue® blood glucose monitor

Preparation

1 Gather equipment: safety automatic lancet.

2 Identify the patient properly. Briefly explain the test to the patient.

3 Clean your hands.

4 Put on gloves.

Procedure

5 Select the site and cleanse it with antiseptic (especially the side of a finger) (**FIGURE 14–4A**).

6 Cleanse the skin with an alcohol wipe (Figure 14–4B) and allow the skin to dry.

7 Without touching the cleansed site, gently massage the finger a few times from base to tip to aid blood flow (Figure 14–4C).

8 Decide on which side of the finger to make the incision.

9 Remove the safety lancet from the protective paper without touching the tip, and as you hold the patient's finger firmly with one hand, make a swift, deep puncture with the retractable safety puncture device (Figure 14–4D).

10 Wipe the first three drops of blood away with clean gauze (Figure 14–4E).

11 Gently massage the finger from base to tip to obtain the needed drop of blood. Do not squeeze the fingertip, because this can cause hemolysis of the blood sample.

12 Apply the Hemocue® microcuvette to the drop of blood. The correct volume is drawn into the cuvette by capillary action (capillary, venous or arterial blood can be used) (Figure 14–4F).

13 Wipe off any excess blood from the sides of the cuvette (Figure 14–4G).

14 Place the microcuvette into the cuvette holder and insert it into the photometer (Figure 14–4H).

15 The laboratory test result is displayed automatically (Figure 14–4I).

PROCEDURE 14–1

Obtaining Blood Specimen for Glucose Testing (Skin Puncture) (continued)

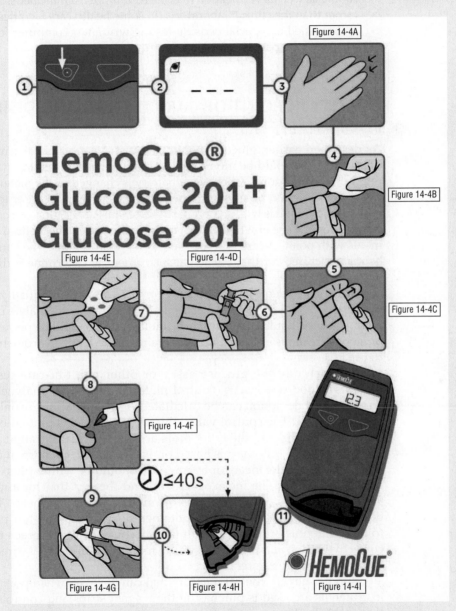

FIGURE 14–4
Courtesy of HemoCue, Inc., Lake Forest, CA.

After The Procedure

16 Discard the safety automatic lancet in the sharps container with biohazard label.

17 Discard the gauze, alcohol wipes, and gloves in biohazardous waste containers.

18 Wash or sanitize your hands.

For these point-of-care testing analyzers, the health care worker needs to

- Carefully read the package insert and user manual.
- Watch an experienced laboratory professional, doctor, or nurse perform the test.
- Strictly follow daily quality control procedures.
- Carefully record the results, including the date, time, and health care worker identification, as well as verification that the results are from the bedside (or patient's home) rather than the clinical laboratory. (In some health care facilities, bedside test results are recorded on special bedside-testing written or computer forms or in a separate section of the patient's medical record.)

QUALITY IN POINT-OF-CARE TESTING AND DISINFECTING POCT ANALYZERS

As described earlier, glucose-monitoring instruments and instruments that measure other analytes should be monitored daily with **quality control material.** These values must also be monitored whenever a battery is changed or the meter is cleaned. The control material should be similar to the patient's specimen in order to determine whether the analytic system is working properly. For example, the glucose control material should be based on the use of whole blood, because this type of body fluid is used for measurements with point-of-care glucose-monitoring instruments. The control material should be manufactured for that particular instrument to determine if the analytic system is working properly.

Many instruments have automatic control or "electronic quality control" (EQC). The purpose of EQC is to test the electronics: the internal and analyte circuits of the instrument. Both the liquid quality control and the EQC should be performed if the analyzer or meter directions indicate that both are required. Some instruments are now designed to use EQC only.

For each day the glucose assay or other point-of-care test is performed on patients' blood specimens, control material should be analyzed so that the mean and standard deviation can be calculated. The calculations usually occur on 20 to 30 control values.[5] The control value obtained each day is plotted on a chart under the appropriate date, and the daily plots are joined with a straight line (**FIGURE 14–5**). Interpretation of this chart is based on the fact that for a normal distribution, 95% of the values about the mean, or average ($\bar{x}$), should be within plus or minus 2 standard deviations (SD) of the mean (average), and the fact that for a normal distribution, 99% of the values are within plus or minus 3 SD of the mean. Tolerance limits are determined by pooling the data obtained during a 30-day test period and referring to the mean plus or minus 2 SD. If a daily control value exceeds the tolerance limits, corrective action *must* occur according to the manufacturer's directions and be documented for future reference.

Another quality control measure that can be taken when point-of-care monitoring instruments are used is purchasing the reagent strips and controls in large quantities that enable health care workers to use constant pools of the same lot number. This leads to reproducibility of the results. In addition, required preventive maintenance of each point-of-care instrument is critical for accurate results.

Some point-of-care testing instruments can store and download calibrators, controls, and patients' results, and can therefore provide a complete instrument log for quality assurance interpretation. **BOX 14–2** provides a list of problems to avoid so that quality results may be obtained.

Routine cleaning of the point-of-care testing instruments is needed to avoid the transmission of nosocomial infections. Using a cleaning tissue with a disinfectant such as 5% bleach solution can minimize the possibilities of transferring microorganisms from one patient to another as the instrument is being used for testing. Also,

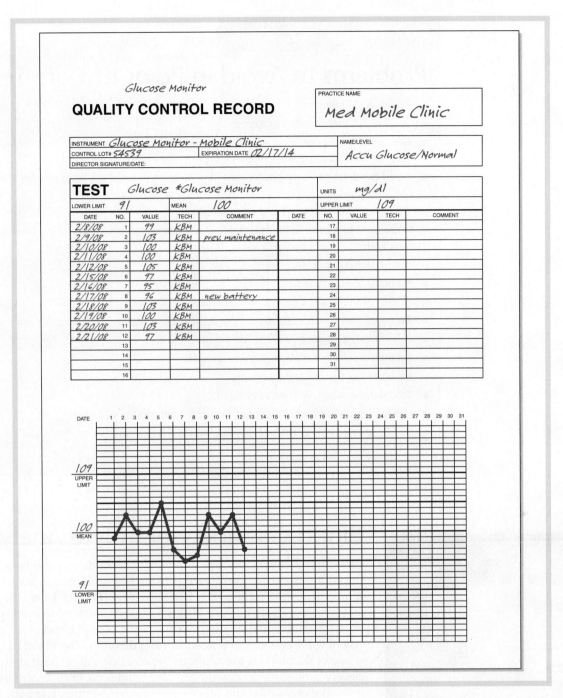

FIGURE 14–5
Quality Control Record

many health care institutions have procedures in place that assign glucose instruments to a single patient during his or her length of stay in the hospital. Also, changing gloves between patients' that are being tested is a *must*—no matter what other precautions are being taken for infection control. It is recommended that the health care worker strictly follow the health care institution's policy to disinfect these analyzers and meters.

BOX 14–2

Problems to Avoid in Point-of-Care Testing

- Patient is misidentified.
- Specimen is inappropriately stored.
- The blood is contaminated with alcohol. (After alcohol is used to cleanse the skin puncture site, the skin must dry completely before puncturing the site.)
- Blood is hemolyzed because the skin puncture site was not dry from alcohol after cleansing the puncture site.
- Wrong volume of specimen is collected.
- Instrument blotting/wiping technique is not performed according to the manufacturer's directions.
- Instrument is not clean.
- Reagents are outdated.
- Timing of the analytic procedure is incorrect.
- Reagents are not stored at the proper temperature, leading to their deterioration.
- Patient has not dieted properly for the procedure.
- Patient's result/time/date/and so on is mislabeled.
- Recording of the result is incorrect.
- Battery for instrument is weak or dead.
- Calibrators and/or controls are not properly used and/or recorded.
- Results are not sent to the appropriate individuals in a timely manner.

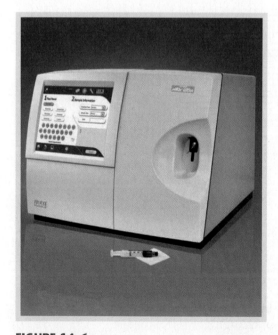

FIGURE 14–6

NOVA Biomedical Stat Profile® pHOx Ultra Analyzer

Courtesy of Nova Biomedical, Waltham, MA.

Blood Gas and Electrolyte Analysis

Blood gas analysis for critical patient care needs can also be accomplished through **patient-focused testing** using instrumentation such as the Nova Biomedical Stat Profile pHOx Ultra analyzer (**FIGURE 14–6**). Blood gas analysis involves measurement of the partial pressure of oxygen (pO_2), partial pressure of carbon dioxide (pCO_2), and pH. The pO_2 and pCO_2 are analyzed whenever a patient has a heart or lung disorder. The blood pH determines whether the blood is too acidic or too alkaline. All of these analytes must be closely monitored in emergency care situations, critical care units, cardiac intensive care units, and other units requiring immediate patient diagnosis and treatment.

In addition to monitoring blood gases, point-of-care instruments such as the Nova Stat Profile pHOx Ultra Analyzer can measure blood **electrolyte** levels—sodium (Na^+), potassium (K^+), chloride (Cl^-), calcium (Ca^{++})—plus saturated oxygen, glucose, magnesium (Mg^{++}), creatinine, lactate, hematocrit, hemoglobin, and total bilirubin levels. These measurements, as well as blood gas analysis, are needed immediately in critical care situations.

These instruments require preventive maintenance and quality control similar to the glucose-monitoring instruments; however, they measure more than one analyte and thus have more complex operational, quality control, and maintenance needs than the glucose monitors. Consequently, a health care professional involved in collecting blood and determining the analytes' results with these instruments needs to be thoroughly trained in their use prior to actually testing patients' blood.

Point-of-Care Testing for Acute Heart Damage

Another cardiac point-of-care test is the ROCHE TROPT sensitive rapid assay from Roche Diagnostics. It is a POC assay to qualitatively measure **troponin T** to detect heart damage. The assay uses whole venous blood (heparin or EDTA).

White Blood Cell Count System

HemoCue WBC System is unique in being a point-of-care test system for the determination of the **white blood cell (WBC) count** for a patient. The analyzer requires only 10 uL of whole blood from a fingerstick or a venous EDTA sample and provides a WBC count within 3 minutes.

Blood Coagulation Monitoring

Similar to glucose monitoring, monitoring blood coagulation (i.e., prothrombin time [PT] and International Normalized Ratio [INR]) through point-of-care testing provides immediate results that can be used in controlling bleeding or clotting disorders in patients.[6,7] A blood coagulation instrument, such as the CoaguChek XS System from Roche Diagnostics Corporation, is a handheld instrument that can measure prothrombin time (PT/INR) results from only 8 microliters of whole blood, providing results in 1 minute (**FIGURE 14–7**).

The CoaguChek XS System can be used by home health care providers or other outpatient clinic providers to monitor long-term anticoagulation therapy in patients. The immediate test results allow rapid dose adjustments. Again, the health care provider using these instruments must be trained appropriately in the preventive maintenance and quality control parameters in order to obtain accurate results. Also, reading the manufacturer's directions is essential. For example, the CoaguChek XS System is calibrated to use the first drop of blood in skin puncture. Also, venous blood can be used for the analysis.

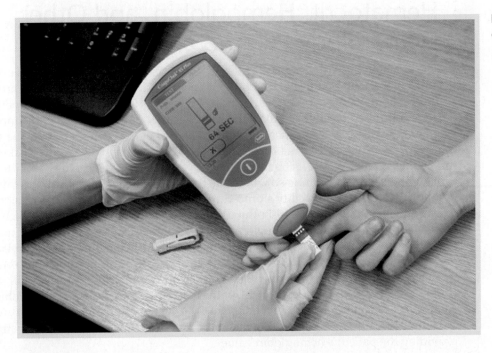

FIGURE 14–7
CoaguChek XS System

Courtesy of Trevor Smith/Alamy

FIGURE 14–8
Actalyke XL Activated Clotting
Time Test (ACT) System

Courtesy of Helena Laboratories Point of Care, Beaumont, TX.

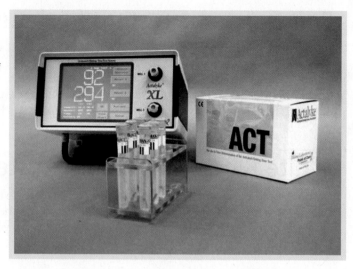

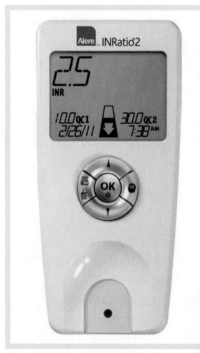

FIGURE 14–9
Alere INRatio2® Meter

Courtesy of Alere: Physician Diagnostics Group

The International Technidyne Corporation (ITC) ProTime Microcoagulation System is a portable battery-operated ProTime testing instrument designed to monitor patients' oral anticoagulation using venous or capillary blood. The blood is collected into the disposable cuvette that is inserted directly into the instrument for measurement of PT/INR.

Another point-of-care coagulation system is the Actalyke Activated Clotting Time Test (ACT) System (**FIGURE 14–8**). The Actalyke XL is designed to monitor heparin therapy during cardiac procedures and dialysis. Actalyke instruments and reagent tubes provide the sensitivity, reliability, and rapidity needed to make timely treatment decisions at the point of care. Yet another POC coagulation system is the Alere INRatio2® Meter (**FIGURE 14–9**), which is used to measure PT/INR for maintenance of proper anticoagulation therapy. These instruments are designed for use at the point of care (i.e., home, intensive care unit, physician's office) to monitor anticoagulation therapy such as heparin or warfarin sodium (Coumadin).

Hematocrit, Hemoglobin, and Other Hematology Parameters

The hematocrit (Hct, packed cell volume [PCV], Crit) represents the volume of circulating blood that is occupied by red blood cells (RBCs). It is expressed as a percentage; thus, a hematocrit value of 38% indicates that 38 mL of each 100 mL of peripheral blood is composed of RBCs. Hematocrit values are obtained to aid in the diagnosis and evaluation of anemia, a less than normal number of erythrocytes, and may be used to evaluate blood volume and total RBC mass. Blood collection usually occurs by skin puncture. For accurate test results, remember not to excessively squeeze the finger to obtain capillary blood because doing so will dilute the sample with tissue fluid. It is important to follow the health care facility's procedure. Plastic microcapillary tubes must be used to avoid the possibility of blood-borne pathogen exposure from a broken tube.

Determining a patient's hemoglobin level is another test to aid in the diagnosis and evaluation of anemia and other blood abnormalities. The hemoglobin test has been determined by the American Medical Association (AMA) to be more accurate than the hematocrit test in diagnosis and treatment. Also, the hemoglobin procedure is a safer method to detect anemia. A point-of-care analyzer that can be used to measure hemoglobin is the HemoCue β-Hemoglobin System (**FIGURE 14–10**). A patient's venous, capillary, or arterial whole blood sample is placed in the microcuvette and inserted into this instrument, providing the patient's hemoglobin value.

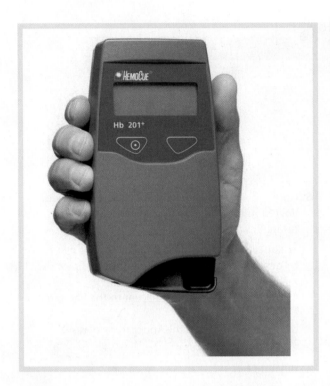

FIGURE 14–10
HemoCue® Hb 201 + Analyzer

Courtesy of HemoCue America, Brea, CA.

Cholesterol Screening

Another laboratory testing procedure that health care providers are performing through point-of-care testing is cholesterol screening. The Chemcard Cholesterol Test provides a semi-quantitative estimate of total cholesterol in 3 minutes using a single drop of whole blood. Using a fingerstick drop of blood, total cholesterol (TC) values can be obtained with the Alere Cholestech LDX System. This instrument can measure a lipid profile including total cholesterol, HDL cholesterol, LDL cholesterol, and triglycerides in 5 minutes and the patient's sample amount is 40 microliters of whole blood. *Total cholesterol* is a fatlike substance that occurs naturally in the body. If total cholesterol accumulates in the bloodstream, the excess amount is deposited in the arteries and leads to arterial blockage and heart disease. The high-density lipoprotein cholesterol, or **HDL cholesterol,** is referred to as the "good cholesterol" because increased blood values protect the patient from heart disease. The low-density lipoprotein cholesterol, or **LDL cholesterol,** is referred to as the "bad cholesterol" since high values are linked to heart disease. **Triglycerides** are fatty acids and glycerol that circulate in the blood and are stored as body fat. The overall patient's results for a lipid profile provide a diagnostic tool for the clinician to identify if the patient may be at risk for heart disease.

Other POCT Tests and Future Trends

Additional point-of-care testing procedures that have evolved include the **hemoglobin A1c** procedure that is a test for maintenance of blood glucose levels and the handheld **Bili*Check*** for measuring bilirubin in newborns. The device is held against the infant's forehead and completes the test in 15 minutes. The measurement is conducted through the skin; no blood is collected.

More point-of-care testing procedures are evolving that will inevitably involve phlebotomists, nurses, patient care technicians, and others who are providing care at the hospital bedside, nursing home, and/or home. For each new procedure, the health care worker must make a point of learning in detail the blood collection requirements, preventive maintenance, quality control, infection control requirements, ethical and legal implications of doing such a test (e.g., HIV testing), record keeping, and calibration requirements in order to provide accurate and precise test results.

Study Questions

For the following questions, select the one best answer.

1 Which of the following is a blood electrolyte measured by point-of-care testing?

a. glucose
b. potassium
c. hemoglobin
d. insulin

2 Diabetes mellitus is caused by the inability of the pancreas to make or to use which substance?

a. glucose
b. cholesterol
c. sodium
d. insulin

3 Which tests can be measured by electrolyte monitoring through point-of-care testing?

a. Na^+, K^+, PT, and APTT
b. pCO_2, pO_2, and Na^+
c. Na^+, K^+, Cl^-, and Calcium
d. pCO_2, Cl^-, HCO_3^-, and pO_2

4 After the safety lancet is used for the skin puncture in the HemoCue Glucose analyzer procedure, what is the next step for glucose measurement?

a. use the first drop of blood for the glucose test
b. use an alcohol pad to remove the first drop of blood
c. wipe the first three drops of blood away with clean gauze
d. squeeze the patient's finger to make a big first drop of blood for the monitor

5 Which of the following POC assays can detect heart damage?

a. chloride
b. troponin T
c. partial pressure of carbon dioxide
d. sodium

6 How can a health care worker increase the blood flow from the skin puncture site for patient testing?

a. squeeze the punctured finger
b. gently massage the area from base to tip of the finger
c. puncture another site adjacent to the first puncture site
d. use a cold pack on the finger to increase the blood flow

7 What do blood gas analyses measure?

a. Na^+ and K^+
b. pCO_2, pO_2, and pH
c. Cl^- and HCO_3^-
d. pCO_2, Na^+, and Cl^-

8 Which tests are measured through blood coagulation monitoring by point-of-care testing?

a. PT and INR
b. PT and pCO_2
c. pO_2 and pCO_2
d. PT, APTT, and pH

9 Which of the following is referred to as the "good cholesterol"?

a. LDL cholesterol
b. HDL cholesterol
c. total cholesterol
d. cholesterol ratio

10 In which of the following organs is insulin produced?

a. gallbladder
b. pancreas
c. liver
d. kidney

Case Study

Ms. Garner, a 50-year-old African American woman with type 2 diabetes, tested her glucose level at home on November 11, 2013, and obtained a glucose reading of 89 mg/dL using a test strip. This value is well within normal limits for blood glucose, but because she was having symptoms of sweating and was feeling lightheaded, Ms. Garner went to her physician the next day. The physician immediately hospitalized her for treatment of uncontrolled diabetes. During the hospitalization, the following glucose meter versus clinical laboratory comparisons were performed:

Date	Glucose Meter Results (mg/dL)	Lab Test Results (mg/dL)
11/12/13	151	351
11/13/13	194	289
11/14/13 (a.m.)	97	192
11/14/13 (p.m.)	99	194

From product performance specifications, health care workers determined that the control comparisons for November 12 through November 14 were outside the acceptable product performance range. The patient indicated that she followed the preventive maintenance schedule described in the documentation packaged with the glucose meter and had purchased the meter, test strips, and controls 2 years ago. The controls were checked occasionally, maybe every month or two.

Questions

1 What is the problem in this case study?

2 What troubleshooting techniques(s) should have been implemented to resolve this problem?

Action in Practice

The bedside request for a hemoglobin measurement on Ms. McGuire was given to Ms. Louise Walker, the health care worker on that hospital floor. Name a possible POCT analyzer that might be used for this POCT procedure on Ms. McGuire and the types of whole blood samples that can be used for the analysis on this instrument.

COMPETENCY ASSESSMENT

Check Yourself

1 List 10 situations that can lead to problems in point-of-care testing.

2 What blood electrolytes can be measured on point-of-care testing instruments?

Competency Checklist: Point-of-Care Testing

This checklist can be completed as a group or individually.

(1) Completed (2) Needs to improve

_____ 1. Describe the procedural steps in POC glucose testing.
_____ 2. Explain the difference between HDL cholesterol and LDL cholesterol.
_____ 3. Describe two types of analytes that aid in the diagnosis and evaluation of anemia and
state which one has been determined to be more accurate in diagnosis and treatment.

REFERENCES

1. Acolet, D., Ahmet, Z., Houang, E., et al. (1994). Enterobacter cloacae in a neonatal intensive care unit: Account of an outbreak and its relationship to the use of third generation cephalosporins. *J Hosp Infect, 28:* 273–286.

2. Centers for Disease Control. (2012).DC. Multiple outbreaks of hepatitis B virus infection related to assisted monitoring of blood glucose among residents of assisted living facilities—Virginia, 2009–2011. *MMWR Morb Mortal Wkly Rep, 61:* 339–343.

3. Clinical and Laboratory Standards Institute (CLSI). (2013). *Point-of-care blood glucose testing in acute and chronic care facilities. Approved guideline,* 3rd ed. Wayne, PA: Author.

4. Clinical and Laboratory Standards Institute (CLSI). (2005). *Glucose monitoring in settings without laboratory support, approved guideline,* 2nd ed. Wayne, PA: Author.

5. Westgard, J., & Klee, G. (2006). Quality management. In C. Burtis, E. Ashwood, & D. Bruns (Eds), *Tietz textbook of clinical chemistry and molecular diagnostics.* St. Louis: Elsevier/Saunders.

6. Plesch, W. & Van Den Besselaar, A. M. H. P. (2009). Validation of the international normalized ratio (INR) in a new point-of-care system designed for home monitoring of oral anticoagulation therapy. *International Journal of Laboratory Hematology, 31:* 20–25. doi: 10.1111/j.1751-553X.2007.00998.x

7. Wurster, M., & Doran, T. (2006). Anticoagulation management: A new approach. *Disease Management, 4:* 201–209.

RESOURCES

Price, C., St. John, A., & Kricka, J. (2010). *Point-of-care testing,* 3rd ed. Washington, DC: American Association for Clinical Chemistry.

St-Louis, P. (2000). Status of point-of-care testing: Promise, realities, and possibilities. *Clin Bio Chem, 33*(6): 427–440.

Tang, Z., Lee, J., Louie, R., & Kost, G. (2000). Effects of different hematocrit levels on glucose measurements with handheld meters for point-of-care testing. *Archives of Path and Lab Med, 124:* 1135–1140.

Chapter 15

Blood Cultures, Arterial, Intravenous (IV), and Special Collection Procedures

Chapter Objectives

Upon completion of Chapter 15, the learner is responsible for doing the following:

1. List the steps and equipment in blood culture collections.

2. Discuss the requirements for the glucose and lactose tolerance tests.

3. Explain the special precautions and types of equipment needed to collect arterial blood gases.

4. Differentiate cannulas from fistulas.

5. List the special requirements for collecting blood through intravenous (IV) catheters.

6. Differentiate therapeutic phlebotomy from autologous transfusion.

7. Describe the special precautions needed to collect blood in therapeutic drug monitoring (TDM) procedures.

8. List the types of patient specimens that are needed for trace metal analyses.

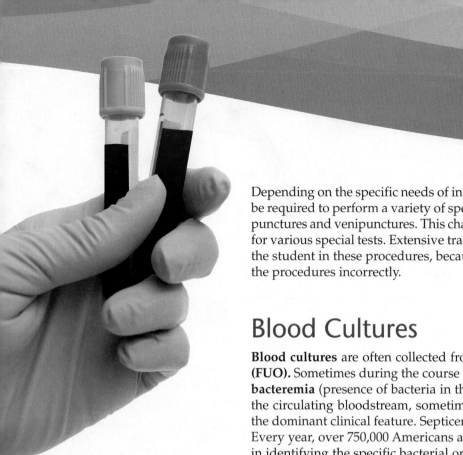

Depending on the specific needs of individual clinical settings, health care workers may be required to perform a variety of special tests or procedures in addition to routine skin punctures and venipunctures. This chapter presents the basic techniques and precautions for various special tests. Extensive training sessions and supervision should accompany the student in these procedures, because the patient can be harmed if students perform the procedures incorrectly.

Blood Cultures

Blood cultures are often collected from patients who have **fevers of unknown origin (FUO).** Sometimes during the course of a bacterial infection in one location of the body, **bacteremia** (presence of bacteria in the blood) or **septicemia** (presence of pathogens in the circulating bloodstream, sometimes called *blood poisoning*) may result and become the dominant clinical feature. Septicemia is a major cause of death in the United States.[1] Every year, over 750,000 Americans are diagnosed with septicemia.[2] Blood cultures aid in identifying the specific bacterial organism causing the infections and should be performed on any patient suspected to have bacteremia.[3] Blood culture collections must be performed with extreme and meticulous care and aseptic techniques. Every precaution should be taken to minimize the percentage of contaminated blood cultures that usually occur because of poor collection technique and skills.[4]

Venipuncture is the method used when collecting blood specimens for blood cultures (see **PROCEDURES 15–1, 15–2, 15–3, 15–4,** and **15–5**). Indwelling catheter collections for blood cultures are not recommended because of high contamination results. Important differences in a blood culture procedure relate to the following:

- The health care worker must explain the procedure in greater detail to the patient.
- The puncture site must be decontaminated prior to collection to ensure skin antisepsis.
- The type of collection tubes used must contain culture media that enable bacteria to grow under laboratory conditions.
- The timing and number of blood cultures obtained must be clearly indicated.

POSSIBLE INTERFERING FACTORS

- If blood culture collections are ordered along with other laboratory tests, blood culture specimens must be collected first. If an evacuated blood collection tube is used prior to the blood culture SPS evacuated tubes or blood culture bottles, the needle can become contaminated and cause false-positive results.
- When the needle enters the venipuncture site, it should not be scraped across the skin, since this can contaminate the needle and therefore the blood cultures. Additionally, a blood culture collection through existing intravenous lines should be avoided.
- The anaerobic blood culture bottle must be inoculated first in all procedures except the butterfly assembly method, because injection of air into the anaerobic bottle can cause the death of some anaerobic microorganisms and result in a false-negative culture.
- Whenever possible, blood cultures should be obtained before initiation of antibiotics. If antimicrobial therapy cannot be avoided prior to collection, special blood culture

bottles must be used. These bottles contain resin beads that neutralize antibiotics already in the patient's blood specimen. If these vials are not gently mixed to neutralize the antibiotics in the blood, the antibiotics can inhibit bacterial growth and cause false-negative blood culture results.

■ Sometimes two sets of blood cultures are ordered, and the second set should be obtained in the same manner as the first, except that the second venipuncture should be at a different site (i.e., the other arm) and/or at a different time (60 minutes later).

■ If using a tube holder/needle assembly for evacuated tubes, there is a possibility that media from the culture bottle might flow backward into the vein (reflux action). This is why most manufacturers recommend that the media collection bottles should not be filled directly from a tube holder/needle assembly. The blood should be collected through a butterfly attached to a tube holder or directly into a syringe.

PROCEDURE 15–1

Site Preparation for Blood Culture Collection

Rationale   To obtain a sterile puncture site because bacteria normally located on the skin can contaminate a blood culture if it is not properly cleaned before the venipuncture.

Equipment

- Personal protective equipment, nonlatex gloves (recommended nitrile, sterile gloves for aseptic technique), clean uniform, and laboratory coat
- Isopropyl alcohol preps
- 2 chlorhexidine gluconate swab sticks (2 packages)
- 2 blood culture bottles (1 for anaerobic microorganisms and 1 for aerobic microorganisms) (2 bottles/set collected; check expiration date for each bottle)
- Sodium polyanethole sulfonate (SPS) evacuated tubes
- Safety needles (21 or 23 gauge) or blood collection set
- Safety sterile syringe or evacuated safety tube assembly and blunt-tipped cannula for syringe and direct-draw holder/adapter
- Sterile gauze pads
- Nonlatex bandages
- Nonlatex disposable tourniquet
- Patient identification labels/requisitions
- Pen
- Plastic "ziplock" specimen bags
- Biohazard waste container

Preparation

1 Identify the patient properly. Explain the test to the patient.

2 Wash or sanitize your hands with an alcohol hand rinse, put on nonlatex gloves, and prepare and assemble equipment and supplies next to the patient. Offer to answer any questions for the patient. Place the tourniquet on the arm.

(continued)

PROCEDURE 15–1

Site Preparation for Blood Culture Collection (continued)

Procedure

3 Locate the vein, loosen the tourniquet, scrub the site of the venipuncture with 70% isopropyl alcohol for 60 seconds to rid the site of excess dirt. Then scrub the site with a chlorhexidine gluconate swab for at least 30 seconds (infants must be older than 2 months of age for a scrub with chlorhexidine). The chlorhexidine swab should initially be placed at the site of needle insertion and then moved outward in concentric circles to a diameter of approximately 2.5 inches, as shown in **FIGURE 15–1**. Scrub with friction.

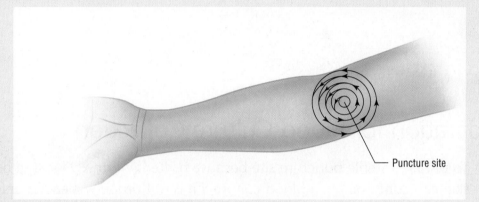

Puncture site

FIGURE 15–1
Arm Preparation for the Collection of Blood Culture Specimens

4 Some health care facilities use a blood culture preparation kit that has a one-step application. The application has chlorhexidine gluconate/isopropyl alcohol antiseptic combined for an effective 30-second cleansing of the venipuncture site (**FIGURE 15–2**).

FIGURE 15–3 shows a blood culture bottle and scrub preparation.

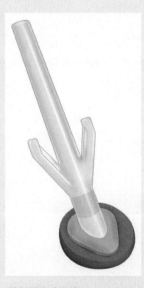

FIGURE 15–2
One-Step 30-Second
Application for Blood Culture
Venipuncture Preparation

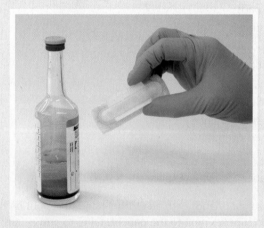

FIGURE 15–3
Blood Culture Bottle and Scrub Preparation

PROCEDURE 15–1

Site Preparation for Blood Culture Collection (continued)

After the Procedure

5 Collect the blood culture by vacuum tube, syringe, or safety butterfly assembly.

Notes

- Research has shown lower blood culture contamination rates in collection sites prepared with iodine tincture or chlorhexidine instead of iodophor (e.g., povidone-iodine).[5,6,7,8]

- Do not touch any area that has been prepped. Allow the area to dry for 1 minute in order for the antiseptic to be effective against skin bacteria. Do not blow on the site to speed drying.

- Removal of the entire metal ring on some manufacturers' bottles introduces air into them and can cause contamination.

- Read the manufacturer's directions on blood culture bottles before using them, because they may vary as to the volume of blood specimen needed and their preparation requirements. If the fill line is not marked, place each bottle on a flat surface and then use a marker to note a "fill-to line." Usually, the fill level is 10 mL/bottle for adults.

  There is a direct relationship between the volume of blood obtained and the yield of a blood culture set. From 40 to 60 mL of blood should be obtained per episode (in other words, 2 to 3 sets with 20 mL per set, and 10 mL per bottle).

- Treat the top of the blood culture bottle as a sterile area, and take care not to contaminate it.

- **Sodium polyanethole sulfonate (SPS)** in the yellow-topped evacuated tube is especially designed for blood culture collections because it inhibits phagocytosis and neutralizes biochemicals that may interfere in the blood culture recovery of microorganisms.

PROCEDURE 15–2

Safety Syringe Blood Culture Collection

Rationale To perform a blood culture collection using a safety syringe.

For the safety *sterile* syringe collections, it is commonly recommended to do an adult collection of 20 mL and transfer the first 10 mL to the anaerobic bottle and the remaining 10 mL to the aerobic bottle.

Equipment

- Personal protective equipment, nonlatex gloves (recommended sterile gloves for aseptic technique), clean uniform, and laboratory coat
- Isopropyl alcohol preps
- 2 chlorhexidine gluconate swab sticks (2 packages)
- 2 blood culture bottles (1 for anaerobic microorganisms and 1 for aerobic microorganisms) (2 bottles/set collected; check expiration date for each bottle)
- Sodium polyanethole sulfonate (SPS) evacuated tubes
- Safety needles (21 or 23 gauge)
- Safety sterile syringe, blunt-tipped cannula (connector), and direct-draw holder/adapter
- Sterile gauze pads
- Nonlatex bandages

(continued)

PROCEDURE 15–2

Safety Syringe Blood Culture Collection (continued)

- Nonlatex tourniquet
- Patient identification labels
- Laboratory requisition and pen
- Plastic "ziplock" specimen bags
- Biohazard waste container

Preparation

1 Identify the patient properly. Explain the test to the patient.

2 Wash or sanitize your hands with an alcohol hand rinse, put on gloves, and prepare and assemble equipment and supplies next to the patient. Offer to answer any questions for the patient. Place the tourniquet on the arm.

Procedure

3 Locate the vein and loosen the tourniquet. Disinfect the rubber septum on the blood culture bottles with 70% isopropyl alcohol and allow it to dry (manufacturers may differ in how to disinfect culture bottles). Scrub the site of the venipuncture with 70% isopropyl alcohol for 60 seconds to rid the site of excess dirt, and then scrub with chlorhexidine gluconate for at least 30 seconds (infants must be older than 2 months of age for a chlorhexidine application). Begin by placing the swab at the site of needle insertion and then move it outward in concentric circles to a diameter of approximately 2.5 inches.

4 Alert the patient before venipuncture. Reapply the tourniquet, anchor the vein, and smoothly insert the needle, bevel up.

5 After the collection of the blood into the safety sterile syringe, activate the safety needle cover and aseptically dispose of the needle into the sharps container without touching the needle.

6 Then place a blunt-tipped cannula (connector) on the syringe tip and attach the blunt-tipped connector to the direct-draw holder/adapter (**FIGURE 15–4**).

7 Starting with the anaerobic microbiology bottle in an upright position, place the blood-transfer device on the bottle, fill to the desired amount, and remove the syringe with the blood-transfer device from the bottle.

8 If anaerobic and aerobic microbiology bottles are to be filled with the patient's blood, fill the aerobic bottle immediately after the anaerobic bottle, and then fill the other blood collection tubes according to the "order of draw." *Never* push on the syringe plunger. Allow the vacuum in the microbiology bottles and tubes to pull the blood into the bottles and tubes.

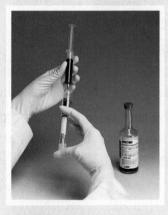

FIGURE 15–4
Courtesy and © Becton, Dickinson and Company Microbiology Systems, Sparks, MD.

9 If only 3 mL or less of blood are collected, place the entire amount in the aerobic bottle.

10 For infants and small children, only 1 to 5 mL of blood can usually be collected for bacterial culture. Use blood culture bottles that are designed specifically for the pediatric patient.[9,10]

PROCEDURE 15–3

Safety Butterfly Assembly Blood Culture Collection

Rationale   To perform a blood culture collection using a safety butterfly.

Equipment

- Personal protective equipment, nonlatex gloves (recommended sterile gloves for aseptic technique), clean uniform, and laboratory coat
- Isopropyl alcohol preps
- 2 chlorhexidine gluconate swab sticks (2 packages)
- 2 blood culture bottles (1 for anaerobic microorganisms and 1 for aerobic microorganisms) (2 bottles/set collected; check expiration date for each bottle)
- Sodium polyanethole sulfonate (SPS) evacuated tubes
- Safety needles (21 or 23 gauge) or blood collection set
- Evacuated safety tube assembly
- Sterile gauze pads
- Nonlatex bandages
- Nonlatex tourniquet
- Patient identification labels
- Laboratory requisition and pen
- Plastic "ziplock" specimen bag
- Biohazard waste container

Preparation

1 Identify the patient properly. Explain the test to the patient.

2 Wash or sanitize your hands with an alcohol hand rinse, put on gloves, and prepare and assemble equipment and supplies next to the patient.

3 Offer to answer any questions for the patient. Place the tourniquet on the arm.

Procedure

4 Locate the vein and loosen the tourniquet. Disinfect the rubber septum on the blood culture bottles with 70% isopropyl alcohol and allow it to dry.

5 Scrub the site of the venipuncture with 70% isopropyl alcohol for 60 seconds to rid the site of excess dirt, and then scrub with the chlorhexidine gluconate for at least 30 seconds (infants must be older than 2 months of age for a chlorhexidine application). Begin with the swab at the site of needle insertion and then move it outward in concentric circles to a diameter of approximately 2.5 inches. Follow the manufacturer's directions for disinfection of blood culture bottles.

6 Alert the patient before venipuncture. Reapply the tourniquet, anchor the vein, and smoothly insert the needle, bevel up.

7 Use a safety butterfly assembly (safety blood collection set) (see Figure 8–13, p. 262) for insertion of the butterfly needle into the venipuncture site after the appropriate skin preparation.

8 It can be helpful to place a strip of tape over the butterfly wings to keep the needle in place as the blood culture bottles are filled with the blood.

(continued)

PROCEDURE 15–3

Safety Butterfly Assembly Blood Culture Collection (continued)

9 Transfer the blood to the microbiology bottles via a direct draw adapter that fits directly over the blood culture bottle (**FIGURE 15–5**).

10 Using this method, blood is transferred to the aerobic bottle first, since the assembly tubing contains air.

11 If only 3 mL or less of blood are collected, place the entire amount in the aerobic bottle.

12 For infants and small children, only 1 to 5 mL of blood can usually be collected for bacterial culture. Use blood culture bottles that are designed specifically for the pediatric patient.[9,10]

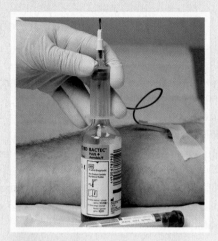

FIGURE 15–5
Blood Culture Collection Using BACTEC Microbiology Bottle with Blood Collection Safety Set

Courtesy and © Becton, Dickinson and Company, Sparks, MD.

PROCEDURE 15–4

Evacuated Tube System for Blood Culture Collection

Rationale To perform a blood culture collection using an evacuated tube system.

Equipment

- Personal protective equipment, nonlatex gloves (recommended sterile gloves for aseptic technique), clean uniform, and laboratory coat
- Isopropyl alcohol preps
- 2 chlorhexidine gluconate swab sticks (2 packages)
- 2 blood culture bottles (1 for anaerobic microorganisms and 1 for aerobic microorganisms) (2 bottles/set collected; check expiration date for each bottle)
- Sodium polyanethole sulfonate (SPS) evacuated tubes
- Safety needles
- Single-use evacuated tube holders
- Sterile gauze pads
- Nonlatex bandages
- Nonlatex tourniquet
- Patient identification labels
- Laboratory requisition and pen
- Plastic "ziplock" specimen bags
- Biohazard waste container

PROCEDURE 15–4

Evacuated Tube System for Blood Culture Collection (continued)

Preparation

1 Identify the patient properly. Explain the test to the patient.

2 Wash or sanitize your hands with an alcohol hand rinse, put on gloves, and prepare and assemble equipment and supplies next to the patient. Offer to answer any questions for the patient. Place the tourniquet on the arm.

Procedure

3 Locate the vein, loosen the tourniquet, scrub the site of the venipuncture with 70% isopropyl alcohol for 60 seconds to rid the site of excess dirt, and then scrub with the chlorhexidine gluconate for at least 30 seconds (infants must be older than 2 months of age for a chlorhexidine application). Initially place the swab at the site of needle insertion and then move it outward in concentric circles to a diameter of approximately 2.5 inches.

4 Alert the patient before venipuncture. Reapply the tourniquet, anchor the vein, and smoothly insert the needle, bevel up.

5 After performing a venipuncture by evacuated tube system, collect blood into the SPS tubes and then fill other tubes, as required (see Chapter 10, "Venipuncture Procedures," for additional information).

Note: Collecting blood directly into blood culture bottles with a needle holder designed for collecting blood into evacuated tubes is *not* recommended because of the risk of reflux of the culture media back into the vein and also because the amount of blood collected into the bottle cannot be controlled.

6 The blood from an SPS tube can be transferred to the blood culture media.

PROCEDURE 15–5

After Blood Culture Collection by the Previous Methods

Procedure

1 At the patient's bedside, label the tubes and/or bottles and label each culture bottle or tube with the site of specimen collection. Ask the patient to double-check his or her name on the labels, if possible.

2 Document the date and time the specimen was obtained and the site of the specimen collection.

3 Discard the safety needle or the evacuated tube holder/needle assembly or butterfly blood collection set in the sharps biohazardous container.

4 Discard blood-soaked gauze pads, contaminated items, and gowns or gloves used in isolation rooms in appropriate biohazardous waste containers, as discussed in Chapter 4.

5 Dispose of gowns and gloves that are not from isolation rooms in the appropriate containers.

6 Wash or sanitize your hands.

7 Thank the patient for cooperating and depart with all specimens and all remaining supplies. Do not leave anything at the patient's bedside.

8 Deliver the blood specimens immediately to the laboratory.

Clinical Alert!

- For any of the blood collection procedures, the venipuncture site *must not* be repalpated after the venipuncture site is prepared for blood collection, even if the gloved forefinger is cleansed.

- Relocating the vein by repalpation after sterilization recontaminates the site. If palpation of the site prior to puncture is anticipated, wear *sterile* gloves.

- Make a mental note of the vein's location in relation to skin features such as a mole, crease, freckles, etc.

- If you must repalpate, do not palpate at the actual venipuncture site.

- Microbiology culture bottles *must* be held upright during the venipuncture collection to avoid reflux of culture media into the patient.

Clinical Alert! Never use the safety butterfly set without a

direct draw adapter for the transfer of blood to the bottles. If the needle is not covered in this transfer of blood to the bottles, the needle poses a risk of accidental needlestick as it is pushed into the bottle.
Also, it is important to check with the manufacturers of blood collection safety-holder/needle devices before attempting blood culture collections, since some of these devices do not accommodate the blood transfer to blood culture bottles. It is important to use a blood-transfer device that is compatible to the safety-holder/needle device to avoid a needlestick injury.

Chlorhexidine does not have to be cleaned from the skin after the venipuncture is complete unless the patient may have an allergic reaction to it.[11] The health care provider must initial the patient identification labels, indicate the time and date of collection on the labels, indicate the site of collection (i.e., right arm, left arm), and attach a label to each vial or tube.

Changing needles should *not* occur after collecting blood for culture, because it can lead to a needlestick injury to the health care worker. Careful skin cleansing plays a critical role in minimizing blood culture contamination.[12] Also, performing a venipuncture at a skin site that is obviously infected increases the chance of contamination of the blood culture.

Glucose Tolerance Test (GTT)

For patients who have symptoms suggesting problems in carbohydrate (i.e., sugar) metabolism, such as diabetes mellitus, the **glucose tolerance test** can be an effective diagnostic tool. When a glucose tolerance test is to be performed, the patient should be given complete instructions about the procedure so that his or her cooperation can be ensured (**BOX 15–1**).

For best results, the patient should follow these standards:

1. Eat normal, balanced meals for at least 3 days prior to the test.
2. Fast for at least 8 hours prior to the beginning of the test.
3. Do *not* drink unsweetened tea, coffee, or any other beverage while fasting or during the procedure.
4. Drink water.
5. Do *not* smoke, chew tobacco or gum (including sugarless gum) while fasting or during the procedure. (*Note:* If a patient is chewing gum before or during this procedure, note this on the requisition form, since chewing gum may interfere with the test results.)
6. Do *not* exercise, even mildly, during the test.
7. Be ambulatory. Glucose tolerance tests should not be performed on nonambulatory patients since inactivity, such as bed rest, reduces glucose tolerance.
8. The patient should *not* take the test if she or he has had an illness in the last two weeks.

The test is performed by first obtaining a fasting blood specimen. The fasting blood specimen should be taken to the laboratory for test results. Then the patient can be given a standard load of glucose (e.g., a liquid drink called Glucola), and subsequent blood and urine samples can be obtained at intervals, usually during a 2- to 3-hour period. If the fasting specimen is abnormal, the physician must be notified before giving the load of glucose. Each specimen is then analyzed for its glucose content. In general, glucose levels should return to normal within 2 hours after ingestion of the glucose. During the test, the patient drinks a standard dose of glucose: 75 grams for adults, or approximately 1 gram per kilogram of body weight for children and small adults. A dose of 75 grams is recommended for diagnosis of gestational diabetes.[13,14] Gestational diabetes

BOX 15–1

Glucose Tolerance Test: Sample Patient Information Card

Introduction

A glucose tolerance test (GTT) has been ordered by your physician. The purpose of a GTT is to test the efficiency of your body's insulin-releasing mechanism and glucose-disposing system.

You must prepare your body for the GTT by changing your eating and medication routines slightly for three days before the test. It is very important that you follow the following instructions in order for accurate results to be obtained.

Basically, you will need to follow these three guidelines to prepare for your GTT test:

1. Your carbohydrate intake must be at least 150 g per day for 3 days prior to the GTT.
2. Do not eat anything for 8 hours before the GTT, but do not fast for more than 12 hours before the test.
3. Do not exercise for 12 hours before the GTT.

Preparation: Medication

Before proceeding with the GTT, you must tell your physician if you are currently using any of the following medications, because they may interfere with test results:

- Alcohol
- Anticonvulsants (seizure medication)
- Blood pressure medication
- Clofibrate
- Corticosteroids
- Diuretics (fluid pills)
- Estrogens (birth control pills or estrogen replacement pills)
- Salicylates (aspirin, pain killers)—only if taken in high doses, such as for rheumatoid arthritis

Preparation: Diet and Exercise

Remember that for 3 days prior to your test, your diet must contain at least 150 g of carbohydrates per day. The following is a list of high-carbohydrate foods:

- **Milk and milk products**—12 g of carbohydrates per serving. One serving is equal to 8 oz of milk (whole, skim, or buttermilk), 4 oz of evaporated milk, or 1 cup of plain yogurt.
- **Vegetables**—5 g of carbohydrates per serving. One serving is equal to one-half cup of any vegetable, excluding starches (e.g., potatoes, corn, or peas).
- **Fruits and fruit juices**—10 g of carbohydrates per serving. One serving is equal to one-half cup of juice, 1 small piece of fresh fruit, or one-half cup of unsweetened canned fruit, with the following exceptions:

Apple juice	$\frac{1}{3}$ cup
Grape juice	$\frac{1}{4}$ cup
Raisins	2 tbsp.
Watermelon	1 cup
Prunes	2 medium
Banana	$\frac{1}{2}$ small
Dates	2
Cantaloupe	$\frac{1}{4}$ 6-inch melon
Honeydew melon	$\frac{1}{8}$ 7-inch melon

(continued)

BOX 15–1 (continued)

- **Breads and starches**—15 g of carbohydrates per serving. One serving is equal to 1 slice of bread or 1 small roll. Other 1-serving sizes include:

Bagel/English muffin	1/2
Tortilla	1
Cooked cereal	1/2 cup
Dry cereal	3/4 cup
Cooked rice, noodles, pasta	1/2 cup
White potatoes, dried beans, and peas	1/2 cup
Yams	1/4 cup
Corn	1/3 cup
Crackers	5 to 6

- **Meats, cheeses, and fats**—These foods contain few or no carbohydrates.
- **Miscellaneous**

Ice cream	1/2 cup	15 g of carbohydrates
Sherbet	1/2 cup	30 g of carbohydrates
Gelatin	1/2 cup	30 g of carbohydrates
Jams, jellies	1 tbsp.	15 g of carbohydrates
Sugar	1 tsp.	4 g of carbohydrates
Carbonated beverage	6 oz	20 g of carbohydrates
Hard candy	2 pcs.	10 g of carbohydrates
Fruit pie	1/6 pie	60 g of carbohydrates
Cream pie	1/6 pie	50 g of carbohydrates
Plain cake	1/10 cake	30 g of carbohydrates
Frosted cake	1/10 cake	38 g of carbohydrates

Preparation: General Health

The following physical conditions should be reported to your doctor because they, too, might affect the results of your test:

- Acute pancreatitis
- Adrenal insufficiency
- Diabetes mellitus
- Hyperinsulinism (excess insulin secretion, resulting in hypoglycemia)
- Hyperthyroidism
- Hypopituitarism (decreased function of pituitary gland)
- Pregnancy
- Stress

If you have any difficulty making the necessary alterations in your diet or medication schedule, please inform your doctor. For accurate test results, these instructions must be followed.

Courtesy of Division of Laboratory Medicine, University of Texas, M. D. Anderson Cancer Center, Houston, TX.

can occur during pregnancy, usually in the second or third trimester (see "Postprandial Glucose Test," p. 467). Commercial preparations are available as flavored drinks to make the glucose more palatable. The patient must start and finish the drink within 5 minutes. Water intake is encouraged throughout the procedure. If the patient vomits at any point in the procedure, the physician should be notified immediately to determine whether the test should be continued or stopped.[13,14,15,16]

When the patient finishes drinking the solution, the time is noted, and 30-, 60-, 120-, and 180-minute blood specimens are obtained.

Examples of timed blood collections for GTT follow:

- Fasting specimen obtained and sent to laboratory (lab result okay to proceed with GTT)
- Glucose load given (i.e., Glucola) at 7:00 AM
- One-half hour specimen at 7:30 AM
- 1 hour specimen at 8:00 AM
- 2 hour specimen at 9:00 AM

The tubes should be labeled with the time as well as "30 minutes," "1st hour," etc. (**FIGURE 15–6**). Upon collection, each specimen should be sent to the laboratory for immediate testing. Venous blood is the preferred specimen for glucose tolerance tests because normal glucose values are determined on venous blood. If serum samples are collected, the serum separator tube should be used. Otherwise, the grey-topped tube may be used for this procedure.

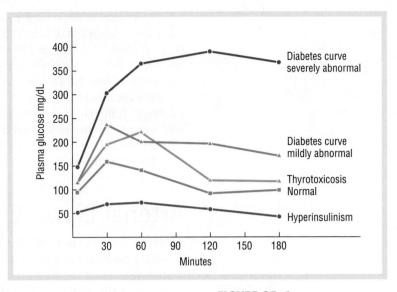

FIGURE 15–6
Graph of Glucose Tolerance Test Results

Postprandial Glucose Test

The two-hour **postprandial glucose test** (meaning after a meal) can be used to screen patients for diabetes (including gestational diabetes) because glucose levels in serum specimens collected two hours after a meal are rarely elevated in normal patients. In contrast, diabetic patients usually have increased values two hours after a meal.

The day of the test, the patient should eat a breakfast of orange juice, cereal with sugar, toast, and milk to provide an approximate equivalent of 75 to 100 g of glucose. A blood specimen is taken two hours after the patient finishes eating breakfast. The glucose level of this specimen is then determined, and the physician can decide whether further carbohydrate metabolism tests (such as a glucose tolerance test) are needed.

Modified Oral Glucose Tolerance Test

The modified oral glucose tolerance test is a variation of the postprandial glucose test in that after a fasting glucose specimen is collected, the patient is given 75 grams (for adults) of glucose and another blood specimen is collected at two hours after the patient has taken the dose of glucose. Again, water intake is encouraged throughout this procedure.

Lactose Tolerance Test

Some people have difficulty digesting lactose, a milk sugar. They appear to lack a lactase enzyme that breaks down the lactose into glucose and galactose. They usually experience gastrointestinal discomfort, followed by diarrhea, after drinking a milk product. These patients usually show no further symptoms if milk is removed from their diet. In order to diagnose this disorder, after overnight fasting, 50 grams of flavored liquid containing lactose can be given to the patient to drink. Tests are then performed to determine whether the patient's body has the ability to break down lactose and absorb it.

The preferred, noninvasive method is the measurement of breath hydrogen content. In this method, breath samples are collected as the patient exhales. The exhaled gases are analyzed for hydrogen, a by-product of bacteria that breaks down the lactose but is not absorbed. This test measures the ability of a person's intestines to digest lactose. It is used to diagnose a deficiency of intestinal lactase (the enzyme used to digest lactose).

A test that is becoming less preferable to the breath hydrogen content test is the **lactose tolerance test.** In this procedure, a solution containing 50 grams of lactose is given to the patient. The standard procedure includes the venipuncture collection of a baseline specimen and 5-, 10-, 30-, 60-, 90-, and 120-minute specimens for plasma glucose measurements. When the results are graphed, the curve should be similar to that obtained from the glucose tolerance test, if the patient has the mucosal lactase enzyme and digests the sugar properly. If the patient is intolerant to lactose, his or her blood glucose level will increase by no more than 20 mg/dl from the fasting sample level. The health care worker should be sure that a bathroom is located near the patient testing area because patients who are lactose intolerant may experience severe discomfort during the testing.

Arterial Blood Gases

Arterial blood gases (ABGs) provide useful information about the respiratory status and the acid-base balance of patients with pulmonary (lung) disease or disorders. The term *arterial blood gas analysis* refers to the measurement of the partial pressures of the physiologically active gases in blood (i.e., pO_2, pCO_2), the blood pH, and the oxygen saturation in hemoglobin. In addition, critically ill patients with other diseases, such as diabetes mellitus, benefit from ABG measurement, which is used to help manage their electrolyte and acid-base balance. Arterial blood rather than venous blood is used because arterial blood has the same composition throughout the body tissues, whereas venous blood has various compositions relative to metabolic activities in body tissues. Capillary blood gases are used for infants, and the procedure is covered in Chapter 13, "Pediatric and Geriatric Procedures."

Arterial puncture to obtain arterial blood for blood gas evaluation requires skill and knowledge of the technique. A health care provider must undergo extensive training on arterial punctures, including demonstration of the procedure, observation, and, under the supervision of a qualified instructor, several performances on patients.

RADIAL ARTERY PUNCTURE SITE

When an ABG analysis is ordered, the experienced health care worker should palpate the areas of the forearm where the artery is typically close to the surface. The **radial artery,** located on the thumb side of the wrist (as shown in **FIGURE 15–7**) is the artery most frequently used for blood collection for ABG analysis.[17]

Using your index and middle fingers, palpate the pulses from the radial artery about 1 inch above the wrist (Figure 15–7). This artery has widespread collateral flow, which means that the hand area is supplied with blood from more than one artery. Arterial blood flows into the hand from both the radial and the ulnar arteries. In addition, the radial artery lies over ligaments and bones of the wrist and can be easily compressed to lessen the chance of a hematoma during the procedure. A drawback to using the radial artery is its small size.

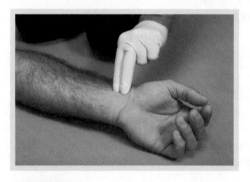

FIGURE 15–7
Locating the Radial Artery

BRACHIAL AND FEMORAL ARTERY PUNCTURE SITES

The **brachial artery** is an alternative site for blood collection for ABG analysis. The brachial artery is in the cubital fossa of the arm, as shown in **FIGURE 15–8**.

Another choice, the **femoral artery,** is the largest artery used in ABG collections. It is located in the groin area of the leg, lateral to the femur bone, as shown in Figure 15–8. Even though the brachial and femoral arteries are larger than the radial artery, they are used less frequently because they lack collateral circulation. A four-year study on blood collections from the brachial artery has demonstrated that

ALERT

Clinical Alert! The pulse of the brachial artery may be felt at the fold of the elbow on the little finger side of the arm. Puncture of a vein is a possibility due to the close proximity of the brachial artery. In particular, the brachial artery lies close to the median nerve, which can be accidentally punctured.

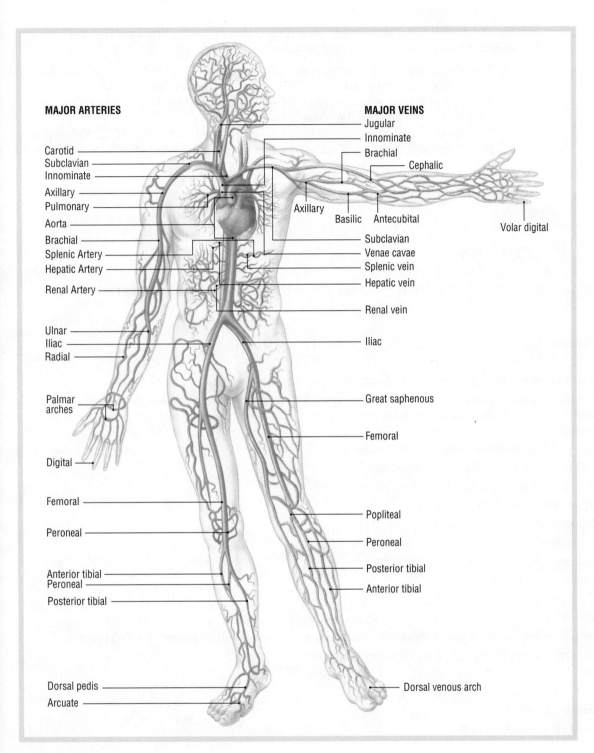

MAJOR ARTERIES

Carotid
Subclavian
Innominate
Axillary
Pulmonary
Aorta
Brachial
Splenic Artery
Hepatic Artery
Renal Artery
Ulnar
Iliac
Radial
Palmar arches
Digital
Femoral
Peroneal
Anterior tibial
Peroneal
Posterior tibial
Dorsal pedis
Arcuate

MAJOR VEINS

Jugular
Innominate
Brachial
Cephalic
Axillary
Basilic   Antecubital
Volar digital
Subclavian
Venae cavae
Splenic vein
Hepatic vein
Renal vein
Iliac
Great saphenous
Femoral
Popliteal
Peroneal
Posterior tibial
Anterior tibial
Dorsal venous arch

FIGURE 15–8
Arteries (in red) in the Arm and Leg

brachial artery puncture is an acceptably safe procedure and a reasonable alternative to radial artery puncture.[18] The femoral artery is sometimes used on patients with cardio-vascular disorders. The possibility of releasing plaque from the inner wall of the artery in geriatric patients, however, is a definite disadvantage of using the femoral artery as a puncture site. Usually, the femoral artery is the last choice for an arterial puncture site, and the health care provider must have expertise in obtaining blood from this artery.

To use the radial artery for blood collection for ABG analysis (**PROCEDURE 15–6**), the health care provider must first perform the modified Allen test to make certain that the ulnar and radial arteries are providing collateral circulation (see Figure 15–9). The **modified Allen test** is performed as follows:

1. The health care worker compresses both arteries with the index and middle fingers, and the patient is asked to tightly clench his or her fist.
2. The patient is then asked to open his or her hand, and the health care provider releases the pressure on the ulnar artery.
3. The blood vessels in the hand should fill with blood within 5 to 10 seconds—if so, the Allen test is positive. If color does not return to the hand after 5 to 10 seconds, the Allen test is negative.

PROCEDURE 15–6

Radial ABG Procedure

Rationale   To perform a blood collection for arterial blood gas analysis using the radial artery.

Equipment

- Chlorhexidine gluconate
- ½ to 1% lidocaine to numb site
- Prefilled heparinized safety syringe, 1 to 5 mL (especially designed *plastic syringe* for collections for ABG analysis)
  (Collection with a plastic syringe requires the sample to be transported at room temperature and analyzed within 30 minutes. If analysis will occur after a 30-minute delay from collection, collect the blood in a *glass syringe* and transport it in slurry of ice water.)
- Safety needles (20 to 22 gauge, for collections for ABG analysis)
- Safety needles (25 to 26 gauge, for lidocaine administration)
- Safety syringe for lidocaine administration (1- or 2-mL plastic syringe)
- Gauze squares to be held on site after puncture
- Plastic bag or cup with crushed ice and water
- Patient identification label
- Laboratory requisition
- Waterproof ink pen
- Alcohol pad
- Adhesive bandage strip
- Oxygen-measuring device to record on laboratory requisition the oxygen concentration on patient receiving oxygen
- Thermometer to record patient's temperature on laboratory requisition
- Mask
- Nonlatex gloves
- Protective laboratory coat or smock
- Biohazardous waste containers for sharps

Preparation

1 Gather and organize the necessary equipment and supplies for a successful arterial puncture.

2 Properly identify and inform the patient of the arterial puncture procedure.

3 Determine that the patient has been in a stable state for at least the previous 30 minutes (i.e., no respiratory changes). In addition, the patient's temperature needs to be taken.

4 Attempt to calm the patient before collecting the specimen if the patient appears anxious. The anxiety can lead to **hyperventilation** (i.e., rapid breathing), which will falsely alter the ABG levels.

5 Before proceeding, determine whether the patient is receiving anticoagulant therapy or is allergic to lidocaine. Record the patient's temperature, oxygen concentration from the respirator (if applicable), and respiratory rate.

PROCEDURE 15–6

Radial ABG Procedure (continued)

Procedure

6 Wash your hands; put on gloves, a facial mask, and a protective laboratory coat; and then palpate the radial artery in the forearm. The radial artery in the patient's nondominant hand is usually the best choice.

7 With the forefinger or first two fingers, press at these sites to find the artery (Figure 15–7). Never use the thumb for palpating because there is a pulse in the thumb that may be confused with the patient's pulse. Avoid any site that has a hematoma or was previously used for an arterial puncture.

8 Position the patient's arm with the wrist slightly extended and rotated. Check for adequate collateral circulation using the modified Allen test.

A CLOSER LOOK

Modified Allen Test

Rationale

To use the radial artery for blood collection for ABG analysis, the health care worker must first perform the modified Allen test to make certain that the ulnar and radial arteries are providing collateral circulation (**FIGURE 15–9**).[19]

Procedure

A Compress the radial and ulnar arteries of the same hand with your index and middle fingers, and ask the patient to tightly clench his or her fist.

B Ask the patient to open his or her hand and release the pressure on the ulnar artery.

C The blood vessels in the hand should fill with blood within 5 to 10 seconds; if so, the Allen test is positive for the presence of good collateral circulation. If color does not return to the hand after 5 to 10 seconds, the Allen test is negative. A negative Allen test indicates the inability of the ulnar artery to supply blood to the hand adequately and shows a lack of collateral circulation. Thus, the radial artery should *not be used* after a negative Allen test, because this artery might be accidentally damaged during puncture, resulting in a total lack of blood flow to the hand. Select an alternate artery if a negative Allen test occurs.

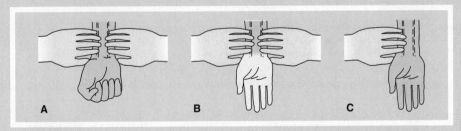

FIGURE 15–9
Modified Allen Test

(continued)

PROCEDURE 15–6

Radial ABG Procedure (continued)

9 After the radial artery site is chosen, clean the area well with the chlorhexidine swab. Do not touch, fan, or blow on the site after it is cleansed.

10 If the patient desires a local anesthetic, fill a 1-mL syringe with lidocaine and inject the lidocaine with the 25- to 26-gauge needle subcutaneously around the anticipated puncture site.

11 No tourniquet is required, because the artery has its own strong blood pressure. Use a prefilled heparinized safety syringe (1 to 5 mL) with a needle to withdraw the sample.

12 Hold the syringe or collection device in one hand as one would hold a dart, pull the skin taut with a finger of the other hand over the artery, and pierce the pulsating artery at a high angle, usually 30 to 45 degrees against the bloodstream (**FIGURE 15–10**). Little or no suction is needed since the blood pulsates and flows quickly into the syringe under its own pressure.

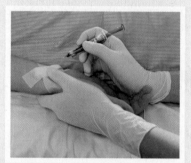

FIGURE 15–10
Completing Arterial Blood Gas Collection

Courtesy of Radiometer America, Inc.

13 When approximately 1 mL of blood is collected, withdraw the needle carefully to avoid introducing bubbles into the syringe. Apply gauze and direct manual pressure on the site for at least 5 minutes.

14 Engage the safety syringe cover to cover the needle exposure, gently mix the blood in the syringe with the heparin, and label the syringe. Mix the blood gently by inverting the syringe at least five times.

15 Before leaving the patient, leave a pressure bandage on the site.

16 If bleeding from the site persists, apply more manual pressure and ring for assistance from the patient's primary nurse. Never leave a patient who is bleeding, particularly after an arterial puncture.

After the Procedure

17 Notify the primary nurse after an arterial puncture is performed so that the area may be checked frequently for deep or superficial bleeding.

18 Discard blood-soaked gauze pads, contaminated items, and gowns or gloves used in isolation rooms in appropriate biohazardous waste containers, as discussed in Chapter 4, "Infection Control."

19 Dispose of gowns and gloves that are not from isolation rooms in the appropriate containers.

20 Wash or sanitize your hands.

21 Thank the patient for cooperating and depart with all specimens and all remaining supplies. Do not leave anything at the patient's bedside.

22 Deliver the blood specimen with the laboratory test request immediately to the laboratory. The delivery should not occur by pneumatic tube due to false alteration of the pO_2 result. Hand delivery within 15 minutes is best for optimal laboratory results.

A negative Allen test indicates the inability of the ulnar artery to supply blood to the hand adequately and shows a lack of collateral circulation. Thus, the radial artery should not be used in a negative Allen test, since this artery might be accidentally damaged during puncture, resulting in total lack of blood flow to the hand.

Arterial blood results for some analytes (e.g., ammonia, glucose, lactic acid, alcohol) may differ from venous blood results because of metabolic activities. Therefore, arterial blood samples should be collected for the blood gas measurements only when specifically requested by the attending physician. In such situations, the requisition must indicate that arterial blood was collected for the analytes.

Therapeutic Drug Monitoring (TDM)

Therapeutic drug monitoring (TDM) is used to monitor the concentration of certain drugs in a patient's bloodstream (BOX 15–2). It is an important laboratory assessment tool in the following circumstances:

- If the drug is highly toxic
- When underdosing or overdosing can have serious consequences
- If the use of multiple drugs may alter the action of the drug being measured
- If individual patients metabolize drugs at different rates
- If the effectiveness of the drug is questionable
- If compliance with medication regimen is a concern

BOX 15–2

Information Required for Therapeutic Drug Monitoring

Laboratory personnel must acquire and document additional information when performing TDM. A health care worker may be asked to obtain the following information:

- Patient's name
- Patient's identification number
- Patient's location
- Test ordered
- Requesting physician
- Collection time and date
- Mode of collection (e.g., venipuncture, central venous catheter collection)
- Whether the order is for a peak level, trough level, or continuous-infusion random level determination
- Time and date of last dose
- Time and date of next dose
- A unit nurse's verification that the dose was administered

Specific specimen guidelines for each drug should be established by pharmacy and laboratory staff and adhered to strictly.

ALERT

Clinical Alert! The time of collection is much more critical for drugs with shorter half-lives (e.g., gentamicin, tobramycin, and procainamide) than for those with longer half-lives (e.g., phenobarbital and digoxin). It is important to note that there are clinical situations that may result in an increased half-life (e.g. heart failure and cirrhosis of the liver). In addition, certain drug levels (e.g., aminoglycosides) in the blood can be falsely altered if collected through a central venous catheter. Also, blood specimens should not be taken from the arm into which drugs or other fluids are being infused.

Often, therapeutic drug monitoring is used for patients taking anticonvulsant drugs, tricyclic antidepressants, digoxin, theophylline, lithium, chemotherapeutic agents such as methotrexate, or antibiotics such as gentamicin.

Laboratory drug monitoring of therapeutic agents is a complex endeavor that requires much coordination among laboratory, nursing, and pharmacy personnel. A basic understanding of the variables, information needed, and definitions of terms is important to obtain accurate laboratory results. For most drugs, plasma, serum, or whole blood is used to determine circulating levels of the drug.[20]

To adequately evaluate the appropriate dosage levels of many drugs, the collection and evaluation of specimens for trough and peak levels are necessary. The *trough level* is the lowest concentration in the patient's blood; that is, the specimen should be collected immediately prior (i.e., not more than 15 minutes) to administration of the drug to ensure that the medication level stays within the therapeutic (effective dosage) range. The *peak level* is the highest concentration of a drug in the patient's blood (**FIGURE 15–11**). The time required to reach the highest concentration varies with the mode of administration (intramuscular injection versus IV infusion) and the rate at which the drug is infused. Generally, the level in the bloodstream drops from peak concentration to zero within five half-lives of the drug if no other dosages are given. Random levels may be appropriate for monitoring the drug dosage if the drug is administered by continuous infusion and if enough time has elapsed for the drug to reach equilibrium.

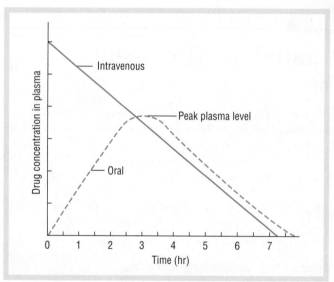

FIGURE 15–11

Drug Concentration over Time in Blood Plasma Following a Single Dose

Several drugs cannot be analyzed from blood collected in serum separator tubes. Blood specimens for therapeutic drug monitoring should be maintained in an upright position during transportation. In addition, because falsely elevated or decreased values have occurred with the use of gel serum separator tubes, this type of evacuated blood collection tube should be evaluated in your own health care facility and determined not to cause interferences. Most TDM assays should be performed on serum/plasma. The Clinical and Laboratory Standards Institute (CLSI) has devised toxicology and drug-monitoring requirements for blood collection containers; these requirements can be helpful to the pharmacy and laboratory personnel who are responsible for establishing specific specimen guidelines for each drug.

Collection for Trace Metals (Elements)

Testing for **trace metals** (elements) involves the use of specially prepared trace-metal-free evacuated blood collection tubes.[21] Tubes and microcollection containers are available with low lead content to use in the blood collection for lead levels. The lead tube tops are tan in color. The royal-blue–topped evacuated tubes are available for blood collection to test for trace elements including antimony, arsenic, cadmium, lead, calcium, chromium, copper, iron, magnesium, manganese, mercury, selenium, and zinc. Specific specimen collection guidelines should be established as part of the clinical laboratory's technical procedures for trace metal testing.

Genetic Molecular Tests

The proper collection of a blood specimen for genetic molecular tests is critical to obtaining accurate results. Special informed consent forms must be signed by the patient prior to performing molecular testing. Lavender-topped tubes or specially designed collection tubes are used for collection of the specimen, depending on laboratory protocol. To screen newborns and infants, please see Chapter 13, "Pediatric and Geriatric Procedures." For cytogenetic testing, peripheral blood samples are usually requested to be collected in a green-topped evacuated tube containing sodium heparin. In addition to the blood specimen, the patient's correct demographics (i.e., vital statistics such as age, place of birth, parents' ethnicity/race) must be obtained, which are more essential for genetic laboratory tests than for other types of assays. The genetic material (e.g., RNA) is viable for approximately 6 to 24 hours, and thus the specimens must be sent to the laboratory immediately. This type of testing is becoming increasingly popular and expansive in genetic assays. Thus, the health care worker needs to stay up-to-date on the necessary blood collection protocols for genetic molecular tests.

Intravenous Line Collections

Intravenous (IV) lines are used to administer medications, blood products, or other fluids because the substances enter directly into the patient's bloodstream and the outcomes are more rapid than that of oral medications (which must be digested first) or because the medications may be too irritating to the tissues for an intramuscular injection. Most health care agencies have policies about who can access the IV lines and who can administer medications.

Drawing blood specimens through **intravenous (IV) catheter** or central venous catheter (CVC) lines requires special techniques, training, and experience. A CVC, also called a **central intravenous line,** is one of numerous **vascular access devices (VADs).** The CVC is usually inserted into the (1) subclavian vein, which is in the chest area below the clavicle; (2) jugular vein; or (3) superior vena cava (see Figure 15–8, p. 469). A dressing covers the tubing that extends above the skin.

Another type of vascular access device is a **peripherally inserted central catheter (PICC),** which is inserted into the cephalic vein or basilic vein of the arm or hand veins (**FIGURE 15–12**). The PICC is usually only used for blood collection when it is first inserted, because it can become easily infected around the area. Its main purpose is to deliver long-term medication, intravenous antibiotics, chemotherapy, and blood product replacement. One general guideline to follow when taking blood specimen collections is that it is usually *not* advisable to collect a blood specimen from the arm in which an IV is connected. This is because the IV fluids may dilute the specimen. Unfortunately, this procedure is sometimes unavoidable, but the health care worker should always follow the health facility's protocols. Refer to Chapter 9 for details regarding blood collection from an arm with an IV.

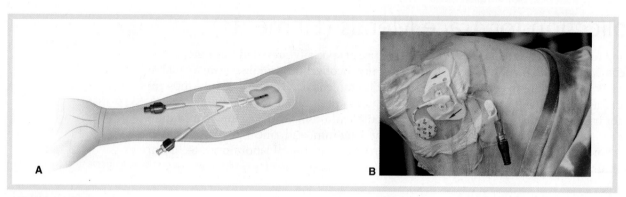

FIGURE 15–12

Inserting the Peripherally Inserted Central Catheter (PICC)

B. Rob Byron/shutterstock

Clinical Alert!

- The IV line is a direct pathway into the patient's bloodstream. Each time the IV system is accessed, the possibility of contamination and infection exists.

- Some facilities do not allow evacuated blood tubes to be used for blood collection through a central venous catheter due to the potential for increased pressure buildup in the catheter.

- Heparin can bind within the catheter and lead to inaccurate coagulation test results when collecting through a CVC.

Collecting Blood Through a Central Venous Catheter

Usually, managers of health care facilities require nursing or laboratory personnel to take specialized training courses prior to allowing them to collect blood from a central venous line (**PROCEDURE 15–7**).[22]

PROCEDURE 15–7

Collecting Blood through a CVC

Rationale   To collect blood for laboratory tests through a central venous catheter.

Equipment

- Personal protective equipment, gloves (recommended sterile gloves for aseptic technique), mask, clean uniform, and laboratory coat
- Laboratory requisition forms and pen
- Evacuated tubes and labels for the specimen
- Transfer device for syringe to evacuated tube blood transfer
- Two 10-mL disposable Luer-Lok syringes filled with sterile normal saline
- One 3-mL disposable Luer-Lok syringe with 3-mL injectable heparinized saline (used for flushing the catheter)
- Two 10-mL disposable syringes with needleless cannula
- Antimicrobial swabs
- Linen protector to provide a clean work area
- A biohazard container for wastes
- Alcohol wipes

Preparation

1 Check the patient's chart for physician's order to collect blood through the CVC.

2 Obtain laboratory requisitions and labels that reflect patient location and tests for which blood is needed.

3 Identify the patient, as described in Chapter 10.

PROCEDURE 15–7

Collecting Blood through a CVC (continued)

4 Explain the test to the patient.

5 Wash or sanitize your hands with an alcohol hand rinse, put on gloves (nonlatex), and prepare and assemble equipment and supplies next to the patient.

Procedure

The procedure may involve the following steps but is subject to differences among hospitals and must be performed by authorized personnel only and under institutional guidelines.[23]

6 Aseptically draw 10 mL of injectable normal saline into a syringe.

7 Provide adequate room and light for the procedure.

8 Position the patient by elevating the bed to a comfortable working level and making the bed flat. Have the catheter hub at or below the level of the patient's heart.

9 If you are authorized to do so, shut off IV fluids infusing through the line and unclamp the most proximal lumen of the multilumen catheter to avoid contamination from IV fluids. Prior to blood collection, stop infusion of IV fluids for at least 2 minutes (depending on the individual facility's protocols) (**FIGURE 15–13**). Swab the cap and hub with antimicrobial swabs for 30 seconds and allow to dry.

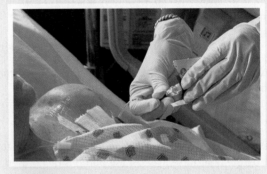

FIGURE 15–13

10 Insert 10 mL saline-filled needleless syringe into the cap; unclamp the catheter (**FIGURE 15–14**).

11 Flush catheter with 5 to 10 mL saline to determine patency (lack of obstruction) of catheter.

12 Clamp catheter, remove syringe, and aseptically insert new needleless 10-mL empty syringe and unclamp catheter.

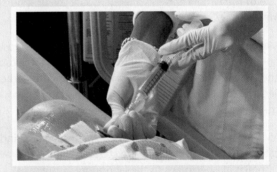

FIGURE 15–14

13 Aspirate (slowly and steadily) 5 mL of blood from catheter for discard. Aspirate 8 to 10 mL of blood if coagulation studies have been ordered (**FIGURE 15–15**). (Confirm these discard amounts with the facility's protocols.) Close clamp, remove syringe with blood, and place in tray in order to discard later in biohazard container.

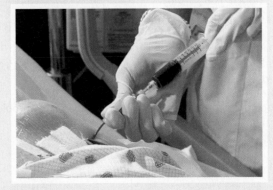

FIGURE 15–15

(continued)

PROCEDURE 15–7

Collecting Blood through a CVC (continued)

14 Swab the cap again with a new antimicrobial swab and insert a 10-mL syringe into the cap and aspirate the required amount of blood. Transfer the blood from the syringe to the appropriate evacuated tubes using the safety transfer device and proper order of draw (see Chapter 10). Dispose of the syringe and transfer device into a biohazardous waste container.

15 Swab the cap to aseptically clean it.

16 Complete an irrigation of the catheter with a second needleless syringe containing 10 mL saline (**FIGURE 15–16**); clamp the catheter and remove the syringe or maintain positive pressure on the syringe plunger with your thumb while withdrawing the syringe from the injection cap to avoid the possibility of occlusion.

17 Some institutions require flushing also with a heparin solution. If so, swab the cap aseptically again and then insert 3-mL syringe filled with 3 mL dilute heparin solution.

18 Unclamp the catheter and gently infuse heparin solution.

19 Change cap. *Note:* Cap should be changed after *each* blood collection.

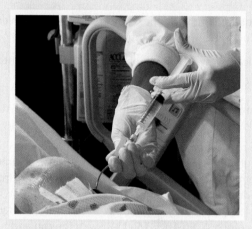

FIGURE 15–16

After the Procedure

20 Determine that IV fluids are infusing properly at the rate set by the unit nurse. *Note:* If the pump is being used, make certain the pump is *on* and the alarm is *on*. If the rate of the IV flow appears altered, notify the unit nurse immediately.

21 Make sure the patient is in a safe and comfortable position, with the bed down, side-rails up, and bedside table and call light accessible to the patient. As mentioned earlier, discard all used equipment and supplies in appropriate containers (**FIGURE 15–17**).

22 Always immediately label the blood specimens and indicate that these specimens were collected by a line draw. Dispatch all specimens to the laboratory in the usual manner.

23 Wash or sanitize your hands.

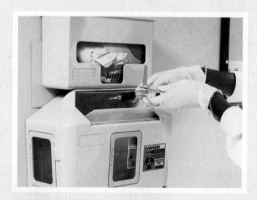

FIGURE 15–17

24 Thank the patient for cooperating and depart with all remaining supplies. Do not leave anything at the patient's bedside.

25 Document completion of the procedure and any problems in the patient's medical record.

Cannulas and Fistulas

A variety of cannulae (a flexible tube in various sizes and shapes) are used in medicine. In patients with kidney disease, one type of **cannula** is a tubular instrument that is used to gain access to venous blood for dialysis or blood collection. Blood should be drawn from the cannula of these patients only by specially trained personnel because the procedure requires special techniques and experience. An arterial cannula is inserted into an artery, usually the radial artery, and is used in major surgeries and critical care units to collect repeated blood samples.

A **fistula** is an artificial shunt in which the vein and artery have been fused through surgery. It is a permanent connection tube located in the arm of a patient undergoing kidney dialysis. Only specialized personnel can collect blood from a fistula. The health care worker should use extreme caution when collecting a blood specimen from these patients and avoid using the arm with the fistula as the site for venipuncture. Also, a tourniquet or blood pressure cuff should not be applied to an arm with a fistula.

Donor Room Collections

Properly trained health care providers may be employed in a regional blood center or a hospital blood donor center to screen and collect blood from donors. This section summarizes the procedure outlined by the AABB, an international organization involved in transfusion therapies.[24] Only an experienced, properly trained health care worker or technologist should be considered for this function because a physical, emotional, or traumatic experience may keep a donor from volunteering in the future.

DONOR INTERVIEW AND SELECTION

Not everyone who wants to donate blood is eligible. The interviewer must determine the eligibility of each potential donor. Careful determination of donor eligibility helps prevent the spread of disease to blood product recipients as well as untoward effects on the potential donor.

The following information on every donor should be kept indefinitely and is initially obtained from every prospective donor, regardless of the acceptability of his or her donation:[25]

1. Date and time of donation
2. Last name, first name, and middle initial
3. Address
4. Telephone number
5. Gender
6. Age and birth date (donors should be at least age 17; however, minors may be accepted if written consent is obtained in accordance with applicable state law; elderly prospective donors may be accepted at the discretion of the blood bank physician)
7. Written consent form signed by the donor (1) allowing the donor to defer from being a donor if he or she has risk factors for HIV, the causative agent of acquired immunodeficiency syndrome (AIDS) or (2) authorizing the blood bank to take and use his or her blood
8. A record of reasons for deferrals, if any
9. Social security number or driver's license number (may be used for additional identification but is not mandatory)
10. Name of patient or group to be credited, if a credit system is used
11. Race (not mandatory, but this information can be useful in screening patients for a specific phenotype [chromosomal makeup])

12. Unique characteristics about a donor's blood (donated blood that is negative for cytomegalovirus or that is Rh-negative group-O blood is used for neonatal patients)

To help minimize the incidence of dizziness, fainting, or other reactions to blood loss, donors are encouraged to eat within 4 to 6 hours of donating blood. Eating a light snack just before the phlebotomy may help prevent these reactions; however, a donor should not be required to eat if he or she does not want to do so.

Blood bank records must link each component of a donor unit (red blood cells, white blood cells, platelets, etc.) to its disposition. If the donation is a "replacement for credit" for a particular patient, the donor must supply the patient's name or the group name that is to be credited.

A brief physical examination is required to determine whether the donor is in generally good condition on the day that he or she is to donate blood. The physical examination entails a few simple procedures easily mastered by the health care worker:

1. **Weight**—The volume of blood donated must be no more than 10.5 mL of whole blood per kilogram of body weight. Also, the anticoagulant in the bag must be modified for a lesser donation.
2. **Temperature**—The donor's oral temperature must not exceed 37.5°C (99.5°F).
3. **Pulse**—The donor's pulse should be regular and strong, between 50 and 100 beats per minute. The pulse should be taken for at least 15 seconds.
4. **Blood pressure**—The systolic blood pressure should measure no higher than 180 mm Hg, and the diastolic blood pressure should be no higher than 100 mm Hg. People with blood pressure outside these limits should be deferred as donors and referred to their physicians for evaluation of a possible health problem (Appendix 4).
5. **Skin lesions**—Both arms should be examined for signs of drug abuse, such as needle marks or sclerotic veins. The presence of mild skin disorders, such as a poison ivy rash, does not necessarily prohibit an individual from donating unless the lesions are in the antecubital area or the rash is particularly extensive. The skin at the site of the venipuncture must be free of lesions.
6. **General appearance**—If the donor looks ill, excessively nervous, or under the influence of alcohol or drugs, he or she should be deferred.
7. **Hematocrit or hemoglobin values**—The hematocrit value must be no less than 38% for donors. The hemoglobin value must be no less than 12.5 g/dl. A fingerstick is commonly used to collect blood for such determinations. The health care worker may use one of the following procedures: Collect blood in a plastic hematocrit tube for centrifuging and reading; measure hemoglobin spectrophotometrically; or use the copper sulfate method, in which the hemoglobin is qualitatively determined. (For further details on the copper sulfate method, please refer to the AABB technical manual.)[24,25]
8. **Extensive medical history**—This history must be taken on all potential donors, regardless of the number of previous donations on record. Most blood bank donor rooms have a simple card listing all the questions to be asked and "yes" or "no" columns that are used to indicate the donor's responses. The health care provider should refer to the protocol of the donor room at the institution's blood bank or the AABB technical manual, which sets guidelines for donor screening and acceptance.

Collection of Donor's Blood

The health care worker in a donor room must operate under the supervision of a qualified, licensed physician. Blood should be collected by using the aseptic technique; a sterile, closed system; and a single venipuncture. If a second venipuncture is needed, an entirely new, sterile donor set is necessary; the first is discarded according to the contaminated material disposal protocol of the institution.

A donor should never be left alone either during or immediately after blood collection. The health care worker should be well versed in donor reactions, equipment safety precautions, first-aid techniques, and location of first-aid equipment in case it is needed in the course of donation. See Appendix 8 for standard operating procedures (SOPS) for donor phlebotomy from the Gulf Coast Regional Blood Center. In Appendix 8, the SOPs pertain to basic donor phlebotomy:

- Selecting the Venipuncture Site
- Routine Arm Scrub
- Whole Blood Venipuncture
- Ending the Blood Draw

"The Gulf Coast Regional Blood Center SOPs are an example of standard operating procedures for donor phlebotomy. These steps are subject to differences among blood collectors and must be performed by authorized personnel only and under institutional guidelines" (Gulf Coast Regional Blood Center, Houston, Texas).

All donated blood is classified and labeled by type, either A, B, AB, or O, and as Rh-positive or Rh-negative. Each unit of donor's blood must be matched to the recipient's blood using blood type and antibody classifications. A special instrument can be used to separate the blood into components (red blood cells, platelets, plasma, etc.) and then to pump the remaining components back into the donor. This procedure is called *apheresis*. It takes several weeks for a donor's body to rebuild and replace his or her donated blood cells and platelets.

Autologous Transfusion

A practice that is frequently used is **autologous transfusion**: The patient donates his or her own blood before anticipated surgery. The reason for this type of transfusion is that the safest blood a recipient can receive is his or her own blood.[25] The autologous transfusion prevents transfusion-transmitted infectious diseases (e.g., HIV, hepatitis) and eliminates the formation of antibodies in the transfused patient.

Therapeutic Phlebotomy

Therapeutic phlebotomy is the intentional removal of blood for therapeutic reasons (**FIGURE 15–18**). It is used in the treatment of some myeloproliferative diseases, such as polycythemia and hereditary hemochromatoisis, or other conditions in which there is an excessive production of blood cells. Records in the blood bank should indicate the

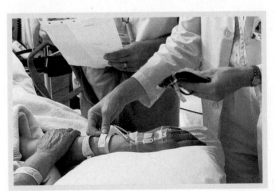

FIGURE 15–18

Therapeutic Phlebotomy Collection

As in other donor collections, health care workers must be experienced and properly trained to collect blood from these patients.

patient's diagnosis, the physician's request for the phlebotomy, and the amount of blood to be taken. The medical director of the blood bank must decide whether the patient is to be bled in the donor room or in a private section of the blood bank. Some health care facilities use locations other than the blood bank for therapeutic phlebotomy because some patients are visibly ill and weak, and their presence may have an adverse psychological effect on the healthy donors in the donor room. When a patient is obviously ill, his or her physician or the medical director of the blood bank should be present during the phlebotomy. Generally, the patient should be bled more slowly than a healthy donor, and the resting period should be extended.

The blood obtained through therapeutic bleeding may be used for homologous transfusion (i.e., blood is transfused from another person) if the unit is deemed suitable by the director of the blood bank. Usually, the blood from patients with hereditary hemochromatosis may be used for homologous transfusion. If it is to be used, the recipient's physician must agree to use the blood from his or her patient, and a record of the agreement should be kept. The unit is then labeled and processed in the usual manner. The label must indicate that the blood is the result of a therapeutic bleed and must include the patient's diagnosis. If the unit is unsuitable for transfusion, the entire unit is disposed of in the usual manner for contaminated wastes.

Study Questions

For the following questions, select the one best answer.

1 Which of the following is the preferred site for blood collection for ABG analysis?

a. brachial artery
b. femoral artery
c. radial artery
d. ulnar artery

2 The reason for performing the modified Allen test is to

a. obtain the oxygen concentration of the patient
b. determine whether the patient's blood pressure is elevated
c. determine that the ulnar and radial arteries provide collateral circulation
d. test for the possibility of a hematoma

3 What is a cannula?

a. the fusion of a vein and an artery
b. a good source of arterial blood
c. an artificial shunt that provides access to arterial blood
d. a tubular instrument used to gain access to venous blood

4 Which of the following is a milk sugar that sometimes cannot be digested by healthy individuals?

a. glucose
b. glucola
c. lactate
d. lactose

5 Which of the following supplies is not needed during an arterial puncture for an ABG determination?

a. heparin
b. tourniquet
c. lidocaine
d. syringe

6 Which of the following evacuated tubes is preferred for the collection of a blood culture specimen?

a. green-topped evacuated tube
b. yellow-topped evacuated tube
c. light-blue–topped evacuated tube
d. pink-topped evacuated tube

7 During a glucose tolerance test, which procedure is acceptable?

a. the patient should be encouraged to drink water throughout the procedure
b. a standard amount of glucose drink is given to the patient, then a fasting blood collection is performed
c. the patient is allowed to chew sugarless gum
d. all the patient's specimens are timed from the fasting collection

8 Blood collection for cadmium and manganese should occur in which of the following evacuated blood collection tubes?

a. tan-topped tube
b. serum separator tube
c. royal-blue–topped tube
d. green-topped tube

9 Autologous transfusion is to prevent which of the following possibilities?

a. antibodies forming in the transfused patient
b. diabetes mellitus developing in the transfused patient
c. antigens forming in the transfused patient
d. polycythemia developing in the transfused patient

10 When blood is drawn from the radial artery for an ABG determination, the needle should be inserted at an angle of no less than

a. 20 degrees
b. 65 degrees
c. 45 degrees
d. 30 degrees

Case Study

Mr. Sanchez has been sent to the laboratory by his physician to have a three-hour glucose tolerance test performed. When he arrives at 10:30 AM, the health care worker, Jessica Sharpe, asks him if he has fasted overnight and been on the prescribed carbohydrate diet for the preceding days. Mr. Sanchez states that he has followed the one-day diet plan and has not eaten or had anything to drink since 9:00 last night. He had only one cigarette this morning around 8:15 and a cup of black coffee, no sugar.

Questions

1 Did Mr. Sanchez follow the proper protocol for the diet plan preceding the glucose tolerance test? What is the protocol that should be followed for the diet plan preceding the glucose tolerance test?

2 The glucose tolerance test requires fasting overnight. Did Mr. Sanchez follow the fasting procedure properly? Please explain.

Action in Practice

An obese male and frequent participant in hometown blood drives boarded the mobile blood donation center, also called the bloodmobile. After passing the screening requirements, he was greeted by the health care worker assigned to collect his blood. The worker, Ms. Chen, was in her first week of training. She was able to palpate the vein but noticed there was some scar tissue. When she performed the needlestick on the donor, Ms. Chen had to manipulate it slightly and go deeper to withdraw blood. As the blood entered the tubing, she noticed it was bright red and appeared to "pulse" into the tubing; she was relieved to have blood flowing into the donor tubing and bag. As the trainer observed, he immediately noticed the circumstance and halted the procedure.

Questions

1 Why did the trainer halt the procedure?

2 What might have happened to the donor who was trying to donate the blood if the procedure had not been stopped?

3 What actions need to be taken with the health care worker?

COMPETENCY ASSESSMENT

Check Yourself

1 List three possible interfering factors in the collection of blood for blood cultures.

2 Explain the differences between homologous transfusion and autologous transfusion.

Competency Checklist: Special Collection

This checklist can be completed as a group or individually.

(1) Completed (2) Needs to improve

_____ 1. Explain the difference between the "peak" and "trough" in therapeutic drug monitoring.

_____ 2. List at least five trace elements and the evacuated collection tube that should be used to collect for trace element testing.

REFERENCES

1. Ruge, D., Sandin, R., Siegelski, S., Greene, J., & Johnson, N. (2002). Reduction in blood culture contamination rates by establishment of policy for central intravenous catheters. *Lab Med, 33*(10): 797–800.

2. Angus, D. C., Linde-Zwirble, W. T., Lidicker, J., Clermont, G., Carcillo, J., & Pinsky, M. R. (2001, July). Epidemiology of severe sepsis in the United States: Analysis of incidence, outcome and associated costs of care. *Critical Care Medicine, 29*(7): 1303–1310.

3. Coburn, B., Morris, A. M., Tomlinson, G., & Detsky, A. S. (2012). Does this adult patient with suspected bacteremia require blood cultures? *JAMA, 308:* 502.

4. Weinstein, M. P. (2003). Blood culture contamination: Persisting problems and partial progress. *J Clin Microbiol,41:* 2275–2278.

5. Schifman, R., & Pindur, A. (1993). The effect of skin disinfection material on reducing blood culture contamination. *Am J Clin Pathol, 99:* 536–538.

6. Little, J. R., Murray, P.R., Traynor , P. S., & Spitznagel, E. (1999). A randomized trial of povidone-iodine compared with iodine tincture for venipuncture site disinfection: Effects on rates of blood culture contamination. *Am J Med, 107:* 119.

7. Strand, C. L., Wajsbort, R. R., & Sturmann, K. (1993). Effect of iodophor vs. iodine tincture skin preparation on blood culture contamination rate. *JAMA, 269:* 1004.

8. Mimoz, O., Karim, A., Mercat, A., et al. (1999). Chlorhexidine compared with povidone-iodine as skin preparation before blood culture. A randomized, controlled trial. *Ann Intern Med, 131:* 834.

9. Forbes, B., Sahm, D., & Weissfeld, A. (2002). *Bailey and Scott's diagnostic microbiology,* 11th ed. St. Louis, MO: Mosby.

10. O'Hara, C., Weinstein, M., & Miller, J. (2003). Manual and automated systems for detection and identification of microorganisms. In Murray, P., Baron, E., Jorgensen, J., Pfaller, M., & Yolken, R. (Eds.). (2003). *Manual of clinical microbiology,* 8th ed. Washington, DC: ASM Press, pp. 185–207.

11. Clinical and Laboratory Standards Institute (CLSI). (2007). *Principles and procedures for blood cultures, approved guideline,* M47-A. Wayne, PA: Author.

12. Andries, W. D. (2012). Blood culture systems: From patient to result. Sepsis—An ongoing and significant challenge. InTech, DOI: 10.5772/50139. Available from *www.intechopen.com/books/sepsis-an-ongoing-and-significant-challenge/blood-culture-systems-from-patient-to-result.* Doi: 10.5772/50139

13. International Association of Diabetes and Pregnancy Study Groups recommendations on the diagnosis and classification of hyperglycemia in pregnancy. (2010). *Diabetes Care, 33*(3): 676–682. PMID: 20190296

14. American Diabetes Association: Executive Summary: Standards of medical care in diabetes. (2012, January). *Diabetes Care,35*(Suppl.1) http://care.diabetesjournals.org.

15. Report of the Expert Committee on the Diagnosis and Classification of Diabetes Mellitus. (2000). *Diabetes Care, 23* (suppl. 1). http://journal.diabetes.org.

16. Follow-Up Report of the Expert Committee on the Diagnosis of Diabetes Mellitus. (2003). *Diabetes Care, 26*(11): 3160–3167.

17. Theodor, A. (n.d.). Arterial blood gases: *UpToDate. www.uptodate.com,* accessed February 26, 2013.

18. Okeson, G. C., & Wulbrecht, P. H. (1998). The safety of brachial artery puncture for arterial blood sampling. *Chest,114:* 748–751.

19. Clinical and Laboratory Standards Institute (CLSI). (2004). *Procedures for the collection of arterial blood specimens, approved standard,* 4th ed. Wayne, PA: Author.

20. Kaplan, L. A., Pesce, A. J., & Kazmierczak, S. C. (Eds.). (2003). Therapeutic drug monitoring. In *Clinical chemistry: Theory, analysis correlation,* 4th ed. St. Louis: Mosby, pp. 1073–1084.

21. Clinical and Laboratory Standards Institute (CLSI). (2001). *Analytical procedures for the determination of lead in blood and urine, approved standard,* C40-A. Wayne, PA: Author.

22. Farjo, L. (2003). Blood collection from peripherally inserted central venous catheters: An institution's effort to evaluate and update its current policy. *J Infusion Nursing, 26*(6): 374–379.

23. Clinical and Laboratory Standards Institute (CLSI). (2007). *Procedures for the collection of diagnostic blood specimens by venipuncture, approved standard,* H3-A6. Wayne, PA: Author.

24. Roback, J., Combs, M., & Grossman, B. (Eds.). (2011). *AABB technical manual,* 17th ed. Bethesda, MD: AABB Publishers.

25. Kleinman, S. (2013). Procedures used for blood donor screening: Protection of potential blood donors and recipients. *UpToDate.* www.uptodate.com.

RESOURCES

Edelman, S., & Henry, R. (2007, January). *Diagnosis and management of Type 2 diabetes.* Professional Communications, Inc., West Islip, NY.

Harmening, D. (2005). *Modern blood banking and transfusion practice.* Philadelphia, PA: F. A. Davis.

McPherson, R., & Pincus, M. (Eds.). (2006). *Henry's clinical diagnosis and management by laboratory methods.* St. Louis, MO: Elsevier Health Sciences.

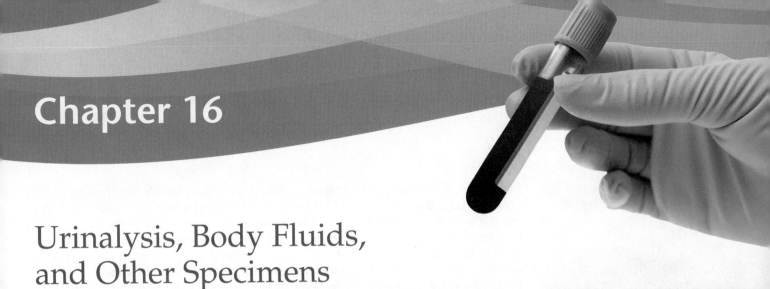

Chapter 16

Urinalysis, Body Fluids, and Other Specimens

Chapter Objectives

Upon completion of Chapter 16, the learner is responsible for doing the following:

1. Identify body fluid specimens, other than blood, that are analyzed in the clinical laboratory, and identify the correct procedures for collecting and/or transporting these specimens to the laboratory.

2. Describe the correct methodology for labeling urine specimens.

3. Identify specimens collected for microbiological, throat, sputum, and nasopharyngeal cultures and the protocol that must be followed when transporting these specimens.

4. List the types of patient specimens that are needed for gastric and sweat chloride analyses.

5. List three types of urine specimen collections and differentiate the uses of the urine specimens obtained from these collections.

6. Instruct a patient on the correct procedure for collecting a timed urine specimen and a midstream clean-catch specimen.

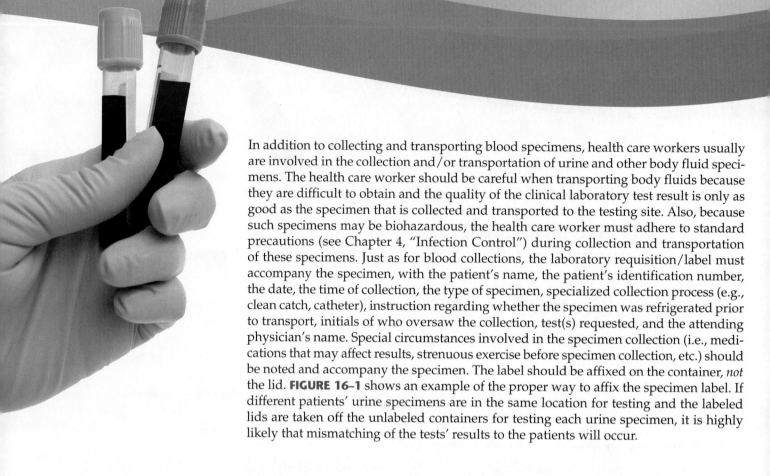

In addition to collecting and transporting blood specimens, health care workers usually are involved in the collection and/or transportation of urine and other body fluid specimens. The health care worker should be careful when transporting body fluids because they are difficult to obtain and the quality of the clinical laboratory test result is only as good as the specimen that is collected and transported to the testing site. Also, because such specimens may be biohazardous, the health care worker must adhere to standard precautions (see Chapter 4, "Infection Control") during collection and transportation of these specimens. Just as for blood collections, the laboratory requisition/label must accompany the specimen, with the patient's name, the patient's identification number, the date, the time of collection, the type of specimen, specialized collection process (e.g., clean catch, catheter), instruction regarding whether the specimen was refrigerated prior to transport, initials of who oversaw the collection, test(s) requested, and the attending physician's name. Special circumstances involved in the specimen collection (i.e., medications that may affect results, strenuous exercise before specimen collection, etc.) should be noted and accompany the specimen. The label should be affixed on the container, *not* the lid. **FIGURE 16–1** shows an example of the proper way to affix the specimen label. If different patients' urine specimens are in the same location for testing and the labeled lids are taken off the unlabeled containers for testing each urine specimen, it is highly likely that mismatching of the tests' results to the patients will occur.

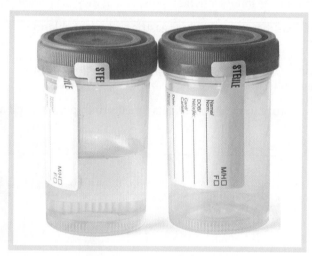

FIGURE 16–1

Urine Collection Container

The label with necessary patient's information should be affixed to the container, *not* the lid.

Source: Sylvie Bouchard/Shutterstock.com

Urine Collection

Routine urinalysis (UA) is one of the most frequently requested laboratory procedures because it can provide a useful indication of body health. It can be performed on a "first morning" specimen or a "random" urine specimen. Various diseases and disorders, such as those listed in **TABLE 16–1**, can be detected through a routine UA. Some of the more common types of urine specimen collections and their uses are provided in **TABLE 16–2**. The routine UA includes a physical, chemical, and sometimes microscopic analysis of the urine sample. The physical properties include color, transparency versus cloudiness, odor, and concentration as detected through a specific gravity measurement.

TABLE 16–1

Abnormal Urine Test Results and Associated Conditions

Abnormal Urine Test Result	Associated Condition
Presence of protein in urine (proteinuria)	Kidney disease; inflammatory disease or disorder
	Prolonged exercise
	Chemical poisoning
Presence of hemoglobin in urine (indicates blood destruction)	Kidney disease; inflammatory disease
	Malaria
	Severe burns
	Chemical poisoning
Presence of bilirubin in urine	Liver disease
	Obstructive jaundice
Presence of glucose in urine (glycosuria)	Diabetes mellitus
Presence of leukocytes in urine (white blood cells)	Infection of the kidney
	Infection of the urinary bladder
	Infection of the urethra
Presence of ketone bodies in urine (ketosis)	Diabetes mellitus
	Starvation
	Vomiting

The chemical analysis for abnormal constituents is determined by using plastic reagent strips impregnated with color-reacting substances that test for the presence of glucose, protein, blood (red blood cells and hemoglobin), white blood cells, ketones, bacteria, bilirubin, and other constituents (**FIGURE 16–2**). The manufacturer's directions must be followed in order to obtain the correct test results.

The plastic reagent strip, which has a separate reagent pad for each chemical test, is dipped into the urine briefly (**FIGURE 16–3**). The color of each reagent pad is compared to a color chart usually shown on the outer label of the reagent strip container.

TABLE 16–2

Types of Urine Specimen Collections and Their Uses

Specimen Type	Reason for Collection	Examples of Uses
Random	This type of specimen is most convenient to obtain.	Routine urinalysis (UA)
First urine of the morning	This urine excretion is the most concentrated.	Protein, nitrate, microscopic analysis: quantitative and qualitative
		Routine urinalysis (UA)
Fasting	Metabolic abnormalities are more easily diagnosed with this type of specimen.	Glucose-level determinations for diabetes mellitus testing
Clean-catch midstream	The specimen is free of contamination.	Culture for bacteria and/or microscopic analysis
Catheter	The **catheter urine specimen** is collected after a catheter is inserted into the bladder, using a sterile procedure.	UA, chemical analysis
Suprapubic	The **suprapubic specimen** is collected through aspirating urine from the bladder.	Culture for bacteria and/or microscopic analysis
Timed (e.g., 2 hour, 4 hour, 24 hour)	The excretion rate of the analyte can be determined.	Creatinine clearance test; urobilinogen determinations; hormone studies
Tolerance test	Timed blood and urine specimens are obtained to detect metabolic abnormalities.	Glucose tolerance test (GTT) and other tolerance tests

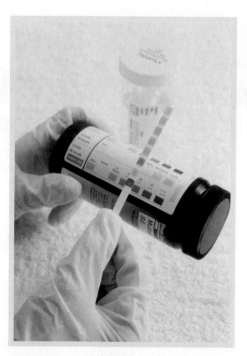

FIGURE 16–2

Chemistry Urine Strip

The chemistry urine strip is used to check urine for ketone bodies and other constituents. The strip is checked against the chart found on the bottle after dipping the strip into the urine.

Courtesy of Photo Researchers, Inc.

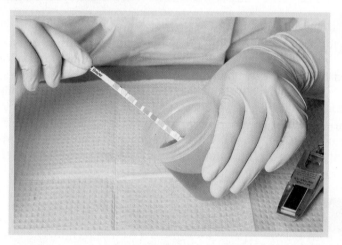

FIGURE 16–3

Dipping the Plastic Urinalysis Strip into the Urine for Chemical Analysis

Caution should be taken during this process because the colors on this chart can be altered if it comes into contact with excess urine on the test strip. The results are reported according to the reagent label specifications (e.g., trace, 1+, 2+, and so on for a positive result, or negative when no reaction occurs). The strip is discarded after it is used one time. As for all types of point-of-care testing, proper storage and quality control monitoring must be used to ensure accurate results.

Other tests that can be performed on urine specimens are the pregnancy, myoglobin, and porphyrin tests. Urine is also the specimen of choice for drug abuse testing, as discussed in Chapter 17. Other laboratory procedures associated with the urinary system include the **creatinine clearance test** to determine the ability of the kidneys to remove creatinine from the blood, and the **blood urea nitrogen (BUN)** test to measure the amount of urea in the blood.

SINGLE-SPECIMEN COLLECTION

The preferred urine specimen for most analyses is the first voided urine of the morning (**FIGURE 16–4**), when urine is the most concentrated. This **first morning specimen** should be collected immediately after the donor wakes up in the morning. This type of urine specimen is also referred to as an *early morning* or **overnight specimen.**

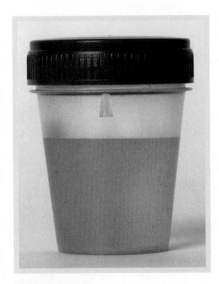

FIGURE 16–4

Single Specimen Collection

Urine is most concentrated in the morning.

Courtesy of Dorling Kindersley Media Library.

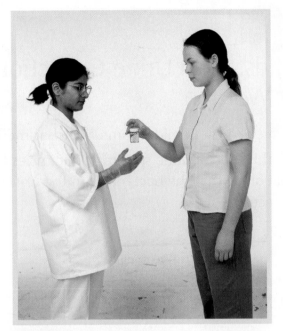

FIGURE 16–5

Patient's Labeled Urine Specimen Given to Health Care Worker

Courtesy of Dorling Kindersley Media Library.

The **random urine specimen** can be collected at any time but with the time recorded on the specimen label. For all urine specimens, the urine collection containers must be clean and dry prior to the collection process. For routine UA procedures, appropriate containers include plastic disposable cups or bags (for infants) with a capacity of 50 mL. The containers must be properly labeled (label on the container, not the lid), free of interfering chemicals, able to be tightly capped, and leakproof (**FIGURE 16–5**).

The specimen should be transported to the UA section promptly for analysis within 1 hour after the patient voids. If transportation or analysis cannot occur within this time period, the urine should be refrigerated.

Another type of single-specimen urine test is the urine **culture and sensitivity (C&S).** This specimen requires a **clean-catch midstream** urine collection. The patient is instructed to void approximately one-third of the urine into the toilet, collect approximately one-fourth in a readily available sterile container, and allow the rest to pass into the toilet.[1]

If a patient asks what a clean-catch urine specimen is, the procedure should be described, stating that this type of specimen is used to detect the presence or absence of infecting organisms. The specimen must be free of contaminating matter that may be present on the external genital areas. Thus, the steps in PROCEDURE 16–1 should be explained to a female patient who is to obtain a clean-catch midstream urine specimen. For a male patient, the process in PROCEDURE 16–2 should be adhered to for obtaining a clean-catch midstream urine specimen.[2]

The urine specimen must be transported to the microbiology section promptly. If it cannot be taken to the area for microbiological culturing within 1 hour of collection, the specimen should be refrigerated to prevent an overgrowth of contaminate bacteria.

Suprapubic aspiration and catheterization is a procedure to obtain uncontaminated bladder urine. This type of urine specimen is collected with sterile technique by aspirating urine from the patient's bladder through the abdominal wall. The urine specimen should be placed in a sterile container for microbiological cultures.

PROCEDURE 16–1

Clean-Catch Midstream Urine Collection Instructions for Women

Rationale   To collect a clean-catch midstream urine specimen.

Collecting this type of urine specimen minimizes the degree of bacterial contamination so that the bacteria from the **urinary tract infection (UTI)** can be detected.

Equipment

- Antiseptic soap and water
- Disinfectant swab or towellettes
- Sterile specimen container with label
- Clean gloves

Preparation

1 Identify the patient by checking at least two forms of identification.

2 Explain the collection procedure to the patient and the importance of thoroughly cleaning her hands and the area thoroughly before the urine collection in order to obtain a good specimen.

Procedure

3 After washing her hands, the woman should separate the skin folds around the urinary opening and clean this area with mild antiseptic soap and water or special towelettes. She should thoroughly cleanse from front to back.

4 Holding the skin folds apart with one hand and after urinating about one-third of urine into the toilet, the patient should urinate into a sterile container until the container is one-quarter to one-half full. The container should not touch the genital area.

5 After collecting the specimen, the patient or health care worker, with gloved hands, should place the lid tightly on the container, taking care not to touch the edges or inside of the container. It must be covered with the lid that was provided after urination. It is extremely important not to touch the inside or lip of the container with hands or other parts of the body.

6 The health care worker (or sometimes the patient) will label the container with the patient's name and the time of collection and deliver it to the requested location.

7 Health care personnel should refrigerate the urine specimen immediately.

8 Both the patient and the health care worker should discard gloves in the appropriate biohazard container and wash their hands after urine collection and handling.

PROCEDURE 16–2

Clean-Catch Midstream Urine Collection Instructions for Men

Rationale   To collect a clean-catch midstream urine specimen.

Collecting this type of urine specimen minimizes the degree of bacterial contamination so that the bacteria from the UTI can be detected.

Equipment

■ Antiseptic soap and water
■ Disinfectant swab or towellettes
■ Sterile specimen container with label
■ Clean gloves

Preparation

1 Identify the patient by checking at least two forms of identification.

2 Explain the collection procedure to the patient and the importance of thoroughly cleaning his hands and the area thoroughly before the urine collection in order to obtain a good specimen.

Procedure

3 For circumcised males, the man should wash his hands and the end of his penis with soapy water or special towelettes using a circular motion and moving from the middle to outside and then let dry. The penis must be cleansed in this manner from the clean area to the dirty area in order to decrease bacterial levels that could contaminate the urine specimen.

4 For uncircumcised males, the man should retract the foreskin and clean the area as directed in the previous step to avoid bacterial contamination from the foreskin area.

5 Both uncircumcised and circumcised males should allow some urine to pass into the toilet. The patient should then collect the urine in the sterile container until it is one-quarter to one-half full. The container should not touch the penis.

6 The health care worker (or sometimes the patient) will label the container with the patient's name and the time of collection and deliver it to the requested location.

7 Health care personnel should refrigerate the urine specimen immediately.

8 Both the patient and health care worker should discard gloves in the appropriate biohazard container and wash their hands after urine collection and handling.

TIMED URINE COLLECTIONS

For some laboratory assays, such as the creatinine clearance test, urobilinogen determinations, electrolytes and hormone studies, 24-hour (or other timed period) urine specimens must be obtained. Some health care institutions still require chemical preservatives for particular timed specimens. The patient and health care worker need to avoid exposure to these preservatives, and the urine container with these preservatives must be kept out of reach of children. Incorrect collection and preservatives are frequent errors affecting timed collections. The health care worker should be aware of the protocol for collecting a 24-hour urine specimen so that he or she can assist other health care professionals and the patient in preventing collection errors. The steps in **PROCEDURE 16–3** should be followed for a 24-hour urine collection.[3]

PROCEDURE 16–3

Collecting a 24-Hour Urine Specimen

Rationale   To collect a 24-hour urine specimen.

Timed urine specimens are required to detect abnormalities involving hormones, kidneys, and other organs and systems of the body.

Equipment

- Wide-mouthed, 3- to 4-liter container with lid
- Preservative, if required
- Label for specimen
- Requisition
- Container with ice, if required

Note: To obtain accurate test results, the laboratory needs the *entire* 24-hour urine specimen.

Preparation

1 Identify the patient by checking at least two forms of identification.

2 Explain the whole procedure to the patient and also provide written directions. Provide instructions in the patient's native language. Explain the importance of handwashing for the urine collection.

3 Give the patient the container and lid. Add any required preservatives to the container before giving it to the patient. Write the preservative and any precautions on the collection container label. Place the label on the container, not on the lid. Include the following information on the label:

- Patient's name
- Patient's identification number
- Starting collection date and time
- Ending collection date and time
- Name of the requested laboratory test

Other information may be required by the facility and/or physician.

Procedure

4 Instruct the patient verbally that the collection of the 24-hour urine specimen begins with emptying the bladder and discarding the first urine passed. The exact time should be written on the container label.

5 Except for the first urine discarded, all urine should be collected during the next 24-hour period. Tell the patient to continue collecting and saving *all* urine samples for the complete 24-hour period.

6 Instruct the patient to close the lid securely and gently mix or invert the bottle after each urine sample is added.

7 Remind the patient to urinate at the end of the collection period and to include this urine in the 24-hour collection. Tell the patient to urinate before having a bowel movement because fecal material in the urine specimen will make the specimen unacceptable for collection.

8 Instruct the patient to refrigerate the entire specimen after adding each collection during the 24-hour period, except in the case of urate testing.

9 Some preservatives for 24-hour urine collection are corrosive if accidentally spilled or if the patient comes in contact with them during collection. Thus, warn the patient of any preservatives in the container.

PROCEDURE 16–3

Collecting a 24-Hour Urine Specimen (continued)

ALERT

> **Clinical Alert!** The timed specimen container may contain a preservative that may burn your skin. Do *not* remove the preservative from the collection container. Keep the container upright so that it does not spill. Urinate into a clean dry plastic container and transfer the urine to the collection container. Do not splash when pouring urine into the bottle. *Keep out of the reach of children. If liquid in bottle is splashed or spilled, wash spill immediately with water.*

10 Inform the patient not to add anything except urine to the container and not to discard any urine during the collection period.

11 A normal intake of fluids during the collection period is desirable unless otherwise indicated by the physician.

12 Some laboratory assays (i.e., 5-hydroxyindolacetic acid-HIAA) require special dietary restrictions; give these instructions to the patient. For example, for the 5-HIAA test, the patient must not eat bananas, pineapple, eggplant, plums, walnuts, avocadoes, or tomatoes 3 to 4 days prior to the time of the 24-hour urine collection, because these foods can lead to false-positive results.

13 If possible, discontinue medications for 48 to 72 hours preceding the urine collection as a precaution against interference in the laboratory assays. The patient should discuss the possible medication interference with his or her physician prior to discontinuing them for the procedure.

14 Transport the 24-hour urine specimen to the clinical laboratory as soon as possible. Place the specimen in an insulated bag or a portable cooler to maintain its cool temperature.

URINE CYTOLOGY

Cytology is the discipline in which body cells are studied to detect various diseases, including inflammatory disorders and cancers. Cytology specimens can be obtained from urine as well as cerebrospinal fluid and other body fluids. A well-established staining procedure for urine and gynecological smears is the Pap (Papanicolaou) stain. It is frequently used to stain a smear from urinary sediment to detect abnormal cells that occur in bladder and urinary tract cancers. A midstream clean-catch specimen is required for the test and should be transported to the laboratory as soon as collection occurs to avoid deterioration of the cells in the urine specimen.

Cerebrospinal Fluid

Cerebrospinal fluid (CSF) is a clear, plasma-like fluid that circulates around the outside of the brain, in cavities within the brain and in the space surrounding the spinal cord. It is obtained by a physician through a spinal tap or lumbar puncture. Cerebrospinal fluid is collected by the medical staff to diagnose meningitis, brain abscess, central nervous system cancers, multiple sclerosis, and other disorders. The fluid is usually collected in three sterile nonglass containers numbered in the order in which they were collected.

1. The first tube is usually sent to chemistry and immunology studies.
2. The second tube is used for clinical microbiology testing for cultures.
3. The third tube is usually used for cytological, cell counts, and a hematology differential.

It is important to be aware of the laboratory procedures within the health care institution, since laboratories differ on which CSF container is used for which test.

   Tests commonly performed on CSF include total protein level, glucose level, cell count, microbiological, chloride level, and cryptococcal antigen determinations.

Wearing gloves, CSF must be immediately transported to the clinical laboratory for STAT analysis. The cells within the CSF will begin to deteriorate within 1 hour of collection. If transportation cannot occur immediately, the CSF specimen for chemistry should be refrigerated and the CSF tube for clinical microbiology and hematology should be kept at room temperature, but processed as soon as possible.[4,5]

Fecal Specimens

Stool (fecal) specimens are commonly collected to detect parasites (e.g., ova and parasites [O&P]), enteric disease organisms (e.g., *Salmonella, Shigella, Staphylococcus aureus*), and viruses. The specimen is collected in a wide-mouthed plastic or waxed cardboard container with a tight-fitting lid. If the patient is to collect the stool specimen at home, he or she should be given a collecting container and instructed to avoid urinating in the container because urine can kill the microorganisms in the collected stool specimen. For children, the container can be placed under the toilet seat so that the child can sit on the toilet. The patient should be instructed to wash the outside of the specimen container after collection and to wash his or her hands thoroughly. The specimen container must be properly sealed to prevent leakage and contamination, because fecal material from patients with infectious intestinal diseases is extremely hazardous. The specimen must be transported to the laboratory immediately and maintained at body temperature (37°C) for detection of parasitic infections.

In addition to the collection of stool specimens for microorganism detection, feces are collected to detect invisible (occult) quantities of blood that do not alter the appearance of the stool. Laboratory determination of occult blood assists in the confirmation of the presence of blood in black stools and can be helpful in detecting gastrointestinal (GI) tract lesions and colorectal cancer. Feces for **occult blood tests** (also known as *stool occult blood test*, **hemoccult test, guaiac smear test, fecal immunochemical test,** and **fecal occult blood test [FOBT]**) are often collected by the patient using special test cards, such as the ForSure FOB-Test (**FIGURE 16–6**) and the ColoScreen-ES (**FIGURE 16–7**). The card can be mailed or brought to the health care facility after collection.

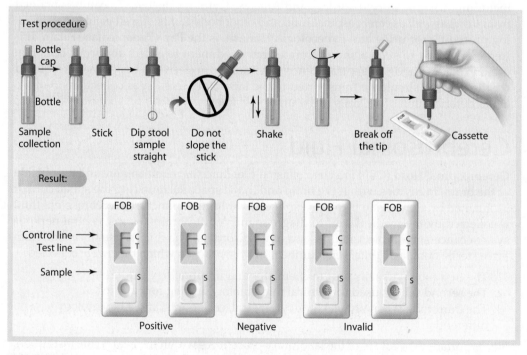

FIGURE 16–6
ForSure FOB-Test

These cards for the occult blood testing usually should be stored at room temperature and protected from heat, light, and chemicals (i.e., iodine, ammonia, bleach, and household cleaners). The health care workers involved in specimen collection and transportation should be aware of the procedural steps for these occult blood tests to instruct the patient for proper collections.[6] Many factors can contribute to false-negative or false-positive test results (e.g., patient's ingestion of aspirin, corticosteroids, ibuprofen, anticoagulants, and/or rare meats).

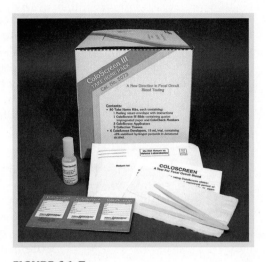

FIGURE 16–7

ColoScreen Take-Home Packs to Test for Occult Blood

Courtesy of Helena Laboratories, Beaumont, TX.

Seminal Fluid

Semen is examined in the clinical laboratory to (1) determine the effectiveness of a vasectomy, (2) investigate the possibility of sexual criminal charges, and (3) assess fertility. Before collection of a semen specimen, the patient should be given clear instructions for proper specimen collection. Semen must be collected in containers that are clean, free of trace detergents and spermicides (chemicals that kill sperms). Specimens must not be exposed to extremes of temperature or light prior to being submitted to the clinical laboratory and should be transported within 2 hours of collection.

Amniotic Fluid

Fluid that bathes the fetus within the amniotic sac is called **amniotic fluid.** It may be collected by a physician when the pregnant patient is at approximately 16 weeks' gestation so that fetal abnormalities can be detected through chromosomal analysis and chemical tests, such as the alpha-fetoprotein (AFP) assay. Occasionally, amniotic fluid is obtained in the last trimester of pregnancy to determine the lung maturity of the fetus. In addition to wearing gloves when transporting amniotic fluid to the laboratory, the health care worker must protect the specimen from light and transport it immediately.

Synovial Fluid

Synovial fluid surrounds the joints as a filtrate of blood plasma and hyaluronic acid produced by the surrounding joint tissue cells. Examination of the synovial fluid is important to identify infectious arthritis from noninfectious arthritis (e.g., osteoarthritis, traumatic arthritis, gout) when inflammation occurs in a joint. The best laboratory results occur when the fluid is collected in three tubes: (1) a sterile heparinized tube for microbiological studies, (2) a sodium heparin or liquid EDTA tube for microscopic examination, and (3) a tube without additive for chemistry and immunology testing.[5] After the specimen is collected by a physician, the fluid needs to be transported promptly to the laboratory at room temperature.

Other Body Fluids

In addition to the fluids just discussed, other types of body fluids that sometimes must be transported to the laboratory include fluid aspirated from body cavities—for example, **pleural fluid** obtained from the lung cavity, **pericardial fluid** from the heart cavity, and **peritoneal fluid** from the abdominal cavity. Other specimens for forensic and toxicology studies are mentioned in Chapter 17.

When receiving any type of body fluid for transportation, the health care worker needs to verify that the container is properly labeled with the patient's name, the patient's identification number, the date, the time of collection, the type of body fluid collected, and the initials of the person who collected the specimen. The containers holding any type of body fluids may be contaminated on the outside, and it is extremely important to wear gloves and other PPE required by the health care facility when transporting them.

Culture Specimens

Other specimens that the health care worker may be requested to transport to the clinical laboratory typically include sputum, throat swabs, sinus drainage, wound tissue, and ear, eye, or skin scrapings for microbiological cultures. The health care worker should be extremely careful while transporting each type of specimen because the specimens can easily become contaminated and may be biohazardous. For safety, the health care worker needs to wear gloves and other PPE required by the health care facility when handling and transporting these specimens in their containers.

BUCCAL SWABS

A health care worker may be asked to collect a **buccal swab** (that is, a sample from the cheek or mouth) from a patient. It involves swabbing the inside of the patient's cheek with a special swab. This provides a relatively noninvasive way to collect DNA samples for testing.

SPUTUM COLLECTION

Sputum (fluid from the lungs containing pus) is collected in a sterile container for microbiology specimens to test for pathogenic organisms, including tuberculosis (**FIGURE 16–8**). Also, sputum can be collected in containers with a preservative for cytology testing (**PROCEDURE 16–4**). The preservative is poisonous, and the patient and health care worker involved in the collection and transportation of this specimen should be aware of this toxic additive.

> **ALERT**
>
> **Clinical Alert!** A sputum specimen obtained in the early morning before eating or drinking provides the best specimen for analysis since it is the most concentrated. The patient needs to remove dentures prior to the collection.

FIGURE 16–8
Collecting a Sterile Sputum Specimen from a Patient

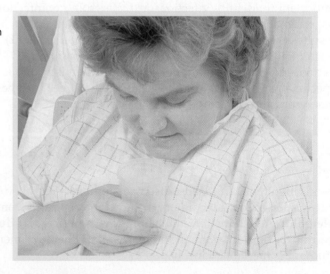

PROCEDURE 16–4

Collecting a Sputum Specimen

Rationale   To perform a sputum collection for microbiologic analysis to diagnose and treat respiratory infections.

Equipment

- Gloves and other PPE required by the health care facility
- Sterile container with or without preservatives as required for laboratory
- Laboratory requisition/label for specimen

Preparation

1 Gather and organize the necessary equipment.

2 Properly identify and inform the patient of the collection procedure.

Procedure

3 Wash your hands and put on gloves, a protective laboratory coat, and a facial mask (if needed to avoid contamination from patient's coughing).

4 A fresh, early-morning specimen resulting from a deep cough is needed for diagnosing infection. The patient must not use mouthwash or gargle before collection. The laboratory usually will not accept saliva, combined specimens, or 24-hour specimens. The specimen must be submitted in a sterile container to be accepted for diagnostic workup.

5 Obtain the specimen in early morning, preferably when first waking up.

6 Instruct the patient to take a deep breath and then **expectorate** (to cough deeply and spit thick matter from the lungs) from a deep cough directly into the sterile container (one to two teaspoons are adequate). Instruct the patient to avoid spitting saliva (**FIGURES 16–9** and **16–10**).

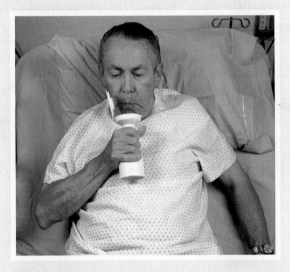

FIGURE 16–9
Instruct the patient to lift the hinged lid of the sputum collection container and expectorate directly into the container and avoid contaminating the outside of the container.

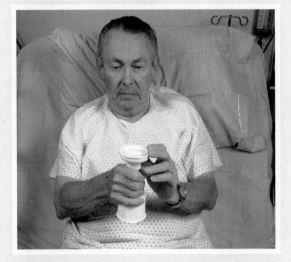

FIGURE 16–10
Instruct the patient to obtain one to two teaspoons of sputum and then close the lid of the container.

(continued)

PROCEDURE 16–4

Collecting a Sputum Specimen (continued)

After the Procedure

7 Thank the patient for cooperating and depart.

8 The container must be free from external contamination. Containers contaminated on the exterior pose a serious health hazard to health care workers and will not be accepted by the laboratory.

9 Wearing gloves and PPE required by the health care facility, transport the container to the laboratory in the appropriately labeled container.

10 Deliver the labeled specimen to the laboratory immediately. If transportation to the laboratory is delayed, refrigerate the labeled specimen until transportation is available.

NASOPHARYNGEAL CULTURE COLLECTIONS

Nasopharyngeal cultures are often performed to detect carrier states of *Neisseria meningitidis*, *Corynebacterium diphtheriae*, *Streptococcus pyogenes*, *Haemophilus influenzae*, and *Staphylococcus aureus*. For infants and children, from whom significant sputum cultures are difficult to obtain, nasopharyngeal cultures may be used to diagnose whooping cough, croup, and pneumonia. These aspirates and washings are collected by medical staff who have education and experience in these invasive collection procedures.

THROAT SWAB COLLECTIONS

Throat swab collections (**PROCEDURE 16–5**) are most commonly obtained to determine the presence of streptococcal infections either by screening methods (commercially available rapid strep tests) or by microbial culture. Because coughing may force organisms from the lower respiratory tract into the nasopharynx, it may be best when performing a throat culture on a child or an infant to stimulate coughing in order to obtain a more significant nasopharyngeal culture. Health care workers should be taught the correct procedures before they are allowed to acquire specimens from patients.

In the clinical microbiology laboratory, the swab is spread out, or "streaked," for distribution of the microorganisms on various agar media that have nutrients to grow pathogenic organisms. A Gram-stained smear (a microscopic method to identify bacteria) is often useful to provide preliminary indications of infection and should be made with the swab by rolling it across a sterile slide before placing it in a transport medium or inoculating agar media plates. The agar media plates are then placed under optimal growth conditions for suspected pathogens.

PROCEDURE 16–5

Collecting a Throat Swab for Culture

Rationale   To perform a throat swab collection for determination of streptococcal infections.

Equipment

- Gloves and other PPE required by the health care facility
- Tongue blade
- Light source
- Sterile culture swab and sterile container
- Laboratory requisition/label

Preparation

1 Gather and organize the necessary equipment.

2 Properly identify and inform the patient of the collection procedure.

Procedure

3 Wash your hands and put on gloves, a protective laboratory coat, and a facial mask (if needed to avoid contamination from patient's coughing).

4 Instruct the patient to open wide his or her mouth, as if to yawn. Direct a light source into the mouth and throat.

5 Using the sterile swab, swab the tonsillar areas, back of the throat, and any areas of inflammation (i.e., redness, white pockets of pus) and/or ulceration (**FIGURE 16–11**).[7] It is important not to contaminate the swab with the oral secretions from the mouth, which may dilute, allow overgrowth, or inhibit the growth of pathogens (disease-causing microorganisms).

6 Place the swab in a special transport medium (**FIGURE 16–12**), or inoculate the fluid on the swab directly onto agar in a petri dish by rolling the swab across a small area of the medium. In some facilities, a rapid strep screening test is performed directly from the throat swab. Follow your facility's protocol for whichever test is ordered.

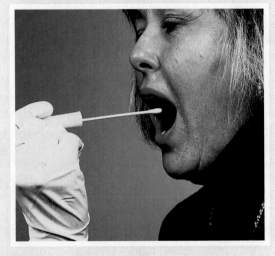

FIGURE 16–11
Obtaining a Throat Culture

After swabbing the throat from side to side, remove the applicator swab, being careful *not* to touch any part of the mouth.

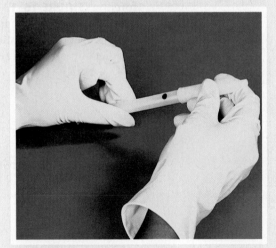

FIGURE 16–12
Specimen Tube for Swab

Place the applicator swab in the specimen tube with caution to avoid contaminating the swab.

(continued)

PROCEDURE 16–5

Collecting a Throat Swab for Culture (continued)

After the Procedure

7 Discard the contaminated tongue blade in the appropriate biohazard waste containers.

8 Thank the patient for cooperating and depart.

9 Wearing gloves and PPE required by the health care facility, transport the swab to the laboratory in the appropriately labeled sterile transport swab container.

10 Any container must be free from external contamination. Containers contaminated on the exterior constitute a serious health hazard to personnel.

11 If transport to the laboratory is delayed, refrigerate the specimen until transportation is available.

SKIN TESTS

On occasion, a nurse or other health care worker may be asked to perform a **skin test.** The health care worker should check the policies of the health care facility prior to performing the procedure. This procedure involves the deliberate exposure of a patient to a substance that may cause significant harm; therefore, the health care worker must be educated in the emergency treatment of allergic reactions or have someone close by with this expertise. Skin tests are simple and relatively inexpensive. They determine whether a patient has ever had contact with a particular antigen and has produced antibodies to that antigen. A wide range of disease states stimulate antibody responses in individuals. Tests range from detection of ragweed and milk allergies in hypersensitive individuals, to detection of tuberculosis (TB) and fungal infections in persons who have had contact with these organisms. The allergy skin test is performed on the patient's forearm (**FIGURE 16–13**) or back using a common procedure called the *prick technique.*[8] The prick skin testing involves application of droplets of allergen extract solutions on the forearm or back, after the skin has been cleaned with a 70% alcohol solution. Each droplet contains a single allergen extract (i.e., specific tree pollen, latex, ragweed).

FIGURE 16–13

Allergy Skin Testing

Courtesy of Andy Crawford/ Dorling Kindersley Media Library.

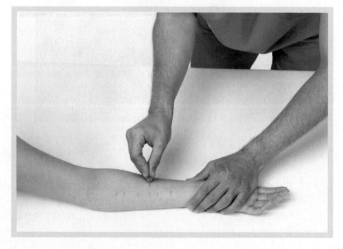

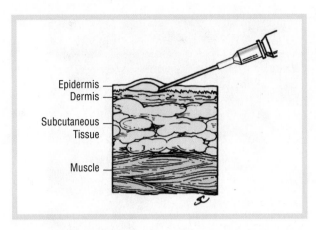

FIGURE 16–14

TB Skin Test

Insert the needle at a 15-degree angle just under the epidermis for intradermal injection of the TB purified protein derivative (PPD) antigen.

The TB skin test can be administered using an automatic device or by pulling 0.1 mL of diluted antigen into a tuberculin syringe. All air bubbles should be expelled by holding the syringe vertically and tapping the sides of the barrel. The volar (palm side) surface of the patient's forearm should be cleaned with alcohol and prepared in the same manner as for a venipuncture (see Chapter 10). The area should be devoid of scars, skin eruptions, tattoos, and excessive hair. Holding the syringe at a slight angle (approximately 15 degrees), the needle should be slipped just under the skin (**FIGURE 16–14**). The plunger should be pulled back slightly to ensure that a blood vessel has not been entered. The fluid may then be slowly expelled into the site, observing for a wheal (blister) formation and blanching at the site. If the wheal does not appear, the injection was given too deeply. The needle should be promptly removed, and only slight pressure applied, with gauze, over the site. Care should be taken that the fluid does not leak onto the gauze or run out of the injection site. The patient should hold the arm in an extended position until the site has time to close and retain the fluid. A bandage should not be used over the site because it may absorb some of the fluid and distort the results of the skin test by causing skin irritation from the adhesive.

The patient should report any reaction, no matter how slight, to the physician. Also, a return visit for proper interpretation of the skin reaction should be scheduled with the physician. At some health care agencies, the patient is asked to note the exact size of the reaction site or to compare his or her reaction with pictures on a prelabeled card that can be mailed back to the institution. When this is the case, patients should be fully informed about how to read positive and negative reactions.

GASTRIC ANALYSIS

Gastric analysis determines how much acid is produced in an individual's stomach. The stomach (gastric) contents are emptied through a gastric tube. The test involves passing a tube through the patient's nose (intubating) and into the stomach (**FIGURE 16–15**). The health care worker may be asked to assist and collect specimens as required. The responsibility for properly intubating the patient usually rests with the physician or the nurse. The health care worker can be present to assist in patient care and to collect any required blood specimens, but under no circumstances should be expected to carry out the procedure unless properly trained. Improper placement of the tube poses a high risk to the patient and could result in a punctured lung if the tube enters the bronchial system instead of the esophagus. The health care worker can and should be responsible for proper labeling of gastric and blood samples when he or she is present and assisting during the procedure.

FIGURE 16-15
Aspirating Gastric Contents from
the Patient

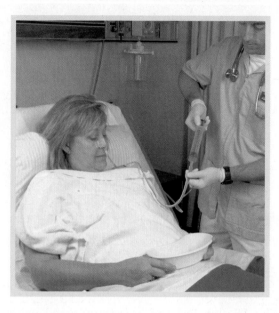

BREATH ANALYSIS FOR PEPTIC ULCERS

Helicobacter pylori is a bacteria that damages the stomach or intestinal lining and is linked to ulcers and stomach cancer. A positive *H. pylori* test, antibody, antigen, or breath test indicates that the patient has been infected with this organism. The health care worker should be aware of the noninvasive testing procedural steps to assist the patient if these are included in his or her responsibilities.

Sweat Chloride by Iontophoresis

The **sweat chloride test** is used as the gold standard in the diagnosis of cystic fibrosis. *Cystic fibrosis* is a genetic disorder of the exocrine glands (relating to glandular secretions released externally through a duct). It is the most common fatal autosomal recessive disease among the Caucasian populations. Primarily affected are the lungs, upper respiratory tract, liver, and pancreas. Patients with cystic fibrosis produce chloride in their sweat at two to five times the level produced by healthy individuals. Sweat chloride testing should be performed on all infants with a positive newborn screen.[9,10,11]

For the laboratory evaluation, pilocarpine hydrochloric acid (HCl) is **iontophoresed** (a painless weak electrical current is used to stimulate drug-carrying ions to pass through intact skin) into the skin of the patient to stimulate sweat production. The sweat is absorbed onto preweighed gauze pads; then the weight of the sweat is determined. The pad is then diluted with deionized water, and the chloride is generally read by titration with a chloridometer or automated analyzer (i.e., ion-selective electrode systematically validated against the chloridometer).

When a health care provider receives an order to perform a sweat chloride test on a patient, he or she should properly prepare for the procedure under the supervision of a clinical laboratory scientist. The collection and analysis should be performed in duplicate for quality assurance of accuracy in testing. The CLSI document, *Sweat Testing: Sample Collection and Quantitative Chloride Analysis, Approved Guideline*, 3rd edition, should be followed as outlined.[12]

Study Questions

For the following questions, select the one best answer.

1 Which of the following can be used in children and infants to diagnose cystic fibrosis?

a. CSF
b. sweat chloride
c. amniotic fluid
d. pericardial fluid

2 Which type of urine specimen is needed to detect an infection?

a. random
b. suprapubic
c. routine
d. 24-hour

3 What does glycosuria refer to?

a. glycogen in body fluids
b. glucose in the urine
c. CSF with increased glucose
d. breakdown of glycogen to glucose

4 Which of the following types of specimens is most frequently collected for analysis?

a. amniotic fluid
b. urine
c. CSF
d. pericardial fluid

5 Which of the following body fluids is extracted from joint cavities?

a. pleural fluid
b. peritoneal fluid
c. synovial fluid
d. pericardial fluid

6 The O&P analysis is requested on which type of specimen?

a. CSF
b. amniotic fluid
c. fecal matter
d. synovial fluid

7 Fetal abnormalities are detected through analysis of which fluid?

a. pleural
b. peritoneal
c. amniotic
d. CSF

8 The FOBT is frequently requested on which type of specimen?

a. CSF
b. fecal matter
c. throat culture
d. seminal fluid

9 Ketosis is frequently detected with which of the following conditions?

a. liver disease
b. diabetes mellitus
c. chemical poisoning
d. infection

10 Which of the following body fluids is obtained from fluid surrounding the heart?

a. synovial fluid
b. pericardial fluid
c. peritoneal fluid
d. CSF

Case Study

Hanna Burkley, the newly hired health care worker in the specimen collection department, was told to gather the equipment for collecting a sputum specimen from a patient and review the instructions for the procedure in order to give the proper instructions to the patient and collect the specimen.

That afternoon, Hanna gathered her gloves and other PPE, as well as the sterile container for the specimen, and went to the patient's room for the collection. Upon arriving at the patient's room, she introduced herself to the patient, put on her gloves, a protective laboratory coat, and a facial mask. Hanna instructed the patient to cough deeply and spit the sputum into the specimen container. Then she thanked the patient and transported the container to the laboratory. Hanna labeled the container when she arrived in the laboratory.

Questions

1 Did Hanna follow the proper protocol for the collection of the sputum specimen collection?

2 What are the procedural steps that should be followed for this collection?

Action in Practice

The physician for Ms. Maria Herrera requested that she should have a urinalysis to detect protein and white blood cells.

Questions

1 Which type of urine specimen should be collected?

2 What is the analytical procedure for detection of protein and white blood cells?

COMPETENCY ASSESSMENT

Check Yourself

1 List five types of specimens other than blood that the health care worker might be requested to transport to the clinical laboratory.

2 Explain the difference between pleural fluid and pericardial fluid.

Competency Checklist: Urinalysis, Body Fluids, and Other Specimens

This checklist can be completed as a group or individually.

(1) Completed (2) Needs to improve

_____ 1. Describe the procedural steps in the throat swab collection.
_____ 2. Explain the difference between sputum and mucus.
_____ 3. Describe the procedural steps for timed urine collection for urobilinogen testing.

REFERENCES

1. Garza, D. (1983). Urine collection and preservation. In Ross, D. L., & Neely, A. E. (Eds.), *Textbook of urinalysis and body fluids.* New York: Appleton-Century-Crofts, p. 61.

2. Meyrier, A., & Zaleznik, D. (2004, August 22). Urine sampling and culture in the diagnosis of urinary tract infection in adults. M. D. Anderson Cancer Center: UpToDate, Version 15.3, www.uptodate.com, accessed November 27, 2007.

3. Clinical and Laboratory Standards Institute (CLSI). (2009). *Urinalysis, approved guideline,* 3rd ed., Document GP16-A3. Wayne, PA: Author.

4. Brunzel, N. (2009, August). *Fundamentals of urine and body fluid analysis.* New York: Elsevier.

5. Karcher, D. S., & McPherson, R. A. (2011). Cerebrospinal, synovial, serous body fluids, and alternative specimens. In *Henry's clinical diagnosis and management by laboratory methods,* 22nd ed. Amsterdam: Elsevier, p. 481.

6. U.S. Preventive Services Task Force (USPSTF). (2009, August). *Screening tests at-a-glance.* CDC Publication #21-1029. www.cdc.gov/screenforlife, accessed July 3, 2012.

7. Becan-McBride, K., & Ross, D. (1988). *Essentials for the small laboratory and physician's office.* Chicago: Mosby-Year Book.

8. Nelson, H. S, Knoetzer J., & Bucher, B. (1996). Effect of distance between sites and region of the body on results of skin prick tests. *J Allergy Clin Immunol, 97:* 596.

9. The Cystic Fibrosis Foundation. (2010, December 17). *Testing for cystic fibrosis.* www.Cff.org/AboutCF/Testing, accessed July 3, 2012.

10. Wagermer, J. S., Sontag, M. K., Sagel, S.D., & Accurso, F. J. (2004). Update on newborn screening for cystic fibrosis. *Curr Opin Pulm Med., 10:* 500.

11. LeGrys, V. A., Yankaskas, J. R., & Quittell, L. M., et al. (2007). Diagnostic sweat testing: The Cystic Fibrosis Foundation guidelines. *J Pediatr, 151:* 85.

12. Clinical Laboratory Standards Institute (CLSI). (2010). *Sweat testing: Sample collection and quantitative chloride analysis, approved guideline,* 3rd ed., Document C34-A3. Wayne, PA: Author.

RESOURCES

Smith, R. A., Cokkinides, V., & Eyre, H. J. (2007). Cancer screening in the United States, 2007: A review of current guidelines, practices, and prospects. *CA Cancer J Clin, 57:* 90–104.

Vaillancourt, S., et al. (2007). To clean or not to clean: Effect on contamination rates in midstream urine collections in toilet-trained Children. *Pediatrics, 119:* 1288–1293.

www.webmd.com The WebMD website provides health information and medical news.

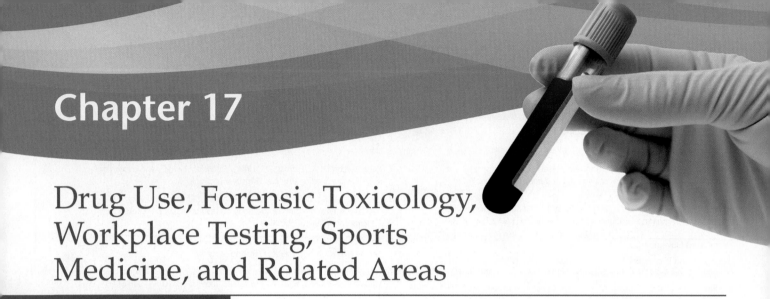

Chapter 17

Drug Use, Forensic Toxicology, Workplace Testing, Sports Medicine, and Related Areas

Chapter Objectives

Upon completion of Chapter 17, the learner is responsible for doing the following:

1. Define toxicology and forensic toxicology.

2. Give five examples of forensic specimens and describe the role of the health care worker in handling or processing them.

3. Describe why drug testing is valuable and explain the role of the health care worker, or "collector," in federal drug-testing programs.

4. Define and describe the function of a chain of custody.

5. Describe how to detect adulteration of urine specimens.

6. List two methods of measuring blood alcohol content and at least three factors that can affect testing.

Overview and Prevalence of Drug Use

The **abuse** (improper use) of or **addiction** (relapsing, compulsive use of, and dependence on, a substance in spite of harmful consequences) to **illicit drugs** is a serious problem in the United States and is monitored by the National Institutes of Health and National Institute on Drug Abuse. Illicit drugs are illegal drugs such as unauthorized marijuana, cocaine, heroin, hallucinogens, and inhalants and the nonmedical use of **over-the-counter (OTC)** or prescription pain relievers, tranquilizers, stimulants, and sedatives. Based on data collected in 2011, BOX 17–1 presents facts about adolescent substance abuse in the United States. However, the problem goes beyond adolescents; millions of Americans are affected by substance abuse each year. This textbook briefly discusses substance abuse because health care workers may be involved in

- Specimen collections for drug testing
- Assisting with the drug screening or analysis
- Detection of specimen **adulteration** (tampering with the specimen)
- Preemployment or random drug-testing programs

Substance abuse and/or addiction have a significant impact on health care (e.g., legal, economic, social, psychological, and patient safety issues) (TABLE 17–1). According to Quest Diagnostics, a leading provider of diagnostic information, job candidates subject to preemployment drug screening tested positive for illicit drugs at a greater rate in the first six months of 2012 than in all of 2011.[1,2] Over the past decade, with improvements in therapy and new drugs (e.g., opioid medications) to treat pain, there has been a rise

---

BOX 17–1

Facts about Substance Abuse[1]

According to the CDC (2011 data), the following data are only a small sampling of the information available:

- For high school seniors, the rate of cigarette use was 18.7 percent; and for eighth-graders it was 6.1 percent.
- For high school seniors, the rate of marijuana use was 22.6 percent; and for eighth-graders it was 8.5 percent.
- Among high school seniors, the rate of alcohol use was 40 percent; and for eighth-graders it was 12.7 percent. Among students in grades 9 through 12, 24.1 percent reported riding with a driver that had been drinking alcohol, and 8.2 percent actually drove while drinking alcohol.
- Among high school seniors, 21.6 percent reported **binge drinking** (five or more alcoholic drinks in a row at least once in a two-week period), and 6.4 percent of eighth-graders reported binge drinking.
- Among high school seniors, alcohol is the most abused substance, followed by marijuana, then prescription-type drugs used nonmedically, hallucinogens, inhalants, and cocaine.

TABLE 17-1

Commonly Abused Drugs
Visit NIDA at www.drugabuse.gov

NIDA — NATIONAL INSTITUTE ON DRUG ABUSE

National Institutes of Health
U.S. Department of Health and Human Services
NIH... Turning Discovery Into Health

Substances: Category and Name	Examples of Commercial and Street Names	DEA Schedule*/ How Administered**	Acute Effects/Health Risks
Tobacco			
Nicotine	Found in cigarettes, cigars, bidis, and smokeless tobacco (snuff, spit tobacco, chew)	Not scheduled/smoked, snorted, chewed	*Increased blood pressure and heart rate/chronic lung disease; cardiovascular disease; stroke; cancers of the mouth, pharynx, larynx, esophagus, stomach, pancreas, cervix, kidney, bladder, and acute myeloid leukemia; adverse pregnancy outcomes; addiction*
Alcohol			
Alcohol (ethyl alcohol)	Found in liquor, beer, and wine	Not scheduled/swallowed	*In low doses, euphoria, mild stimulation, relaxation, lowered inhibitions; in higher doses, drowsiness, slurred speech, nausea, emotional volatility, loss of coordination, visual distortions, impaired memory, sexual dysfunction, loss of consciousness/increased risk of injuries, violence, fetal damage (in pregnant women); depression; neurologic deficits; hypertension; liver and heart disease; addiction; fatal overdose*
Cannabinoids			
Marijuana	Blunt, dope, ganja, grass, herb, joint, bud, Mary Jane, pot, reefer, green, trees, smoke, sinsemilla, skunk, weed	I/smoked, swallowed	*Euphoria; relaxation; slowed reaction time; distorted sensory perception; impaired balance and coordination; increased heart rate and appetite; impaired learning, memory; anxiety; panic attacks; psychosis/cough; frequent respiratory infections; possible mental health decline; addiction*
Hashish	Boom, gangster, hash, hash oil, hemp	I/smoked, swallowed	
Opioids			
Heroin	*Diacetylmorphine:* smack, horse, brown sugar, dope, H, junk, skag, skunk, white horse, China white; cheese (with OTC cold medicine and antihistamine)	I/injected, smoked, snorted	*Euphoria; drowsiness; impaired coordination; dizziness; confusion; nausea; sedation; feeling of heaviness in the body; slowed or arrested breathing/constipation; endocarditis; hepatitis; HIV; addiction; fatal overdose*
Opium	*Laudanum, paregoric:* big O, black stuff, block, gum, hop	II, III, V/swallowed, smoked	
Stimulants			
Cocaine	*Cocaine hydrochloride:* blow, bump, C, candy, Charlie, coke, crack, flake, rock, snow, toot	II/snorted, smoked, injected	*Increased heart rate, blood pressure, body temperature, metabolism; feelings of exhilaration; increased energy, mental alertness; tremors; reduced appetite; irritability; anxiety; panic; paranoia; violent behavior; psychosis/weight loss; insomnia; cardiac or cardiovascular complications; stroke; seizures; addiction*
Amphetamine	*Biphetamine, Dexedrine:* bennies, black beauties, crosses, hearts, LA turnaround, speed, truck drivers, uppers	II/swallowed, snorted, smoked, injected	**Also, for cocaine**—*nasal damage from snorting*
Methamphetamine	*Desoxyn:* meth, ice, crank, chalk, crystal, fire, glass, go fast, speed	II/swallowed, snorted, smoked, injected	**Also, for methamphetamine**—*severe dental problems*
Club Drugs			
MDMA (methylenedioxymethamphetamine)	Ecstasy, Adam, clarity, Eve, lover's speed, peace, uppers	I/swallowed, snorted, injected	**MDMA**—*mild hallucinogenic effects; increased tactile sensitivity, empathic feelings; lowered inhibition; anxiety; chills; sweating; teeth clenching; muscle cramping/ sleep disturbances; depression; impaired memory; hyperthermia; addiction*
Flunitrazepam***	*Rohypnol:* forget-me pill, Mexican Valium, R2, roach, Roche, roofies, roofinol, rope, rophies	IV/swallowed, snorted	**Flunitrazepam**—*sedation; muscle relaxation; confusion; memory loss; dizziness; impaired coordination/addiction*
GHB***	*Gamma-hydroxybutyrate:* G, Georgia home boy, grievous bodily harm, liquid ecstasy, soap, scoop, goop, liquid X	I/swallowed	**GHB**—*drowsiness; nausea; headache; disorientation; loss of coordination; memory loss/ unconsciousness; seizures; coma*
Dissociative Drugs			
Ketamine	*Ketalar SV:* cat Valium, K, Special K, vitamin K	III/injected, snorted, smoked	*Feelings of being separate from one's body and environment; impaired motor function/anxiety; tremors; numbness; memory loss; nausea*
PCP and analogs	*Phencyclidine:* angel dust, boat, hog, love boat, peace pill	I, II/swallowed, smoked, injected	**Also, for ketamine**—*analgesia; impaired memory; delirium; respiratory depression and arrest; death*
Salvia divinorum	*Salvia, Shepherdess's Herb, Maria Pastora, magic mint, Sally-D*	Not scheduled/chewed, swallowed, smoked	**Also, for PCP and analogs**—*analgesia; psychosis; aggression; violence; slurred speech; loss of coordination; hallucinations*
Dextromethorphan (DXM)	Found in some cough and cold medications: Robotripping, Robo, Triple C	Not scheduled/swallowed	**Also, for DXM**—*euphoria; slurred speech; confusion; dizziness; distorted visual perceptions*
Hallucinogens			
LSD	*Lysergic acid diethylamide:* acid, blotter, cubes, microdot, yellow sunshine, blue heaven	I/swallowed, absorbed through mouth tissues	*Altered states of perception and feeling; hallucinations; nausea*
Mescaline	*Buttons, cactus, mesc, peyote*	I/swallowed, smoked	**Also, for LSD and mescaline**—*increased body temperature, heart rate, blood pressure; loss of appetite; sweating; sleeplessness; numbness; dizziness; weakness; tremors; impulsive behavior, rapid shifts in emotion*
Psilocybin	Magic mushrooms, purple passion, shrooms, little smoke	I/swallowed	**Also, for LSD**—*Flashbacks, Hallucinogen Persisting Perception Disorder*
			Also, for psilocybin—*nervousness; paranoia; panic*
Other Compounds			
Anabolic steroids	*Anadrol, Oxandrin, Durabolin, Depo-Testosterone, Equipoise:* roids, juice, gym candy, pumpers	III/injected, swallowed, applied to skin	**Steroids**—*no intoxication effects/hypertension; blood clotting and cholesterol changes; liver cysts; hostility and aggression; acne; in adolescents—premature stoppage of growth; in males—prostate cancer, reduced sperm production, shrunken testicles, breast enlargement; in females—menstrual irregularities, development of beard and other masculine characteristics*
Inhalants	*Solvents (paint thinners, gasoline, glues); gases (butane, propane, aerosol propellants, nitrous oxide); nitrites (isoamyl, isobutyl, cyclohexyl):* laughing gas, poppers, snappers, whippets	Not scheduled/inhaled through nose or mouth	**Inhalants** *(varies by chemical)*—*stimulation; loss of inhibition; headache; nausea or vomiting; slurred speech; loss of motor coordination; wheezing/cramps; muscle weakness; depression; memory impairment; damage to cardiovascular and nervous systems; unconsciousness; sudden death*

Substances: Category and Name	Examples of Commercial and Street Names	DEA Schedule*/ How Administered**	Acute Effects/Health Risks
Prescription Medications			
CNS Depressants			
Stimulants	For more information on prescription medications, please visit http://www.nida.nih.gov/DrugPages/PrescripDrugsChart.html.		
Opioid Pain Relievers			

* Schedule I and II drugs have a high potential for abuse. They require greater storage security and have a quota on manufacturing, among other restrictions. Schedule I drugs are available for research only and have no approved medical use; Schedule II drugs are available only by prescription (unrefillable) and require a form for ordering. Schedule III and IV drugs are available by prescription, may have five refills in 6 months, and may be ordered orally. Some Schedule V drugs are available over the counter.

** Some of the health risks are directly related to the route of drug administration. For example, injection drug use can increase the risk of infection through needle contamination with staphylococci, HIV, hepatitis, and other organisms.

*** Associated with sexual assaults.

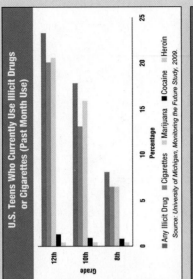

U.S. Teens Who Currently Use Illicit Drugs or Cigarettes (Past Month Use)

Source: University of Michigan, Monitoring the Future Study, 2009.

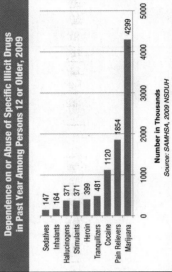

Dependence on or Abuse of Specific Illicit Drugs in Past Year Among Persons 12 or Older, 2009

	Number in Thousands
Sedatives	147
Inhalants	164
Hallucinogens	371
Stimulants	371
Heroin	399
Tranquilizers	481
Cocaine	1120
Pain Relievers	1854
Marijuana	4299

Source: SAMHSA, 2009 NSDUH

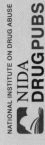

NATIONAL INSTITUTE ON DRUG ABUSE

DRUGPUBS

RESEARCH DISSEMINATION CENTER

Order NIDA publications from DrugPubs:
1-877-643-2644 or 1-240-645-0228 (TTY/TDD)

Revised March 2011
Reprinted April 2012

Principles of Drug Addiction Treatment

More than three decades of scientific research show that treatment can help drug-addicted individuals stop drug use, avoid relapse and successfully recover their lives. Based on this research, 13 fundamental principles that characterize effective drug abuse treatment have been developed. These principles are detailed in *NIDA's Principles of Drug Addiction Treatment: A Research-Based Guide*. The guide also describes different types of science-based treatments and provides answers to commonly asked questions.

1. **Addiction is a complex but treatable disease that affects brain function and behavior.** Drugs alter the brain's structure and how it functions, resulting in changes that persist long after drug use has ceased. This may help explain why abusers are at risk for relapse even after long periods of abstinence.

2. **No single treatment is appropriate for everyone.** Matching treatment settings, interventions, and services to an individual's particular problems and needs is critical to his or her ultimate success.

3. **Treatment needs to be readily available.** Because drug-addicted individuals may be uncertain about entering treatment, taking advantage of available services the moment people are ready for treatment is critical. Potential patients can be lost if treatment is not immediately available or readily accessible.

4. **Effective treatment attends to multiple needs of the individual, not just his or her drug abuse.** To be effective, treatment must address the individual's drug abuse and any associated medical, psychological, social, vocational, and legal problems.

5. **Remaining in treatment for an adequate period of time is critical.** The appropriate duration for an individual depends on the type and degree of his or her problems and needs. Research indicates that most addicted individuals need at least 3 months in treatment to significantly reduce or stop their drug use and that the best outcomes occur with longer durations of treatment.

6. **Counseling—individual and/or group—and other behavioral therapies are the most commonly used forms of drug abuse treatment.** Behavioral therapies vary in their focus and may involve addressing a patient's motivations to change, building skills to resist drug use, replacing drug-using activities with constructive and rewarding activities, improving problemsolving skills, and facilitating better interpersonal relationships.

7. **Medications are an important element of treatment for many patients, especially when combined with counseling and other behavioral therapies.** For example, methadone and buprenorphine are effective in helping individuals addicted to heroin or other opioids stabilize their lives and reduce their illicit drug use. Also, for persons addicted to nicotine, a nicotine replacement product (nicotine patches or gum) or an oral medication (bupropion or varenicline), can be an effective component of treatment when part of a comprehensive behavioral treatment program.

8. **An individual's treatment and services plan must be assessed continually and modified as necessary to ensure it meets his or her changing needs.** A patient may require varying combinations of services and treatment components during the course of treatment and recovery. In addition to counseling or psychotherapy, a patient may

require medication, medical services, family therapy, parenting instruction, vocational rehabilitation and/or social and legal services. For many patients, a continuing care approach provides the best results, with treatment intensity varying according to a person's changing needs.

9. **Many drug-addicted individuals also have other mental disorders.** Because drug abuse and addiction—both of which are forms of mental disorders—often co-occur with other mental illnesses, patients presenting with one condition should be assessed for the other(s). And when these problems co-occur, treatment should address both (or all), including the use of medications as appropriate.

10. **Medically assisted detoxification is only the first stage of addiction treatment and by itself does little to change long-term drug abuse.** Although medically assisted detoxification can safely manage the acute physical symptoms of withdrawal, detoxification alone is rarely sufficient to help addicted individuals achieve long-term abstinence. Thus, patients should be encouraged to continue drug treatment following detoxification.

11. **Treatment does not need to be voluntary to be effective.** Sanctions or enticements from family, employment settings, and/or the criminal justice system can significantly increase treatment entry, retention rates, and the ultimate success of drug treatment interventions.

12. **Drug use during treatment must be monitored continuously, as lapses during treatment do occur.** Knowing their drug use is being monitored can be a powerful incentive for patients and can help them withstand urges to use drugs. Monitoring also provides an early indication of a return to drug use, signaling a possible need to adjust an individual's treatment plan to better meet his or her needs.

13. **Treatment programs should assess patients for the presence of HIV/AIDS, hepatitis B and C, tuberculosis, and other infectious diseases, as well as provide targeted risk-reduction counseling to help patients modify or change behaviors that place them at risk of contracting or spreading infectious diseases.** Targeted counseling specifically focused on reducing infectious disease risk can help patients further reduce or avoid substance-related and other high-risk behaviors. Treatment providers should encourage and support HIV screening and inform patients that highly active antiretroviral therapy (HAART) has proven effective in combating HIV, including among drug-abusing populations.

This chart may be reprinted. Citation of the source is appreciated.

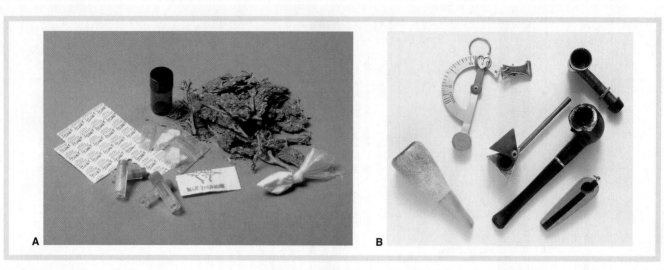

FIGURE 17–1

Illicit Drugs and Accessories

A. Illegal drugs come in tablets, vials, packets, and dried leaves. B. Pipes and weighing scales for illicit drug use.

Courtesy of Dorling Kindersley Media Library.

in the rate of prescription drug use, abuse, addictions, and deaths from lethal overdoses[3] (**FIGURE 17–1**).

Alcohol (which is not categorized as an illicit drug) is the most commonly abused substance, and adolescents use alcohol and tobacco more than any other drugs. These are often referred to as **gateway drugs** because these two substances often "open the gate" to more serious substance abuse problems and addictions. Most addictions develop during adolescence (**FIGURE 17–2**).

The development of smaller collection devices, screening techniques, clinical laboratory automation, molecular advances, and computer technology has increased the variety of laboratory testing options available for the diagnosis and treatment of drugs of abuse and analysis of specimens in remote locations or from crime scenes. The following sections will provide basic guidelines and resources for further information.

FIGURE 17–2

Alcohol Is the Most Commonly Abused Substance.

Courtesy of Dorling Kindersley Media Library.

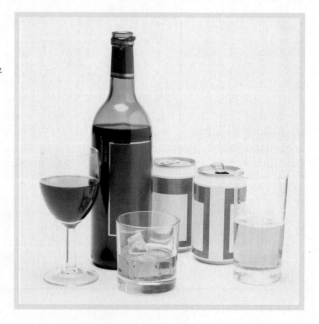

Health care workers who are responsible for collecting specimens for drug testing must ensure the specimen's integrity whether they work in a private health facility or in federal workplace drug-testing programs. All workplace drug-testing programs have numerous legal ramifications that require a high degree of vigilance by workers involved in the process. The major responsibilities for the specimen "collector," a term used in federal guidelines, include:

- Identification of both the donor and the specimen
- Prevention of specimen adulteration or substitution
- Tamper-proofing the collected specimen
- Initiation and accountability for the chain of custody
- Accurate and comprehensive documentation

Drug Analysis: Rationale, Methods, and Interferences

A drug **metabolite** is the compound produced when the body processes the drug. Identifying these metabolites is the focus of drug analysis because the metabolites are usually present in the body longer than the parent drug. For example, use of marijuana produces a large number of metabolites in the body, whereas amphetamines do not have any metabolites because the drug normally passes through the body unchanged in its chemical structure. Positive testing means that the individual has used the substance recently, although the so-called **window of detection** can vary with each drug. The window of detection is the period of time after using the drug that it is detectable. This time period is affected by the[2]

- Amount and type of drug taken
- Frequency of use
- Method that the drug was taken (inhaled, oral, injected)
- Rate the drug is metabolized in the body
- Cutoff concentration of the testing procedure
- User's physical condition (hydration, etc.)
- Body fat
- Other pathologic conditions (such as kidney disease)

The most common tests detect five specific drugs: amphetamines, cocaine, marijuana, opiates, and phencyclidine (PCP). Alcohol analysis is usually done separately. Urine drug tests are most common because they are the least expensive and minimally invasive to the person being tested. However, there are limitations to all drug tests and the specimens on which testing is performed. Refer to **BOX 17–2** for examples of specimens for drug testing and forensic analysis. For example, drug tests on urine can usually detect marijuana use within the past week; cocaine, heroin, and other hard drugs within the past 2 days, and alcohol use within the past several hours. Tests on hair can detect drug use over longer periods of time (approximately 10 to 90 days), depending on the length of the hair. However, they are more expensive and time consuming to perform and can be affected by hair treatments.

Drug tests do *not* measure the frequency of drug usage or the degree of impairment the person has, nor do drug tests determine if an individual has a disorder that requires treatment or a prescription. In addition, the testing cannot distinguish between prescription, over-the-counter, or illicit street drugs. For example, an over-the-counter pain reliever with codeine cannot be distinguished from illicit opiates.[3]

BOX 17–2

Drug Testing and Forensic Analysis

Specimens for Drug Testing
Urine (most common) (**FIGURE 17–3**)
Venous blood
Hair
Saliva
Breath
Nails
Sweat

Specimens for Forensic Analysis
(FIGURE 17–4)

- Anorectal swabs
- Arterial or venous blood
- Bones
- Capillary blood
- Clothing and fabrics (carpet, bed linens, etc.)
- Dried blood stains
- Hair
- Nails: nail scrapings or clippings
- Saliva, gastric fluid, bile
- Skin, sweat
- Sperm, semen residue
- Teeth: oral swabs
- Urine
- Vaginal swabs[4,5,6]

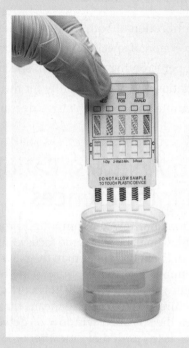

FIGURE 17–3
Urine (or Drug) Specimens

GIPhotoStock/Science Source

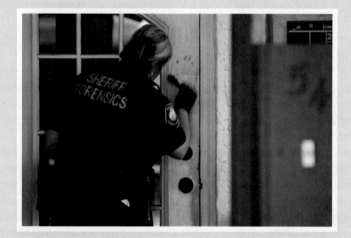

FIGURE 17–4
Crime Scene

© ZUMA Press, Inc./Alamy

Drug analysis uses two main methodologies: **qualitative tests,** often used for screenings that give only a positive or negative result, and **quantitative tests** that provide a definitive amount or level. Examples of each follow.

Point-of-care (POC) immunoassays (IAs) are often used for screening because of their low cost and rapid turnaround time; however, these tests are subject to many interfering factors such as ingestion of food products and drugs that resemble the analyte being tested. Their cutoff levels are high so that false-negative results may occur. In addition, POC tests can detect positivity or negativity for a class of drugs, but not distinguish specific drugs.[4]

Thin layer chromatography (TLC) is an older type of technology that is less commonly used and requires extensive skill in analysis. It can be used to test for multiple drugs; however, interfering substances can affect testing.

Gas chromatography (GC)–mass spectrometry (MS) has the highest degree of specificity for drug detection and is often used to confirm screening results; however, it is more expensive and time consuming to use. Mass spectrometry results are drug-specific and very sensitive and have become the industry standard.[4,5]

The following ingested substances can interfere with drug tests:

- Poppy seeds contain trace amounts of morphine and codeine.
- Coca leaf tea contains trace amounts of cocaine.
- Golden seal tea may cause false-negatives for tetrahydrocannibinol (THC) if tested by IA.
- Mahuang/ephedrine may cause false-positives for amphetamines if tested by IA.
- Ibuprofen may cause false-positives for barbiturates, benzodiazepines, and cannabinoids if tested by IA.
- Salicylates can cause false-negatives for cocaine if tested by IA.
- Dextromethorphan may cause false-positives for PCP and opiods if tested by IA.
- Fluconazole may cause false-negatives for cocaine by GC-MS.
- Narcotic analgesics such as hydrocodone and oxycodone can cause false-positives for opiates if tested by IA.[3]

Forensic Toxicology Specimens

Toxicology is the scientific study of poisons (including drugs), how they are detected, their actions in the human body, and the treatment of the conditions they produce. **Forensic specimens** are those substances involved in civil or criminal legal cases. **Forensic toxicology** involves testing specimens for poisons or drugs of abuse in legal cases.

In toxicologic analysis, very small amounts of analytes are usually found in the blood, urine, or other specimens obtained for analysis. Thus, the type of specimen (e.g., venous blood, arterial blood, urine, hair, meconium) and the materials and equipment used for collecting specimens for toxicologic analysis can greatly affect analytic results. The glass or plastic collection tube, cover, or both may contain materials that will contaminate and/or react with or absorb the analytes. Even oils or bacteria from dirty fingers that handle specimens may cause contamination. Thus, for toxicologic specimens, the health care worker must strictly adhere to the facility's laboratory guidelines for collection of these types of specimens.

Extensive training, experience, and supervision are required for collecting specimens for forensic analyses. Box 17–2 includes the types of specimens that may be used for forensic toxicology studies or other medical applications of a criminal investigation.

Forensic laboratory analysis is different from other types of laboratory analyses in the following ways:[6,7]

- Specimens are diverse, ranging from vaginal swabs in rape cases to contact lenses found on a sofa at a crime scene to blood clots from a subdural hematoma caused by a head injury.

- Specimens may be decomposing or have been exposed to the elements (rain, mud, mixed blood from multiple individuals).

- Specimens may be available in only trace amounts from a crime scene (a single hair or one smudge of blood).

- Specimens are often from autopsy procedures for **postmortem** (after death) testing to determine the cause of death and/or provide additional forensic evidence. Refer to **BOX 17–3** for greater details about forensic information from an autopsy.

- Forensic scientists must perform analyses in all types of environments, and their results must be able to stand up to the most intense judicial scrutiny.

Crime laboratories are involved in analyzing trace evidence (evidence found at the scene of the crime or on a person, such as fingerprints, shoe impressions, hairs, fibers, paint chips, glass fragments, soil samples); firearms and toolmarks (to analyze bullets and tool markings); drug chemistry (identification of drugs); toxicology (carbon monoxide, poisonings, drugs); arson and fire debris; biology and serology (semen stains, vaginal swabs from sexual assaults, crime scene specimens, DNA analysis); documents (paper, ink, type of printing, gum marks); and computers.[5]

DNA testing is particularly helpful because of its accuracy in identification. Many highly publicized trials hinge on the outcome of DNA testing, and inmates have been released because of a wrongful conviction proven by DNA testing. In sexual assault cases, only 20 to 45 percent of the victims show signs of bodily injuries; therefore, laboratory evidence is vital to support the victim's claims. In general, DNA analysis is useful for the following reasons:

- It is the same in all cells of the body (except eggs and sperm cells, which contain one-half of the DNA).

- It stays the same throughout life.

BOX 17–3

Forensic Information from an Autopsy

Forensic pathology is a fascinating field that has become popularized by television and movies because of the key role it plays in resolving criminal investigations and civil litigation. Forensic pathology involves anatomic or structural alterations of the body and clinical analysis that involves laboratory testing on body fluids and tissues.

During an autopsy, the forensic pathologist does a "gross examination" to determine the following:[7]

- Height and weight
- Color of hair, eyes, and skin
- Physical marks such as wounds, scars, tattoos, etc.
- Any other unusual physical features

The clinical portion of the autopsy includes:

- Dissection and measurement of internal organs
- Taking samples from tissues (brain, liver, lungs) for microscopic examinations
- Taking samples such as blood, fluid from the eye (vitreous humor, urine, bile, stomach contents for analysis)
- Selecting samples for toxicology testing, testing for infectious diseases, and other laboratory tests such as DNA typing

■   It is present in most cells.

■   It differs from one person to another, except in the case of identical twins.

All specimens must be labeled using permanent markers with the victim's name, sample, site, and, if possible, an identification number for reference. The evidence must pass directly from the medical examiner to the individuals who will process specimens, using a chain of custody signature process (described next). This provides a complete documentation system of all individuals who handle the specimen from the moment it is obtained until it is tested and stored or destroyed.

Chain of Custody

The primary difference between a clinical laboratory and forensic laboratory is that forensic laboratories are legally accountable for documentation of the handling of evidence within the organization. This documentation begins the moment that the specimens are received from the medical examiner's (county coroner) office. The **chain of custody** is a process for maintaining control of and accountability for each specimen from the time it is collected to the time of disposal. This process documents the identity of each individual who handles the specimen and each time a specimen is transferred in the chain. A chain of custody form is also required, which indicates specific identification of the patient, subject, or decedent (a deceased person); the individual who obtained and processed the specimen; and the date, location, and signature of the subject documenting that the specimen in the container is the one that was obtained from the person identified on the label. The specimen must be placed in a specimen transfer bag that is permanently sealed until it is opened for analysis. The seal ensures the "tamper-evident" transfer of contents until they reach the destination for analysis.[8]

Similar to the ability of workers to ensure the proper identification and accurate labeling requirements in a clinical laboratory, specially trained, experienced health care workers would also be able to handle the additional requirements for chain of custody specimens. Actually, many clinical laboratories also use the chain of custody—for example, with in-house drug-testing programs.

In contrast to the clinical laboratory, forensic specimens are accepted in any condition; that is, the specimens are often clotted and/or submitted in nontraditional containers, frequently after timing delays or exposure to the elements. Health care workers must cross-check that the requisitions from the medical examiner's office, as well as the name, age, sex, case number, and types of specimens collected, match up with the labeled evidence.[4]

Workplace Drug Testing

Workplace drug-testing programs initially began when the Department of Health and Human Services (HHS) established guidelines for federal drug-testing programs, as well as standards for certification of laboratories engaged in urine drug testing for federal agencies such as the U.S. Department of Transportation (DOT), Department of Defense (DOD), Nuclear Regulatory Commission (NRC), and the Department of Energy (DOE). Currently, the Department of Transportation, Office of Drug and Alcohol Policy and Compliance, provides standards for testing of specimens, quality assurance and quality control, the chain of custody form called the **Custody and Control Form (CCF),** personnel, and the reporting of results. Refer to **FIGURE 17–5** to view the Federal Drug Testing Custody and Control Form. **BOX 17–4** summarizes the rationale and procedures associated with drug-testing programs. The DOT guidelines and forms apply only to DOT-required testing. Other employers (nonfederal) or state programs may use these collection and testing procedures and may use forms similar to the federal CCF, but they must not use the federal CCF nor imply that they are conducting tests using DOT authority. The DOT guidelines

FEDERAL DRUG TESTING CUSTODY AND CONTROL FORM

Dyna Diagnostics Toxi Health Laboratory
1777 North Meade Street
South City, KS 60609

SPECIMEN ID NO. **0000001**

ACCESSION NO.

OMB No. 0930-0158

STEP 1: COMPLETED BY COLLECTOR OR EMPLOYER REPRESENTATIVE

A. Employer Name, Address, I.D. No.

ACME Transit
55 Broadway Road
Springfield, NE 99919
ID# 73765201

B. MRO Name, Address, Phone No. and Fax No.

Dr. Randall Clark
655 Main Street
Omaha, NE 99876
Phone: 372-885-9604 Fax: 372-885-9027

C. Donor SSN or Employee I.D. No. _123-45-6789_

D. Specify Testing Authority: ☐ HHS ☐ NRC ☒ DOT – Specify DOT Agency: ☐ FMCSA ☐ FAA ☐ FRA ☒ FTA ☐ PHMSA ☐ USCG

E. Reason for Test: ☐ Pre-employment ☒ Random ☐ Reasonable Suspicion/Cause ☐ Post Accident ☐ Return to Duty ☐ Follow-up ☐ Other (specify) _____

F. Drug Tests to be Performed: ☒ THC, COC, PCP, OPI, AMP ☐ THC & COC Only ☐ Other (specify) _____

G. Collection Site Address:

Geturco
4301 Powers Rd.
Smithfield, NE 99724

Collector Phone No. _505-403-1655_
Collector Fax No. _505-403-1919_

STEP 2: COMPLETED BY COLLECTOR (make remarks when appropriate) Collector reads specimen temperature within 4 minutes.

| Temperature between 90° and 100° F? ☒ Yes ☐ No, Enter Remark | Collection: ☒ Split ☐ Single | ☐ None Provided, Enter Remark | ☐ Observed, Enter Remark |

REMARKS

STEP 3: Collector affixes bottle seal(s) to bottle(s). Collector dates seal(s). Donor initials seal(s). Donor completes STEP 5 on Copy 2 (MRO Copy)

STEP 4: CHAIN OF CUSTODY - INITIATED BY COLLECTOR AND COMPLETED BY TEST FACILITY

I certify that the specimen given to me by the donor identified in the certification section on Copy 2 of this form was collected, labeled, sealed and released to the Delivery Service noted in accordance with applicable Federal requirements.

SPECIMEN BOTTLE(S) RELEASED TO:

X _Richard K. Anderson_
Signature of Collector

Richard K. Anderson
(PRINT) Collector's Name (First, MI, Last)

7, 13, 12   10:17 AM/PM
Date (Mo/Day/Yr)   Time of Collection

FedEx - UPS Co.
Name of Delivery Service

STEP 5: COMPLETED BY DONOR

I certify that I provided my urine specimen to the collector; that I have not adulterated it in any manner; each specimen bottle used was sealed with a tamper-evident seal in my presence; and that the information provided on this form and on the label affixed to each specimen bottle is correct.

X _Roberta Gomez_
Signature of Donor

Roberta Gomez
(PRINT) Donor's Name (First, MI, Last)

7, 13, 12
Date (Mo/Day/Yr)

Daytime Phone No. _555-494-3131_   Evening Phone No. _555-617-4424_   Date of Birth _12, 22, 77_
(Mo/Day/Yr)

After the Medical Review Officer receives the test results for the specimen identified by this form, he/she may contact you to ask about prescriptions and over-the-counter medications you may have taken. Therefore, you may want to make a list of those medications for your own records. THIS LIST IS NOT NECESSARY. If you choose to make a list, do so either on a separate piece of paper or on the back of your copy (Copy 5). – DO NOT PROVIDE THIS INFORMATION ON THE BACK OF ANY OTHER COPY OF THE FORM. TAKE COPY 5 WITH YOU.

STEP 6: COMPLETED BY MEDICAL REVIEW OFFICER - PRIMARY SPECIMEN

In accordance with applicable Federal requirements, my verification is:

☐ NEGATIVE ☐ POSITIVE for: _____
　　　☐ DILUTE

☐ REFUSAL TO TEST because – check reason(s) below: ☐ TEST CANCELLED
　　　☐ ADULTERATED (adulterant/reason): _____
　　　　　☐ SUBSTITUTED
　　　　　　☐ OTHER: _____

REMARKS: _____

X _____
Signature of Medical Review Officer

(PRINT) Medical Review Officer's Name (First, MI, Last)

_____/_____/_____
Date (Mo/Day/Yr)

STEP 7: COMPLETED BY MEDICAL REVIEW OFFICER - SPLIT SPECIMEN

In accordance with applicable Federal requirements, my verification for the split specimen (if tested) is:

☐ RECONFIRMED for: _____   ☐ TEST CANCELLED

☐ FAILED TO RECONFIRM for: _____

REMARKS: _____

X _____
Signature of Medical Review Officer

(PRINT) Medical Review Officer's Name (First, MI, Last)

_____/_____/_____
Date (Mo/Day/Yr)

COPY 4 - EMPLOYER COPY

A

FIGURE 17–5

Federal Drug Testing

A. Custody and Control Form.

Federal Transit Administration Drug and Alcohol Program

UNEVENTFUL URINE COLLECTION – Did the collector ...

☐ Require employee to provide positive identification (Part 40.61(c)).

☐ Explain basic collection procedure, show employee instructions on back of CCF (Part 40.61(e)).

☐ Direct the employee to remove outer clothing (jacket, hat) and to leave these garments and other personal items (briefcase, purse, etc.) in a mutually agreeable location (Part 40.61(f)).
  - ○ Advises employee that failure to comply constitutes a refusal to test.
  - ○ Allows employee to keep wallet (40.61(f)(2)).

☐ Direct employee to empty pockets and display items in them (Part 40.61(f)(4)).
  - ○ If no potential adulterants are found, allow employee to return items to pockets.

☐ Use the Federal Drug Testing Custody and Control Form (OMB No. 0930-0158) (40.45(a)).

☐ Complete Step 1 of CCF (Part 40.63(a)).
  - ○ Ensure that the name and address of the HHS-certified lab or HHS-certified IITF are on the top of the CCF.
  - ○ Ensures that the Specimen ID at the top of the CCF matches the Specimen ID on labels/seals.
  - ○ Checks the Specify Testing Authority (DOT) and the Specify DOT Agency checkboxes.
  - ○ Checks the Reason for Test box (Pre-Employment, Random, Post-Accident, etc.).
  - ○ Checks the Drug Tests to Be Performed box (THC, COC, PCP, OPI, AMP for DOT).

☐ Instruct employee to wash/dry hands and not to wash hands again until delivering specimen to collector (Part 40.63(b)).

☐ Ensure collection container is selected and unwrapped in presence of employee (Part 40.63(c)).

☐ Secure urination facility before the collection (If single-toilet room with a full-length privacy door) (Parts 40.41 & 43).
  - ○ Secures any water sources or make them unavailable to employees (e.g., turn off water inlet, tape handles to prevent opening faucets).
  - ○ Ensures that the water in the toilet tank contains bluing agent.
  - ○ Ensures that soap, disinfectants, cleaning agents, or other possible adulterants are not present.
  - ○ Inspects the site to ensure that no foreign or unauthorized substances are present.
  - ○ Tapes or otherwise securely shuts any movable toilet tank or puts bluing agent in the tank.
  - ○ Ensures that undetected access (e.g., through a door not in your view) is not possible.
  - ○ Secures areas and items (e.g., ledges, trash receptacles, paper-towel holders, under-sink areas, drop-down ceiling panels) that appear suitable for concealing contaminants.

☐ Direct employee to go into room used for urination and instruct employee to:
  - ○ Provide at least 45 ml of urine.
  - ○ Not flush the toilet.
  - ○ Return specimen to the collector as soon as the void is complete.
  - ○ Allow only the employee into the room used for urination (40.41(d)(1)).

☐ Check that the specimen:
  - ○ Contains at least 45 ml of urine. If not, follow shy bladder procedure (Part 40.65(a)).
  - ○ Reads temperature strip within 4 minutes (Part 40.65(b)).

☐ Mark appropriate box in Step 2 of CCF (Yes = between 90 and 100 degrees).

☐ Check specimen for signs of tampering (Part 40.65).

☐ Check specimen for unusual color, foreign objects/material, or other signs of tampering (odor).

☐ Mark box in Step 2 of the CCF indicating a split specimen collection (Part 40.71(b)(1)).

☐ Pour at least 30 ml of urine into the primary specimen bottle (Part 40.71(b)(2)).

☐ Pour at least 15 ml of urine into the secondary specimen bottle (Part 40.71(b)(3)).

☐ Secure the lids or caps on the specimen bottles (Part 40.71(b)(4)).

☐ Place the tamper-evident seals on the specimen bottles (Part 40.71(b)(5)).
  - ○ Dates the specimen bottle seals, after affixed to the bottle (Part 40.71(b)(5)).
  - ○ Ensures that the <u>employee</u> initials specimen bottle seals (Part 40.71(b)(7)).

☐ Direct employee to read and sign certification statement on Copy (MRO) 2, Step 5 of CCF and to provide date of birth, printed name, day and evening contact telephone numbers (Part 40.71(a)(1)).

☐ Print collector name in Copy 1, Step 4 of CCF; record the date and time of collection; sign statement; enter actual name of delivery service transferring the specimen to laboratory (Part 40.73(a)(2)).

☐ Ensure that all copies of the CCF are legible and complete (Part 40.73(a)(3)).

☐ Remove Copy 5 of the CCF and give it to the employee (Part 40.73(a)(4)).

☐ Place specimen bottles and Copy 1 of CCF in plastic bag and secure both pouches of plastic bag (Part 40.73(a)(5)-(a)(6)).

☐ Advise employee that he/she may leave the site (Part 40.73(a)(7)).

☐ Place plastic bag in shipping container and seal container as appropriate (Part 40.73(a)(8)(i)-(ii)).

☐ Recheck the urination facility, performing all steps as was done prior to the collection to ensure the site's continued integrity.

☐ Conduct the collection for only one employee at a time (40.43(d)(1)).

For additional information, go to www.fta.dot.gov (Click on SAFETY & SECURITY)

B

FIGURE 17–5 (*continued*)

B. Checklist for Uneventful Urine Collection.

BOX 17–4

Drug Testing in the Workplace

Workplace drug-testing programs are used for one or more of the following reasons:

- To comply with federal regulations
- To comply with customer or contract requirements and insurance carrier requirements
- To minimize the chances of hiring employees who are drug users/abusers
- To reinforce a "no drug use" policy
- To identify users and refer them for assistance
- To establish reasons for disciplinary actions
- To improve safety and the health of employees, and to reduce addiction

The types of industries that are required by the Department of Transportation to participate in antidrug programs include:

- Aviation, highway, railroad, mass transit, pipeline, hazardous materials transport, maritime, and other safety-sensitive industries.

Situations in which drug testing is appropriate or necessary include the following:

- **Preemployment testing**—Job offers are made only after a negative drug test.
- **Prepromotion tests**—Employee testing takes place prior to getting a promotion.
- **Annual physical tests**—As a result of physical exams, users/abusers can be identified so they can be referred for assistance and/or disciplinary action.
- **Reasonable suspicion/for-cause tests**—Employees who show signs of being impaired or have documented patterns of unsafe work practices can be identified.
- **Random tests**—Random testing, which involves testing at unpredictable times, is commonly used in safety- or security-sensitive jobs.
- **Postaccident/injury tests**—Used to determine if drugs or alcohol were a factor in an employee being involved in an incident and/or accident.
- **Treatment follow-up or clearance to return to work**—Periodic testing is done for employees after they have participated in a rehabilitation program.
- **Compliance with investigations of child or elder abuse**
- **Operation of company vehicles when drug/alcohol use is suspected**

The consequences of testing positive are serious and involve important aspects for the employer and employee:

- Employees must be knowledgeable of the consequences of testing positive. For example, actions might include paid or unpaid leave, referral to an employee assistance program, automatic discharge, disciplinary actions, and/or appeals procedures.

Testing procedures:

- Institutional procedures for drug testing are normally a part of the workplace drug-testing program with which employees must be familiar.
- Information may include where specimens will be collected and tested, how results will be reported, the chain of custody, the drugs and cutoff levels used to determine if a test is positive or negative, and the confirmatory tests used if the initial test is positive.
- The time to detect drugs is dependent on metabolic rate, dose of the drug, how it was taken, and the cutoff concentrations used by each laboratory. Drugs are generally detectable for several days.
- Employees should be aware and thoroughly trained in all of the procedures.[8]

BOX 17–5

Guidelines for Federal Drug Testing Custody and Control Form

The Federal Drug Testing Custody and Control Form (CCF) (Figure 17–5) must be used to document the handling and storage of specimens from the time a donor gives the specimen to the collector to the final disposition of the specimen. The CCF is obtained from the approved collection sites or laboratories performing the testing. Collectors must be trained and evaluated using federal guidelines. In general, training includes:

1. Knowing the identification processes—including name, identification, and contact information of the employer, the medical review officer (MRO), and the donor; the reason for the test (e.g., random, preemployment); and tests to be performed.
2. Giving the donor instructions about specimen collection and handling—including sealing the specimen after the collector records the temperature, and noting if it is a split or single or second specimen, if it was an "observed" collection and why, and if no collection was obtained and why (e.g., unable to urinate or "shy bladder").
3. Monitoring and documenting all circumstances that might indicate adulteration or substitution of the specimen.
4. Assuring that copies of the CCF go to the correct destinations (including the employee being tested).

are discussed in **BOX 17–5** because they do apply to many industries; however, special training and evaluation is required to be authorized for federal drug testing. **TABLE 17–2** indicates the classes of drugs that are tested and the drug concentration cutoff levels. These levels, developed by the Department of Health and Human Services, Substance Abuse and Mental Health Services Administration, determine whether a test is positive or negative and have been proven to be accurate, reliable, and defensible in court.[1,2]

The collector is the key to the success of a drug-testing program and is the one individual with whom all donors will have direct, face-to-face contact: "A collector is a trained individual who instructs and assists a donor at a collection site, receives and makes an initial inspection of the urine specimen provided by a donor, and initiates and completes the Federal Drug Testing Custody and Control Form (CCF)."[8] If the collector does not ensure the integrity of the specimen and adhere to the collection process, the specimen may not be considered a valid piece of evidence. If a specimen is reported positive for a drug or metabolite, the entire collection process must be able to withstand the closest scrutiny and all challenges to its integrity.[8] Figure 17–5 indicates the basic format of the DOT CCF, and Table 17–2 indicates drug cutoff concentrations used by certified laboratories to test urine specimens.

As with other types of specimens, the collector for an employee drug-testing program must appropriately identify the individual being tested. Acceptable forms of identification include:

1. A photo identification (driver's license, employee badge issued by the employer, picture identification issued by a federal, state, or local government agency), or
2. Identification by an employer or employer representative, or
3. Any other identification allowed under an operating administration's rules.[8]

   Unacceptable forms of identification include:

1. Identification by a coworker
2. Identification by another safety-sensitive employee
3. Use of a single nonphoto identification card (e.g., Social Security card, credit card, union or other membership cards, pay vouchers, voter registration card)
4. Faxed or photocopies of identification document.[8]

TABLE 17-2

Drug Cutoff Concentrations

The following cutoff concentrations are used by certified laboratories to test urine specimens collected by federal agencies and by employers regulated by the Department of Transportation.

Effective Date: October 1, 2010

Reference: Federal Register, November 25, 2008 (73 FR 7 1858), Section 3.4

Initial test analyte	Initial test cutoff concentration	Confirmatory test analyte	Confirmatory test cutoff concentration
Marijuana metabolites	50 ng/mL	THCA[1]	15 ng/mL
Cocaine metabolites	150 ng/mL	Benzoylecgonine	100 ng/mL
Opiate metabolites Codeine/Morphine[2]	2000 ng/mL	Codeine	2000 ng/mL
		Morphine	2000 ng/mL
6-Acetylmorphine	10 ng/mL	6-Acetylmorphine	10 ng/mL
Phencyclidine	25 ng/mL	Phencyclidine	25 ng/mL
Amphetamines[3] AMP/MAMP[4]	500 ng/mL	Amphetamine	250 ng/mL
		Methamphetamine[5]	250 ng/mL
MDMA[6]	500 ng/mL	MDMA	250 ng/mL
		MDA[7]	250 ng/mL
		MDEA[8]	250 ng/mL

[1] Delta-9-tetrahydrocannabinol-9-carboxylic acid (THCA)
[2] Morphine is the target analyte for codeine/morphine testing.
[3] Either a single initial test kit or multiple initial test kits may be used provided the single test kit detects each target analyte independently at the specified cutoff.
[4] Methamphetamine is the target analyte for amphetamine/methamphetamine testing.
[5] To be reported as positive for methamphetamine, a specimen must also contain amphetamine at a concentration equal to or greater than 100 ng/mL.
[6] Methylenedioxymethamphetamine (MDMA).
[7] Methylenedioxyamphetamine (MDA).
[8] Methylenedioxyethylamphetamine (MDEA).

Tampering with Specimens

The Department of Transportation and many other employers use split urine specimen collections for drug testing. This is accomplished after the individual being tested provides the collector with approximately 45 mL of urine in an acceptable container. The collector must inspect the specimen immediately to check for signs of tampering, such as unusual color, presence of foreign objects or material, or temperature that is outside the required range (32° to 38°C/90° to 100°F). The collector must check the temperature no later than 4 minutes after the individual being tested comes out of the restroom and hands over the specimen. The collector, not the individual being tested, then pours at least 30 mL of urine from the collection container into a specimen bottle and places the cap on the bottle. This will be the primary specimen, or "A" bottle. The collector, not the individual being tested, then pours at least 15 mL of urine into a second bottle and places the cap on it. This will be the "B" bottle used for the split specimen.

Drug users have become very imaginative in devising ways to avoid a positive drug test result. Adulteration is a means of tampering with the specimen, usually urine, to make the specimen test negative for drugs. It occurs in two ways: The person ingests substances to alter his or her own urine or the person adds or substitutes substances for urine at the time of collection. Water is the most common substance added to the specimen or ingested to dilute the urine so that the drug concentrations are below the detection limit. Other substances that have been added to urine include liquid soap, bleach, salt, ammonia, vinegar, baking soda, UrinAid (glutaraldehyde), Klear (potassium nitrite), lemon juice, and cologne.[2,8]

Detecting and deterring adulterants in urine can occur by:

- Sensory examination (odor and color) of the urine—for example, bleach odor, foaming, or turbidity can be a sign of a liquid soap additive.

- Taking urine temperature within 4 minutes after the donor provides the specimen. Urine samples for drug testing contain a temperature strip affixed to the container.

- Simple tests such as specific gravity (it should not be less than 1.003 or greater than 1.025), urine creatinine (less than 20 mg/dL), and electrolytes (to determine values outside the physiologic range). Klear can be detected as a strong positive nitrite in a urine specimen with no bacteria present.

- Adding bluing to the toilet water, and preventing the patient from taking unneeded items into the collection stall.

- Direct observation of devices used to tamper with the specimen (tubing connected to a heated urine container and worn under clothing).

If tampering is suspected or observed, the health care worker may request another specimen and, in some cases, conduct another collection procedure under direct observation. Federal guidelines are extensive and extremely strict about the circumstances for these measures; however, there are situations when they are required (**BOX 17–6**).

Drug Testing in the Private Sector

Many private-sector employers, including hospitals and clinics, also have workplace drug-testing procedures in place, and the testing guidelines may vary slightly from the federal standards. However, private industries often elect to use laboratories that comply with the federal standards. For purposes of this review, the federal guidelines are discussed. Employees may be tested without prior notice; therefore, the collection procedure, processing, analysis, and reporting are strict and well defined. Also, private employers may request that the certified laboratory test for several drugs or drug classes other than those required by the federal agencies, or they may use different testing levels for initial or confirmatory tests.

BOX 17–6

DOT's 10 Steps to Collection Site Security and Integrity

1. Pay careful attention to the individual employee being tested.
2. Ensure that there is no unauthorized access into the collection areas and that undetected access (e.g., through a door not in view) is not possible.
3. Make sure that employees show proper picture ID.
4. Make sure employees empty pockets; remove outer garments (coveralls, jacket, coat, hat); leave briefcases, purses, and bags behind; and wash their hands.
5. Maintain personal control of the specimen and CCF at all times during the collection.
6. Secure any water sources or otherwise make them unavailable to the employee (e.g., turn off water inlet, tape handles to prevent opening faucets, secure tank lids).
7. Ensure that the water in the toilet and tank has a bluing (coloring) agent in it. Tape or otherwise secure shut any movable toilet tank top or put bluing in the tank.
8. Ensure that no soap, disinfectants, cleaning agents, or other possible adulterants are present.
9. Inspect the site to ensure that no foreign or unauthorized substances are present.
10. Secure areas and items (e.g., ledges, trash receptacles, paper towel holders, under sink areas, ceiling tiles) that appear suitable for concealing adulterants

Office of Drug and Alcohol Policy and Compliance, U.S. Department of Transportation, www.dot.gov, accessed July 8, 2013.

Drug Use in Sports

The use of drugs and performance-enhancing substances in sports has become more prevalent and highly publicized in recent years. Drug use occurs at many levels of competitive sports, including collegiate (e.g., National Collegiate Athletic Association [NCAA]) and professional (e.g., National Basketball Association [NBA], Major League Baseball [MLB], the National Football League [NFL]), and the Olympics.

The NCAA Drug-Testing Program tests more than 10,000 student athletes annually. The program involves urine collection on specific occasions and laboratory analyses for substances on a list of banned-drug classes developed by the NCAA Executive Committee. The list is regularly updated and consists of substances that are performance-enhancing and/or potentially harmful to the student athlete. Many nutritional/dietary supplements are not well regulated and contain chemical substances banned by the NCAA. Since the U.S. Food and Drug Administration (FDA) does not regulate the supplement industry, impure supplements may lead to positive NCAA drug tests and the loss of the athlete's eligibility to compete. The NCAA banned drugs (and substances that are chemically related to these classes) include this partial list:[9]

- Stimulants, such as amphetamines (Adderall), caffeine (guarana), cocaine, ephedrine, fenfluramine (Fen), methamphetamine, methylphenidate (Ritalin), phentermine (Phen), synephrine (bitter orange), methylhexaneamine, "bath salts" (mephedrone), etc.
- Anabolic steroids, sometimes listed as a chemical formula like 3,6,17-androstenetrione, boldenone, clenbuterol, DHEA(7-keto), nandrolone, stanozolol, testosterone, etc.
- Alcohol and Beta blockers (banned for rifle competition only)
- Diuretics (water pills) and other masking agents
- Street drugs, such as heroin, marijuana, tetrahydrocannabinol (TCH), synthetic cannabinoids (spice, K2), etc.
- Peptide hormones and analogues, including growth hormone (hGH), human chorionic gonadotropin (hCG), erythropoietin (EPO), etc.
- Anti-estrogens, such as tamoxifen, etc.
- Beta-2 agonists, including bambuterol, formoterol, etc.

BLOOD DOPING AND THE USE OF ERYTHROPOIETIN (EPO)

The NCAA and the International Olympic Committee (IOC) prohibit the practice of "blood doping," whereby whole blood, packed red blood cells, or blood substitutes are injected intravenously in athletes who try to increase their oxygen-carrying capacity and thereby increase endurance by overloading their system with erythrocytes or drugs such as recombinant human erythropoietin (rHuEPO), a genetically engineered protein almost identical to the natural EPO. Naturally occurring EPO increases the body's production of red blood cells, thereby increasing the oxygen-carrying capacity. The administration of rHuEPO is given to individuals for legitimate medical treatment of renal failure and for anemia secondary to renal failure. However, it has also been associated with serious cardiovascular problems, iron overload, strokes, and deaths. Although EPO is hard to detect, recent advances in blood and urine testing are becoming strong deterrents and testing methods can tell the difference between rHuEPO and natural EPO.

Neonatal Drug Testing

Pregnant women who use drugs pass the drugs to their unborn child. Many health problems are associated with neonatal drug exposure, including premature birth, low birth weight, impaired neurological functioning, and a higher risk of abuse and neglect.[10] Neonatal drug exposure is determined by using the maternal history, newborn clinical symptoms, and laboratory toxicology testing of the mother and infant. Cocaine is the drug most often identified in neonatal drug testing. Other drugs include opiates (including heroin, morphine, codeine, and other narcotics such as hydromorphone and hydrocodone), amphetamine and methamphetamines, and phencyclidine (PCP).

Urine is the specimen most often used for neonatal drug exposure. Collection is possible by using neonatal urine collection bags and collecting the urine during the first 24 hours after birth. If the infant's urine is positive, it generally means that the mother used drugs 24 to 72 hours prior to childbirth. **Meconium,** the first intestinal discharge of a neonate, is greenish and consists of epithelial cells, mucus, and bile. Meconium is also used for drug analysis; the specimen is easier to collect than urine. Since meconium accumulates in the fetal bowel at approximately 16 weeks of gestation, a positive result indicates drug exposure to the neonate months before the birth. Other specimens used are amniotic fluids, cord blood, and gastric fluid; however, they are less suitable because of poor recovery of drugs from these samples.[10]

Blood Alcohol and Breath Testing

The number of deaths caused by drunk drivers is significant because the rate of fatal crash risk is 6 to 10 times higher (depending on age) when an individual is driving with an alcohol level at the legal limit.[11] It is a crime in all 50 states (and most countries) to drive a vehicle (and in some states, a bicycle or boat) while under the influence of alcohol and/or drugs. The drugs need not be illegal and can be prescription or over-the-counter (OTC) medications. There are many terms that refer to the condition whereby mental and motor skills are impaired. These terms include *alcohol-impaired driving,* **driving under the influence (DUI)** *of alcohol, driving while intoxicated (DWI), drunk driving, drinking and driving,* and *drink-driving.* Most countries have specified legal limits for **blood alcohol content (BAC),** or the concentration of alcohol in blood. It is usually expressed as a percentage. For example, the legal limit of BAC in the United States is 0.08 percent, or 80 mg per 100 mL. Drivers under the age of 21 are not allowed to drive with any detectable blood alcohol.

Individuals with a BAC of 0.08 percent or greater are subject to fines and/or imprisonment and/or having their license revoked. In some states, convicted drunk drivers are required to use an interlock, a breath device linked to the ignition of their vehicle so that if the BAC limit is exceeded, the ignition will not start.

There are hundreds of analyzers and methods for testing alcohol levels in blood, breath, and urine. As with all testing devices, there is variability in the methodology, accuracy, and reliability of each. The most accurate BAC is tested using a standard blood specimen, either from a venipuncture or fingerstick and can be performed on a variety of analyzers. However, health care workers who collect these specimens should recall from Chapter 10 that alcohol preps *should not* be used to cleanse a puncture site if testing for blood alcohol because of the possibility that the residual alcohol from the pad will cause a false positive or an elevation in the test results.

Patient variables that affect the blood alcohol content include:

- Gender (men and women are slightly different in the ways they process alcohol)
- Weight or amount of body fat
- Amount of alcohol ingested
- Other foods ingested
- Time elapsed since the ingestion
- Effects of other drugs in the body

How many drinks does it take to get to the legal limit? There is no definitive answer to this question because of differences in physiological and individual alcohol tolerance, but there are several smart phone apps and online calculators (see additional resources at the end of the chapter) that "estimate" the number based on standard assumptions for alcohol content and these individual characteristics. Generally speaking, using the number of drinks to estimate intoxication is not useful information (**BOX 17–7**).

BOX 17–7

Sobriety Tests

If a law-enforcement officer suspects that you are driving under the influence (swerving, speeding, failing to stop, caused injury, etc.), you may be stopped, and he or she may ask you to do one of the following field sobriety tests:[11,12]

- Perform a balance test by walking a straight line (heel to toe), or standing on one leg, or standing feet together and leaning the head back to look up at the sky while holding arms out to the side, or checking finger-to-nose hand coordination (**FIGURE 17–6**).

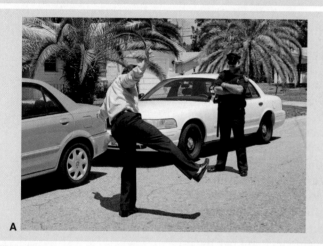 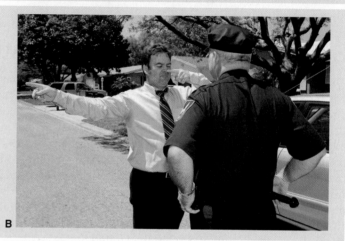

FIGURE 17–6

Field Sobriety Test

A. Balance test. **B.** Finger-to-nose hand coordination.

© Lisa F. Young/Fotolia

- Perform a speech test by reciting a line of letters, the alphabet, numbers, or counting backwards.
- Look for pupil enlargement or constriction.

If you fail these tests, the officer may ask you to take a chemical test or may arrest you. State regulations vary about whether you are given a choice of test to take (blood, breath, or urine). And in most states, refusal to cooperate with the testing can result in penalties such as suspension of your driver's license.

Breathalyzers (devices into which the person breathes) are often used in the field by law-enforcement personnel because they are economical, easy to use, less invasive than a venipuncture, portable, and provide fast results. Since measurements taken from breath are not actually blood levels, they are a calculated ratio of the alcohol content in the breath to estimates of alcohol in the blood. (The same is generally true for urine test results that estimate BAC.) Thus, there is a higher risk of inaccurate results and they may not be admissible in court. In some cases, handheld breathalyzers are used only as a pass–fail, field sobriety test to help determine probable cause for an arrest. Breath tests are affected by

- Ambient temperature
- Individual breathing patterns (hyperventilation or after exercising)
- Diet
- Fever

Future Trends

In the United States, the demand for faster, more sophisticated drug detection is significant. Thus, the technology field is rapidly developing specialized tests and testing panels for drugs of abuse. Employers in the transportation industry, homeland security, health care, and criminal justice systems are demanding rapid onsite testing. At the same time, drug users have become more sophisticated at finding ways to alter test results. Unfortunately, many products available on the Internet describe their ability to adulterate drug test results. Future technology will therefore be aimed at better, faster drug detection methods while tightening the ability to adulterate specimens.

Study Questions

For the following questions, select the one best answer.

1 Which of the following is an example of an illicit drug?

   a. tobacco

   b. alcohol

   c. heroin

   d. valium

2 Forensic toxicology is the

   a. study of hair and nails

   b. performance of urine drug screens

   c. study of toxins in legal cases

   d. acquisition of specimens for criminal cases

3 Gateway drugs include

   a. alcohol and tobacco

   b. marijuana and crack

   c. heroin and cocaine

   d. ecstasy and LSD

4 Forensic specimens are those involved in which of the following?

   a. routine testing for diabetes

   b. legal cases/criminal investigations

   c. urine screening for preemployment physicals

   d. random drug screens

5 What is the purpose of a chain of custody process?

   a. maintain control of the donor who gives the specimen

   b. account for a specimen from point of collection to final disposition

   c. specimen identification

   d. provide privacy to the donor

6 Urine specimen containers used in federal workplace testing usually have which of the following?

   a. designated area for a fingerprint

   b. temperature strips

   c. aliquot identification

   d. confidentiality notices

7 A bluing color agent is used to

   a. detect adulteration in a urine specimen

   b. indicate a positive result on a drug screen

   c. distinguish one forensic specimen from another

   d. indicate a negative result on a drug screen

8 In a clinical laboratory, a low-cost, rapid analytical method used for drug screening is

   a. immunoassay

   b. thin layer chromatography

   c. gas chromatography

   d. molecular analysis

9 An example of a field sobriety test is:

   a. diabetic screen

   b. NCAA drug screen

   c. blood alcohol level

   d. balance test

10 An employee in the airline industry may be screened for drugs in which of the following circumstances?

   a. randomly

   b. upon retirement

   c. when going on vacation

   d. when renewing a driver's license

Case Study 1

Identity in Workplace Drug-Testing Programs A health care worker is assigned to be the collector in a federal drug-testing program. Jake Washington, a new employee, shows up for a urine drug screen with his friend. Jake has a jacket and sweater on and is carrying a backpack. When the collector begins the process for specimen collection, she suggests that the friend wait in a chair nearby and then asks Jake for a photo identification card. He states that he has not yet been given an ID card and that he does not have a driver's license with him. Jake offers that he has a copy of his old college identification card. His friend overhears the conversation and says, "I can vouch for him—I've known him for five years." Jake then adds, "Yeah, he knows me well, so could we just go ahead and collect the specimen?" Both Jake and his friend seem nervous.

Questions

1 What should the collector do to identify the employee?

2 What concerns are apparent in this situation?

Case Study 2

Time and Temperature for Urine Drug Tests Lisa, an airline employee who was involved in an accident, was sent to provide a urine specimen for drug testing. After the proper identification procedures and use of the correct specimen container, Lisa walked out of the bathroom with her specimen and gave it to the health care worker for further processing. The health care worker was busy answering the telephone and trying to catch up with paperwork and before she knew it, 10 minutes had elapsed before she remembered to process the urine specimen.

Questions

1 What did the health care worker do wrong?

2 What factors is the health care worker supposed to check after the urine specimen is provided?

Action in Practice

Did you know that hair contains a record of what was consumed by an individual? Trace amounts of ingested substances can become part of the hair's composition. This is particularly important in forensic hair analysis because poisons such as lead or arsenic can be detected. Hair analysis can detect what and how long ago something was ingested, so the longer the hair length, the longer the record of what was consumed by that individual.

Questions

1 What might the health care worker's role be in forensic hair analysis?

2 Does the length of time after collecting the forensic hair specimen make any difference?

COMPETENCY ASSESSMENT

Check Yourself

1 What are the most commonly used drugs by adolescents?

2 Name one example of each of the following drug categories:

Stimulant

Depressant

Cannabinoid

Opioid

Inhalant

Competency Checklist

This checklist can be completed as a group or individually.

(1) Completed (2) Needs to improve

_____　1.　List five specimens that might be used in a forensic evaluation.
_____　2.　Name three ways that substance abuse affects health care.
_____　3.　Name the three specimens used for measuring or estimating BAC.
_____　4.　Describe at least five steps for ensuring a safe specimen collection site for a workplace drug program.
_____　5.　Describe three ways a health care worker can tell if a urine specimen for drug testing has been adulterated.

REFERENCES

1. Centers for Disease Control and Prevention. (2012). Health, United States, 2012, Trend Tables, Use of Selected substances among high school seniors, 10th graders, and 8th graders, by sex and race: United States, selected years 1980–2011, www.cdc.gov, accessed July 5, 2013.

2. Get the Facts: Drug Testing, Basic Data. (n.d.), DrugWarFacts.org, accessed July 5, 2013.

3. U.S. Department of Health and Human Services. (2011, October). Drug testing welfare recipients: Recent proposals and continuing controversies, http://aspe.hhs.gov/hsp/11?DrugTesting/ib.pdf, accessed July 6, 2013.

4. Owens, G. T. (2013, June 4). Mass spectroscopy-confirmed UDT (urine drug testing) for monitoring controlled substances has become a standard of care. *Advance for Med. Lab. Professionals*, www.laboratorian.advanceweb.com, accessed July 8, 2013.

5. Neerman, M. F. (2006). Drugs of abuse: Analyses and ingested agents that can induce interference or cross-reactivity, *Lab Med, 37*(6): 358–361.

6. Daniel, P. J. (2007). Career alternatives: A phlebotomist in forensics? *Lab Med, 38*(5): 271–272.

7. American Association for Clinical Chemistry. (2010, June 3, and 2012, May 7). Lab tests online, the world of forensic laboratory testing, forensic pathology and autopsies, http://labtestsonline.org, accessed July 8, 2013.

8. U.S. Department of Transportation, Office of Drug and Alcohol Policy and Compliance. (2010, October 1). Urine specimen collection guidelines, www.dot.gov, accessed July 8, 2013.

9. National Collegiate Athletic Association (NCAA). (n.d.). 2012–2013 NCAA banned drugs, www.ncaa.org, accessed July 8, 2013.

10. Soo, V. A. (2000, July 3). Neonatal drug testing. *Adv Med Lab Professional*, pp. 19–23, http://laboratorian.advanceweb.com, accessed July 8, 2013.

11. Insurance Institute for Highway Safety. (2013, March). Highway loss data institute, Q and A: Alcohol, www.iihs.org/research/qanda/alcohol_general.aspx, accessed July 8, 2013.

12. Field Sobriety Tests. (n.d.). Field sobriety tests: Standardized and non-standardized, http://fieldsobrietytests.org, accessed July 8, 2013.

RESOURCES

www.bloodalcoholcalculator.org Online blood alcohol content (BAC) calculator

www.cdc.gov/nchs/hus.htm Centers for Disease Control and Prevention

www.dot.gov U.S. Department of Transportation

www.drivinglaws.org Drunk Driving Laws

www.thecommunityofconcern.org Community of Concern

www.ignitioninterlockdevice.org Information about interlock devices for vehicles

www.drugabuse.gov National Institute on Drug Abuse

www.samhsa.gov U.S. Department of Health and Human Services—Substance Abuse and Mental Health

www.safety-devices.com/breathalyzer.htm Company that markets numerous types of digital breathalyzer devices

Appendix Contents

Appendix 1

NAACLS Phlebotomy Competencies and Matrix

The National Association for Accreditation of Clinical Laboratory Sciences (NAACLS) is an international agency for accreditation and approval of educational programs in clinical laboratory sciences. The approval process involves a comprehensive analysis of each program including administrative, financial, organizational, and curriculum requirements. A Self-Study Template is available from the NAACLS website, www.naacls.org, and proposes that phlebotomy programs seeking approval should provide documentation for the following areas related to Curriculum Requirements.

A. Instructional Areas

1. Describe all prerequisite coursework required for admission to the program.
2. Describe how the curriculum addresses the following components of education across all major areas of instruction:

    a. variety of collection techniques
    b. contact with various patient types in a variety of settings
    c. a minimum of 100 hours of applied experiences and a minimum of 100 unaided collections
    d. guarantees the same level of learning experience for each student.

3. Using the NAACLS phlebotomy-specific matrix, identify where items are addressed in the curriculum. (Refer to the matrix below.)
4. Discuss how items in the matrix are included within courses, or approached as topics in separate courses.

B. Learning Experiences

1. Discuss learning experiences provided to achieve entry level competencies. Suggested documents include
    a. lectures
    b. student laboratories
    c. class discussions
    d. case studies
    e. other learning activities utilized

C. Evaluations

1. Describe the evaluation systems(s) utilized by the program to assess the effectiveness of instruction, frequency of use of the various evaluation tools, and how the results of evaluation are utilized in program evaluation and revision

While NAACLS criteria are important for educators and program administrators, the competencies are also important for students' understanding of professional responsibilites and expectations. This textbook is designed to support and enhance the learning experiences and evaluations provided in an accredited phlebotomy program curriculum. The matrix below simply cross-references the NAACLS competencies with chapters in two phlebotomy textbooks in which the topic or related topics are covered. It also provides a brief overview of the depth of coverage (beginning, intermediate, or advanced) in the context of a curriculum for phlebotomists. Even though some of the text discussions are not exhaustive, this matrix provides an overview of where material can be obtained and a basis from which students and instructors can seek out further information. Also, in relation to evauations, every chapter provides multiple forms of evaluation (study questions, case studies, and specific competency assessment checklists) that involve various levels of cognitive ability (recall, decision-making, etc). In addition, Appendix 13 provides a Competency Assessment Tracking Sheet for documenting progress. Students and instructors are strongly encouraged to utilize all methods to help achieve professional competency.

Depth of Coverage: B = Beginning/Basic   I = Intermediate   A = Advanced

NAACLS Entry Level Competencies		*Phlebotomy Simplified, 2ed*	Chapter(s) where related topics are found	*Phlebotomy Handbook, 9ed*	Chapter(s) where topics are found
A.	Demonstrate knowledge of the health care delivery system and medical terminology	B	1, 2, 3	B-I	1, 2, 6, 7, Appendices 2, 3
B.	Demonstrate knowledge of infection control and safety.	B	4, 8, 9	I-A	4, 5, 10, 11, Appendix 5
C.	Demonstrate basic understanding of the anatomy and physiology of body systems and anatomic terminology in order to relate major areas of the clinical laboratory to general pathologic conditions associated with the body systems.	B	3	I-A	6, 7, Appendix 4
D.	Demonstrate basic understanding of age specific or psycho-social considerations involved in the performance of phlebotomy procedures on various age groups of patients	B	9, 10, Appendix 4	I-A	13, 14, Appendices 7, 12
E.	Demonstrate understanding of the importance of specimen collection and specimen integrity in the delivery of patient care	B-I	2, 5	I-A	1, 3, 9, 10, 11, 12, 15, 16, 17
F.	Demonstrate knowledge of collection equipment, various types of additives used, special precautions necessary and substances that can interfere in clinical analysis of blood constituents.	B	6, 8	A	7, 8, 9, 10, 11, 12, 13, 15, 16, 17
G.	Follow standard operating procedures to collect specimens via venipuncture and capillary (dermal) puncture.	B	6, 8, 9, 10	B-I-A	8, 9, 10, 11, 13, 15, Appendices 6, 8
H.	Demonstrate understanding of requisitioning, specimen transport, and specimen processing.	B	1, 5	I-A	1, 2, 12
I.	Demonstrate understanding of quality assurance and quality control in phlebotomy.	B	1	B-I-A	1, 14, Appendices 9, 10, 11
J.	Communicate (verbally and nonverbally) effectively and appropriately in the workplace.	I	1	I-A	2, 3

Competencies reprinted with permission from the National Association for Accreditation of Clinical Laboratory Sciences (NAACLS). Adopted 2012, Revised 1/2014, www.naacls.org, accessed February 18, 2014.

Appendix 2

Finding a Job

Finding a job that is a good fit for both the applicant and the employer is a time-consuming, often challenging process. However, the time and effort spent researching and applying for a position can have a positive payoff in terms of job satisfaction, salary, benefits, environment, and personal gratification. The keys to finding the right job are to spend time searching, be prepared with documentation and questions during an interview, and keep an open mind. Here are some essential factors to think about. This list can be used as a checklist for your application process.

Places to Seek Employment	Newspaper, professional journals, and online postings
	Health care organizations
	Friends and relatives
	College career centers, faculty, and advisors
	Bulletin boards and electronic bulletin boards
	Employment agencies
Contacting an Employer	Check employer's website.
	Call for an appointment.
	Send a cover letter (see example on p. 537).
	Send a resume (see example on p. 538).
	Complete a job application (usually online at the employer's website).
Cover Letter/Email	Be neat and use correct spelling.
	State where you heard about the job.
	State the specific job for which you are applying.
	State why you are qualified for this position.
	Give a brief summary of your education, experience, and qualifications.
	Refer to your resume.
	Request an interview.
	Give your name, address, and phone number.

Resume	List name, address, phone number(s), and e-mail address. Avoid using silly email addresses such as toughguy@xyz.123. If needed, consider getting an email account just for your job search. For your phone(s), record professional sounding voice messages.
	Do *not* list personal data such as age, marital status, height, weight, religion, national origin, etc. Employers should consider hiring you solely on your job qualifications. Do *not* send a picture. Do *not* use abbreviations.
	Keep in mind that employers can and do review applicants' websites and/or social networking websites; use good judgment about how much and what types of information you reveal, if any. If needed, review postings on all your social media profiles while considering that an employer might see them. Many applicants provide the public URL of their LinkedIn professional profiles. Many applicants also use their personal websites to post their resumes.
	Career plans. (Provide one to three concise statements about your short-term and long-term career goals.)
	Education. (Unless it is noted otherwise, list the most recent first, followed in reverse chronological order; only list high school and beyond.)
	Work experience. (Unless it is noted otherwise, list the most recent first, followed in reverse chronological order; part time or full time, dates, duration of employment. Do *not* leave gaps in employment dates, briefly state reasons for any gap [e.g., returned to school, worked temporary jobs, left for family responsibilities].)
	Mention specific accomplishments and/or leadership activities at work or in community affairs
	Special skills and abilities. (List non–English language skills, computer skills with particular software, telephone expertise, use of special equipment, experience with specific patient populations, etc.)
	Volunteer activities. (Provide any community service, membership in service organizations, etc.)
	Interests. (Mention sports, music, art, hobbies, etc.)
	Reference names and contact information can be provided on request. (Always ask permission of those you use as references before providing their contact information. Avoid using relatives and social friends as references because they may not know enough about your work skills and experience.)
Interview	Be well groomed and do not chew gum. Dress neatly and professionally; keep makeup and accessories to a minimum; avoid strong aftershave or perfumes. Turn off/silence your cellular phone.
	Consider taking a briefcase or notebook. Request business cards of those you meet. Offer your own business card. If you do not have one, print a generic card with your contact information. Take notes of key duties and major points made during the interview.
	Arrive *on time* or a few minutes early.
	Greet the interviewer with your name and a smile.
	Shake hands firmly.
	Stand until you are asked to sit.
	Answer questions truthfully and sincerely.
	Prepare a few questions about the organization and the job.

For example, about the organization:

What are the future plans for this department and organization?

How would someone with my background fit into these plans?

How would you describe the organizational culture?

What are some of the challenges that this department faces?

About the job:

Could you describe the training program for this job?

Is this a new or replacement job?

To whom does this position report?

Is there a career ladder or path for this position?

Avoid discussing personal problems.

Be enthusiastic, smile, and maintain eye contact.

Do not criticize former employers or teachers.

Thank the interviewer for his or her time and leave promptly.

After the Interview

Send a thank-you letter or e-mail to the interviewer.

If something in your application changes, make the employer aware of it immediately.

Making a Decision

List advantages and disadvantages of your choices. Rank them based on responsibilities, salary, location, working conditions, benefits, career goals, and your "gut feeling" of the work environment.

If you have an offer, it is acceptable to contact other potential employers to ask about their time frames for a decision. If necessary, it is acceptable to let them know you already have a firm offer.

Once your decision is made, inform all those who helped you in your job search (including references) and thank them for their assistance.

Resources

www.quickstudy.com   Provides a variety of educational products for medicine, health, and business, and free downloads targeted to college students.

Sample of a Cover Letter for a Job Inquiry

(For email, use the same content without the letter-based format.)

Jane Doe
8200 West Jersey Avenue
Lubbock, Texas 79452
555-799-9999
jdoe@nnn.com

March 6, 2014

Ms. A. D. Jones
Director, Laboratory Services
Muncy Hospital
P.O. Box 22333
San Antonio, Texas 78277

Dear Ms. Jones,
I am responding to an advertisement in the *San Antonio Press* on February 28, 2014, for an entry-level phlebotomy technician. I graduated from Lamar High School in 2011. Since then, I have worked part-time and been a part-time student at the Community College. I recently completed a phlebotomy training program, and my goal is to utilize my skills while pursuing additional studies in laboratory sciences.

I have enclosed my resume, which includes a list of skills and experience. I believe that I am well qualified for this position because of my work with adults and children coupled with my organizational skills. I hope to arrange an interview as soon as is convenient for you. Please feel free to contact me at 555-799-9999 to schedule an interview or for additional information. Thank you.

Sincerely,
Jane Doe

Sample Resume

Jane Doe
8200 West Jersey Avenue
Lubbock, Texas 79452
555-799-9999
jdoe@nnn.com

Career Plans	To become an experienced phlebotomist while continuing my education in laboratory sciences
Experience	*2012–present* Community college phlebotomy student and part-time library assistant; responsibilities include clerical duties (filing, answering multiple telephone lines, word processing), greeting customers, and providing assistance in locating reference materials.
	2011–2012 Part-time caretaker for three children; responsibilities included carpooling, providing after-school snacks, assistance with homework, monitoring activities.
	2010–2011 Part-time employee at ABC Grocery; responsibilities included assisting customers in locating products, restocking groceries, checking out grocery items at cash register, assisting with inventory.
Education	*2011* Graduated from Lamar High School
	Elected captain of the varsity soccer team
Skills/Strengths	Excellent communication skills in Spanish
	Computer skills include proficiency with MAC and PC word processing, Internet research, Excel, and PowerPoint
Interests	Reading, camping, art, youth group, Girl Scouts
References	Available on request

Appendix 3

International Organizations

The following organizations have international interests in phlebotomy practices and/or offer certifications in this or related fields. Many countries have professional groups that are concerned about phlebotomy practices but do not have formal contacts. Global interest in this field is expected to continue to grow.

American Society for Clinical Pathology (ASCP)
Board of Certification (BOC)
33 West Monroe, Suite 1600
Chicago, IL 60603-5617
1-800-267-2727
Outside U.S.: 312-541-4890
www.ascp.org/Board-of-Certification/International

International Healthcare Worker Safety Center
(Global Initiative for Healthcare Worker Safety—for policy and legislation)
1224 Jefferson Park Avenue
Suite 400, Blake Center
Charlottesville, VA 22903
434-924-5159
www.healthsystem.virginia.edu/internet/epinet/

International Organization for Standardization (ISO)
1, ch. de la Voie-Creuse
Case postale 56
CH-1211 Geneva 20,
Switzerland
Tel.: +41 22 749 01 11
www.iso.org

The Joint Commission International (also has offices in Dubai and Singapore)
1515 West 22nd Street, Suite 1300W
Oakbrook Terrace, IL 60523
www.jointcommissioninternational.org

World Health Organization
Avenue Appia 20
CH-1211 Geneva 27
Switzerland
Tel.: +41 22 791 2111
Fax.: +41 22 791 3111
www.who.int/en/

Appendix 4

The Basics of Vital Signs

Vital signs are indicators of the body's functioning, using measures of temperature, pulse, and respiration rate (TPR) as well as blood pressure. The body is considered to be in homeostasis when vital signs are within normal limits. Vital signs that are not within normal limits indicate a clinical problem. Health care workers often have responsibilities that involve measurement of vital signs. Accuracy in the measurement and recording of results is critical to proper treatment decisions for each patient.

Temperature

Temperature is a measure of body heat and is influenced by factors that cause the body to retain heat (such as exercise, ingestion of food, exposure to hot temperatures, illness, infection, excitement, and anxiety) or to lose heat (such as sleep, fasting, exposure to cold, certain illnesses, decreased muscle activity, depression, and mouth breathing).

Several types of thermometers (instruments used to measure temperature) are available, including the following:

- **Glass thermometer**—This type of thermometer has a hollow glass tube with calibration lines marking the outside; it is filled with mercury. Mercury is heat sensitive and rises up the hollow tube when exposed to the heat of the patient. The patient's temperature is then read when the mercury stops rising after several minutes. Glass thermometers are specially designed to take temperatures orally or rectally. Those designed for taking oral temperature should not be used to take rectal temperature, and vice versa.

- **Aural thermometer**—Primarily used for babies and children an aural thermometer has a sensor and is placed in the ear to measure temperature. It can also be used if the patient is having trouble breathing, which would make using an oral thermometer uncomfortable for the patient.

- **Chemically treated or plastic thermometer**—Temperature is measured by a color change on a strip of treated paper/plastic. The treated strip is placed on the skin and disposed of after one use.

- **Electronic/digital thermometer**—Widely used today, this type of thermometer has a probe that can be covered with a disposable protective shield after each use. Temperature is read easily and quickly from a digital screen. The manufacturer's instructions should be closely followed. (**PROCEDURE A4–1.**)

Four sites are used to take body temperature:

1. **Oral** (by mouth)—This is the safest, most common, convenient, and comfortable site to take temperature. Normal oral temperature is 98.6°F or 37°C. (See Procedure A4–1.)

2. **Rectal** (by insertion 1.5 inches into the rectum)—The most accurate temperature is from this site. This site is used when use of the mouth is difficult—for example, when patients have trouble breathing, are weak or confused, are being given oxygen, or have paralysis of the face caused by stroke or accident. Normal rectal temperature is 99.6°F or 38°C.

3. **Aural** (ear canal)—This, too, is a safe and accurate site for patients who are less than age 6 or have the same conditions listed for the use of rectal thermometers. Normal aural temperature is 98.6°F or 37° C. (**PROCEDURE A4–2.**)

4. **Axillary** (in the armpit)—The axillary temperature is the least accurate and should be used only when other sites are not easily accessed due to clinical conditions. Normal axillary temperature is 97.6°F or 36.4°C. (**PROCEDURE A4–3.**)

PROCEDURE A4–1

Taking Oral Temperature

Rationale   This is the most common way to take a patient's temperature. This procedure allows the health care worker to record the patient's temperature along with other vital signs.

Equipment

- Plastic covers (disposable)
- Electronic/digital thermometer
- Disposable gloves
- Marking pen

Preparation

1 Follow standard precautions prior to, during, and after the procedure.

2 Prepare and assemble equipment by placing plastic covers near the thermometer. (Remember that the blue probes are for oral and the red for rectal.) Note that several types of thermometers are commercially available.

3 Identify the patient properly and explain the procedure.

4 Place the clean plastic cover over the thermometer probe.

Procedure

5 Insert the probe under the tongue gently. Position the thermometer to the side of the lips (**FIGURES A4–1A** and **A4–1B**).

6 Hold in place for 15 seconds or until a sound is emitted to indicate that the body temperature is displayed.

7 Read the temperature (**FIGURE A4–1C**).

8 Remove plastic cover and discard (**FIGURE A4–1D**).

9 Record temperature and, if elevated, report to appropriate personnel.

10 Position patient for comfort and thank him or her for cooperating.

11 Wash hands and return thermometer to storage place.

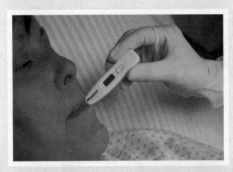

FIGURE A4–1A

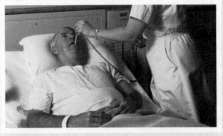

FIGURE A4–1B

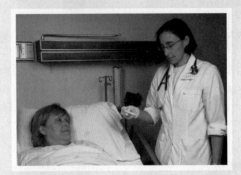

FIGURE A4–1C

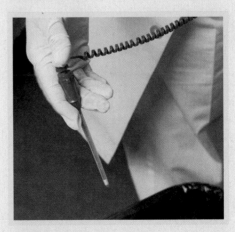

FIGURE A4–1D

PROCEDURE A4–2

Taking Aural Temperature

Rationale   To take a patient's aural temperature.

Equipment

- Probe covers (disposable)
- Aural electronic thermometer
- Disposable gloves
- Marking pen

Procedure

1   The steps for taking aural temperature are essentially the same as for oral procedures.

2   Assemble the aural electronic thermometer using a disposable probe cover (**FIGURE A4–2A**).

3   Insert the aural thermometer gently into the ear canal and hold it for 15 seconds or until a signal is emitted (**FIGURE A4–2B**).

4   Record the temperature and remove and discard the plastic sheath.

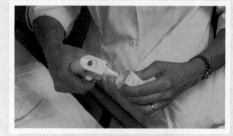

FIGURE A4–2A

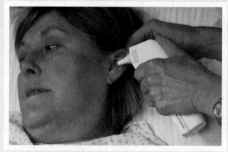

FIGURE A4–2B

PROCEDURE A4–3

Taking Axillary Temperature

Rationale   To take a patient's axillary temperature.

Equipment

- Plastic covers (disposable)
- Chemically treated strips or electronic/digital thermometer
- Disposable gloves
- Marking pen

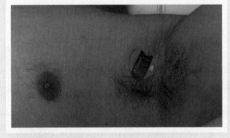

FIGURE A4–3A

Procedure

1 The steps for taking axillary temperature are similar to oral procedures, except the device may differ. Use chemically treated strips on the axillary site (**FIGURE A4–3A**).

2 Alternatively, digital or other thermometer models can be used. Insert the thermometer into the axilla (armpit) and keep it there for approximately 5 minutes (**FIGURE A4–3B**).

3 When taking an axillary temperature on a child, it is helpful to involve the parent in the process if possible. In **FIGURE A4–3C**, note that the patient is sitting up to facilitate comfort.

4 Record the temperature and discard the plastic cover.

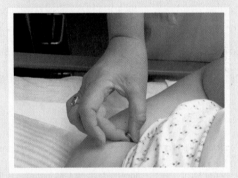

FIGURE A4–3B

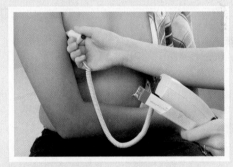

FIGURE A4–3C

PULSE

Pulse is the number of times the heart beats in one minute. It is a measure of how well blood is circulating through the body and is taken by placing fingers over an artery and squeezing gently against the bone. The pulsating feeling is actually pressure of the blood against the wall of the artery as the heart contracts and relaxes (**PROCEDURE A4–4**). Pulse or pressure points are indicated in **FIGURE A4–4A**. The pulse rate should be the same at all pulse points. The most common site to count the pulse rate is at the radial artery near the wrist.

Average pulse rates are as follows:

Age	Rate per Minute
Before birth	140–150
At birth	90–160
First year of life	115–130
Childhood	80–115
Adult	60–80

Artery Checkpoint	Site/Use	
Temporal	Temple area of the head. Used to control bleeding from the head and scalp and to monitor circulation.	
Facial	Under ear, near jaw. Monitor circulation.	
Carotid	Neck. In an emergency (*cardiac arrest*), most readily accessible site.	
Brachial	Antecubital space of the elbow. Most common site used to check blood pressure.	
Radial	Radial (*thumb side*) of the wrist. Most common site for taking a pulse.	
Femoral	Groin area. Monitor circulation.	
Popliteal	Behind the knee. Monitor circulation.	
Posterior tibial	Inner side of heel. Monitor lower limb circulation.	
Dorsalis pedis	Upper surface of the foot. Monitor lower limb circulation.	

Labels on figure: Temporal, Facial, Carotid, Brachial, Radial, Femoral, Popliteal, Posterior tibial, Dorsalis pedis

FIGURE A4–4A
Pulse or Pressure Points

PROCEDURE A4–4

Assessing Peripheral Pulse Rate[1]

Rationale   To measure the number of heart beats per minute and to assess whether pulse rhythm is regular or irregular and whether blood is adequately circulating in the extremities.

The patient's peripheral pulse rate is reported along with other vital signs.

Equipment
- Timer or watch with second hand or indicator
- Pen

PROCEDURE A4–4

Assessing Peripheral Pulse Rate (continued)

Preparation

1 Introduce yourself to the patient and identify the patient properly.

2 Explain what you are going to do.

3 Perform hand hygiene.

4 Position the patient in a comfortable position. Provide for patient privacy.

Procedure

5 Place your fingers on the patient's radial artery at the base of his or her thumb (or other pulse point) (**FIGURE A4–4B**). Do not use your own thumb to measure pulse.

6 Alternative sites include the carotid artery (neck) and the dorsalis pedis or posterior tibial arteries (foot) (**FIGURES A4–4C**, **FIGURES A4–4D**, and **A4–4E**).

7 Count the number of pulsations that occur within one minute.

8 Record the pulse rate immediately.

9 Wash your hands and thank the patient for cooperating.

10 Record the pulse rate on other necessary records.

11 Report any unusual observations, irregular rhythm intervals, or abnormal rates immediately.

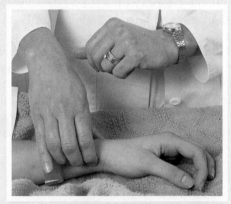

FIGURE A4–4B

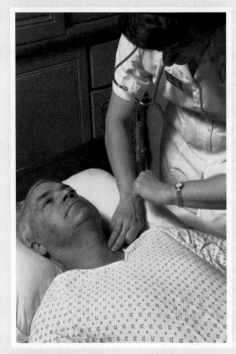

FIGURE A4–4C

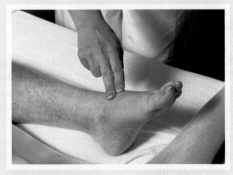

FIGURE A4–4D

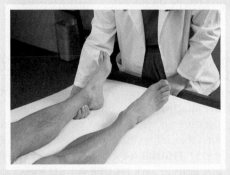

FIGURE A4–4E

Blood Pressure

Blood pressure is the force of blood pushing against the walls of blood vessels and is measured and reported using two numbers, one for the systolic pressure and one for the diastolic pressure. *Systolic* blood pressure (SBP) is exerted when the heart is contracting and is the greater force on the wall of the arteries. *Diastolic* blood pressure (DBP) is the lesser force exerted on the walls of the arteries as the heart relaxes between contractions. Many factors can increase blood pressure, including exercise, eating, stimulant drugs, and anxiety. Factors that decrease blood pressure include hemorrhage, inactivity, fasting, suppressant drugs, and depression.

Normal blood pressure is measured by an instrument called a sphygmomanometer, or blood pressure (BP) cuff. Values on the instrument relate to "millimeters of mercury" (mm Hg) in a tube at certain points. There are three types of sphygmomanometers: mercury (now almost obsolete because of the hazardous nature of mercury), aneroid (cloth-covered bladder that fills with air as the bulb is squeezed and inflated), and electronic/digital. When taking blood pressure, one must do two important things simultaneously—listen to the heartbeat and watch the pressure gauge—to take a reading at precise moments. (**PROCEDURE A4–5.**)

PROCEDURE A4–5

Taking Blood Pressure

Rationale   To determine arterial blood pressure (BP). The patient's blood pressure is reported along with other vital signs.

Equipment

- Alcohol pads
- Stethoscope
- Sphygmomanometer (digital readout, round pressure gauge, or mercury column)
- Supplies to record the measurement

Preparation

1 Introduce yourself to the patient and identify the patient properly.

2 Explain what you are going to do. Plan to take two measurements.

3 Perform hand hygiene.

4 If possible, position the patient in a seated, comfortable chair for at least 5 minutes. It is preferable for the feet to be on the floor and the arm supported at heart level.

5 Use a properly calibrated and validated instrument. Make sure that the blood pressure cuff is the correct size (encircling the upper arm). There are standard sizes that fit infants, small children, and adults and larger cuffs for obese patients or for taking the BP on the leg.

Procedure

6 Support the patient's arm on a firm surface if possible. Wrap the blood pressure cuff according to the manufacturer's instructions around the upper arm and directly over the brachial artery. For adults, the lower border of the cuff is approximately 1 inch (2.5 cm) above the antecubital space. Note that there are several types of sphygmomanometers, all of which are attached to a blood pressure cuff used around the arm to inflate with air, and with different readouts: digital, round pressure gauge, or older types using a mercury column. **FIGURE A4–5A** shows a digital readout and what happens when the cuff is inflated and then deflated. **FIGURE A4–5B** shows an aneroid sphygmomanometer and blood pressure cuff. **FIGURE A4–5C** shows a blood pressure monitor that registers systolic and diastolic pressures and often other vital signs as well. **FIGURE A4–5D** shows an older-style mercury column.

PROCEDURE A4–5

Taking Blood Pressure (continued)

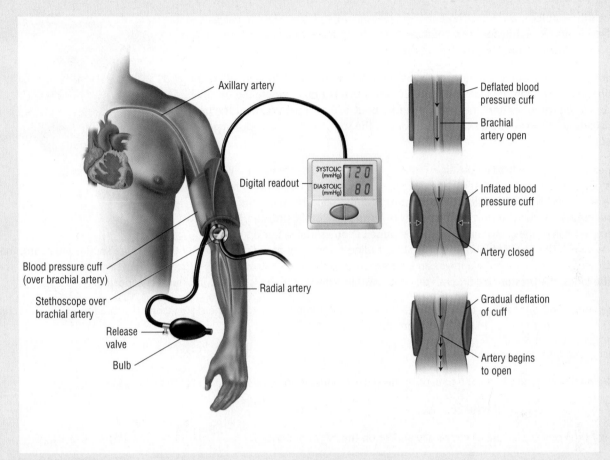

Axillary artery

Digital readout

SYSTOLIC (mmHg) 120
DIASTOLIC (mmHg) 80

Blood pressure cuff (over brachial artery)

Stethoscope over brachial artery

Radial artery

Release valve

Bulb

Deflated blood pressure cuff

Brachial artery open

Inflated blood pressure cuff

Artery closed

Gradual deflation of cuff

Artery begins to open

FIGURE A4–5A

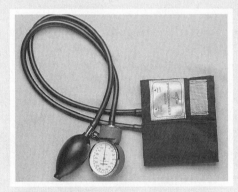

FIGURE A4–5B

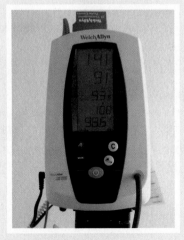

FIGURE A4–5C

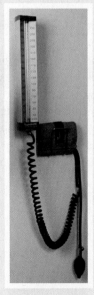

FIGURE A4–5D

(continued)

PROCEDURE A4–5

Taking Blood Pressure (continued)

7 Clean the earpieces on the stethoscope and place in your ears so that the ear attachments tilt slightly forward. The sounds are heard more clearly when the ear attachments follow the direction of the ear canal.

8 Place the stethoscope amplifier over the artery distal to the cuff, and then inflate the cuff until the sphygmomanometer reads 30mm above the point where the brachial pulse disappeared (or until the pressure reads about 170mm). At this point the brachial artery collapses, the flow of blood stops so the sound of the pulse disappears (**FIGURE A4–5E**).

9 Open the valve slowly to let the air out of the cuff. At first, blood enters only at peak systolic pressure and the stethoscope picks up the sound of blood pulsing through the artery. As air is removed from the cuff, the sounds change because the artery is opening. When the cuff pressure decreases to less than diastolic pressure, blood flow becomes continuous, and the sound of the pulse becomes muffled or disappears completely. The systolic blood pressure (SBP) reading is the point at which the first of two or more sounds are heard, that is the sound when the pulse appears and corresponds to the peak systolic pressure (the first number reported). When the pulse fades, the pressure reading has reached diastolic level (DBP) and is the second number reported.

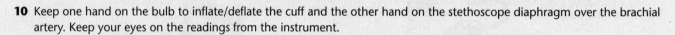

FIGURE A4–5E

10 Keep one hand on the bulb to inflate/deflate the cuff and the other hand on the stethoscope diaphragm over the brachial artery. Keep your eyes on the readings from the instrument.

11 Record readings and repeat if possible.

12 Wash your hands and thank the patient for his or her cooperation.

13 Clean the earpieces on the stethoscope, and put equipment away.

14 Record the blood pressure electronically and/or on the necessary documents.

15 Report any abnormal results to the appropriate personnel.

Special Notes

- *Infants:*—Use a pediatric stethoscope with a small diaphragm. The lower edge of the cuff can be closer to the antecubital space of an infant.
- *Children:*—Use appropriately sized equipment. Explain the steps of the process and what it will feel like. Demonstrate on a doll.
- *Elderly:*—Skin may be fragile, so do not leave the cuff on longer than necessary. If the patient has arm contractures, use other sites or methods for taking the pressure. Remember that various positions (lying or standing) may have an effect on blood pressure, especially if the patient is on medication for hypertension.[1]
- Blood pressure changes frequently and is an important vital sign. Health care workers must be accurate in their measurements and recording of results, and report any abnormalities immediately.

TABLE A4–1

Classification of Blood Pressure for Adults[2]

BP Classification	SBP (mm Hg) (top number)	And/Or	DBP (mm Hg) (bottom number)
Normal	Less than 120	And	Less than 80
Prehypertension	120–139	Or	80–89
Stage 1 Hypertension	140–159	Or	90–99
Stage 2 Hypertension	160 or higher	Or	100 or higher

The systolic blood pressure, the higher value, is reported first, and the diastolic blood pressure, the lower value, is reported second. The average normal adult reading of 120/80 is read as "120 over 80." Normal systolic pressure ranges between 90 and 140 mm Hg; normal diastolic pressure ranges between 60 and 90 mm Hg. Blood pressure above the normal range is considered to be hypertension or high blood pressure; conversely, readings below the normal range are considered to be hypotension or low blood pressure.[2] Refer to **TABLE A4–1.**

RESPIRATION RATE

Respiration rate is the measure of how many times a patient breathes in and out in one minute. Inspiration or inhalation is the intake of air and expiration or exhalation is the breathing out of gases from the lungs into the atmosphere. Normally, breathing occurs automatically and effortlessly with inspiration lasting about 1 to 1.5 seconds and expiration lasting 2 to 3 seconds. The rise of the chest (inhaling) and the fall of the chest (exhaling) count as one respiration. Normal adult respiration rate is between 12 to 20 respirations per minute. Newborns, infants, and children have higher respiration rates. Factors that cause the respiration rate to increase are exercise, stress or anxiety, respiratory diseases, medications, pain, increased environmental temperature, altitude, and heart disease. Conversely, factors that cause the rate to decrease are lower environmental temperature, relaxation, depression, head injury, or medications. Any abnormalities (short shallow breaths, difficulty breathing, irregular breathing, cessation of breathing, bubbling or wheezing sounds) should be reported immediately.

REPORTING/RECORDING VITAL SIGNS

Temperature, pulse, and respiration (TPR) are most often reported in that order. Blood pressure is the fourth vital sign and is usually reported in a designated location in the patient's electronic medical record/medical chart near the other vital signs. A common notation for TPR would be 98.6/73/15, meaning oral temperature of 98.6, a pulse rate of 73, and respiration rate of 15. (**PROCEDURE A4–6.**) Rectal temperatures are indicated by the letter *R* (in a circle), axillary temperatures by *AX* next to the reading, and sometimes aural temperatures by a *T* next to the reading—for example, 99.6R, or 97.6AX, or 98.6T.

Accurate reading and reporting of vital signs is an important function that all members of the health care team rely on. Abnormal results should be reported immediately.

PROCEDURE A4–6

Assessing Respiration Rate

Rationale   To record the number of respirations (inhale and exhale = 1 respiration) per minute.

Equipment

- Watch or timer with seconds indicated

Preparation

1 Introduce yourself to the patient and identify the patient properly.

2 Explain what you are going to do. Plan to take two measurements.

3 Perform hand hygiene.

4 Position the patient in a seated, comfortable chair or slightly reclining. Provide for patient privacy.

Procedure

5 Since some patients alter their breathing patterns when they are aware that it is being measured, it is best to keep the patient calm and count respirations while the patient's attention is elsewhere, such as while his or her temperature is being taken or just after taking the pulse but while still holding the pulse point. Experienced personnel can do it simultaneously while taking the pulse.

6 If the respirations are regular, count the number of respirations for 30 seconds and multiply by 2. If the respirations are irregular, count the number of respirations in 60 seconds. The rise and fall of the chest indicates one respiration. Also record the depth of inhalation (normal, shallow, or deep) and the rhythm of the respirations (regular or irregular). Sometimes it helps to visualize each respiration if the patient holds one arm across his or her chest.

7 Record the measurement and assessments and proceed to take and record other vital signs.

8 Thank the patient for his or her cooperation prior to leaving.

References

1. Berman, A., Snyder, S. J., Kozier, B., & Erb, G. (2008). *Fundamentals of nursing, concepts, process, and practice*, 8th ed. Upper Saddle River, NJ: Pearson Prentice Hall.
2. National Heart Lung and Blood Institute (NHLBI). (n.d.) What is High Blood Pressure. *www.nhlbi.nih.gov*, accessed February 19, 2014.

Appendix 5

Centers for Disease Control and Prevention (CDC) Guideline for Hand Hygiene in Health Care Settings

Strong evidence suggests that hand hygiene can reduce the serious and preventable risks associated with transmission of infections from one person to another. The following recommendations and guidelines are excerpted from the complete CDC report and promote improved hand hygiene and hand antisepsis to reduce transmission of pathogens to patients and health care workers. The complete guideline and report are available for free at www.cdc.gov/mmwr/PDF/rr/rr5116.pdf. The World Health Organization and The Joint Commission International have also established suggested actions and guidelines for hand hygiene. These recommendations overlap with the CDC recommendations and are not listed here; however, many resources and publications are available at their respective websites: www.jointcommission.org and www.who.int/en/.

Part A: Recommendations to Improve Hand-Hygiene Practices

www.cdc.gov.

CATEGORIES

These recommendations are designed to improve hand hygiene practices of health care workers and to reduce transmission of pathogenic microorganisms to patients and personnel in health care settings. This guideline and its recommendations are not intended for use in food processing or food-service establishments, and are not meant to replace guidance provided by the Food and Drug Administration's Model Food Code.

As in previous Centers for Disease Control and Prevention (CDC)/Healthcare and Infection Control Practices Advisory Committee (HICPAC) guidelines, each recommendation is categorized on the basis of existing scientific data, theoretical rationale, applicability, and economic impact. The CDC/HICPAC system for categorizing recommendations is as follows:

Category IA. Strongly recommended for implementation and strongly supported by well-designed experimental, clinical, or epidemiologic studies.

Category IB. Strongly recommended for implementation and supported by certain experimental, clinical, or epidemiologic studies and a strong theoretical rationale.

Category IC. Required for implementation, as mandated by federal or state regulation or standard.

Category II. Suggested for implementation and supported by suggestive clinical or epidemiologic studies or a theoretical rationale.

No recommendation. Unresolved issue. Practices for which insufficient evidence or no consensus regarding efficacy exist.

RECOMMENDATIONS

1. Indications for handwashing and hand antisepsis
   a. When hands are visibly dirty or contaminated with proteinaceous material or are visibly soiled with blood or other body fluids, wash hands with either a nonantimicrobial soap and water or an antimicrobial soap and water (IA).
   b. If hands are not visibly soiled, use an alcohol-based hand rub for routinely decontaminating hands in all other clinical situations described in items 1c–j (IA). Alternatively, wash hands with an antimicrobial soap and water in all clinical situations described in items 1c–j (IB).
   c. Decontaminate hands before having direct contact with patients (IB).

   d. Decontaminate hands before donning sterile gloves when inserting a central intravascular catheter (IB).

   e. Decontaminate hands before inserting indwelling urinary catheters, peripheral vascular catheters, or other invasive devices that do not require a surgical procedure (IB).

   f. Decontaminate hands after contact with a patient's intact skin (e.g., when taking a pulse or blood pressure, and lifting a patient) (IB).

   g. Decontaminate hands after contact with body fluids or excretions, mucous membranes, nonintact skin, and wound dressings even if hands are not visibly soiled (IA).

   h. Decontaminate hands if moving from a contaminated body site to a clean body site during patient care (II).

   i. Decontaminate hands after contact with inanimate objects (including medical equipment) in the immediate vicinity of the patient (II).

   j. Decontaminate hands after removing gloves (IB).

   k. Before eating and after using a restroom, wash hands with a nonantimicrobial soap and water or with an antimicrobial soap and water (IB).

   l. Antimicrobial-impregnated wipes (i.e., towelettes) may be considered as an alternative to washing hands with nonantimicrobial soap and water. Because they are not as effective as alcohol-based hand rubs or washing hands with an antimicrobial soap and water for reducing bacterial counts on the hands of health care workers, they are not a substitute for using an alcohol-based hand rub or antimicrobial soap (IB).

   m. Wash hands with nonantimicrobial soap and water or with antimicrobial soap and water if exposure to *Bacillus anthracis* is suspected or proven. The physical action of washing and rinsing hands under such circumstances is recommended because alcohols, chlorhexidine, iodophors, and other antiseptic agents have poor activity against spores (II).

   n. No recommendation can be made regarding the routine use of nonalcohol-based hand rubs for hand hygiene in health care settings. Unresolved issue.

2. Hand-hygiene technique

   a. When decontaminating hands with an alcohol-based hand rub, apply product to palm of one hand and rub hands together, covering all surfaces of hands and fingers, until hands are dry (IB). Follow the manufacturer's recommendations regarding the volume of product to use.

   b. When washing hands with soap and water, wet hands first with water, apply an amount of product recommended by the manufacturer to hands, and rub hands together vigorously for at least 15 seconds, covering all surfaces of the hands and fingers. Rinse hands with water and dry thoroughly with a disposable towel. Use towel to turn off the faucet (IB). Avoid using hot water, because repeated exposure to hot water may increase the risk of dermatitis (IB).

   c. Liquid, bar, leaflet, or powdered forms of plain soap are acceptable when washing hands with a nonantimicrobial soap and water. When bar soap is used, soap racks that facilitate drainage and small bars of soap should be used (II).

   d. Multiple-use cloth towels of the hanging or roll type are not recommended for use in health-care settings (II).

3. Surgical hand antisepsis

   a. Remove rings, watches, and bracelets before beginning the surgical hand scrub (II).

   b. Remove debris from underneath fingernails using a nail cleaner under running water (II).

   c. Surgical hand antisepsis using either an antimicrobial soap or an alcohol-based hand rub with persistent activity is recommended before donning sterile gloves when performing surgical procedures (IB).

   d. When performing surgical hand antisepsis using an antimicrobial soap, scrub hands and forearms for the length of time recommended by the manufacturer, usually 2 to 6 minutes. Long scrub times (e.g., 10 minutes) are not necessary (IB).

   e. When using an alcohol-based surgical hand-scrub product with persistent activity, follow the manufacturer's instructions. Before applying the alcohol solution, prewash hands and forearms with a nonantimicrobial soap and dry hands and forearms completely. After application of the alcohol-based product as recommended, allow hands and forearms to dry thoroughly before donning sterile gloves (IB).

4. Selection of hand-hygiene agents

   a. Provide personnel with efficacious hand-hygiene products that have low irritancy potential, particularly when these products are used multiple times per shift (IB). This recommendation applies to products used for hand antisepsis before and after patient care in clinical areas and to products used for surgical hand antisepsis by surgical personnel.

   b. To maximize acceptance of hand-hygiene products by health care workers, solicit input from these employees regarding the feel, fragrance, and skin tolerance of any products under consideration. The cost of hand-hygiene products should not be the primary factor influencing product selection (IB).

c. When selecting nonantimicrobial soaps, antimicrobial soaps, or alcohol-based hand rubs, solicit information from manufacturers regarding any known interactions between products used to clean hands, skin care products, and the types of gloves used in the institution (II).

d. Before making purchasing decisions, evaluate the dispenser systems of various product manufacturers or distributors to ensure that dispensers function adequately and deliver an appropriate volume of product (II).

e. Do not add soap to a partially empty soap dispenser. This practice of "topping off" dispensers can lead to bacterial contamination of soap (IA).

5. Skin care

a. Provide health care workers with hand lotions or creams to minimize the occurrence of irritant contact dermatitis associated with hand antisepsis or handwashing (IA).

b. Solicit information from manufacturers regarding any effects that hand lotions, creams, or alcohol-based hand antiseptics may have on the persistent effects of antimicrobial soaps being used in the institution (IB).

6. Other aspects of hand hygiene

a. Do not wear artificial fingernails or extenders when having direct contact with patients at high risk (e.g., those in intensive care units or operating rooms) (IA).

b. Keep natural nails tips less than 1/4-inch long (II).

c. Wear gloves when contact with blood or other potentially infectious materials, mucous membranes, and nonintact skin could occur (IC).

d. Remove gloves after caring for a patient. Do not wear the same pair of gloves for the care of more than one patient, and do not wash gloves between uses with different patients (IB).

e. Change gloves during patient care if moving from a contaminated body site to a clean body site (II).

f. No recommendation can be made regarding wearing rings in health care settings. Unresolved issue.

7. Health care worker educational and motivational programs

a. As part of an overall program to improve hand-hygiene practices of health care workers, educate personnel regarding the types of patient care activities that can result in hand contamination and the advantages and disadvantages of various methods used to clean their hands (II).

b. Monitor health care workers' adherence with recommended hand-hygiene practices and provide personnel with information regarding their performance (IA).

c. Encourage patients and their families to remind health care workers to decontaminate their hands (II).

8. Administrative measures

a. Make improved hand-hygiene adherence an institutional priority and provide appropriate administrative support and financial resources (IB).

b. Implement a multidisciplinary program designed to improve adherence of health personnel to recommended hand-hygiene practices (IB).

c. As part of a multidisciplinary program to improve hand-hygiene adherence, provide health care workers with a readily accessible alcohol-based hand-rub product (IA).

d. To improve hand-hygiene adherence among personnel who work in areas in which high workloads and high intensity of patient care are anticipated, make an alcohol-based hand rub available at the entrance to the patient's room or at the bedside, in other convenient locations, and in individual pocket-sized containers to be carried by health care workers (IA).

e. Store supplies of alcohol-based hand rubs in cabinets or areas approved for flammable materials (IC).

Reference

CDC: Guideline for Hand Hygiene in Health Care Settings. (2002, October 25). *Morbidity and Mortality Weekly Report,* p. 51 (RR-16). Complete report available at www.cdc.gov/handhygiene

Resource

www.cdc.gov/handhygiene This public site provides vast information about hand hygiene, including basics, training, guidelines, and measurements of adherence.

Part B: Antimicrobial Spectrum and Characteristics of Hand-Hygiene Antiseptic Agents

Group	Gram-Positive Bacteria	Gram-Negative Bacteria	Mycobacteria	Fungi	Viruses	Speed of Action	Comments
Alcohols	+++	+++	+++	+++	+++	Fast	Optimum concentration 60–95%; no persistent activity
Chlorhexidine (2% and 4% aqueous)	+++	++	+	+	+++	Intermediate	Persistent activity; rare allergic reactions
Iodine compounds	+++	+++	+++	++	+++	Intermediate	Causes skin burns; usually too irritating for hand hygiene
Iodophors	+++	+++	+	++	++	Intermediate	Less irritating than iodine; acceptance varies
Phenol derivatives	+++	+	+	+	+	Intermediate	Activity neutralized by nonionic surfactants
Triclosan	+++	++	+	−	+++	Intermediate	Acceptability on hands varies
Quaternary ammonium compounds	+	++	−	−	+	Slow	Used only in combination with alcohols; ecologic concerns

Note: + + + = excellent; + + = good but does not include the entire bacterial spectrum; + = fair; — = no activity or not sufficient.

Hexachlorophene is not included because it is no longer an accepted ingredient of hand disinfectants.

Appendix 6

Common Laboratory Assays, Tube Requirements, and Reference Intervals

The information in this appendix contains general guidelines for common laboratory tests for which phlebotomists may perform venipunctures. Keep in mind that in practice, there is significant variability among laboratories and health facilities about which tubes should be used for different tests. *There is no single standard or guide available for tube selection.* Tube selection can be based on the types of patients (pediatric, geriatric, normal adult), the specific testing methodology used during the examination/analytical phase, and the different manufacturers of the test tubes purchased. Each laboratory should have protocols in place for tube selection that are based on an evaluation for suitability and safety and well-established reference intervals. *In the following table, reference intervals are provided for illustration and educational purposes only and are not intended to be comprehensive or definitive. Test tube requirements and reference intervals were taken from several sources and should not be used for patient evaluation.*

Key to specimen tube top/color

Light blue top

Royal blue top

Green top

Gray top

Pink top

Lavender top

Red top or gold top

Tan top

White top

Yellow top

Yellow–Red top

Common Laboratory Assays and the Required Types of Specimens and Anticoagulants

Test Name/Abbreviation	Specimen Type and Tube (Stopper Type/Color)	Reference Interval (Conventional Units)	Conversion Factor (Multiply By)	Reference Interval (SI Units)
ABO group and Rh typing	Whole blood (pink)	Reported as A, B, O, or AB and Rh pos/neg		
Acid phosphatase	Serum (speckled/red) or plasma (green)	0.0–0.6 U/L	1.0	0.0–0.6 U/L
Activated partial thromboplastin time (APTT or PTT; also see Partial thromboplastin time)	Plasma (light blue)	Variable due to testing methods		
Adrenal cortical antibody	Serum (speckled)			
Adrenocorticotropic hormone (ACTH)	Plasma (lavender) Critical frozen	Less than 120 pg/mL	0.22	Less than 26 pmol/L

(continued)

Test Name/ Abbreviation	Specimen Type and Tube (Stopper Type/Color)	Reference Interval (Conventional Units)	Conversion Factor (Multiply By)	Reference Interval (SI Units)
Alanine aminotransferase (ALT) (SGPT)	Serum (red) or plasma (green)			0.15–1.1 ukal/L
Albumin	Serum (speckled) or plasma	3.8–5.0 g/dL	10	38–50 g/L
Alcohol (ethanol)	Serum (red) or plasma (gray, lavender)	Less than 100 mg/dL	0.2171	Less than 21.7 mmol/L
Aldosterone	Serum (speckled) or plasma (green) Collect at 8:00 AM. Patient should be on normal diet two weeks prior to test. Patient should be recumbent for at least 30 minutes prior to blood collection.	7–30 ng/dL	0.0277	0.19–0.83 nmol/L
Alpha-Globin gene analysis	Whole blood (lavender)	Reporting of gene analysis		
Alpha 1 Antitrypsin	Blood (red)	95–300 mg/dl		
Alpha 1 Fetoprotein	Blood (gold)	Tumor marker cut off at 44 ng/ml or ug/L		
Aluminum	Blood (royal blue)	Varies due to tissue storage		
Ammonia	Blood (green)	15–110 ug/dl		
Amylase	Blood (red top/gold top)	25–125 U/L		200–240 nmol/L
Antibody to hepatitis A virus (anti-HAV), B core antigenx (Anti-HBc), BE antigen, B surface antigen (Anti-HBs)	Serum (red, speckled, gold) or plasma (lavender)			
Antibody identification	Whole blood (pink)	Reporting varies depending on antibodies tested		
Antistreptolysin O test	Serum (red) Perform test immediately or refrigerate immediately			
Arterial blood gases (ABG) (See Blood gases)				
Aspartate aminotransferase (AST) (GOT) (SGOT)	Serum (red) or plasma (green)	6–40 IU/L		0.25–0.75 ukal/L
Basic metabolic panel (BMP)	Plasma (green) or serum (red/gold)	Several chemistry tests covering certain body systems		
Bilirubin, conjugated	Serum (speckled) Protect blood from light	Less than 0.3 mg/dL	17.1	Less than 5μ mol/L
Bilirubin, total		0.1–1.2 mg/dL	17.1	2–21 μmol/L
Blood cell count, CBC survey (WBC, RBC, Hgb, Hct, MCV, MCH, MCHC)	Plasma (lavender)	Refer to reference intervals in Chapter 7		
Blood cell count, differential	Blood smear or Plasma (lavender)			
Blood cell count, eosinophil	Plasma (lavender)			
Blood cell count, erythrocyte (RBC)	Plasma (lavender)			
Blood cell count, leukocyte (WBC)	Plasma (lavender)			
Blood cell count, platelets	Plasma (lavender)			
Blood cell count, reticulocyte	Plasma (lavender)			

Test Name/ Abbreviation	Specimen Type and Tube (Stopper Type/Color)	Reference Interval (Conventional Units)	Conversion Factor (Multiply By)	Reference Interval (SI Units)
Blood culture (BC)	Whole blood (2 yellow) or 2 BC vials—anaerobic and aerobic	Negative for microorganisms		
Blood gases, arterial (ABG)	Arterial blood (heparinized syringe)			
base excess (BE)		–3.3 to +2.3 mmol/L	1	–3.3 to +2.3 mmol/L
pCO_2		35–45 mmHg	1	35–45 mmHg
pO_2		80–100 mmHg	1	80–100 mmHg
pH		7.35–7.45	1	7.35–7.45
Bicarbonate		21–28 mmol/L	1	21–28 mmol/L
BUN (blood urea nitrogen)	Serum (speckled or red)	8–23 mg/dL	0.357	2.9–8.2 mmol/L
Calcitonin (CALCIT)	Blood (green)	Cutoff of 5ng/L		
Calcium, ionized	Whole blood (green), serum (red) *Deliver immediately*	4.6–5.8 mg/dL	0.25	1.15–1.27 mmol/L
Calcium, total	Serum (speckled or red)	9.2–11.0 mg/dL	0.25	2.3–2.7 mmol/L
Carbon dioxide (CO_2) venous	Serum (speckled or red)	24–30 mmol/L	1	24–30 mmol/L
Cardiac troponins (cTnl, cTnT)	Serum (speckled)			
Carotene	Serum red or gold	50-300 ug/dl		
Chemistry screen (T. protein, Alb, Ca, Glu, BUN, Creat, T.bil, Alk p'tase, AST ALT, potassium, creatinine, chloride, sodium, CO_2)	Serum (speckled or red) or plasma (green)	Refer to reference intervals in Chapter 7		
Chlamydia antibodies	Serum (red or gold); must use aseptic technique and refrigerate serum	Negative for bacterial antibodies		
Chloride	Serum (speckled or red)	95–103 mEq/L	1	95–103 mmol/L
Cholesterol (total)	Serum (speckled) (*fasting*)	140–200 mg/dL	0.025	3.6–5.2 mmol/L
Chromium	Plain royal blue top	0.05 to 0.5 mcg/mL		
Chromosome analysis	Sterile plasma (green)	Chromosomal abnormalities are reported		
Complete blood count (CBC)	Plasma (lavender)	See reference ranges in Chapter 7		
Copper	Plain royal blue top	70–150 ug/dL; 11–24 umol/L		
Cortisol (am)	Serum (red) or plasma (green)	5–23 µg /dL	27.6	138–635 nmol/L
Creatinine	Serum (speckled or red) or plasma (green)	0.6–1.2 mg/dL	88.4	53–106 µmol/L
Creatine kinase	Plasma (light green)	24–174 U/L		24–174 U/L
C-reactive protein	Serum (red)	0–1.0 mg/dL		0–10 mg/L
Cyclosporine (CYCLO)	Whole blood (lavender)	Therapeutic ranges differ at different health care facilities		
D-dimer (D-D$_{1M}$)	Plasma (blue)	Highly variable due to testing methods		
Differential (DIFF)	Whole blood (lavender)	White blood cells classified; red blood cells reviewed for abnormalities; and platelets reviewed and estimated		
Drug screen	Serum (red)	Depends on drugs tested		
Electrolytes (Na, K, Cl, HCO$_3$)	Plasma (green) or serum (red)	Refer to reference intervals in Chapter 7		
ESR (sedimentation rate, sed rate)	Plasma (lavender)	Refer to reference intervals in Chapter 7		
Ethanol (alcohol)	Whole blood (gray) or serum (red)	Less than 100 mg/dL	0.2171	Less than 21.7 mmol/L

(continued)

Test Name/ Abbreviation	Specimen Type and Tube (Stopper Type/Color)	Reference Interval (Conventional Units)	Conversion Factor (Multiply By)	Reference Interval (SI Units)
Factor assays	Plasma (blue) test not valid if patient on hepanin	Depends on test methods		
Fasting blood glucose (FBG)	Plasma (gray) or whole blood (green)	70–110 mg/dL	0.0556	3.0–6.1 mmol/L
Febrile agglutinin (FEBR AB)	Serum (red)	Antibody screen for *Salmonella, Rickettsia, Brucella,* and *Francisella tularensis*		
Ferritin	Serum (speckled or red) orplasma (green)	Men: 15–200 ng/mL	1	15–200 µg/L
		Women: 12–150 ng/mL	1	12–150 µg/L
Fibrinogen	Plasma (blue)	200–400 mg/dL	0.01	2–4 g/L
Fluorescent treponemal antibody absorption (FTA-ABS)	Serum (red)	Identifies syphilis infection		
Folate, serum	Serum (speckled or red)	More than 2.3 ng/dL	2.265	More than 5.0 nmol/L
Gamma-glutamyl transpeptidase (GGT or GT)	Serum (red)	Less than 0.63 ukal/L		
Gentamycin (GENT)	Blood (red)	Therapeutic ranges Peak: 5–10 mg/L Trough: 1–2mg/L		
Glucose (fasting)	Plasma (green) or serum (red)	70–110 mg/dL	0.0556	3.0–6.1 mmol/L
Glucose-6-phosphate dehydrogenase (G-6-PD)	Whole Blood (Yellow)	8–8.6 units/gram of hemoglobin		
Glycohemoglobin Alc (see Hemoglobin Alc)				
Haptoglobin	Blood (speckled)	60–270 mg/dL	0.01	0.6–2.7 g/L
HDL (High Density Lipoprotein) (HDL)	Serum (red)	35–80 mg/dL		
Hematocrit (HCT)	Plasma (lavender)	Men: 41.5–50.4%	0.01	0.415–0.504 volfraction
		Women: 35.9–44.6%	0.01	0.359–0.446 volfraction
Hematology profile (Hct, Hgb, WBC, RBC, MCV, MCH, MCHC)	Plasma (lavender)	Refer to reference intervals in Chapter 7		
Hemoglobin	Plasma (lavender)	12–18 g/dL	10	120–180 g/L
Hemoglobin Alc	Blood (red)	3.6–5.3% of Hb		
Hepatitis B surface (HBsAb) Antibody	Serum (red)	Negative		
Hepatitis B surface (HBsAg) Antigen	Serum (red)	Negative		
INR/PT	Plasma (blue)	Depends on methodology used		
Iron binding capacity (IBC)	Serum/plasma	250–400 µg/dL	0.179	44.8–71.6 µmol/L
Iron profile (total)	Serum (speckled or red) *Avoid hemolysis*	60–150 µg/dL	0.179	10.7–26.9 µmol/L
Lactate dehydrogenase (LD) and LD isoenzymes (LD-1)	Serum (speckled or red) or plasma (green)	5–200 U/L	1.0	5–200 U/L
Lactic acid (on ice)	Blood (gray) *Avoid hemolysis*	5–20 mg/dL	0.111	0.6–2.2 mmol/L
Lead, blood	Blood (royal blue) or (lavender)	Less than 10 µg/dL	0.048	Less than 0.48 µmol/L

Test Name/ Abbreviation	Specimen Type and Tube (Stopper Type/Color)	Reference Interval (Conventional Units)	Conversion Factor (Multiply By)	Reference Interval (SI Units)
LDL Cholesterol	Serum (red)	2–3.4 mmol/L		
Lipase	Serum (red) or plasma (green)	7–60 U/L		
Lipid profile	Serum (red) or plasma (green)	Reference intervals are variable depending on methods used		
Lithium (therapeutic)	Serum (speckled or red)	0.5–1.4 mEq/L	1	0.5–1.4 mmol/L
Magnesium, serum	Serum (red)	1.3–2.1 mEq/L	0.5	0.65–1.05 mmol/L
Malaria Prep	Blood (purple)	Reported as negative or if positive, as malaria species		
Mononucleosis screen (mono-test)	Serum (red) or plasma (lavender)	Reported as negative or positive		
Osmolality, serum	Blood (speckled)	280–295 mOsm/kg	1	280–295 mmol/kg
Partial thromboplastin time (PTT) (APTT)	Blood (blue) *Indicate if patient on anticoagulant*	Reference intervals are variable depending on methods used		
Platelet aggregation (Plt. Agg)	Blood (light-blue) and blood (lavender)	Adults: >65% aggregation		
Platelet count	Plasma (lavender)	$150–400 \times 10^3/mm^3$	10^6	$150–400 \times 10^9 L$
Potassium (K)	Blood (Green)	3.5—5.0 mmol/or mEq/L		
Pregnancy test (HCG)	Serum (red)	Less than 3 mIU/mL nonpregnant female	1.0	Less than 3 IU/L
Prostatic specific antigen (PSA)	Serum (red)	Less than 4 ng/mL	1.0	Less than 4 ng/mL
Protein, total	Blood (speckled)	6–7.8 g/dL	10	60–78 g/L
Prothrombin time (PT)	Plasma (light blue)	10–13 sec (varies between labs)		
Red blood cell count (RBC)	Blood (lavender)	Men: $4.5–5.9 \ 10^6/mm^3$	10^6	$4.5–5.9 \ 10^{12}/L$
		Women: $4.5–5.1 \ 10^6/mm^3$	10^6	$4.5–5.1 \ 10^{12}/L$
Reticulocyte count	Plasma (lavender)	Refer to reference intervals in Chapter 7		
Rheumatoid factor (RF)	Serum (red)	Negative		
Sedimentation rate (ESR) (erythrocyte sedimentation rate)	Plasma (lavender)	Refer to reference intervals in Chapter 7		
Sodium, blood	Blood (green)	136–142 mEq/L	1	136–142 mmol/L
Thyroid studies (T_3, T_4, TSH)	Serum (speckled or red)	Reference ranges vary with methods used		
Triglycerides (fasting)	Serum (speckled or red) or plasma (green)	10–90 mg/dL	0.01129	0.11–2.15 mmol/L
Troponin I (cardiac)	Serum (speckled or red) or plasma (green)	Less than 0.6 ng/mL	1.0	Less than 0.6 µg/L
Troponin T (cardiac)	Serum (speckled)	Less than 0.2 ng/mL	1.0	Less than 0.2 µg/L
Urea nitrogen (BUN)	Serum (speckled)	Refer to reference intervals in Chapter 7		
Uric acid	Serum (speckled or red)	Refer to reference intervals in Chapter 7		
WBC count/differential	Plasma (lavender)	Refer to reference intervals in Chapter 7		
Zinc	Serum (blue)	50–150 µg/dL	0.153	7.7–23 µmol/L

Resources

1. American Medical Association. (1998). *Manual of Style,* 9th ed. Baltimore: Williams and Wilkins.
2. Medical Laboratory Observer (MLO). (2013–2014). Clinical Laboratory Reference (CLR), Table of Reference Intervals, 2013–2014. www.clr-online.com, accessed March 24, 2014.
3. Kaplan, L. A., & Pesce, A. J. (2010). *Clinical chemistry: Theory, analysis, correlation,* 5th ed. Missouri, MO: St. Louis.

Appendix 7

Guide for Maximum Amounts of Blood to Be Drawn from Patients Younger than Age 14

The reduction of blood loss during venipuncuture procedures is especially important for children and infants. Special care is needed to avoid iatrogenic anemia caused by excessive venipuncture procedures in a short amount of time. This is an example of a guide from one hospital to assist in monitoring blood loss due to venipuncture.

Patient's Weight		Maximum amount to be drawn at any one time (mL)	Maximum amount of blood (cumulative) to be collected during a given hospital stay (one month or less) (mL)
Pounds	Kilograms		
6–8	2.7–3.6	2.5	23
8–10	3.6–4.5	3.5	30
10–15	4.5–6.8	5	40
16–20	7.3–9.1	10	60
21–25	9.5–11.4	10	70
26–30	11.8–13.6	10	80
31–35	14.1–15.9	10	100
36–40	16.4–18.2	10	130
41–45	18.6–20.5	20	140
46–50	20.9–22.7	20	160
51–55	23.2–25.0	20	180
56–60	25.5–27.3	20	200
61–65	27.7–29.5	25	220
66–70	30.0–31.8	30	240
71–75	32.3–34.1	30	250
76–80	34.5–36.4	30	270
81–85	36.8–38.6	30	290
86–90	39.1–40.9	30	310
91–95	41.4–43.2	30	330
96–100	43.6–45.5	30	350

Courtesy of Memorial Hermann Hospital Laboratory, with permission.

Standard Operating Procedures (SOPs) for Donor Phlebotomy

These standard operating procedures are examples for donor phlebotomy. The steps are subject to differences among blood collectors and must be performed by authorized personnel only and under institutional guidelines. *These SOPs are reprinted with permission from the Gulf Coast Regional Blood Center,* www.giveblood.org

Selecting the Venipuncture Site

Scope

To provide instructions for selecting a suitable venipuncture site while using either Donor-ID or a manual Donor Record.

Materials

- Applicable Blood Donation Record (Donor Record)
- Donor-ID system and peripherals
- Handgrip
- Tourniquet or pressure cuff

Procedure

SELECTING THE VENIPUNCTURE SITE

Step	Action
1	Make sure that the donor's arm(s) are suitable for donating.
2	**If using Donor-ID:** • Select the appropriate option to indicate which arm(s) will be used for the procedure in **Screen [PBAR]**, "Arm Selection." • Click **<Left Arm>** or **<Right Arm>**. • Check the box for "Check arms" on **Screen [PBPR]**, "Prepare Arm."
3	Have the donor recline on the bed.
4	Apply a tourniquet or pressure cuff snugly around the donor's arm.
5	Have the donor squeeze a handgrip from time to time.
6	Select a vein for venipuncture. *Avoid areas that are scarred or have pits or dimples related to prior phlebotomies, since these areas are harder to clean and to remove bacteria.* *You may mark the vein so that you can easily find the vein later.*
7	**If you cannot find a suitable vein:** Ask another phlebotomist and/or consult with your supervisor for help.
8	Loosen the tourniquet or blood pressure cuff.
9	**If no one can find a suitable vein:** • Defer the donor per the applicable deferral SOP. • Record in the Comments section of the Donor Record "could not locate suitable vein" (or a similar statement) along with your initials,

Step	Action
	ID number, and the date.
10	Perform a ChloraPrep arm scrub procedure per the applicable phlebotomy SOP.

REQUIRE ASSISTANCE IN DONOR-ID

Step	Action
11	Check the box for "Prepare Donor for Draw" on **Screen [PBPR]**, "Prepare Arm," once you select a suitable vein and clean the arm.
12	Click **<Continue>** on **Screen [PBPR]**.
13	**If the initial phlebotomist cannot complete the procedure and/or a different phlebotomist performs an adjustment:** • Click <Require Assistance> on Screen [PBPR], "Prepare Arm." • Ask for assistance from another phlebotomist. • On an additional handheld, have the second phlebotomist prepare the donor per this phlebotomy SOP and click <Continue>. • Click <Check Status> on Screen [PBBE].
14	Click **<Begin Draw>** on either handheld to perform the venipuncture according to the applicable phlebotomy SOP.

ChloraPrep Arm Scrub

Scope

To provide instructions on performing the arm scrub of the venipuncture site with the ChloraPrep 1.5 mL Frepp applicator.

Materials

- ChloraPrep 1.5 mL Frepp Applicator
- Sterile gauze

Procedure

PERFORMING THE ARM SCRUB

Step	Action
1	Open the sterile blister pack of the ChloraPrep applicator.
2	Remove the applicator using an aseptic technique.
3	Squeeze the side handles together to break the ampoule. ***When the ampoule breaks, solution will flow into the foam head, and you may stop squeezing the handles.***
4	Place the applicator foam head on the venipuncture site and press down once or twice to prime the applicator.
5	For at least 30 seconds, apply the solution in a back, forth, up, and down motion to the venipuncture site, in a 2.5-inch diameter area.
6	Allow the ChloraPrep solution to air dry on the venipuncture site for at least 30 seconds. ***This allows time for the ChloraPrep to properly clean the site.***
7	Discard the used applicator.
8	Do not touch or repalpate the area after you clean it.
9	Do not wipe the cleaning solution from the cleaned area.
10	**If the cleaned area is touched or otherwise compromised:** Repeat the entire arm scrub procedure.

IF NOT PERFORMING THE VENIPUNCTURE RIGHT AWAY

Step	Action
11	You may cover the venipuncture area with sterile gauze—after 30 seconds has elapsed—if you do not perform the venipuncture right away.

Step	Action
12	When handling the gauze: • Apply the gauze carefully to avoid contaminating the intended venipuncture site. • Avoid applying pressure while applying and removing the gauze. • Pick up the gauze only along its edges. • Uncover the venipuncture site by removing the gauze and placing it on the donor's arm away from the cleaned area with the ChloraPrep side of the gauze facing upward.

Whole Blood Venipuncture

Scope	To provide instructions on venipuncture for whole blood products while using either Donor-ID or a manual Donor Record.

Materials
- Appropriate blood collection bags
- Gauze
- Handgrip
- Hemostat
- Tape
- Tourniquet or blood pressure cuff

Procedure

Step	Action
1	During the collection process, the donor should be in a reclining position. *If the donor cannot be in a reclining position, contact the Medical Director for help.*
2	Check for a hemostat applied to the blood tubing between the donor needle and the Y-junction.
3	Apply enough pressure with the tourniquet or the blood pressure cuff to help identify the suitable vein in the arm.
4	Have the donor squeeze the handgrip.
5	Check for a loose loop tied in the blood tubing between the Y-junction and sampling site and another loop between the cannula and primary bag.
6	Check that the blood bag is properly placed on the weighing device.
7	Check that the sample pouch is hanging downward and not resting on any surface.
8	Remove the cover from the needle by holding the hub and twisting the cover.
9	Retract the skin firmly below the scrubbed area.
10	Insert the needle through the skin and into the vein in one smooth motion.
11	While holding the needle hub stable, release the hemostat. *You may change which hand holds the needle hub, if it is easier for you this way.*
12	Tell the donor to unclench his or her fist.

Step	Action
13	Watch for blood flow into the sample pouch.
14	Engage the needle guard by sliding the device up the tubing and over to cover two thirds of the needle hub. *In adverse collection conditions (ex. fine veins), leave the needle guard down the tube behind the hub during the collection and engage at the end of collection.* *Document in the Comments section of the manual Donor Record or GC302 when the needle guard is not used.* *If applicable, record the difficult condition per the phlebotomy SOP instructions for difficult stick documentation.*
15	Tape the needle guard and tubing to the donor's arm over the guard's raised arrow.
16	Cover the venipuncture site with the gauze.
17	Ask the donor to open and close his or her hand slowly and repeatedly during the collection.
18	Loosen and readjust the tourniquet, if needed, for the donor's comfort.

Ending the Blood Draw

Scope

To provide instructions for ending the blood draw while using either Donor-ID or a manual Donor Record.

Materials

- Applicable Blood Donation Record (Donor Record)
- Form GC2000, Quality Improvement Report (QIR)
- Job Aid JA1623, Classification and Treatment Of Adverse Reactions
- Label LC3-020, Quarantined Component Tag
- Label LC26-007, DIN (or BUI) Labels
- Crimper and grommets, or heat sealer
- Donor-ID system and peripherals
- Handgrip
- Hemostat

Procedure

CLOSING THE UNIT TUBING LINE

Step	Action	
1	Instruct the donor to stop squeezing the handgrip.	
2	Clamp the unit tubing closed with a hemostat above the Y-junction.	
3	Tighten the loop in the tubing to form a white knot about one inch below the cannula.	
4	Check that you pulled the knot tight.	
5	**If using the heat sealer instead of the white knot method:** Perform two heat seals on the tubing approximately one inch below the cannula. Check that the heat seals are intact.	**If using the crimper and grommets instead of the white knot method:** Place two grommets on the tubing approximately one inch below the cannula. Close the grommets with the crimper. Check that you closed the grommets correctly.
6	Release the tourniquet or blood pressure cuff.	

IF USING DONOR-ID

Step	Action
7	Click **<Phlebotomy>** on the handheld "Home" screen.
8	Login to Donor-ID on **Screen [DILI]**, "Login."
9	Locate the donor by name on **Screen [PBVS]**, "Screened Donor Selection," and verify the length of the collection procedure.
10	Scan the Visit ID/DIN from either the donation's blood bags or storage container(s) or select the donor by name on **Screen [PBVS]**, "Screened Donor Selection."
11	Verify the information displayed on **Screen [PBVD]**, "Verify Donor Identity," matches the donor's.

If the donor displayed on the screen is correct:	If the donor displayed on the screen is incorrect:
Click **<Continue>** and continue with the donation process.	Click **<Back>** to return to **Screen [PBVS]** to select a different donor.

Step	Action
12	Click the **<Complete Draw>** link on **Screen [PBMN]**, "Options for Completed Donor."
13	On **Screen [PBCO]**, "Complete Draw:" Click the **<Complete Draw>** button. *Draw Time stops when the <Complete Draw> button is clicked.*
14	End the draw and remove the needle from the donor's arm per the applicable phlebotomy SOP.
15	Scan the ID number of the collection device used during the procedure (weight monitor, shaker, HOMS Scale, etc.), on **Screen [PBTS]**, "Identify Trip Scale" and click **<Continue>**.
16	Select the related completion code and click **<Continue>**. *For help with assigning completion codes, refer to the applicable phlebotomy SOP for the given completion code.*
17	Select the related donor reaction code and click **<Continue>**. *Assess the donor's symptoms as instructed in Job Aid JA1623, Classification and Treatment Of Adverse Reactions.*
18	**If the donor has an adverse reaction:** Refer to the applicable phlebotomy SOP.
19	Print the phlebotomy labels per the applicable phlebotomy SOP.
20	Complete the phlebotomy procedure in the handheld.
21	Provide the donor with the post donation instructions per the applicable phlebotomy SOP.

REQUIRING ASSISTANCE IN DONOR-ID

Step	Action
22	**If the initial phlebotomist cannot complete the procedure and/or a different phlebotomist is needed to assist in the procedure:** • Click **<Complete Draw>** on **Screen [PBMN]**, "Options for Completed Donor." • Click **<Require Assistance>** on **Screen [PBCO]** "Complete Draw." • Ask for assistance from another phlebotomist. • On an additional handheld, have the second phlebotomist end the draw and remove the needle per the applicable subsection of this SOP and click **<Continue>**. • Click **<Check Status>** on **Screen [PBBE]**.
23	Click **<Complete Draw>** on either handheld to record the stop time according to the applicable phlebotomy SOP.

IF USING A MANUAL DONOR RECORD

Step	Action
24	For the "Stop Time," record when the phlebotomy procedure ended (in military time), along with your employee ID number.
25	Remove the needle from the donor's arm per the applicable phlebotomy SOP.
26	Verify the donor record matches the donor and the donation's blood bags or storage containers.
27	Record the following phlebotomy information in the "Phlebotomy 1" area of the Donor Record right after you perform the related procedure step. *If you perform a double stick apheresis procedure, refer to the applicable phlebotomy SOP.*
28	For "Reaction," mark the donor reaction, if applicable: • **M:** Mild • **MO:** Moderate • **SEV:** Severe • **HE:** Hematoma • **INJ:** Injury *Assess the donor's symptoms as instructed in Job Aid JA1623, Classification and Treatment Of Adverse Reactions.*

Step	Action
29	For "Completion Code," mark the completion code, if applicable: • **QNS:** Quantity not sufficient, 1-day deferral • **Q51:** Quantity not sufficient, 56-day deferral • **OD:** Overdraw • **DIFF:** Difficult stick • **SD:** Slow draw • **Q:** Quarantined unit • **ICP:** Incomplete platelets *For help with assigning completion codes, refer to the applicable phlebotomy SOP for the given completion code.*

DOCUMENTATION AND LABELING REVIEW

Step	Action
30	At the donor's bed, check that the bar-coded DIN numbers are identical and present in each of these locations: • The Donor Record • The primary and satellite bags • The sample tubes • The sample pouch • Any applicable special tags and labels • Any applicable procedural records *The phlebotomist will perform the final check for the presence of matching DIN labeling on the bags, sample tubes, the Donor Record, and forms.*
31	**If a bar code is missing:** Notify the supervisor or designee. Have him or her witness as you apply a bar code to the applicable area.
32	**If you cannot correct a labeling problem at the bedside:** • Start an investigation to find the cause of the problem. • Attach a Quarantined Component Tag LC3-020 to the unit(s) related to the problem. • Begin a Quality Improvement Report (QIR) Form GC2000.
33	Check that the related documents are complete, correct, and legible.

Appendix 9

Units of Measurement and Symbols

In 2001, The Joint Commission revealed concern about the use of medical abbreviations that can easily be misinterpreted, especially if they are handwritten. The Joint Commission has now integrated the issue into a performance standard relating to information management. It involves a list of "Do Not Use" abbreviations, acronyms, and symbols. This recommendation is to prevent confusion among caregivers when communicating test orders, medication orders, and/or results. In addition, the Institute for Safe Medication Practices (ISMP) has also published error-prone abbreviations, symbols, etc. The aim is to eliminate misinterpretations of written information. Selected recommendations from both have been incorporated into this appendix as they may apply to phlebotomy practices; however, this list is not exhaustive. For more comprehensive information, consult these organizations' websites (both of which were acccessed July 31, 2013):

www.jointcommission.org

www.ismp.org

Be particularly mindful when you are handwriting data or reading handwritten information. The following symbols are often misread and can lead to errors in patient care. If you find symbols that are unclear, ask for clarification prior to proceeding with any type of phlebotomy procedure.

Do Not Use	Better Options for Use
a	alpha
Å	angstrom
@	can be mistaken for the number two (2); instead write "at"
amp	ampere (unit of electric current)
&	should be a written word, "and"
c	centi- (10^{-2})
°C	degrees centigrade or Celsius (unit of temperature)
cc	cubic centimeter (same as mL); it should not be abbreviated
cd	candela (unit of luminous intensity)
cm	centimeter
cu mm	cubic millimeter
d	deci- (10^{-1})
D/C	"discharge" should not be abbreviated
D/C	"discontinue" should not be abbreviated
decimal point	Always use a zero before a decimal point when the measurement is less than a whole unit so the reader notices the decimal point (for example: .5 mL might be mistaken for 5 mL; instead, write 0.5 mL)
dl	deciliter (1/10 of a liter)

Do Not Use	Better Options for Use
°F	degrees Fahrenheit (unit of temperature)
g or gm	gram (1/1000 of a kilogram, unit of mass)
G%	grams in 100 mL
h	hecto- (10^2)
hpf	high-power field on microscope
IU	"international unit" should not be abbreviated
k	kilo- (10^3)
°K	degrees Kelvin (thermodynamic temperature)
kg	kilogram (1000 g, or 2.2 lb)
l	liter (1000 ml, unit of volume)
Latin abbreviations	Use the exact meaning of words rather than Latin abbreviations. (For example: instead of the terms *q.i.d., q.o.d., t.i.d.,* refer to "once daily, every other day, three times per day," respectively, and they should be written as such.)
less than (<)/ greater than (>)	should be written words, "less than" or "greater than"
lpf	low-power field on microscope
m	meter (unit of length)
m	milli- (10^{-3})
mcg	microgram (1/1000 mg)
mCi	millicurie

Do Not Use	Better Options for Use
mEq or meq	milliequivalent
mg	milligram (1/1000 g)
mg%	milligrams in 100 mL (same as dl)
min	minutes
mL	milliliter (1/1000 L, same as a cubic centimeter)
mm	millimeter (1/10 cm)
mm³	cubic millimeter
mm Hg	millimeters of mercury
mmole	millimole
mol, M	mole (unit of substance)
mOsm	milliosmol
N	normality
n	nano- (10^{-9})
ng	nanogram (1/1000 mg)
p	pico- (10^{-12})
periods	Do not use a terminal period after a symbol for a unit of measurement because it may be interpreted as another symbol (for example: 7 ml. might be mistaken for 7 mL1, which is meaningless; instead, write 7 mL)
pg	picogram (1/1000 ng)

Do Not Use	Better Options for Use
QNS	quantity not sufficient
sec or s	second (unit of time)
sp g	specific gravity
spacing	Use adequate space between numbers and letter symbols so that they will not run together (for example: 8mL might be mistaken as 8001 if the "m" is mistaken for zeros; instead write 8 mL)
TPN	total parenteral nutrition
TPR	temperature, pulse, respirations
trailing zeros	Do not use a zero alone *after* a decimal point because the reader may not notice the decimal point when interpreting a medication order (for example: 3.0 mL might be mistaken for 30 mL; instead, write 3 mL); exceptions may occur for reporting laboratory results, imaging studies, or the size of lesions
U (unit)	Formerly written as "U"; it should not be abbreviated because it is mistaken for zero (0), four (4), or "cc"; instead write unit
WNL	within normal limits
WNR	within normal range
wt	weight
w/v	weight/volume

Appendix 10

Formulas, Calculations, and Metric Conversion

Area	square meter (sq m or m^2)
Blood Volume	Total blood volume = weight (kg) × average blood volume per kg (defined by age)
Clearance	liter/second (L/s)
Mass	kilogram/liter (kg/L)
Substrate	mole/liter (mol/L)
Density	kilogram/liter (kg/L)
Dilutions	Final concentration = Original concentration × dilution 1 × dilution 2, and so on.
Hematology Math	Mean corpuscular volume (MCV) = average volume of red blood cells (RBCs); expressed in cubic microns μm^3 or femtoliters (fL) $MCV = \dfrac{Hct \times 10}{RBC \text{ count (in millions)}}$ Hct = hematocrit value
	Mean corpuscular hemoglobin (MCH) = Average weight of hemoglobin in RBC; expressed in picograms (pg) $MCH = \dfrac{hgb\ (g) \times 10}{RBC \text{ count (in millions)}}$ hgb = hemoglobin value
	Mean corpuscular hemoglobin concentration = Hemoglobin concentration of average RBC $MCHC = \dfrac{hgb\ (g)}{Hct} \times 100\%$
	RBC distribution width (RDW) = numerical expression of variation of RBC size, dispersion of RBC volumes about the mean $RDW = \dfrac{SD \text{ (standard deviation) of RBC size}}{MCV}$
Metric Conversions: Length or Distance	1 inch (in) = 2.54 centimeters (cm) 1 foot (ft) = 30.48 centimeters (cm) 39.37 inches (in.) = 1 meter (m) (Note: 1 meter is slightly more than 3 feet.) 1 mile (mi) = 1.61 kilometers (km)
Mass or Weight	1 ounce (oz) = 28.35 grams (g) 1 pound (lb) = 453.6 grams (g) 2.205 pounds (lb) = 1 kilogram (kg)
Volume	1 fluid ounce (fl oz) = 29.57 milliliters (mL) (Notes: cubic centimeter, cc, is interchangeable with milliliter, mL, for example, 1 cc = 1 mL; 1 ounce is about 30 mL = 30 cc) 1.057 quarts (qt) = 1 liter (liter or L) 1 gallon (gal) = 3.78 liters (liter or L)
Military Time	See Appendix 11
Pressure	Pascal (Pa) = (kg/m)s^2
Quality Control Math: Variance (s^2)	$s^2 = \dfrac{(x - \bar{x})^2}{n - 1}$
Standard deviation(s)	$s = \sqrt{s^2}$
% Coefficient of variation	$\% CV = \dfrac{s}{\bar{x}} \times 100$

Relative Centrifugal Force (rcf)	Measures force of centrifugation acting on blood components and allowing them to separate. Can be used to calibrate centrifuges. $rcf = 1.118 \times 10^{-5} \times 4 \times n^2$ r = rotating radius (centimeters) n = speed of rotation (revolutions per minute) Centrifuges should be calibrated and maintained according to manufacturers' instructions.
Specific Gravity (sp g)	$sp\ g = \dfrac{\text{wt of solid or liquid}}{\text{wt of equal volume of } H_2O \text{ at } 4°C}$

Temperature:
   Celsius or Centigrade
   Kelvin
   Fahrenheit
      (see also Appendix 5)
	$°C = K - 273.15;\ °C = °F - 32 \times 0.555$
	$°K = °C + 273.15 \text{ or } 5/9(°F) + 255.35$
	$°F = (°C \times 1.8) + 32$

Volume	deciliter (dL) = 1/10 of a liter 10 dL = 1L centiliter (cL) = 1/100 of a liter 100 cL = 10dL = 1L milliliter (mL) = 1/1000 of a liter 1000mL = 100 cL = 10dL = 1L

Fahrenheit and Celsius Selected Comparisons

Fahrenheit (Degrees)	Celsius/Centigrade (Degrees)
32	0
95	35
96	35.5
96.8	36
98.6	37
99.6	37.5
100.4	38
102.2	39
104	40

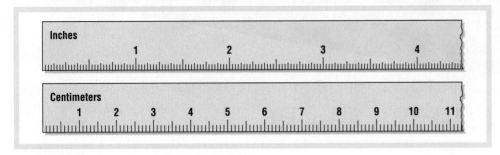

FIGURE A10–1
Comparison of Standard and Metric Units of Length

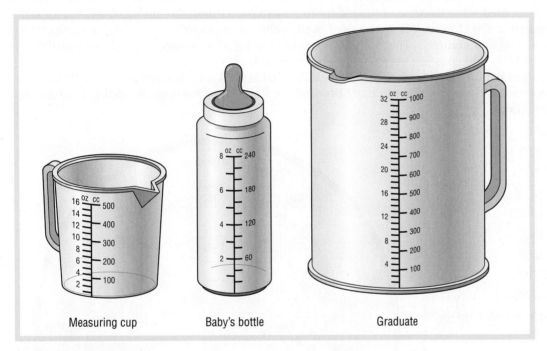

FIGURE A10–2
Graduated Measuring Containers for Fluid Ounces and Cubic Centimeters

Appendix 11

Military Time (24-Hour Clock)

Military time uses a 24-hour time clock and eliminates the need for the AM (or A.M.) and PM (or P.M.) designations that are used in civilian or Greenwich time (12-hour time clock). The 24-hour clock is particularly useful in health care settings so that confusion is eliminated when documenting time for treatment procedures, specimen collections, tests, drug administration, surgical procedures, and so on. It is important that all health care workers understand and use it correctly.

Military time is expressed by four numerals: The first pair is *hours* (00 to 24), and the second pair is *minutes* (00 to 59). Each day begins at midnight, 0000, and ends just before midnight the next day, 2359.

The first 12 hours are equivalent in Greenwich and military time; that is, 3:00 A.M. is equivalent to 0300 in military time, but conversion of afternoon and evening times from a 12-hour clock to military time requires adding 12 to each hour (2:00 P.M. is 1400 in military time).

Examples:
- 1:00 a.m. = 0100
- 5:00 a.m. = 0500
- 10:00 a.m. = 1000
- 11:00 a.m. = 1100
- 12:00 noon = 1200
- 1:00 p.m. = 1300
- 4:00 p.m. = 1600
- 9:00 p.m. = 2100
- 10:00 p.m. = 2200
- 12:00 midnight = 2400/0000

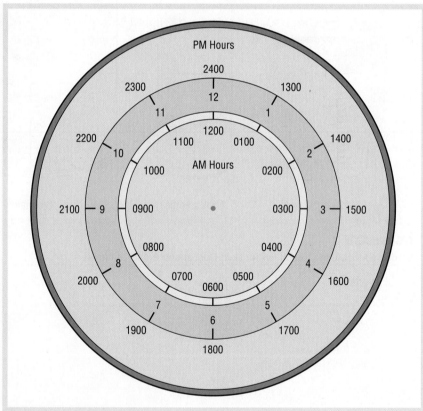

FIGURE A11–1
24-Hour Clock (Military Time)

Military time is usually stated in terms of hundreds (e.g., 1500 is stated as "fifteen hundred hours"; 0300 is stated as "zero three hundred").

Reference

Badasch, S. A., & Chesebro, D. S. (2000). *Introduction to health occupations, today's health care worker,* 5th ed. Upper Saddle River, NJ: Prentice Hall Health.

Appendix 12

Basic Spanish for Specimen Collection Procedures

For individuals who are interested in using languages in their workplace, there are numerous multilanguage dictionary websites and apps available that are reasonably priced or sometimes free. There are also educational programs specifically designed for medical translators and health care workers who want to converse in numerous languages. Phlebotomists are encouraged to learn new languages and use them professionally at work.

The following Spanish translations present the health care worker with a basic means of communicating with patients who speak Spanish. Before speaking with patients, the health care worker should practice using these phrases with someone who knows the correct pronunciation, or take courses for medical translation, etc. Otherwise, the patient may become even more confused. Remember that in Spanish, the letter *h* is always silent. Also, if a word ends in *a*, it is usually feminine gender; if it ends in *o*, it is masculine. Another alternative is to have the key phrases printed on cards that the health care worker may point to or use as a reference when he or she is communicating with the patient. Also, use your hands when speaking; pantomime, point, or use facial expressions to assist in communicating your message. The ultimate goal is to make sure that the patient understands.

English	Spanish
one, two, three, four, five	uno, dos, tres, cuatro, cinco
six, seven, eight, nine, ten	seis, siete, ocho, nueve, diez
twenty, thirty, forty, fifty	veinte, treinta, cuarenta, cincuenta
sixty, seventy, eighty, ninety, one hundred	sesenta, setenta, ochenta, noventa, ciento/cien
Hello	Hola
Good day	Buenos dias/Buendia
Good morning	Buenos dias
Good afternoon	Buenas tardes
Good evening	Buenas noches
mother, father, sister, brother	madre/mama, padre/papa, hermana, hermano
son, daughter, husband, wife	hijo, hija, esposo/marido, esposa/marida
infant/baby	Niño/niña
grandfather, grandmother	abuelo, abuela
friend	amigo/amiga
Mister, Mrs., Miss	Señor, Señora, Señorita
doctor	doctor/medico
technician	técnico
nurse	enfermera
alcohol	alcohol
fasting	enayunas
gloves	guantes
needle	aguja

English	Spanish
sterile	estéril
syringe	jeringa
tourniquet	torniquete
pathology	patología
procedure	procedimiento
hematology	hematología
complete blood count (CBC)	biometría hemática complete
blood bank	banco de sangre
coagulated	coagulado
reports	reportes
specimen	muestra
tubes	tubos
My name is . . .	Me llamo . . ./Mi nombre es . . .
I work in the laboratory.	Trabajo en el laboratorio.
I speak . . .	Hablo . . .
We are going to analyze	Vamos analizar
. . . your blood.	. . . su sangre.
. . . your urine.	. . . su orina.
. . . your sputum.	. . . su esputo.
Do you understand?	¿Entiende usted (ud.)?
I do not understand.	No entiendo.
Please (pls.)	Por favor (p.f.)
Thank you.	Gracias.
You are welcome.	De nada.
Speak slower, pls.	Hable mas despacio, p.f.
Repeat, pls.	Haga me el favor de repetir, p.f.
Can you hear me?	¿Puede oírme?
Can you speak?	¿Puede hablar?
Relax.	Relajese.
What is your name?	¿Como se llama?
What is your address?	¿Que es su domicillo?
What is your birth date?	¿En que fecha nacio?
How old are you?	¿Cuantos años tiene ud.?
Have you been here before?	¿Ha estado ud. aquí antes?
Who is your doctor?	¿Quien es su doctor?
Your doctor wrote the order.	El doctor/la doctora escribio la orden.
Here is the bathroom.	Aquí esta el baño.
Here is the call light.	Aquí esta la luz de emergencia.
You may not eat/drink anything except water.	No debe de comer/beber nada solamente agua.
You may not smoke.	No puede fumar.
Have you had breakfast?	¿Ya tomo el desayuno?
We need a blood/urine/stool sample.	Necesitamos una muestra de su sangre/orina/del excremento.
Please stay in bed.	Por favor, quédese en la cama.

English	Spanish
Do you have any allergies or are you sensitive to any substances? . . . like latex?	¿Tiene usted alergias o es sensible anormal a ciertas sustancias? . . . como el latex?
Have you fainted during blood drawing?	¿Se ha ud desmayado cuando le extrajeron sangre?
Please do not eat after midnight.	Por favor, no coma después de medianoche.
Please	Haga me el favor de
. . . make a fist.	. . . cerrar el puño.
. . . bend your arm.	. . . doblar el brazo.
. . . roll up your sleeve.	. . . levantarse la manga.
. . . open your hand.	. . . abrir la mano.
. . . sit down here.	. . . sientese aquí.
. . . change your position.	. . . cambiarse de posición.
. . . turn over.	. . . voltearse.
. . . change to the left.	. . . cambiarse a la izquierda.
. . . change to the right.	. . . cambiarse a la derecha.
I am going to lift your sleeve.	Voy levantar la manga.
I need to	Necesito
. . . take a blood sample.	. . . sacar una muestra de sangre.
. . . stick/prick your finger.	. . . picarle su dedo.
. . . two tubes of blood.	. . . dos tubos de sangre.
Open your hand.	Abra la mano.
It will hurt a little.	Le va a doler un poquito.
Please do not move.	No se mueva, por favor.
This is done quickly.	Esto se hace rapido.
The needle will stay in your arm while I am collecting the blood sample.	La aguja se quedara en su brazo durante el tiempo necessario para obtener la muestra.
Could you confirm that these tubes are labeled with your name/identity?	¿Podria ud confirmar que estos tubos estan etiquetados con su nombre/identidad?
I am finished. Thank you.	Ya termine. Gracias.
Press this gauze on your arm/finger until I can make sure that the bleeding has stopped.	Comprese esta banda en su brazo/su dedo hasta que pare la sangre.
I am going to put a bandage on you.	Voy a ponerle una cinta adhesiva/un curita/un bandaid.
Are you lightheaded?	¿Esta usted mareado/mareada?
Do you feel as if you are going to faint?	¿Se siente como si se va a desmayar?
Do you feel all right?	¿Se siente bien?
You must lie down.	Necesita acostarse.
Collect the midstream portion of the urine in the container or bottle.	Coleccione la porción del medio de la orina en el vaso.
Void a little, then put urine in this cup.	Orine un poco, luego ponga la orina en esta taza.

Resources

Joyce, E. V., & Villanueva, M. E. (2000). *Say it in Spanish, a guide for health care professionals*, 2nd ed. Philadelphia: W. B. Saunders.

Many dictionaries and translators are also available online and as apps for mobile devices.

Appendix 13

Competency Assessment Tracking Sheet

Student Name: _____

All concepts presented in this textbook are important to phlebotomists; it is vital that the information is clearly understood. Use this tracking sheet to monitor your own progress. If your competency level "needs improvement," review the information in the text again, ask questions of qualified health care educators, and seek out help or clarification before trying the competency assessment again. Do not indicate that you have completed the competency assessment until you have done so at an "acceptable" level. Be honest with yourself. Know your strengths and weaknesses so that you can improve your knowledge and practices, and have a better chance at achieving possible certification in phlebotomy or a related field.

Title of Exercise or Procedure	Date Completed	Competency Level Acceptable	Competency Level Needs Improvement
Chapter 1			
Basics of Phlebotomy Practice and the Clinical Laboratory			
1. List at least five service areas/departments that are commonly found in large health care facilities.			
2. List three ways in which laboratory test results are used.			
3. Name at least five departments/sections common in clinical laboratory/clinical pathology.			
4. List at least three types of laboratory personnel other than phlebotomists.			
5. Name 10 types of locations where phlebotomy services can be performed.			
6. Describe at least three clinical duties of a phlebotomist.			
7. Describe at least three technical duties of a phlebotomist.			
8. Describe at least three clerical duties of a phlebotomist			
9. Describe at least five character traits of a phlebotomist.			
10. Name at least three professional organizations for phlebotomists and other laboratory personnel.			
Quality Basics			
1. Provide three examples of external stakeholders (customers).			
2. Provide eight examples of internal stakeholders (customers).			
3. List five examples of how a phlebotomist may have a negative effect on quality and/or patient outcomes.			
4. List 10 examples of quality improvement assessments that could be monitored for phlebotomy services.			
5. Describe at least eight examples of preexamination/preanalytical factors that affect phlebotomy services.			
6. Describe the difference between a flowchart and a cause-and-effect diagram.			
7. Give two examples of basic QC measures.			

Title of Exercise or Procedure	Date Completed	Competency Level Acceptable	Competency Level Needs Improvement
Chapter 2			
Cultural Competency			
1. I have enough knowledge about the cultures of other racial, religious, and ethnic groups.			
2. I periodically attend multicultural events, social events, and classes or seminars about generational or cultural diversity.			
3. I never use degrading language or terms.			
4. I do not stereotype people based on their group, gender, etc.			
5. I value cultural differences.			
6. I give equal attention to all coworkers and patients regardless of race, religion, ecomonic status, and physical ability.			
7. I am not afraid to ask people who use biased language or behaviors to refrain from doing so.			
Telephone Communication			
1. The telephone is answered on the first or second ring.			
2. The correct greeting is used. ("Good morning," give name and/or department, "How may I help you?")			
3. Words and statements are enunciated and easy to understand.			
4. A professional tone of voice is used.			
5. A moderate volume is used for talking.			
6. A moderate pace is used with appropriate pauses.			
7. The caller is placed on hold after he or she states the reason for the call.			
8. The caller is not left on hold for more than 30 seconds.			
9. Messages are clearly and accurately written.			
10. Spellings and phone numbers are repeated for accuracy.			
11. There is a polite ending to the conversation. ("Good-bye," "Thank you," etc.).			
12. The caller is allowed to hang up first.			
Handwritten Communication			
1. Write a short paragraph (5 to 10 sentences) about the last time you had a blood test. The reader should evaluate:			
a. the clarity of the message			
b. the readability of the handwriting			
c. how well the description of the scene was understood.			
2. Practice writing your full name, and initials 10 times very quickly. The reader should evaluate the			
a. legibility of each letter in each of the 10 names			
b. legibility of each letter in each of the 10 initials			
Computer Components			
Point to and define each of the following computer components and peripherals.			
1. Computer monitor			
2. Keyboard			
3. Printer			
4. Bar code reader (if available)			
5. Scanner			
6. Fax/Scan			
7. Modem			
8. CPU			

Title of Exercise or Procedure	Date Completed	Competency Level Acceptable	Competency Level Needs Improvement
9. Data storage units			
10. Software used on that computer			
Chapter 3			
Ethical, Legal, and Regulatory Issues			
1. Describe four methods for protecting health information.			
2. List six lawsuit prevention tips for minimizing risks.			
Chapter 4			
Infection Control			
1. Describe or identify four pieces of personal protective equipment in the blood collection area.			
2. List the personal protective equipment required to enter an isolation room for droplet precautions.			
Chapter 5			
Safety and First Aid			
1. Describe the steps in providing "bleeding aid" to a victim.			
2. Describe four protective measures for chemical use.			
Chapter 6			
Prefixes			
Write the definitions of the prefixes listed.			
Word Roots			
Write the definitions of the roots listed.			
Suffixes			
Write the definitions of the suffixes listed.			
Identifying Medical Terms			
Write the medical terms for the definitions listed.			
Spelling			
Write the correct spelling of misspelled terms listed.			
Directional Terms			
Define the directional terms listed.			
Body Systems			
Name and correctly spell the organ systems described in this chapter, their functions, and at least two methods used in the clinical laboratory to evaluate the system.			
Chapter 7			
The Cardiovascular and Lymphatic Systems			
Describe the properties of arteries, veins, and capillaries and the blood that comes from each blood vessel.			
List and describe the major structures and functions of the cardiovascular and lymphatic systems. Give examples of common laboratory tests and disorders of these systems.			
Blood Flow and the Hemostatic Process			
1. Verbally describe the flow of blood through the body. Try to begin at the right atrium of the heart and end at the aorta.			
2. Verbally describe the hemostatic process.			
Chapter 8			
Blood Collection Equipment			
1. Describe the use of the BMP LeukoChek in blood collection.			
2. List three safety butterfly needles.			
3. Explain how the BD Blood Transfer Device works.			

Title of Exercise or Procedure	Date Completed	Competency Level Acceptable	Competency Level Needs Improvement
Chapter 9			
Preanalytical Complications			
1. Describe how to collect blood from the patient's arm that has an inserted IV line.			
2. Explain why petechiae occurs in some patients.			
Chapter 10			
Patient Identification			
1. List three ways to confirm a patient's identity.			
2. List three methods *that would not be reliable* for confirming a patient's identity.			
Preparing for the Patient Encounter			
1. The health care worker demonstrates a positive, professional appearance.			
2. The health care worker demonstrates positive body language, including a pleasant facial expression and good posture before beginning the patient encounter.			
3. The health care worker has protective equipment, phlebotomy supplies, test requisitions, a writing pen, and appropriate patient information before beginning the venipuncture process.			
4. The health care worker can describe what to do if he or she cannot identify the patient correctly or if information is incomplete.			
5. The health care worker asks questions about latex allergies and likelihood of fainting.			
6. The health care worker looks for signs of patient understanding of the procedure by offering to answer any questions the patient may have.			
Use of a Tourniquet and Site Selection			
1. A clean latex-free tourniquet is used by stretching ends of the tourniquet around the patient's arm about 3 inches (7.6 cm) above the venipuncture area (antecubital area). The tourniquet is applied tightly but not painfully to the patient. It is not left on more than 1 minute.			
2. The antecubital area is palpated appropriately (not too hard, not too soft, not too much).			
3. Veins are located and identified appropriately. One or more options can easily be identified in the antecubital area.			
4. When it is time to release the tourniquet, the partial loop should allow for easy release by the health care worker using only one hand, because the other hand will be holding the needle and tubes.			
5. Practice applying the tourniquet on the lower arm to identify dorsal hand veins.			
6. Palpate and identify the best option for venipuncture on the dorsal side of the hand.			
7. Release the tourniquet during the appropriate time frame.			
Cleansing the Puncture Site			
1. After the site is selected, it is decontaminated with a commercially packaged alcohol pad.			
2. The site is rubbed with moderate pressure applied to the alcohol pad, working in concentric circles from the inside out.			
3. Adequate time is allotted for the site to dry.			
Performing a Venipuncture			
1. After greeting and identifying the patient, decontaminating hands, donning gloves, and preparing equipment in the presence of the patient, the health care worker offers to answer any questions for the patient.			
2. The health care worker prepares equipment according to the manufacturer's instructions, including attaching a needle onto the appropriate holder.			

Title of Exercise or Procedure	Date Completed	Competency Level Acceptable	Competency Level Needs Improvement
3. The patient's arm is positioned properly.			
4. A clean tourniquet is applied and potential sites are checked by palpating the vein.			
5. If a suitable vein is not felt, the tourniquet is removed and applied to the other arm.			
6. Practice warming the site or lower the arm farther in a downward position to pool venous blood.			
7. An appropriate site is selected and cleaned with an alcohol pad in a circular motion from inside to outside. It is allowed to air dry.			
8. The patient is asked to "please close your fist."			
9. The patient is told that he or she will "feel a stick" or "please remain still while I begin the procedure; you will feel a slight prick."			
10. The patient's arm is held below the site, pulling the skin slightly with the thumb.			
11. The needle assembly and arm are held appropriately.			
12. The needle is parallel to the vein and at the appropriate angle.			
13. The patient is instructed to open his or her fist after blood begins to flow, and the tourniquet is released at the appropriate time.			
14. Evacuated tubes are pushed into the holder in an appropriate manner.			
15. Evacuated tubes are filled in the correct order and until the blood flow stops in each tube.			
16. Each tube is removed from the holder with a gentle twist-and-pull motion and replaced with the next tube.			
17. Tubes are gently mixed/inverted in one hand while holding the needle apparatus and waiting for another tube to fill.			
18. When all tubes have been filled the needle is withdrawn in an appropriate manner.			
19. Bleeding is adequately controlled.			
20. The safety device is activated according to the manufacturer's instructions.			
21. The patient is instructed to apply pressure to the site using the gauze.			
Order of Draw			
Practice numbering the tubes in the correct order of collection for a venipuncture:			
1. Lavender closure used for hematology tests (CBC), yellow closure used for blood cultures, serum closure used for many chemistry tests			
2. Heparin (green), serum (red speckled), coagulation (light blue)			
3. Blood cultures, coagulation, hematology			
4. Coagulation, serum protein			
5. Heparin, EDTA, serum cholesterol, coagulation			
6. Using a butterfly method: coagulation, hematology			
Leaving the Patient			
1. The health care worker rechecks the puncture site to see whether the bleeding has stopped or if the patient wants a bandage.			
2. The health care worker asks whether the patient is feeling faint.			
3. The health care worker labels all specimens appropriately and reconfirms specimen and patient identity.			
4. Used supplies are discarded appropriately.			
5. Hands are decontaminated after the procedure.			
6. Specimens are readied for transport in a secure fashion.			
7. The health care worker thanks the patient before leaving the room (inpatient setting) and escorts patient to exit point (outpatient setting).			

Title of Exercise or Procedure	Date Completed	Competency Level Acceptable	Competency Level Needs Improvement
Chapter 11			
Capillary Blood Collection			
1. Performs patient identification and assessment appropriately.			
2. Prepares the appropriate supplies and puncture device.			
3. Performs hand hygiene and gloving techniques.			
4. Positions the patient appropriately.			
5. Selects the correct finger.			
6. Cleanses the site appropriately.			
7. Uses warming devices or other methods to improve blood flow to the site.			
8. Uses a self-retracting puncture device to make an incision across the fingerprint, and then discards the puncture device.			
9. Wipes away the first drop of blood.			
10. Collects the appropriate specimen in the correct order.			
11. Applies appropriate pressure to produce additional drops of blood.			
12. Applies gentle pressure to stop the bleeding.			
13. Handles the specimens appropriately (e.g., gentle mixing).			
14. Discards all waste in appropriate containers.			
15. Labels the specimens appropriately and prepares them for transport.			
16. Checks the patient status and reconfirms sample labels/identity are correct.			
17. Thanks the patient for cooperating.			
Making Blood Smears for Microscopic Analysis			
1. Using a practice sample of blood, the phlebotomist is able to make 50 suitable blood smears.			
2. Using blood from a capillary puncture on a patient, the phlebotomist wipes away the first drop of blood.			
3. The glass slide is touched to the finger about 0.5 to 1 inch from the end.			
4. The second slide (the spreader) is placed in front of the drop, which allows the drop of blood to spread along the width of the slide.			
5. The spreader is pushed evenly toward the other end of the slide, causing the blood to flow evenly across the glass.			
6. The blood smear is in the shape of a feathered edge.			
7. The slide is allowed to air dry.			
8. The slide is labeled appropriately.			
Chapter 12			
After Venipuncture, Before Delivery to the Laboratory			
1. Name the steps after a venipuncture but before delivering the specimen to the laboratory.			
2. Name analytes that are photosensitive.			
3. Name analytes that are thermolabile.			
4. Name analytes that must be warmed.			
Centrifugation Issues			
1. Name specimens that do not require centrifugation.			
2. Describe the importance of centrifugation time and speed.			
3. Describe why tubes should be balanced in a centrifuge.			
4. Describe the differences in centrifugation practices between serum specimens and plasma specimens.			

Title of Exercise or Procedure	Date Completed	Competency Level Acceptable	Competency Level Needs Improvement
Postcentrifugation			
1. List three factors that affect analyte stability.			
2. List the causes of hemolysis in a blood specimen.			
3. Describe the lag time between the centrifugation and the removal or separation of serum/plasma from cells.			
4. Describe three methods of storage for blood specimens and the temperatures for each.			
5. Define the term *aliquot* and the reasons for preparing a sample aliquot.			
Chapter 13			
Pediatrics and Geriatrics			
1. List blood collection equipment necessary for a capillary blood gas collection from a newborn infant.			
2. Identifies four physical problems that are common in the elderly that can challenge blood collection efforts.			
3. List three important considerations in blood collection from within an elderly patient's home.			
Chapter 14			
Point-of-Care Testing			
1. Describe the procedural steps in POC glucose testing.			
2. Explain the difference between HDL cholesterol and LDL cholesterol.			
3. Describe two types of analytes that aid in the diagnosis and evaluation of anemia and state which one has been determined to be more accurate in diagnosis and treatment.			
Chapter 15			
Special Collection			
1. Explain the difference between the "peak" and "trough" in therapeutic drug monitoring.			
2. List at least five trace elements and the evacuated collection tube that should be used to collect for trace element testing.			
Chapter 16			
Urinalysis, Body Fluids, and Other Specimens			
1. Describe the procedural steps in the throat swab collection.			
2. Explain the difference between sputum and mucous.			
3. Describe the procedural steps for timed urine collection for urobilinogen testing.			
Chapter 17			
Drug Use, Forensic Toxicology, Workplace Testing, Sports Medicine, and Related Areas			
1. List five specimens that might be used in a forensic evaluation.			
2. Name three ways that substance abuse affects health care.			
3. Name the three specimens used for measuring or estimating BAC.			
4. Describe at least five steps for ensuring a safe specimen collection site for a workplace drug program.			
5. Describe three ways a health care worker can tell if a urine specimen for drug testing has been adulterated.			

Appendix 14

Answers to Study Questions, Cases Studies, and Competency Checklists

Chapter 1 Phlebotomy Practice and Quality Assessment

STUDY QUESTIONS

1. d	5. d	8. b
2. c	6. b	9. c
3. a	7. a	10. b
4. c		

CASE STUDY ANSWERS

Case Study 1

1. There are a multitude of possible causes for the missing laboratory results. However, in solving problems such as this, it helps to consider the laboratory workflow pathway. Errors could have occurred in the preexamination phase, examination phase, or postexamination phase. (Refer to Figure 1–2, p. 7.) Wherever the error occurred, it was not appropriately communicated or followed up.

2. Negative effects for the patient could include a major personal inconvenience, wasted time, delay of a potentially important clinical procedure, additional absences from work, lost income, and inconvenience for family members or friends.

3. It is likely that the patient would be angry and frustrated by this situation. In addition, the patient's physician, therapists, and others may also have been inconvenienced by the situation.

Case Study 2

1. It appears that on Saturdays, Sundays, and Mondays the interruptions are at the highest level. The data also suggest that requests for assistance by the nursing staff are also at a peak during these days. In addition, it seems troublesome that some patients are placed in the wrong room, again, mostly on weekends.

2. Although it is hard to speculate about the specific causes, the data clearly indicate that there might be a communication issue with the nursing staff and the phlebotomist during the weekend and Mondays. Perhaps this means that the interruptions are more prevalent because of a single nurse and/or phlebotomist who usually work on those days. In addition, the issue of patients having the wrong room assignments might be a clerical or nursing issue that could easily be cleared up by closer monitoring of the check-in/admission procedures for patients.

3. The solution may be as simple as checking with the nursing and phlebotomy staff who work those days to see if there is a specific communication issue or task that is not being adequately addressed on those days and finding ways to get the specific task addressed. The room assignment problem should probably be addressed with the nursing or clerical staff for a prompt resolution so as to avoid confusion for the patient, family and other visitors, and health care workers. Involving health care workers to be participants in the process of data collection will help them accept solutions to problems.

COMPETENCY CHECKLIST: BASICS OF PHLEBOTOMY PRACTICE AND THE CLINICAL LABORATORY

Refer to pages 2–8.

COMPETENCY CHECKLIST: QUALITY BASICS

Refer to pages 22–31.

Chapter 2 Communication, Computer Essentials, and Documentation

STUDY QUESTIONS

1. c	5. c	8. b
2. c	6. a	9. a
3. d	7. c	10. b
4. a		

CASE STUDY ANSWERS

Case Study 1

1. Any member of the health care team who cares for the patient can access the EMR if authorized with the necessary passwords. Some health care facilities authorize the phlebotomist to have access to this information; other facilities do not.

2. In this situation, the nurse is revealing information about the abnormal chest x-ray that may be upsetting to the patient. Since the phlebotomist does not need to be directly involved with this aspect of the health assessment, it would be best if he or she could give the nurse and patient some private time to go over the abnormal results. The phlebotomist can come back a few minutes later to collect the blood specimen.

3. The patient has a right to privacy and confidentiality and knowledge about who has access to her medical information. Normally, the hospital would have a consent form that should be signed by the patient prior to entering or accessing information in the electronic system.

4. This situation may be somewhat uncomfortable for the patient and the phlebotomist because there is no need for the phlebotomist to hear about the abnormal result. However, the phlebotomist could simply ask: "Would you like some privacy while you discuss the results? I can come back in a few minutes." It might be that the patient would prefer to get the blood specimen taken care of and she would not mind discussing the chest x-ray during the procedure. However, it is probably best to have her undivided attention during the venipuncture procedure. Take verbal cues from both the patient and nurse and act responsibly and professionally.

Case Study 2

1. The fact that Elizabeth does not speak Spanish or that Mrs. Rodriguez does not speak English well is a major barrier to effective communication between them. This barrier needs to be addressed before a successful and comfortable scenario can be achieved. In addition, having so many family members present, including the child, may also be a distraction.

2. Mrs. Rodriguez obviously wants or needs a support group of her family members to be with her during this encounter. Perhaps she is fearful or nervous about the procedure, or she may believe that her family can help her understand what is going to happen. She may believe that if any major medical decisions need to be made, her family members can help her make them.

3. As mentioned in Chapter 1, communication strategies may involve the following:
   a. Seek the assistance of a translator.
   b. Utilize written instructions in Spanish for reinforcing the messages.
   c. Show empathy through body language and facial expressions.
   d. Show respect for privacy.
   e. Build trust by trying to explain carefully using a model, symbols, or body language.
   f. Establish rapport with the patient and her family members.
   g. Listen actively to the patient and her family members.
   h. Provide as much feedback as possible.

4. In this case, one or more of the family members may be able to help with the translation of various parts of the conversation. Even the child may be able to assist with some basic translations and information. They may hold Mrs. Rodriguez's hand or comfort her as the procedure is taking place. If possible, let them participate in helping her relax.

5. Elizabeth may want to familiarize herself with medical terms in Spanish. She could use the translations in Appendix 12 to practice basic requests for venipuncture and urinalysis. She might also take a medical terminology course in Spanish. In addition, Elizabeth could find out more about Hispanic cultures and the diversity among Hispanic cultures through their music, literature, and popular media.

COMPETENCY CHECKLIST: CULTURAL COMPETENCY

Refer to pages 53–54.

COMPETENCY CHECKLIST: TELEPHONE COMMUNICATION

Refer to pages 49–50.

COMPETENCY CHECKLIST: HANDWRITTEN COMMUNICATION

Refer to page 57.

COMPETENCY CHECKLIST: COMPUTER COMPONENTS

Refer to pages 60–63.

Chapter 3 Professional Ethics, Legal, and Regulatory Issues

STUDY QUESTIONS

1. c	5. c	8. c
2. a	6. a	9. a
3. d	7. b	10. d
4. b		

CASE STUDY ANSWER

The health care worker who is going to collect blood from this patient should check the patient's arms for the fragility and scarring of her veins from so many previous venipunctures. He or she should collect the blood specimen with a butterfly needle and perform the venipuncture in an area of the vein that is not scarred from previous venipunctures, if possible. Then, the patient's arm should be checked frequently for at least 5 to 15 minutes after the venipuncture to make certain that she has not developed a hematoma from continued bleeding of the vein into the surrounding tissues as a result of the coumadin therapy.

ACTION IN PRACTICE ANSWERS

1. The first question that Mr. Johnson should ask about professional liability insurance at University Hospital is: "Does this hospital carry liability insurance on its employees?"

2. Three other questions that he should pose could be from following:

    a. Is adequate dollar value coverage provided? In recent lawsuits, total damages of $1 million or more have been awarded against physicians.

    b. What are the coverage limitations? How much does one have to lose if sued?

    c. What are the procedures that must be followed for the policy to provide coverage? Some policies state that divulging the amount of coverage or the fact of coverage voids the policy.

    d. The health care worker should not assume that the lawyers representing the hospital, laboratory, or clinic will have his best interests at heart. The attorney's first obligation is to serve those who have hired him or her. There have been cases in which the hospital was cleared of all charges, but the health care professional was held liable for damages.

COMPETENCY CHECKLIST: ETHICAL, LEGAL, AND REGULATORY ISSUES

For Answer 1: p. 88.
For Answer 2: p. 93.

Chapter 4 Infection Control

STUDY QUESTIONS

1. c	5. b	8. b
2. b	6. a	9. b
3. c	7. a	10. b
4. c		

CASE STUDY ANSWERS

1. Even though Sally was tired, she had a job to do. Her fatigue might have contributed to her inability to draw blood from Mr. Gilmore on the first try; however, there is no way to substantiate that. She probably did the procedure correctly except that she should have discarded the first needle and holder immediately after she used it. At that time she would have noticed that the biohazard container was full, and she could have notified the appropriate person for a replacement. Sally should not have stuffed the other needles into the full biohazard container! However, she took the appropriate action by notifying her supervisor immediately of her injury.

2. Sally would have to review the exposure control plan, OSHA standards, universal precautions, and safety procedures for disposing of contaminated waste.

3. Aside from a thorough review of the procedures mentioned in Question 2, Sally would benefit from going to classes on the importance of being rested and healthy for work. In addition, it appears she needs additional practice on patients who are difficult to draw. She may benefit from observing other experienced health care workers while they perform difficult draws.

ACTION IN PRACTICE ANSWERS

1. The pathogen is *Staphylococcus.*

   The reservoir was another person infected with this bacteria.

   The portal exit is contaminated skin.

   The mode of transmission is a tourniquet with the *Staphylococcus* on it.

   The portal of entry is the contaminated tourniquet on the skin of the next host.

   The susceptible hosts are elderly individuals.

2. The tourniquet that is being used for all of these elderly individuals needs to be thrown away! Latex-free "disposable" tourniquets need to be used and each elderly patient needs a new disposable tourniquet for blood collection.

COMPETENCY CHECKLIST: INFECTION CONTROL

For answer 1: p. 114.

For answer 2: p. 117.

Chapter 5 Safety and First Aid

STUDY QUESTIONS

1. c	5. b	8. b
2. c	6. b	9. b
3. a	7. d	10. d
4. a		

CASE STUDY ANSWERS

1. The chemical name for bleach is sodium hypochlorite.
2. The safety data information should include:
   a. The blue health quadrant has a number 2 and the red flammability hazard has a number 0.
   b. After skin contact with bleach, immediately wash with water and soap and rinse thoroughly.
   c. Sodium hypochlorite (bleach) needs to be tightly sealed and stored in a cool, dry place with good ventilation.
3. The SDS for bleach has more information (i.e., ecological information) than the MSDS.

ACTION IN PRACTICE ANSWERS

1. Maddie seemed so pleased that she successfully communicated with Ms. Hernandez that she forgot to be meticulous about checking the specimen integrity. Maddie should have carefully placed each specimen in a leak-proof plastic container in an upright position in the carrying container with absorbent material. She also should have securely locked the container and placed it in a safer place in her car, perhaps the floor.
2. Maddie should be careful not to touch the contaminated area. She should report the spill immediately and find out the appropriate procedures for spill clean-ups and decontamination procedures.

COMPETENCY CHECKLIST: SAFETY AND FIRST AID

Refer to p. 151, and pp. 145–148.

Chapter 6 Medical Terminology, Anatomy, and Physiology of Organ Systems

STUDY QUESTIONS

1. b	5. b	8. b
2. c	6. b	9. a
3. d	7. d	10. b
4. a		

CASE STUDY ANSWERS

Case Study 1

1. Common sense suggests that the health care worker can empathize with the patient for the condition on her arm and proceed with evaluation of alternative sites for venipuncture, including using the other arm or a fingerstick procedure. (Alternative venipuncture sites are covered in later chapters.) The health care worker cannot really make judgments about the cause of the dermatitis and should be especially cautious since Rosa's arm could be infectious and contagious. The health care worker should refrain from making any judgments or comments about the cause of the condition or the appearance of the site.

2. The health care worker can factually report the condition of the patient's skin to either the nurse or the doctor by using the correct terminology (e.g., "I noticed a red rash extending about 10 centimeters along the patient's right forearm. It was slightly distal to the antecubital area where I would normally collect her blood specimen. The patient indicated it was itching and that she had recently been on a camping trip. I am evaluating other sites for blood collection.") In addition, the health care worker may make a notation about the condition of Rosa's arm on the laboratory information system (e.g., "Red rash on right forearm so blood collection was from the left arm.")

Case Study 2

1. Dorsal or posterior refers to the "back side" of the hand (the side with fingernails). The ventral or anterior side would be the front of the hand (the palm side).

2. Supine means lying on the back, face upward.

3. An orthopedic condition would be related to bone or joint disorders.

COMPETENCY CHECKLIST: PREFIXES

1. without, lack of	6. up	11. similar, same	16. one-thousandth	21. bad
2. away from	7. before	12. slow	17. against	22. bad, difficult
3. toward	8. half	13. bad	18. ten	23. within
4. both	9. self	14. water	19. outside, beyond	24. upon, above
5. without, lack of	10. many	15. a hundred	20. below, deficient	25. one

COMPETENCY CHECKLIST: ROOT WORDS

1. vessel	6. hairlike	11. cell	16. red	21. vein
2. to choke	7. pulse	12. skin	17. blood	22. muscle
3. artery	8. heart	13. electricity	18. necrosis of an area	23. vein
4. artery	9. heart	14. to cast, to throw	19. fat	24. vein
5. fatty substance, porridge	10. vessel	15. serum	20. study	25. lung

COMPETENCY CHECKLIST: SUFFIXES

1. pain
2. immature cell, germ cell
3. urine
4. surgical puncture
5. cell
6. bursting forth
7. pain
8. surgical excision
9. vomiting
10. a weight, mark, record
11. to write, record
12. incision
13. inflammation
14. attraction
15. destruction, separation
16. enlargement, large
17. formation
18. resemble
19. to view
20. to view
21. condition of
22. disease
23. deficiency
24. surgical fixation
25. to eat
26. to speak

COMPETENCY CHECKLIST: IDENTIFYING MEDICAL TERMS

1. arthritis
2. distal
3. hematology
4. hyperglycemia
5. oncology
6. thermometer
7. urology
8. antecubital
9. chemotherapy
10. arteriosclerosis
11. dermatitis
12. dermatology
13. hepatitis
14. osteochondritis
15. hematology

COMPETENCY CHECKLIST: SPELLING

1. hematology
2. phlebotomy
3. oncology
4. proximal
5. leukemia
6. peripheral
7. hematology
8. thoracic
9. antecubital
10. millimeter

COMPETENCY CHECKLIST: DIRECTIONAL TERMS

1. above
2. toward the midline
3. near point of reference
4. toward the back
5. in front of
6. back side
7. toward the sides of the body
8. away from point of reference
9. toward the midline
10. front side

COMPETENCY CHECKLIST: BODY SYSTEMS

(Refer to Figure 16–10, p. 499)

1. Integumentary
2. Skeletal
3. Muscular
4. Nervous
5. Endocrine
6. Respiratory
7. Digestive
8. Urinary
9. Reproductive

Chapter 7 The Cardiovascular and Lymphatic Systems

STUDY QUESTIONS

1. a
2. a
3. b
4. b
5. c
6. d
7. b
8. d
9. d
10. c

CASE STUDY ANSWERS

Case Study 1

1. This patient has some clinical signs of a heart attack (myocardial infarct); however, there are other conditions that may cause chest pains (indigestion, pneumonia, etc.). Given the information, it is likely that the doctor has ordered laboratory tests to diagnose heart damage—for example, cardiac enzymes or biomarkers. The anticoagulant therapy and bruising on Mike's arm are likely indicators that he bleeds easily and his blood coagulation ability may be compromised. The doctor may also order some coagulation tests as well.

2. The patient indicated that he is being treated with anticoagulant therapy and the arm bruises are signs that he might bleed more than usual after the venipuncture. The health care worker must be especially careful after the venipuncture to assure that bleeding has stopped.

Case Study 2

1. Both the circulatory and lymphatic systems are responsible for transportation of blood/fluid to various tissues of the body. In addition, they are similar because they filter and remove pathogens and other foreign substances from the body.

2. The axillary lymph nodes are near the breast, so it is likely that some or all of the nodes have been removed during her mastectomy. Removal of the axillary lymph nodes causes loss of the lymph drainage capabilities on that side.

3. Never collect blood specimens from the mastectomy side regardless of the time elapsed after a mastectomy. Once removed, the lymph nodes do not grow back. The health care worker should collect the blood specimen from the antecubital area of the other arm.

CHECK YOURSELF

Properties	Arteries	Veins	Capillaries
Thickness of vessel wall	Thickest	Thinner than arteries	Thinnest walls to allow gas exchange
Direction of blood flow	From heart/lungs to tissues	From tissues to heart	From arteries to veins
Color of blood	Bright red—oxygenated	Dark red—deoxygenated	Medium red because blood is a mixture of both arterial and venous blood
Ease of stopping blood flow	Blood flows in spurts and is more difficult to control	Relatively easy to stop blood flow with pressure	Easy to stop blood flow and it often stops by itself

COMPETENCY CHECKLIST: TERMS RELATED TO THE CARDIOVASCULAR AND LYMPHATIC SYSTEMS

1. h
2. i
3. k
4. y
5. n
6. m
7. p
8. o
9. u
10. q
11. r
12. t
13. a
14. f
15. g
16. c
17. d
18. v
19. s
20. x
21. j
22. e
23. l
24. b
25. a

COMPETENCY CHECKLIST: STRUCTURES AND FUNCTIONS OF THE CARDIOVASCULAR AND LYMPHATIC SYSTEMS

Answers are found throughout the chapter.

COMPETENCY CHECKLIST: BLOOD FLOW AND THE HEMOSTATIC PROCESS

Refer to pages 210–212 and 233–235.

Chapter 8 Blood Collection Equipment for Venipuncture and Capillary Specimens

STUDY QUESTIONS

1. a	5. a	8. c
2. d	6. b	9. b
3. a	7. d	10. d
4. b		

CASE STUDY ANSWERS

1. The gray-topped vacuum blood collection tube could not be used to collect for the CK and other enzyme assays since the additive in the tube, sodium fluoride, destroys many enzymes.

2. The purple-topped vacuum blood collection tube containing EDTA is the tube of choice for the complete blood count.

3. The pink-topped vacuum blood collection tube is the tube used for blood bank collections.

ACTION IN PRACTICE ANSWERS

1. Ms. Brannon will need a tan-topped tube to collect blood for lead testing; a lavender-topped tube for CBC testing; and a light-blue–topped tube for PT testing.

2. The tan-topped tube has EDTA as the anticoagulant; the lavender-topped tube has EDTA; and the light-blue–topped tube has sodium citrate.

COMPETENCY CHECKLIST: BLOOD COLLECTION EQUIPMENT

Refer to pages 255, 259.

Chapter 9 Preexamination/Preanalytical Complications Causing Medical Errors in Blood Collection

STUDY QUESTIONS

1. c	5. c	8. b
2. a	6. b	9. a
3. c	7. b	10. a
4. d		

CASE STUDY ANSWERS

1. The health care provider should have collected a red-topped "dummy" tube prior to the collection into the light-blue–topped vacuum plastic tube and then collected the blood into the red-speckled–topped vacuum plastic tube. The plastic serum tubes (i.e., speckled-topped) contain a clot activator that may interfere with the coagulation tests and must be collected after the light-topped vacuum tube.

2. Because of the possibility of hemolysis with a 25-gauge needle, the health care worker should have used a 23-gauge needle.

ACTION IN PRACTICE 1 ANSWER

The tourniquet must be immediately released as well as immediately discontinuing the venipuncture. The health care worker must make certain that the patient is not continuing to have pain in her arm and hand from the venipuncture. Reassurance from Ms. Suzuki stating that she is okay, the health care worker can have a second attempt for the venipuncture, preferably from a different location. Any other reaction can bring professional liability to the health care worker.

ACTION IN PRACTICE 2 ANSWERS

1. The health care worker needs to make certain on which side the patient had the mastectomy and then collect from a vein in the other arm.

2 and 3. Often when a mastectomy is performed, lymph nodes are also removed from the area adjacent to the malignant site. Once they have been removed, they never grow back. Since lymph nodes function to move lymph fluid throughout the body, the absence of lymph nodes causes fluid buildup in that region of the body. Although the swelling probably is not significant after five years, even a minor fluid buildup might have a dilution effect on the blood specimen if it were collected from that side of the body. Also, with the absence of lymph nodes on that side, the patient is more susceptible to infectious organisms entering in this area; therefore, venipuncture should not occur on that side.

CHECK YOURSELF

1. Green-topped tubes cannot be underfilled since inaccuracies may result in some chemistry analysis (e.g., amylase, lipase, potassium, ALT, AST) due to the excessive amount of heparin in the partially filled tube.

2. For example, plasma cholesterol, iron, lipid, protein, and potassium levels will be falsely elevated if the tourniquet pressure is too tight or prolonged. Significant elevations may be seen with as short as a 3-minute application of the tourniquet (the recommended time for tourniquet application is no longer than 1 minute at a time). In addition, some enzyme levels can be falsely elevated or decreased because of tourniquet pressure that is too tight or prolonged.

COMPETENCY CHECKLIST: PREANALYTICAL COMPLICATIONS

Refer to pages 291–290.

Chapter 10 Venipuncture Procedures

STUDY QUESTIONS

1. a	5. c	8. b
2. d	6. d	9. a
3. b	7. d	10. a
4. a		

CASE STUDY ANSWERS

Case Study 1

1. There were multiple problems in this case. It is likely that Sarah did not follow the procedures related to how many times one health care worker can puncture one patient. Perhaps she was overly confident as well. Whatever the case, she should not have stuck the patient if she could not palpate a safe vein; she should not have stuck the patient more than twice; she should have warmed the site for a longer period of time; and she should have notified her supervisor about the incident, documented it, and indicated the reason for not being able to collect the blood.

2. Sarah should review all procedures and policies related to blood collection practices, especially those related to patient safety. She should review phlebotomy practices for mastectomy patients and frail patients and methods to improve site selection.

3. Sarah needs substantial advice and retraining about basic patient safety, customer service and satisfaction, phlebotomy procedures, and handling unusual phlebotomy circumstances, and she should apologize to the patient formally.

Case Study 2

1. It is likely that the health care worker hit a nerve near the basilic vein. Since this is not the first or preferred vein of choice (the median cubital vein is preferable), the risks of hitting a nerve are greater. The health care worker should have evaluated these risks as he was choosing a puncture site. He should have checked both arms to select a low-risk puncture site. Since it was at the end of the work shift, George might have been in more of a hurry and perhaps did not evaluate all veins carefully.

2. The health care worker should know the symptoms of nerve damage from a venipuncture (e.g., sharp, shooting pain). He should have discontinued the procedure immediately by withdrawing the needle. Instead he tried to continue the procedure. It is hoped that this patient did not suffer permanent nerve damage and/or file a legal claim, both of which are possible in this case. George should be counseled about how to handle phlebotomy complications in the future.

COMPETENCY CHECKLIST: PATIENT IDENTIFICATION

Refer to pages 315–319.

COMPETENCY CHECKLIST: PREPARING FOR THE PATIENT ENCOUNTER

Refer to page 319.

COMPETENCY CHECKLIST: USE OF A TOURNIQUET AND SITE SELECTION

Refer to pages 319–326.

COMPETENCY CHECKLIST: CLEANSING THE PUNCTURE SITE

Refer to pages 328–329.

COMPETENCY CHECKLIST: PERFORMING A VENIPUNCTURE

Refer to pages 330–339.

COMPETENCY CHECKLIST: ORDER OF DRAW

Refer to pages 343–345.

COMPETENCY CHECKLIST: LEAVING THE PATIENT

Refer to page 345–348.

Chapter 11 Capillary Blood Specimens

STUDY QUESTIONS

1. c
2. d
3. c
4. d
5. c
6. c
7. b
8. b
9. d
10. c

CASE STUDY ANSWERS

Case Study 1

1. The preferred site for the health care worker to perform the skin puncture would be on the third or fourth finger of the left hand.

2. The reason the health care worker should consider the mastectomy information important is that lymph nodes may have been removed from the patient's right side during the mastectomy. Once this has occurred, the patient should never have blood collected from that side. Even though some mastectomy surgeries are less extensive than others, the health care worker should follow CLSI recommendations, which state that blood specimens should not be collected from the side with a mastectomy. The only exception is if the patient's physician gives approval to do so.

Case Study 2

1. Health care workers have several good options available to them in this case: use of a venipuncture method with a winged-infusion set or use of the skin puncture method. Since this child has a keen awareness and dislike of needles, the health care worker can consider giving the patient a choice after explaining that the butterfly needle is a small one that is less painful. However, this may be the ideal case for using a skin puncture procedure to obtain capillary blood specimens. The use of a chemical warmer would help increase the likelihood of successful and complete specimen acquisition.

2. Since hematology tests are frequently performed on capillary blood specimens, and in light of the fact that the patient hates needles, it seems appropriate for the health care worker to perform a skin puncture on the nondominant hand of the child. The appropriate size/depth of the puncture device should be used to avoid complications induced by hitting the bone during a deep puncture.

COMPETENCY CHECKLIST: CAPILLARY BLOOD COLLECTION

Refer to pages 367–371.

COMPETENCY CHECKLIST: MAKING BLOOD SMEARS FOR MICROSCOPIC ANALYSIS

Refer to pages 372–374.

Chapter 12 Specimen Handling, Transportation, and Processing

STUDY QUESTIONS

1. c
2. d
3. d
4. a
5. b
6. b
7. a
8. d
9. a
10. c

CASE STUDY ANSWERS

Case Study 1

1. When blood cells are exposed to serum for prolonged time periods, some analytes, including potassium, undergo significant changes. In addition, if blood specimens to be tested for potassium are chilled, the cells tend to leak potassium into the plasma or serum, causing significantly elevated levels. In this case, either or both of these circumstances could have resulted in the elevated potassium level.

2. Separating the serum/plasma from cells within two hours will maintain the specimen in a stable condition for potassium testing. The health care worker can play a vital role in noticing which tests have been requested, making sure that specimens are transported to the laboratory in a timely manner and processed appropriately. In this case, the blood specimen for potassium should not be chilled.

Case Study 2

1. The mistake that the intern made was to shake the tubes. She had the right idea that they needed to be mixed, but they should have been gently inverted 5 to 10 times, not shaken vigorously. This is the likely cause of the hemolysis that also resulted in delays reporting results, and a needless additional venipuncture to the patient.

2. As mentioned previously, it could have been prevented by gently mixing the specimen instead of the vigorous shaking that occurred.

3. The patient can be told the truth in an apologetic manner—that is, that the specimen was hemolyzed during the handling of the specimen tubes and could not be tested. It should be explained that it would have resulted in erroneous test results if the specimen had been used. The patient should be told that a new specimen is necessary for accurate results. Extend an apology for the rough handling of the specimen and thank the patient for his or her cooperation.

COMPETENCY CHECKLIST: AFTER VENIPUNCTURE, BEFORE DELIVERY TO THE LABORATORY

Refer to page 403 and Box 12-1, p. 391.

COMPETENCY CHECKLIST: CENTRIFUGATION ISSUES

Refer to page 403 and Box 12-1, p. 391.

COMPETENCY CHECKLIST: POSTCENTRIFUGATION

Refer to page 393.

Chapter 13 Pediatric and Geriatric Procedures

STUDY QUESTIONS

1. b	5. a	8. a
2. a	6. c	9. b
3. a	7. a	10. a
4. b		

CASE STUDY ANSWERS

1. The coagulation tube (light-blue evacuated tube) needs to be collected first for the PT/INR. A "dummy" red topped tube should be collected prior to the light-blue topped tube since a butterfly needle with the tubing will be the needle of choice for the venipuncture. The serum tube should be collected next for the potassium. The EDTA tube for the hemoglobin test is collected as the last tube.

2. The elderly person is most likely to have fragile veins and thus it is best to collect the blood by venipuncture using a butterfly needle and small vacuum tubes to decrease the impact of the vacuum pressure on his fragile veins.

3. Treat this elderly individual with the utmost respect and dignity. It is important to establish eye contact. Be sensitive to the patient's needs and smile. Probably speak with a louder voice since he most likely has an inability to hear as well as younger individuals.

ACTION IN PRACTICE ANSWERS

1. Blood collected from a baby for a bilirubin determination should be collected in an amber microcollection tube or a tube covered with foil so that the microcollection tube is not exposed to light. Light breaks down bilirubin. Also, the specimen should not be exposed to heat because it also breaks down bilirubin.

2. Because bilirubin breaks down in the presence of light or exposure to heat, the longer the exposure to light or heat, the more bilirubin will be broken down with a resultant false decreased laboratory value.

COMPETENCY CHECKLIST: PEDIATRICS AND GERIATRICS

Refer to pages 415, 434, and 433.

Chapter 14 Point-of-Care Collections

STUDY QUESTIONS

1. b	5. b	8. a
2. d	6. b	9. b
3. c	7. b	10. b
4. c		

CASE STUDY ANSWERS

1. The problem in this POCT glucose testing case is that the patient's meter was reading outside the control range, but the patient had not checked the control values to determine that the control result was out of range. If the control is out of range, most likely the patient's result is out of range. Also, the controls were two years old and probably beyond the expiration date to use them.

2. The phlebotomist, the nurse, and other health care workers involved in the POCT glucose testing for this patient should troubleshoot for the following:

   a. Test strips and controls that are within appropriate expiration dates and stored at correct temperature

   b. Instrument blotting and wiping technique performed according to the manufacturer's directions

   c. Correct timing of the analytic procedure

   In this case, the control solution had expired on April 23, 2012.

ACTION IN PRACTICE ANSWER

The HemoCue Beta-Hemoglobin Analyzer can be used to measure hemoglobin by POCT. This analyzer can measure hemoglobin using venous, capillary, or arterial blood.

COMPETENCY CHECKLIST: POINT-OF-CARE TESTING

Refer to pages 444–445, 451, and 450.

Chapter 15 Blood Cultures, Arterial, Intravenous (IV), and Special Collection Procedures

STUDY QUESTIONS

1. c	5. b	8. c
2. c	6. b	9. a
3. d	7. a	10. d
4. d		

CASE STUDY ANSWERS

1. No, Mr. Sanchez did not follow the proper protocol. Maybe he was not given the instructions or did not remember them. For best results, the patient should:

   a. Eat normal, balanced meals for at least three days prior to the test.

   b. Fast for 8 to 12 hours prior to the beginning of the test.

c. *Not* drink unsweetened tea, coffee, or any other beverage (besides water) during fasting or during the procedure.

d. Drink water.

e. *Not* smoke, *not* chew tobacco, nor chew gum (including sugarless gum) during the fasting time or during the procedure. (*Note:* If a patient is chewing gum before or during this procedure, note this on the requisition form since chewing gum may interfere in the test results.)

f. *Not* exercise, even mild exercise, during the test.

g. Be ambulatory. Glucose tolerance tests should not be performed on nonambulatory patients since inactivity such as bed rest reduces glucose tolerance.

2. The patient had fasted beyond the 12-hour limit in addition to smoking and drinking coffee just prior to the scheduled blood collection. Also, he did not carry out the three-day diet plan as required. He will need to be rescheduled for the GTT and provided with verbal as well as written instructions for the procedure in order to obtain accurate laboratory test results.

ACTION IN PRACTICE ANSWERS

1. The health care worker punctured a deep artery. This was evident by the bright red color of the blood and the pulsating action as it was collected into the tubing.

2. If the supervisor had not halted the procedure, the puncture may have bled excessively either subcutaneously (hematoma) or on the surface of the skin, especially since a larger bore-sized needle is used for blood donations. Bleeding from an artery is more difficult to stop than bleeding from a vein. Excessive blood loss might also have caused other complications such as syncope, as well as hazards associated with the health care worker's exposure to blood. In addition, deeper manipulation of the needle may have resulted in nerve damage.

3. The health care worker probably needs further training and education about blood donor collections and the hazards associated with her technique. She should be supervised more closely until she demonstrates competence in a variety of donor collections.

COMPETENCY CHECKLIST: SPECIAL COLLECTION

Refer to pages 473–474, 475.

Chapter 16 Urinalysis, Body Fluids, and Other Specimens

STUDY QUESTIONS

1. b	5. c	8. b
2. b	6. c	9. b
3. b	7. c	10. b
4. b		

CASE STUDY ANSWERS

1. Ms. Burkley missed the following important steps: (a) forgot the laboratory requisition and specimen label; (b) did not properly identify and inform the patient of the collection procedure; (c) collected the specimen in the afternoon rather than the morning when the possibility to identify infectious microorganisms is more likely; (d) did not wash her hands before placing her gloves on her hands; and (e) did not label the specimen at the patient's bedside.

2. On pages 498–499, the procedural steps are provided, including the need to collect a sputum specimen in the early morning before the patient has anything to eat or drink.

ACTION IN PRACTICE ANSWERS

1. The first urine of the morning is preferred for these tests, but a random urine sample can also be used.

2. The chemistry urine strip has the color-reacting substances that test for the presence of protein and white blood cells.

COMPETENCY CHECKLIST: URINALYSIS, BODY FLUIDS, AND OTHER SPECIMENS

Refer to pages 500–502, 498, and 493–495.

Chapter 17 Drug Use, Forensic Toxicology, Workplace Testing, Sports Medicine, and Related Areas

STUDY QUESTIONS

1. c	5. b	8. a
2. c	6. b	9. d
3. a	7. a	10. a
4. b		

CASE STUDY ANSWERS

Case Study 1

1. Acceptable forms of identification in a federal workplace drug testing program include the following: a photo identification (driver's license; employee badge issued by the employer; or any other picture identification issued by a federal, state, or local government agency); identification by an employer or employer representative; or any other identification allowed under an operating administration's rules. Unacceptable forms of identification are by a coworker or by another safety-sensitive employee, a single nonphoto card, or faxed or photocopied identification documents. In this case, the collector would need to contact a supervisor to ascertain if anyone else in the company who knows the employee could act as the employer representative and possibly identify him. The collector should not proceed until positive identification is produced. All circumstances should be documented.

2. Several concerns in this situation cause suspicion of an attempt to tamper with the specimen:

   a. The employee lacks a positive identification and could be faking his identity. Even the friend could be the real employee.

   b. The employee could be hiding substances in his jacket or sweater that might be used to add to the specimen. He must remove all outer clothing prior to collecting the specimen.

   c. The backpack could also harbor substances. It must be placed in a secure location while the employee is collecting the specimen.

   d. Since both the employee and his friend seem nervous, other unforeseen circumstances may have been planned in an adulteration attempt.

   The collector must be careful and document all observations and actions in a factual manner.

Case Study 2

1. The health care worker is supposed to check the temperature of the specimen as soon as the employee hands over the specimen, but no later than 4 minutes after the employee comes out of the restroom. The health care worker's actions were inappropriate because she did not check the temperature of the specimen within 4 minutes.

2. The health care worker should have checked the temperature within 4 minutes and noted whether the specimen was within the acceptable temperature range of 32° to 38°C or 90° to 100°F. In addition, the health care worker should have checked that there was an adequate specimen volume for testing (45 mL for DOT collections). She should also have inspected the specimen for adulteration or substitution (blue specimen, bleach smell, excessive foaming when shaken). If a specimen showed signs of tampering, the health care worker should follow strict guidelines about follow-up procedures.

ACTION IN PRACTICE ANSWERS

1. The health care worker might be involved in the following:

    a. Chain-of-custody documentation, including cross-checking that the requisition, sex, and case number match the labeled evidence.

    b. Transferring the hair specimen into the proper container for analysis.

2. The length of time after collection should not have an effect on whether the hair specimen should be tested. Instead, the most important aspect relates to the legal accuracy of the documented times/dates related to handling, processing, and testing. If hair analysis results are accurately reported, but the documentation in the chain-of-custody is not accurate, then the results may be disqualified from a court case.

CHECK YOURSELF

Refer to Table 17–1, pages 510–511, for answers.

COMPETENCY CHECKLIST

Refer to pages 514, 509–512, 525, 523, and 522–523.

Glossary

ABO blood group system a method by which red blood cell antigens are classified (e.g., individual's blood cells with type A antigens have type A blood; those with B antigens have type B blood, etc.).

abuse improper use of illicit drugs.

accession number a term sometimes used for the laboratory-generated unique identification number assigned to blood specimens from a specified collection time. It enables careful tracking of multiple specimens from the same patient.

accuracy a "quality control" term that refers to how close a laboratory result is to the actual value. Accuracy is measured by comparing test results in a specified laboratory to results obtained from an established standard. False-positive or false-negative results represent test results that are *not* accurate. Accuracy is typically used with the term *precision* to assess the quality and effectiveness of a particular analytic procedure.

acid citrate dextrose (ACD) an additive commonly used in specimens collected for blood donations to prevent clotting. It ensures that the red blood cells maintain their oxygen-carrying capacity.

acidosis a pathologic condition existing when the blood pH decreases to less than 7.35.

active listening a set of skills that enables one to become a more effective listener. The skills include concentrating on the speaker, getting ready to listen by clearing one's mind of distracting thoughts, using silent pauses when appropriate, providing reassuring feedback, verifying the conversation that took place, keeping personal judgments to oneself, paying attention to the body language of the person speaking, and maintaining eye contact.

acute care health care delivered in a hospital setting that is associated with a hospital stay of usually less than 30 days.

addiction the continuing, compulsive use of a substance in spite of negative effects on the user.

additives substances (gels, clotting activators, or anticoagulants) that are added in small amounts to specimen collection tubes to alter the specimen so as to make it appropriate for laboratory analysis or handling.

administrative law a type of law that is initiated by the executive branch of government. Federal agencies write regulations that enforce laws created through the legislative body.

adrenals endocrine glands that produce hormones as a result of emotional changes such as fright or anger. Hormone production causes an increase in blood pressure, widened pupils, and heart stimulation.

adulteration the means of tampering with a specimen, usually urine, to make the specimen test negatively for drugs. Water is the most common substance added to the specimen or ingested to dilute the urine so that drug concentrations are below the detection limit.

aerobic microbes that live only in the presence of oxygen.

age-specific care considerations providing services that are age-appropriate and considerate (e.g., special considerations are needed for different ages of children [toddler versus teen] and also for geriatric patients). Factors typically relate to age-related fears/concerns, communication styles, procedures for comforting the patient, and safety.

airborne precautions use of protective devices that reduce the spread of airborne droplet transmission of infectious agents such as rubeola, varicella, and *Mycobacterium tuberculosis*.

alcohol colorless liquid that can be used as an antiseptic.

aliquot a portion of a blood sample that has been removed/separated from the primary specimen tube.

alkalosis a pathologic condition that results when the blood pH increases to more than 7.45. In serious cases, it can lead to coma.

Allen test a procedure used prior to drawing specimens (for ABGs) from the radial artery. It assures that the ulnar and radial arteries are providing collateral circulation to the hand area. Basically, it entails compressing the arteries to the hand and emptying the hand of arterial blood, then releasing the compression to see if the circulation is immediately restored. A negative test would indicate that collateral circulation is not sufficient and an alternative artery (brachial or femoral) should be used for ABG collections.

alveolar sacs grapelike structures in the lungs that allow for diffusion between air and blood.

Alzheimer's disease (AD) a disease that causes loss of intellectual abilities and mood disorders such as depressions and combativeness. It is more prevalent in the elderly.

ambulatory care health care services that are delivered in an outpatient, or nonhospital, setting. It implies that the patients are able to ambulate, or walk, to the clinic to receive their services.

American Hospital Association (AHA) nonprofit group or alliance of member hospitals and health care organizations that promote the interests of hospitals. Annual state and national conferences are held each year to discuss important legislation, financial considerations, regulations, and accreditation issues that affect hospitals. The AHA is an advocacy group for health care organizations, particularly hospitals.

American Nurses Association (ANA) professional organization for nurses.

American Society for Clinical Laboratory Science (ASCLS) professional organization for laboratory personnel that provides continuing education and conference activities.

American Society for Clinical Pathology (ASCP) professional organization that certifies many types of laboratory personnel through the Board of Certification (BOC) based on their passing a certification examination. Certification maintenance review through educational and experiential processes is also performed by the ASCP. The organization offers clinical and research conferences, many types of continuing education activities, and ongoing certification programs.

Americans with Disabilities Act (ADA) federal regulation prohibiting discrimination against individuals with disabilities and ensuring equal opportunities to these individuals.

amniotic fluid fluid from the amniotic sac (i.e., the membranes that hold a developing embryo and fetus).

amphetamines a type of drug in tablet or capsule form that are "stimulants."

anabolism a body function whereby cells use energy to make complex compounds from simpler ones. It allows the synthesis of body fluids (e.g., sweat, tears, saliva, etc.).

analyte a substance being analyzed (i.e., a chemical analysis).

analytic phase the phase in laboratory testing whereby the specimen is actually assessed or evaluated, and results are confirmed and reported. Also called the examination phase.

anatomic pathology major area of laboratory services whereby autopsies are performed and cytology procedures and surgical biopsy tissues are analyzed.

anatomy study of the structural components of the body.

anemia medical condition whereby there is a reduction in hemoglobin, thus lowering the O_2 carrying capacity of blood cells.

anesthetic an agent that produces partial or complete loss of sensation. Used as pain relief.

aneurism a weakness in the wall of an artery or the chamber of the heart that causes a dilation or partial balloon effect (i.e., protrusion of the weakened area).

anterior surface region of the body characterized by the front (or ventral) area and including the thoracic, abdominal, and pelvic cavities.

anticoagulant substance introduced into the blood or a blood specimen to keep it from clotting.

antigen a marker on the surface of cells that identifies it as being "self" or "donor"; identifies the type of cell; stimulates the production of specific antibodies; or stimulates cells to react in specific ways.

antiglycolytic agent an additive used in blood collection tubes that prevents glycolysis.

antimicrobial chemical or therapeutic agent that destroys microorganisms such as bacteria, viruses, and fungi.

antiseptic hand rub applying/rubbing a waterless antiseptic product onto all surfaces of the hands to reduce the number of microorganisms present; the hands are rubbed until the product has dried.

antiseptic hand wash washing hands with soap and water or other detergents containing an antiseptic agent.

antiseptics chemicals (e.g., 70 percent isopropyl alcohol, chlorhexidine, iodine, hexachlorophene, chlorooxylenol, quarternary ammonium compounds, and triclosan) used to clean human skin by inhibiting the growth of microorganisms.

aorta the largest artery in the body.

arterial blood gases (ABGs) analytical test that measures oxygen and carbon dioxide in the blood. Provides useful information about respiratory status and the acid–base balance of patients with pulmonary disorders.

arterialized capillary blood capillary specimens obtained from warmed sites. Since the pressure in arterioles is greater than in the venules, the capillaries tend to fill with a larger volume of arterial blood than venous blood.

arteries highly oxygenated blood vessels that carry blood away from the heart.

arterioles smaller branches of arteries.

ascites fluid accumulation in the peritoneal cavity.

asepsis see *aseptic techniques*

aseptic techniques a degree of cleanliness that prevents infection and the growth of microorganisms. The technique to achieve this condition includes frequent handwashing, use of barrier garments and personal protective equipment (PPE), waste management of contaminated materials, use of cleaning solutions, following standard precautions, and using sterile procedures when necessary.

assault a legal term referring to the unjustifiable attempt to touch another person or the threat to do so in circumstances that cause the other person to believe that it will be carried out, or to cause fear. An assault may be permissible if proper consent has been given (e.g., consent to obtain a blood specimen).

assessments a quality improvement measurement term referring to both the analytic (quantitative) and nonanalytic (qualitative) components of health care. In the clinical laboratory, assessments are used to ensure test sensitivity, specificity, precision and accuracy, and/or effective communication styles, timeliness, etc.

atria two of the four chambers of the heart.

autologous transfusion a patient donates his or her own blood or blood components for use later; this is the safest type of transfusion (i.e., using one's own blood). It prevents transfusion-transmitted infectious diseases and eliminates the formation of antibodies from other donors.

automated retractable skin-puncture device a single-use apparatus that pierces the skin with a lancet that automatically retracts into a protective casing.

bacteremia presence of bacteria in the blood; an infection of the blood.

bar codes series of light and dark bands of varying widths that relate to alphanumeric symbols. They can correspond to the patient's name and/or identification numbers.

basal state for phlebotomy procedures, this refers to the patient's condition in the early morning, approximately 12 hours after the last ingestion of food. In hospitals, most laboratory tests are analyzed on basal state specimens.

basilic vein vessel of the forearm that is acceptable for venipuncture.

basophils a type of granulocyte (white blood cell). Basophilic granules stain dark purple or black with basic dyes, and their nuclei are often S-shaped.

battery a complex legal term referring to the intentional touching of another person without consent, and/or beating or carrying out threatened physical harm. Battery always includes an assault, and is therefore commonly used with the term in *assault and battery*.

beliefs doctrine or faith of a person or group (i.e., spiritual orientation, family bonds, etc.).

bevel slanted surface at the end point of a needle.

BiliCheck a point-of-care test for bilirubin levels in newborns.

binge drinking consuming five or more alcoholic drinks in a row at least once in a two-week period.

bioethics moral issues, dilemmas, or problems that are the result of modern medical practices, health care services, clinical research, and/or technology (often bioethical issues involve "life-and-death" situations). *Bio* refers to "life" and *ethics* refers to a branch of philosophy dealing with the distinction between right and wrong.

bleeding-time test test for assessing platelet plug formation in the capillaries. It is no longer a common procedure but is sometimes performed with other coagulation tests. It utilizes an automated, sterile incision-making instrument to puncture the skin, and then the blood-clotting process is timed. Phlebotomists must be specially trained to perform this procedure accurately.

blind visually impaired or low vision; refers to all people who need alternative techniques to do the same tasks that a sighted person can do normally.

blood circulating fluid and cells in the cardiovascular system. In this textbook, blood refers to human blood, human blood components, and/or products made from human blood.

blood alcohol content (BAC) the concentration of alcohol in blood.

blood-borne pathogens (BBPs) pathogenic microorganisms, including hepatitis B virus and human immunodeficiency virus, that if present in blood, can cause disease in humans.

blood cultures tests that aid in identifying the specific bacterial organism causing infections in the blood. In the case of a patient who is experiencing fever spikes, it is recommended that the blood culture specimens be collected before and after the fever spike, when bacteria are most likely present in the peripheral circulation. Care must be taken by the phlebotomist not to contaminate the specimen, so special preparation of the collection site is required.

blood-drawing chair chair or recliner specifically designed to hold a patient comfortably and safely in a proper position during and after a blood collection procedure. The design typically includes a moveable armrest on both sides of the chair.

blood gas analysis see *arterial blood gases*.

blood pressure assessment of the functioning of the cardiovascular system using an instrument called a sphygmomanometer or blood pressure cuff. It is measured as systolic pressure when the heart receives blood, and diastolic pressure when the heart's ventricles relax.

blood urea nitrogen (BUN) analytic testing procedure to determine the amount of urea in the blood.

blood vessels key component of the circulatory system, these vessels transport blood throughout the body.

blood volume the total amount of blood in an individual's body. This is particularly important in pediatric phlebotomies because withdrawing blood can cause a significant decrease in the total blood volume of a small infant, thus resulting in anemia. Blood volume is based on weight and can be calculated for any size person.

body cavities four areas of the body that house vital organs, glands, blood vessels, and nerves. The human body has the following cavities: cranial, spinal, thoracic, and abdominal-pelvic.

body planes imaginary dividing lines of the body that serve as reference points for describing distance from or proximity to the body. Body planes include the sagittal, frontal, transverse, and medial planes.

brachial artery an artery located in the cubital fossa of the arm and used as an alternative site for ABG collections. Phlebotomists must be specially trained to perform collections from this site.

Braille traditional writing system for sightless individuals; consists of patterns of raised dots read by touch.

breach of confidentiality releasing a patient's laboratory test results without authorization to do so.

breach of duty a legal term referring to an infraction, violation, or failure to perform.

breathalyzer devices whereby a person breathes into the sampling mechanism; typically used for assessing alcohol levels in the body.

buccal swab a swabbing of the inside of the patient's cheek or mouth with a special swab.

buffy coat The white blood cells and platelets that form a thin white layer above the red blood cells in blood specimens that contain anticoagulants.

butterfly needle the most commonly used intravenous device. It is a stainless steel beveled needle and tube with attached plastic wings on one end and a Luer fitting attached to the other. Most butterfly needles come with safety sheaths for needlestick protection after use. Also referred to as a blood collection set or winged infusion set.

butterfly system can be used for difficult venipunctures due to small or fragile veins. The needle is typically smaller, and has a thin tubing with a Luer adapter at the end so that it can be used on a syringe or an evacuated tube system during venipuncture. Most have needle safety devices such as retractable needles and/or needle coverings/sheaths. Also called a winged infusion system or scalp needle set.

calcaneus heel bone.

cannula a tube that can be inserted into a cavity or blood vessel and used as a channel for transporting fluids. The term is most commonly used in dialysis for patients with kidney disease. The cannula is used to gain access to venous blood for dialysis or for blood collections. Specialized training and experience are required to draw blood from a cannula.

capillaries microscopic blood vessels that carry blood and link arterioles to venules.

capillary action a term used when referring to microcollection procedures that indicates the free flowing movement of blood into the capillary tube without the use of suction.

capillary blood a specimen from a skin puncture that contains a blend of blood from venules, arterioles, and tissue fluid.

capillary blood gas analysis using microcollection methods on infants (usually the heel site) to collect specimens for blood gas analyses; these analytical tests measure oxygen and carbon dioxide in the blood. Provides useful information about respiratory status and the acid-base balance of patients with pulmonary disorders.

capillary tubes disposable narrow-bore pipettes that are used for pediatric blood collections and/or microhematocrit measures. The tubes may be coated with anticoagulant such as heparin, and for safety reasons are usually made of plastic.

cardiac (striated involuntary) muscles muscles that make up the wall of the heart.

cardiopulmonary resuscitation (CPR) the method used to revive the heart and/or breathing of a patient whose heart or respiration has stopped. It is advisable for health care workers to be appropriately trained in the use of CPR.

cardiovascular body system that provides for rapid transport of water, nutrients, electrolytes, hormones, enzymes, antibodies, cells, and gases to all cells of the body.

cartilage substance similar to bone except that cells are surrounded by a gelatinous material that allows for flexibility.

catabolism chemical reactions in the body that break down complex substances into simpler ones while simultaneously releasing energy. The process provides energy for all body functions.

catheter urine specimen urine specimen collected after a catheter is inserted into the bladder, using a sterile procedure.

cause-and-effect diagrams (Ishikawa) a quality improvement tool that uses diagrams to identify interactions between equipment, methods, people, supplies, and reagents.

Celsius scale temperature scale named after Anders Celsius, a Swedish astronomer; see *centigrade*.

Centers for Disease Control and Prevention (CDC) federal agency responsible for monitoring morbidity (disease) and mortality (death) throughout the country.

Centers for Medicare and Medicaid Services (CMS) a federal agency that oversees financing and regulation of the health care industry. The CMS is responsible for Medicare, Medicaid, Health Insurance Portability and Accountability (HIPAA), and Clinical Laboratory Improvement Amendments (CLIA). This includes oversight or clinical laboratories.

centigrade thermometer based on a 100-degree range from 0 as the freezing point to 100 as the boiling point for water.

central intravenous line central venous catheter (CVC), a commonly used vascular access device; see *vascular access devices*.

central processing unit (CPU) the main controller of the computer.

centrifugal force the amount of force directing parts (such as cells) outward from the center of rotation when spinning in a centrifuge.

centrifugation phase period of time when a blood specimen is inside the centrifuge.

centriole a cellular structure that plays a role in cellular division.

cephalic vein vein of the forearm that is acceptable for venipuncture.

cerebrospinal fluid (CSF) fluid that surrounds the brain and meninges within the spinal column.

chain of custody process for maintaining control and accountability of a specimen from the point of collection to its final disposition. The process documents the identity of each individual who handles the specimen and each time a specimen is transferred.

chain of infection the process by which infections are transmitted; components include the source of the infection (nonsterile items, contaminated equipment or supplies, etc.), the mode of transmission (direct contact, airborne, medical instruments, etc.), and the susceptible host (patient).

circulatory system body system referring to the heart, blood vessels, and blood; responsible for transporting oxygen and nutrients to cells and transports carbon dioxide and wastes until they are eliminated; transports hormones, regulates body temperature, and helps defend against diseases.

citrate-phosphate-dextrose (CPD) anticoagulant additive typically used for specimens collected for blood donations.

citrates type of anticoagulant additive for blood collection tubes; prevents the blood-clotting sequence by removing calcium and forming calcium salts.

civil law different from criminal law; in civil law, the plaintiff sues for monetary damages.

clean-catch midstream a urine specimen that is used for detecting bacteria and/or for microscopic analysis. Normally, the specimen should be free of contamination because the patient should be instructed to clean and decontaminate themselves prior to urination. The urine specimen should be collected into a sterile container. Urine should be voided and the specimen should be collected mid-urination.

cleanse/decontaminate cleaning the skin surface area with 70 percent isopropyl alcohol prior to a venipuncture or a fingerstick removes dirt and microorganisms from the surface area of the skin and reduces the chances of transmitting an infection.

clinical decisions decisions made by physicians based on medical standards of practice, diagnostic testing (e.g., laboratory tests and x-rays), a patient's history, and observation of signs and symptoms.

Clinical and Laboratory Standards Institute (CLSI) nonprofit organization that recommends quality standards and guidelines for clinical laboratory procedures.

clinical laboratory a workplace where analytic procedures are performed on blood and body fluids for the detection, monitoring, and treatment of disease.

Clinical Laboratory Improvement Amendments of 1988 (CLIA 1988) federal guidelines that regulate all clinical laboratories across the United States. Regulations apply to any site that tests human specimens, including physicians' laboratory offices, or screening tests done at the patient's bedside.

clinical pathology major area of laboratory services where blood and other types of body fluids and tissues are analyzed.

clinical record see *medical records.*

cloud computing computer network that can be a wide area network (WAN) for numerous groups of users or local area network (LAN) within an organization

coagulation a phase in the blood-clotting sequence in which many factors are released and interact to form a fibrin meshwork, or blood clot.

cocaine an addictive, illegal "street drug" made from leaves of the coca plant.

communicable disease category of diseases resulting from the transmission of infectious microorganisms to individuals by direct or indirect contact or as an airborne infection.

competency statement performance expectations that include entry-level skills, tasks, and roles performed by the designated health care worker.

computer storage the amount of information/data that can be retained.

computerized patient records (CPRs) computerized version of a medical/clinical record.

confidentiality the protected right and duty of health care workers not to disclose any information acquired about a patient to those who are not directly involved with the care of the patient.

contact precautions protective measures that reduce the risk of transmission of serious diseases such as respiratory syncytial virus (RSV), herpes simplex, wound infections, and others through direct or indirect contact.

contaminated the presence or anticipated presence of blood or potentially infectious materials on an item or surface.

contaminated sharps objects that can penetrate the skin, including needles, scalpels, broken glass, broken capillary tubes, and exposed wires.

contamination presence of blood or potentially infectious substances on an item or surface.

continuing education (CE) educational programs often required/recommended by certifying or licensing agencies to update health care workers or help them maintain competency in practice.

continuous quality improvement (CQI) a theoretical framework and management strategy to improve health care structures, processes, outcomes, and customer satisfaction. It is ongoing and involves all levels of the administrative structure of an organization.

coronary arteries oxygenated vessels that supply blood to the myocardium (muscle) of the heart. If blood flow through these arteries is decreased (i.e., angina [choking action]), it induces a heart attack.

creatinine clearance test analytic procedure to determine whether or not the kidneys are able to remove creatinine from the blood.

criminal actions legal recourse for acts against the public welfare; these actions can lead to imprisonment of the offender.

critical test result a term that should be defined by each health care organization and typically includes test results that are abnormal, STAT test results, or other results that require an immediate response.

critical value a laboratory result that indicates a pathophysiologic state at such variance with normal as to be life threatening; these values should be defined and reported to the patient's physician as soon as possible. Also called a "panic value."

cross-match testing laboratory analysis that involves exposure of a donor's blood to a patient's blood to see if they are compatible or incompatible.

culture a system of values (individualism, importance of education and financial security), beliefs (spiritual, family bonding), and practices (food, music, traditions) that stem from one's concept of reality. Culture influences decisions and behaviors in many aspects of life.

culture and sensitivity (C&S) microbiologic test to determine the growth of infectious microorganisms in bodily specimens (e.g., urine), and to determine which antibiotics are most effective on the microorganism.

Custody and Control Form (CCF) part of the chain of custody process that requires specific documentation related to donor identification procedures; specimen collection steps; security for the collector, the donor, and the specimen; and tampering with the specimen.

cyanotic bluish in color due to oxygen deficiency.

cytoplasm structure within a cellular membrane; contains mostly water with dissolved nutrients and other structures or organelles of the cell.

date of birth (DOB) a patient's age; personal information (i.e., birthday) included in a patient's medical record and on laboratory test requests.

decontamination use of physical or chemical means to remove or destroy blood-borne pathogens on a surface (including skin) or item so that pathogens are no longer able to transmit disease. Prior to venipuncture, decontamination involves cleaning with a sterile swab or sponge to prevent microbiological contamination of either the patient or the specimen. This is usually accomplished with a sterile swab containing 70 percent isopropyl alcohol (or isopropanol).

deep anatomical term meaning far from the surface of the body.

defendant individual (e.g., a health care worker) against whom a legal action (civil or criminal) or lawsuit is filed.

dehydrated lacking water or fluid

delta checks quality control that allows for detection of clinically significant changes in laboratory results.

deoxyribonucleic acid (DNA) molecule containing thousands of genes that make up an individual's genetic code. Often referred to as a double helix, DNA is inherited from parents and carries the code for an individual's characteristics such as eye or hair color, height, etc.

Department of Health and Human Services (HHS) federal agency involved in many aspects of health delivery, regulation, and monitoring. One responsibility is the establishment of scientific and technical guidelines for federal drug-testing programs and standards for certification of laboratories engaged in urine drug-testing for federal agencies.

Department of Transportation (DOT) federal agency responsible for the transportation industry in the United States. It develops drug-testing guidelines for specified types of transportation personnel and standards for testing specified categories of drugs.

deposition a legal term referring to the testimony of a witness that is recorded in a written legal format.

diabetes mellitus metabolic disease in which carbohydrate utilization is reduced due to a deficiency in insulin and characterized by hyperglycemia, glycosuria, water and electrolyte loss, ketoacidosis, and, in serious conditions, coma. In milder forms of noninsulin-dependent diabetes mellitus, dietary regulation may keep the disorder under control.

diastolic pressure the second measure reported in a blood pressure measurement.

differential (diff) a laboratory test that enumerates and categorizes white blood cells and any abnormalities present.

digestive system body system referring to organs in the gastrointestinal (GI) tract that break down food chemically and physically into nutrients that can be absorbed by the body's cells and allow the elimination of waste products of digestion.

discovery a legal term referring to the right to examine the witness(es) before a trial; it consists of oral testimony under oath and includes cross-examination by lawyers.

disease a specific, measurable condition characterized by specific clinical symptoms, patient history, and laboratory or radiology results.

disinfectants chemical compounds used to remove or kill pathogenic microorganisms; typically used on medical instruments or countertops.

disorder a generic term referring to any pathologic condition of the mind or body.

disposable sterile lancet sterile sharp device, preferably retractable, used in skin puncture collections to penetrate the skin at specified depths (e.g., no more than 2.0 mm for infant heelsticks).

distal anatomical term meaning distant or away from point of attachment.

diurnal rhythms variations in the body's functions or fluids that occur during daylight hours or every 24 hours (e.g., some hormone levels decrease in the afternoon). Also referred to as circadian rhythms.

dizziness lightheadedness, unsteadiness, loss of balance.

dorsal surface region of the body characterized by the back (or posterior) area and including the cranial and spinal cavities.

double bagging practice of using two trash bags for disposing of waste from patients' rooms, particularly those patients in isolation.

driving under the influence (DUI) driving while intoxicated (DWI), drunk driving, drinking and driving, or drink-driving; alcohol levels in the body cause impairment of mental and motor skills.

droplet precautions used to reduce the transmission of diseases such as pertussis, meningitis, pneumonia, and rubella. These diseases can be transmitted through contact of the mucous membranes of the eye, mouth, or nose with large-particle droplets that occur through sneezing, coughing, or talking.

drug screening analytic methods (often qualitative) to detect rapidly the presence or absence of illicit drugs.

edema swelling

edematous condition in which tissues contain excessive fluid; it often results in localized swelling.

efficacy ability to obtain the desired clinical outcome.

electrolytes function to maintain the body's acid-base balance; sodium, potassium, chloride, calcium, phosphate, magnesium.

electronic medical record (EMR) computerized version of a medical/clinical record. Also referred to as electronic health record (EHR).

e-mail electronic mail often used in health care facilities. Guidelines for using e-mail, including a patient's consent to use e-mail, are now required of health care facilities.

embolus a small plug of material (thrombus or bacteria) that can occlude (block) a blood vessel.

endocrine glands ductless glands that release their secretions (hormones) directly into the bloodstream.

endocrine system glandular system of the body that includes pituitary, thyroid, parathyroid, thymus, adrenals, ovaries, and testes. Functions include communication, control, and integration of bodily functions.

endoplasmic reticulum cell structure that acts as a transport channel between the cell membrane and the nuclear membrane.

engineering controls devices that isolate or remove blood-borne pathogen hazards from the workplace (e.g., needleless devices, shielded needle devices, plastic capillary tubes, etc.). "Work practice" controls are activities that reduce the risk of exposure (e.g., "no-hands" procedures for discarding sharps, etc.).

Environmental Protection Agency (EPA) federal agency that, among its other responsibilities, regulates the disposal of hazardous substances and monitors and regulates disinfectant products.

eosinophils a type of granulocyte. Eosinophilic granules stain orange-red with acidic dyes. Their nuclei normally have two lobes.

erythrocytes see *red blood cells.*

erythropoiesis production of erythrocytes, or red blood cells.

erythropoietin (EPO) hormone produced in the kidney that initiates the production of red blood cells.

ethanol ethyl alcohol, a colorless liquid found in alcoholic drinks made by fermentation of sugar in grains.

ethics a branch of philosophy that deals with distinguishing right from wrong and with moral consequences of human actions.

ethylenediamine tetra-acetic acid (EDTA) anticoagulant additive used to prevent the blood-clotting sequence by removing calcium and forming calcium salts. It prevents platelet aggregation and is useful for platelet counts and platelet function tests. Fresh EDTA samples are also useful for making blood films or microscopic slides, because there is minimal distortion of platelets and white blood cells.

eutectic mixture of local anesthetics (EMLA) a topical anesthetic (pain reliever) that is an emulsion of lidocaine and prilocaine and can be applied to intact skin.

evacuated tube tubes designed for blood specimen collections; the vacuum inside the tube creates gentle suction when a double sided needle is inserted (one side into a patient's vein and the other side into the tube) thus enabling blood to flow directly from the vein into the tube.

evacuated tube system method of blood collection using double-sided needles whereby the needle is attached to a holder/adapter and allows for multiple specimen tube fills and changes without blood leakage.

evidence a legal term referring to materials (e.g., tubes, needles, safety devices, waste containers, log books, lab reports, etc.) submitted during a legal case to prove or disprove a lawsuit.

examination (analytical phase) the phase in laboratory testing whereby the specimen is actually assessed or evaluated, and results are confirmed and reported.

exocrine glands glands that secrete fluids through channels or ducts (e.g., sweat, saliva, mucus, digestive juices).

expectorate to cough deeply and spit thick matter from the lungs.

expert witness a legal term referring to a witness who is specially qualified or has expertise in certain areas pertaining to the case.

expiration date for laboratory reagents, supplies, or equipment, it is the date designated by the manufacturer after which the product is no longer suitable for use.

exposure control plan a document required in health facilities that details the process for medical treatment, prophylaxis, and/or follow-up after an employee has been exposed to potentially harmful or infectious substances (e.g., in the case of a needlestick injury).

exposure incident specific eye, mouth, mucous membrane, skin that is not intact, or parenteral contact with blood or potentially infectious materials that occurs on the job.

extrinsic factors substances involved in the clotting process that are stimulated when tissue damage occurs.

fainting see *syncope.*

false imprisonment a legal term referring to the unjustifiable detention of an individual without a legal warrant for his or her arrest.

Farenheit temperature scale where the freezing point of water is 32° and the boiling point is 112°; normal body temperature is 98°.

fasting abstinence from nutritional support such as food and beverages.

fasting blood tests tests performed on blood taken from a patient who has abstained from eating and drinking (except water) for a particular period of time.

fax machines facsimiles are often used to transmit health care information. Guidelines for their use and confidentiality of patient information are required.

feathered edge a term used to describe blood smears on microscopic slides; it is a visible curved edge that thins out smoothly and resembles the tip of a bird's feather.

fecal immunochemical test newer than the FOBT, the immunochemical technology specifically detects hemoglobin in stool samples; some studies suggest that it is more sensitive in detecting cancer.

fecal occult blood test (FOBT) feces are collected to detect invisible (occult) quantities of blood that do not alter the appearance of the stool. Laboratory determination of occult blood assists in the confirmation of the presence of blood in black stools and can be helpful in detecting gastrointestinal (GI) tract lesions and colorectal cancer. Feces are often collected by the patient using special test cards, such as ColoScreen-ES. Also called stool occult blood test, hemoccult, and Guaiac smear test.

felony a legal term referring to a public offense that may require a jail sentence.

femoral artery located in the groin area of the leg and lateral to the femur bone, it is the largest artery used as an alternative site for ABG collections. Phlebotomists must be specially trained to perform collections from this site.

fevers of unknown origin (FUO) indicates the patient has an undiagnosed infection, which usually results in ordering blood cultures.

fibrin substance that forms a blood clot.

fibrinogen protein present in plasma that is converted to fibrin in the presence of thrombin and calcium. Fibrin forms the blood clot.

fibrinolysis the final phase of the hemostatic process whereby repair and regeneration of the injured blood vessel occur and the clot slowly begins to dissolve or break up (lyse).

first morning specimen urine specimen collected immediately after waking up in the morning. Also known as early morning specimen; see *overnight specimen*.

fistula an artificial shunt or passage, commonly used in the arm of a patient undergoing kidney dialysis; the vein and artery are fused through a surgical procedure. Only specially trained personnel can collect blood from a fistula.

flea a tiny magnetic steel wire drawn back and forth along the length of the collection tube several times to mix the specimen.

fomites inanimate objects that can harbor infectious agents and transmit infections (e.g., toilets, sinks, linens, door knobs, glasses, phlebotomy supplies, etc.).

Food and Drug Administration (FDA) federal agency responsible for safety, clinical efficacy, and medical efficacy of the country's food and drug supply. This includes equipment and supplies used in blood collection.

forensic specimens specimens that are involved in civil or criminal legal cases, including specimens for analysis of drugs of abuse.

forensic toxicology study of poisons or drugs of abuse in legal cases.

fraud deliberate deception or cheating either by conduct or words.

frontal plane imaginary line running lengthwise on the body from side to side, dividing the body into anterior and posterior sections.

full disclosure explains the full nature of the research and any risks (e.g., blood collection problems) and benefits to the participant.

gastric analysis gastric fluid analysis to determine gastric function. Involves passing a tube through the patient's nose and into the stomach. It requires specialized training.

gastrointestinal system body system that breaks down food chemically and physically into nutrients that can be absorbed and transported throughout the body to be used for energy by all body cells, and to eliminate the waste products of digestion through the production of feces. See also *digestive system*.

gateway drugs drugs such as tobacco and alcohol, the use of which may lead to the use and abuse of "harder" drugs.

gauge number the size (diameter) of the internal bore (opening) of a needle. The larger the number, the smaller the bore size, and vice versa.

gauze loosely woven material used for bandages that are sterile or chemically clean.

genes located on a chromosome, it is a unit of heredity capable of reproducing itself exactly during cell division; it is made of segments of DNA.

genome an organism's full DNA sequence of genes.

geriatric an elderly patient.

gestational diabetes diabetes that begins during pregnancy (often the second or third trimester). It occurs in 1 to 4 percent of pregnancies and usually subsides after delivery.

global harmonization the worldwide development of consistent hazardous materials classification and transportation regulations.

Global Harmonization System (GHS) worldwide development of hazardous materials classification and transportation regulations that are consistent among all countries. The change to the **GHS** requires the use of sanctioned safety data sheets (SDS).

glucose tolerance test (GTT) diagnostic test for detecting diabetes. The test is performed by obtaining blood and urine specimens at timed intervals after fasting, then after ingesting glucose. Each specimen is analyzed for its glucose content to determine if the glucose level returns to normal within 2 hours after ingestion. Diabetic patients' glucose is metabolized differently and may need to be analyzed up to 5 hours after ingestion. Special instructions are needed for the patient, and special training for the phlebotomist should occur if they will be collecting such specimens.

glycolysis the breakdown or metabolism of glucose by blood cells.

glycolytic inhibitor an additive used in blood collection tubes that prevents glycolysis.

Golgi apparatus cell structure that stores proteins.

granulocytes (basophils, neutrophils, eosinophils) mature leukocytes (white blood cells) in the circulating blood; when stained and viewed microscopically, granules are present.

Guaiac smear test see *fecal occult blood test (FOBT)*.

hand hygiene a term that applies to handwashing (with nonantimicrobial soap and water), antiseptic hand washing, antiseptic hand rub (with waterless antiseptic), or surgical hand antisepsis.

hardware a computer, the programmable machine; the brain of the machine that executes activities.

HazCom the OSHA Hazard Communication Standard, in addition to mandating labels, this Right to Know law requires chemical manufacturers to supply Material Safety Data Sheets (MSDSs) for their chemicals.

HDL cholesterol high-density lipoprotein (HDL) cholesterol, referred to as the "good cholesterol."

health care–associated (hospital acquired, or nosocomial) infections (HAIs) infections acquired after admission into a health facility.

Health Insurance Portability and Accountability Act (HIPAA) 1996 federal law, expanded in 2000, to protect security, privacy, and confidentiality of personal health information.

health literacy written, spoken, or conceptual knowledge of health information.

heart a key organ of the cardiovascular system, it is the pump that forces blood throughout the body.

heelstick pediatric phlebotomy procedure that requires puncturing one of specified areas of an infant's heel.

hematocrit a commonly ordered laboratory test to assess the circulatory system; it describes the concentration of red blood cells and therefore provides an indirect measure of the oxygen-carrying capacity of the blood.

hematology the study of blood and blood-forming tissues.

hematoma a localized leakage of blood into the tissues or into an organ. In phlebotomy, it can occur as a result of blood leakage during the vein puncture, thereby causing a bruise.

hematopoiesis the process of blood cell formation that occurs in the bone marrow.

hematopoietic blood-forming.

hemoccult test see *fecal occult blood test (FOBT)*.

hemoconcentration increased localized blood concentration of large molecules such as proteins, cells, and coagulation factors. This can be caused by excessive application of a tourniquet.

hemoglobin (Hgb) the molecules that carry oxygen and carbon dioxide in the red blood cells.

Hemoglobin A1c point-of-care testing procedure for maintenance of blood glucose levels using an analyzer.

hemolysis rupture or lysis of the blood cells.

hemorrhage excessive or uncontrolled bleeding.

hemostasis maintenance of circulating blood in the liquid state and retention of blood in the vascular system by prevention of blood loss.

HEPA filtration standard air filtration system comonly used in clinical laboratories. HEPA stands for "high efficiency particulate air."

heparin an anticoagulant that prevents blood clotting by inactivating thrombin and thromboplastin, the blood-clotting chemicals in the body.

heparin or saline lock part of a vascular access device, a heparin or saline lock is put in place to be used for medication administration or blood collection. It must be "flushed" routinely to prevent clot formation in the line. Generally speaking, heparin locks are no longer widely used; however, if they are used, blood from this site should not be used for coagulation studies due to possible contamination of the specimen with residual heparin.

histograms bar graphs often used as quality improvement tools.

holder (adapter) plastic apparatus needed for specimen collection using the evacuated tube method. The adapter/holder secures the double-pointed needle: one end of the needle goes into the patient's vein, and the other end of the needle is placed an evacuated tube.

Hollander test involves gastric fluid to determine gastric function in terms of stomach acid production. It uses insulin to stimulate gastric secretions. Special training is required prior to assisting with this procedure.

home health care provision of health care services in a patient's home under the direction of a physician.

homeostasis means literally "remaining the same"; it is a normal state that allows the body to stay in a healthy balance by continually compensating with necessary changes. Also called steady-state condition.

hormones body substances secreted from glands that play a role in growth and development, fluid and electrolyte balance, energy balance, and acid-base balance.

Hospital- or health care-acquired infections (HAIs) see *health care–associated infections*

Hospital Infection Control Practices Advisory Committee interdepartmental committee that monitors infection rates and other indices that assess transmission of infections.

human immunodeficiency virus (HIV) a virus spread by sexual contact or exposure to infected blood.

HVAC refers to heating, ventilation, and air conditioning. These are vital components to the infrastructure of a clinical laboratory.

hyperglycemia increased blood sugar (i.e., as in patients with diabetes).

hyperventilation a condition whereby chemoreceptors in the brain cause a faster and deeper rate of respiration in order to blow off excess carbon dioxide.

hypobilirubinemia abnormally low levels of bilirubin in the blood.

hypothyroidism when referring to infantile hypothyroidism, a disorder that may be congenital and results in defective development of an embryo.

hypoxia a condition in which body tissues are not receiving enough oxygen.

iatrogenic anemia refers to anemia caused by the medical treatment a patient has received—for example, collecting an excessive volume of blood in multiple samples may cause anemia.

icteric relating to jaundice; a yellowish color sometimes seen in serum specimens.

illicit drugs illegal drugs, including opiates, cocaine, amphetamines, etc.

illness a subjective, nonmeasurable term for any departure from wellness (pain, suffering, distress).

immunology the study of diseases of the immune system; allergic disorders.

implanted port type of vascular access device (VAD) surgically implanted beneath the skin; it is a small chamber attached to an indwelling line. Access to these ports must be by specially trained personnel and specially designed noncoring needles.

implied consent a complex legal term that varies from state to state in its interpretation. Basically it entails conditions when immediate action is required to save a patient's life or to prevent impairment of a patient's health (i.e., medical emergency care operates with the notion of implied consent in many cases).

incision a cut into the skin. The term is used to describe the puncture made by an automatic skin puncture device.

infection a disease caused by microorganisms (bacteria, viruses, etc.).

infection control programs guidelines designed to address surveillance, reporting, isolation procedures, education, and management of community-acquired and health-care-associated infections.

inferior vena cava one of the two large veins that bring oxygen-poor blood to the heart from the lower trunk of the body (e.g., legs).

inflammation characterized by redness, heat, swelling, pain, or loss of function; it is the body's defensive response to injuries, infections, or allergies.

informed consent a complex legal term; basically it refers to voluntary permission by a patient to allow touching, examination, and/or treatment by health care workers after they have been given information about the procedures and potential risks and consequences. It allows patients to decide what may be performed on or to their bodies.

inpatients hospitalized patients.

insulin a chemical produced by the pancreas that is released into the bloodstream to facilitate glucose absorption from the blood into the tissues where it is used for energy. When insulin is not produced (as in diabetes mellitus), blood glucose levels increase because it cannot be absorbed into the tissues.

integumentary system body system referring to skin, hair, sweat and oil glands, teeth, and fingernails; involved in protective and regulatory functions.

intensive care unit (ICU) area where patients are more critically ill, require additional monitoring, and are more susceptible to infections.

International Normalized Ratio a numeric ratio for clot-based coagulation tests that are reported in seconds or units based on seconds.

International Organization for Standardization (ISO) a nongovernmental network of standards institutes from 155 countries that develop standards for manufacturing and service industries.

interstitial space between tissues and/or organs.

interstitial (tissue) fluid naturally occurring liquid forming between gaps/layers of tissue; a small component of a capillary blood specimen.

intravenous (IV) catheter vascular access device inserted into a blood vessel for administration of medications, nutrients, and blood collection.

intrinsic system part of the coagulation process that involves the clotting factors contained in the blood.

invasion of privacy a legal term referring to objectionable or personal intrusion on an individual such that it is offensive (e.g., the publishing of confidential information).

iodine used to make tincture of iodine (2 percent solution), which is used as a skin disinfectant. However, many people are allergic to iodine.

iontophoresis a painless weak electrical current is used to stimulate drug-carrying ions to pass through intact skin.

isolation procedures methods used to protect individuals (health care workers) from patients with infectious diseases. Formally divided into two types (category-specific and disease-specific), guidelines now combine isolation practices for moist and potentially infectious body substances, to be used for all patients. The current categories of isolation are based on the mode of transmission and include airborne, droplet, and contact precautions.

jaundice a yellowish discoloration of the skin and/or tissues due to a buildup of bile pigments.

The Joint Commission independent, nonprofit organization that sets quality standards for health care.

judicial law legal processes designed to resolve disputes.

laboratory information systems (LIS) dedicated hardware and software for clinical laboratories and/or anatomical pathology.

lactose tolerance test a test to determine lactose intolerance. Some individuals have difficulty digesting lactose, a milk sugar. This test is similar to the glucose tolerance test (which is usually performed one day before) and requires timed testing for lactose after fasting, then after ingestion of lactose at 1-, 2-, and 3-hour intervals.

lancet/lancing device a sharp apparatus (similar to a needle) used to puncture skin to acquire a capillary blood specimen.

lateral directional term meaning toward the sides of the body.

latex allergy reaction to certain proteins in latex rubber, a natural ingredient in some varieties of gloves. Allergic reactions range from skin redness, rash, hives, or itching to respiratory symptoms and, in rare instances, shock.

law societal rules or regulations designed to protect society and resolve conflicts; laws are rules that must be observed.

LDL cholesterol low-density lipoprotein (LDL) cholesterol, referred to as the "bad cholesterol" since high values are linked to heart disease.

leukocytes see *white blood cells*.

liable a legal term that refers to a legal obligation when damages are concerned.

light sensitive photosensitivity; refers to laboratory specimens; some chemical constituents (bilirubin, vitamin B_{12}, carotene, folate, and urine porphyrins) decompose if exposed to light and therefore should be protected/covered during transportation and handling.

lipemic when referring to serum, it is a cloudy or milky appearance, usually due to a temporarily elevated lipid level after the ingestion of fatty foods.

liter 1000 mL; unit of volume.

lithium iodoacetate antiglycolytic agent and anticoagulant; not to be used for hematology testing or enzymatic determinations.

litigation process a legal action to determine a decision in court. Many malpractice cases are negotiated and settled out of court.

long-term care health care services that are provided for more than 30 days. Usually it is related to chronic conditions (e.g., rehabilitation or services for the elderly in nursing homes).

Luer adapter a device for connecting the needle to the syringe; provides secure fit when locked in place.

lymphatic system body system responsible for maintaining fluid balance, providing a defense against disease, and absorption of fats and other substances from the bloodstream.

lymphedema swelling caused by lymph accumulation in the tissues.

lymphocytes type of white blood cell that is nongranular in appearance; plays a role in immunity and in the production of antibodies.

lymphostasis obstruction and/or lack of flow of the lymph fluid.

lysosomes cell structures that release digestive enzymes into vacuoles, or small pouches, for digestion of food particles.

malice a legal term referring to a reckless disregard for the truth (e.g., knowing that a statement is false).

malpractice a legal term referring to improper or unskillful care of a patient by a member of the health care team, or any professional misconduct, unreasonable lack of skill, or infidelity in professional or judiciary duties; often described as "professional negligence."

marijuana drug derived from the hemp plant, cannabis, that when smoked or eaten causes mood alterations and changes in sensory perceptions and cognitive coordination.

mastectomy removal of breast tissue.

Material Safety Data Sheets (MSDSs) required information about any chemical used in the workplace; MSDSs generally list information about a chemical, precautionary measures, and emergency information about accidental exposures to the chemical.

meconium the first intestinal discharges of the newborn infant, greenish in color; consists of epithelial cells, mucus, and bile.

medial directional term meaning toward the midline of the body.

median cubital vein vein in the antecubital area that is most commonly used for venipuncture.

Medicaid a shared federal- and state-funded program designed to provide health insurance for individuals with low income.

medical records definitive documents (paper or electronic) that contain a chronological log of a patient's care. It must include any information that is clinically significant or relevant to the patient's care.

Medicare federal program designed to provide health insurance for the elderly and members of special groups.

megakaryocytes large cells located in the bone from which platelets are formed.

melanin pigment in the skin that provides color and protects underlying tissues from absorbing ultraviolet rays.

meninges protective membranes that cover the brain and spinal cord.

menstrual cycle menstruation normally begins during puberty (9 to 17 years of age). The monthly menstrual flow lasts between 3 and 7 days and contains normal, hemolyzed, or sometimes agglutinated red blood cells, disintegrated endometrial cells, and glandular secretions.

metabolic acidosis a pathologic condition that occurs when the kidneys cannot eliminate acidic substances (e.g., in diabetes mellitus). It can result in kidney (renal) failure and death.

metabolic alkalosis a pathologic condition that results from excessive vomiting or an abnormal secretion of certain hormones that causes excess elimination of hydrogen ions (from CO_2).

metabolism an important bodily function that allows the formation or breakdown of substances (e.g., proteins) for the purpose of using energy.

metabolite a compound produced when the body processes an illicit drug.

microbiology the study of microbes; microbiologic tests typically use specialized media to detect the growth of infectious microbes from bodily specimens.

microcollection process by which small amounts of blood are collected in small containers or tubes using specially designed devices.

microcontainers specialized collection devices designed for small quantities of blood; some containing anticoagulants. These devices are typically used for pediatric or geriatric patients with fragile or inaccessible veins, and/or for fingersticks.

microorganisms living organisms that are too small to see with the naked eye such as bacteria, viruses, fungi, etc.

misdemeanor a legal term referring to many types of criminal offenses that are not serious enough to be classified as felonies.

misrepresentation use of misleading information or distortion of facts.

mitochondria cell structure that produces energy for the cell.

mode of transmission the method by which pathogenic agents are transmitted (e.g., direct contact, air, medical instruments, other objects, and other vectors).

modified Allen test see *Allen test*.

monocytes type of white blood cell that is nongranular and also plays a role in defense.

monocytosis an increase of monocytes in the blood.

motor neurons nerve cells that transmit impulses to muscles from the spinal cord or the brain.

Multidrug resistant organisms (MDRO) bacteria that are resistant to antibiotics such as methicillin-resistant Staphylococcus aureus (MRSA), vancomycin-resistant enterococci (VRE), and highly resistant gram negative bacteria (HRGNB).

multiple-sample needles used with the evacuated tube method of blood collection, these needles are attached to a holder/adapter and allow for multiple specimen tube fills and changes without blood leakage.

muscular system body system referring to all muscles of the body.

nanotechnology the manipulation of matter, including blood samples, on an atomic or molecular scale.

National Fire Protection Association (NFPA) international nonprofit membership organization that develops codes, standards, training, and education on fire prevention and public safety.

National Phlebotomy Association (NPA) professional organization for phlebotomists that offers continuing educational activities and a certification examination for phlebotomists.

needleless system a device that does not use needles for procedures that are normally associated with needle use. This includes collection of bodily fluids or withdrawal of body fluids after initial venous or arterial access is performed. It includes any procedure that has the potential for occupational exposure to blood-borne pathogens from contaminated sharp objects.

needlestick skin puncture using a retractable puncture device.

negligence a legal term referring to the failure to act or perform duties according to the standards of the profession.

neonatal screening typically refers to mandatory (required by law) laboratory testing of infants for specified disorders such as PKU and hypothyroidism. There is wide variability in what tests are required by each state.

neonate a newborn infant; term used during the first 28 days after birth.

nervous system body system that includes organs that provide communication in the body, sensations, thoughts, emotions, and memories.

neurons specialized nerve cells that transmit nerve impulses.

neutrophilia an increase of neutrophils in the blood.

neutrophils a type of granulocyte. Neutrophilic granules stain bluish with neutral dyes, and their nuclei generally have two or more lobes.

nitrile gloves hand protection used by health care workers in lieu of latex gloves; nitrile butadiene rubber is very different from natural latex and provides a safe alternative for workers who develop allergies to latex gloves.

nosocomial infections see *health care–associated infections*.

nucleolus cell structure located inside the nucleus, aids in cellular metabolism and cellular reproduction.

nucleus cell structure that is the cell's control center; it governs the functions of each individual cell (e.g., growth, repair, reproduction, and metabolism).

obese, obesity an unhealthy abundance of body fat.

occluded veins closed or constricted veins.

occult blood invisible quantities of blood that do not alter the appearance of the stool.

occult blood test analysis that detects hidden (occult) blood in the stool. See *fecal occult blood test*.

occupational exposure contact via skin, eye, mucous membranes, or parenteral with potentially infectious materials as a result of an individual's work duties.

Occupational Safety and Health Administration (OSHA) an agency of the U.S. Department of Labor requiring employers to provide a safe work environment, including measures to protect workers exposed to biological and occupational hazards. OSHA is also responsible for responding to complaints, monitoring employer practices, and imposing sanctions (fines or closure) on employers who are noncompliant.

opiates drugs derived from opium.

order of draw the order in which a blood specimen is aspirated into collection tubes. The order of draw varies according to the type of venipuncture method used, the types of tubes/additives needed for testing, and each manufacturer's specifications.

organelles small structures within cells.

organ systems groups of organs that have common functions.

osteochondritis inflammation of the bone and its cartilage.

osteomyelitis inflammation of the bone due to bacterial infection.

osteoporosis a condition in which the bone becomes porous and at a higher risk of fracturing. This is due to reduced mineral density in bone and is more common in postmenopausal women than in men.

outcomes used as a quality improvement term to refer to what is accomplished for the patient (e.g., healing, return to wellness, or return to normal functions). Poor patient outcomes have been described as the "5 Ds": death, disease, disability, discomfort, and dissatisfaction.

ova and parasites (O&P) laboratory analysis performed on stool specimens that determines the presence of parasitic microorganisms or eggs of parasitic organisms.

overnight specimen see *first morning specimen*.

over-the-counter (OTC) refers to pharmaceuticals that are available without a prescription.

oxalates anticoagulants that prevent blood-clotting sequence by removing calcium and forming calcium salts.

pace (of voice) the rate of speed and urgency of the voice.

palmar anatomical term for the palm side/surface of the hand.

panic value see *critical value*.

parental involvement during pediatric phlebotomy procedures, a parent's support and presence during the procedure is often helpful in reducing stress/anxiety for the patient. On the other hand, some parents are reluctant to be involved, so the phlebotomist must assess each situation to determine the level of parental involvement that would optimize the phlebotomy encounter.

parenteral refers to the piercing of the skin barrier or mucous membranes via needlesticks, bites, cuts, or abrasions; often refers to delivering medications by piercing mucous membranes or skin through needle stick injections, IVs, etc.

Parkinson's disease a neurological disease characterized by muscular tremors and rigidity of movement.

pathogenesis the origin of a disease.

pathogenic agents include disease-causing bacteria, fungi, viruses, or parasites that are transmitted by direct contact, air, medical instruments, other objects, or vectors.

pathology the study of all aspects of disease and abnormal conditions of the body.

Patient Care Partnership The American Hospital Association's 2003 revision to the Patient's Bill of Rights. The key elements involve a patient's rights to high-quality hospital care, a clean and safe environment,